FOR REFERENCE

Do Not Take From This Room

D1472158

VITAL STATISTICS OF THE UNITED STATES

VITAL STATISTICS OF THE UNITED STATES

BIRTHS, LIFE EXPECTANCY, DEATHS, AND SELECTED HEALTH DATA
SEVENTH EDITION, 2016

Shana Hertz Hattis

Bernan Press

Lanham • Boulder • New York • London

BOCA RATON PUBLIC LIBRARY
BOCA RATON, FLORIDA

Published by Bernan Press
An imprint of The Rowman & Littlefield Publishing Group, Inc.
4501 Forbes Boulevard, Suite 200, Lanham, Maryland 20706
www.rowman.com
800-462-6420

Unit A, Whitacre Mews, 26-34 Stannary Street, London SE11 4AB

Copyright © 2016 by Bernan Press

All rights reserved. No part of this publication may be reproduced, stored in a retrieval system, or transmitted in any form or by any means, electronic, mechanical, photocopying, recording, or otherwise, without the prior permission of the publisher.

ISBN: 978-159888-854-6

eISBN: 978-159888-855-3

ISSN: 1549-8603

∞™ The paper used in this publication meets the minimum requirements of American National Standard for Information Sciences Permanence of Paper for Printed Library Materials, ANSI/NISO Z39.48-1992.

Printed in the United States of America

CONTENTS

TABLES

TABLES

INTRODUCTION

Bernan Press is pleased to present a comprehensive collection of birth, mortality, and health data in the seventh edition of *Vital Statistics of the United States: Births, Life Expectancy, Deaths, and Selected Health Data.* This volume provides valuable information compiled by various government agencies including the Centers for Disease Control (CDC) and its National Center for Health Statistics (NCHS) and National Vital Statistics System (NVSS), the U.S. Census Bureau, and the Bureau of Labor Statistics (BLS).

Until 1993, the federal government published *Vital Statistics of the United States* in several thick-bound volumes. However, between the last publication of the federal volume and the first *Vital Statistics* edition from Bernan Press, nothing comparable was offered. During this time, the CDC continued to compile its information as periodical reports and news releases, and Bernan took this opportunity to streamline this information into a cohesive, inclusive volume.

This edition builds upon the groundwork laid by previous editions in the areas of birth, mortality, health, and marriage and divorce. Each part is preceded by highlights of salient data. These sections also contain a diverse array of information about their tables and figures. Notes and definitions and source information are also provided for all four parts.

The Birth section, in many instances, provides final data through 2014. This section covers many aspects of natality, including birth and fertility rates, number of children, births to unmarried women, maternal health, methods of delivery, demographic characteristics of mothers, medical visits by pregnant women, and infant health status.

The Mortality section focuses on deaths and death rates, generally through 2030, as told through various medical, demographic, and social characteristics. Especially detailed are the tables on causes of death, which are shown by leading causes of death, age, sex, Hispanic origin, race, and (to a lesser extent) state of residence. Death rates are also given by marital status and level of educational attainment, and special tables are provided for infant mortality.

The Health section, the largest in the book, offers a collection of statistics concerning health and disease. While health is not a traditional component of vital statistics, its importance to this volume cannot be overstated. Health data provides the user with an even deeper picture of births and deaths in the United States. For example, a user interested in cerebrovascular disease-related deaths may glean useful information from tables about incidence and survival rates. This chapter shows selected data on several topics, including determinants and measures of health, use of addictive substances, ambulatory care, inpatient care, health personnel, health expenditures, and health insurance.

The Marriage and Divorce section provides marriage and divorce rates by state and demographic characteristics. This chapter also provides statistics on marriages ending in widowhood and number of marriages for U.S. residents.

About the Editor

Shana Hertz Hattis is an editor with over a decade of experience in statistical and government research publications. Past titles include *State Profiles: The Population and Economy of Each U.S. State, Housing Statistics of the United States,* and *The United States Government Internet Directory.* She earned her bachelor of science in journalism and master of science in education degrees from Northwestern University.

PART 1

BIRTH

PART 1: BIRTHS

Figure 1-1. Live Births and Fertility Rates, 1930–2014

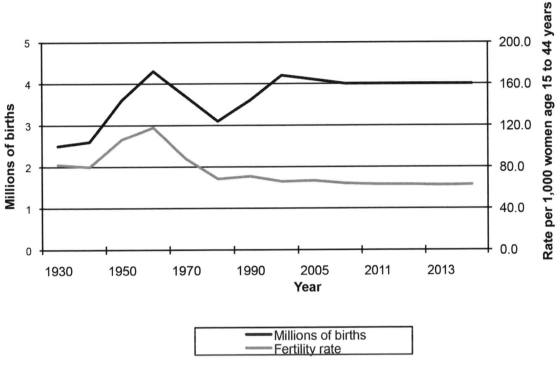

HIGHLIGHTS

- According to preliminary results, there were 3,988,076 births in the United States in 2014, up from 3,932,181 in 2013. Births increased for two racial groups: 7.5 percent for Asian or Other Pacific Islanders and 0.1 percent for non-Hispanic Blacks. Births increased for all races except for American Indian and Alaska Natives; the number also increased for those of Hispanic ethnicity. (Table 1-1)

- The preliminary birth rate for teenagers age 15 to 19 years fell to 24.2 births per 1,000 females. From 1991 to 2014, this rate has declined 60.8 percent, and from 2011 to 2014, it declined 22.7 percent. (Table 1-5)

- In 2014, 40.2 percent of all births were to unmarried women, down from 41.0 percent in 2009. The numbers varied significantly by state. Utah had the lowest number of births to unmarried woman at 18.6 percent, followed by Colorado at 22.4 percent. Mississippi had the highest percentage of births to unmarried women of any state at 54.0 percent. The Northern Marianas had the highest percentage of births to unmarried women of any state or territory at 72.1 percent. (Table 1-38)

Table 1-1. Selected Characteristics, by Race and Hispanic Origin of Mother, 2013 and 2014

(Number, rate, percent.)

Race and His-panic origin of mother	Number		Birth rate		Fertility rate		Total fertility rate		Percent of births to unmarried women	
	2013	2014	2013	2014	2013	2014	2013	2014	2013	2014
All Races and Origins [1]	3,932,181	3,988,076	12.4	12.5	62.5	62.9	1,857.5	1,862.5	40.7	40.2
Non-Hispanic White[2]	2,129,196	2,149,302	10.7	10.8	58.7	59.5	1,751.0	1,762.5	29.3	29.2
Non-Hispanic Black[2]	583,834	588,891	14.4	14.4	64.6	64.5	1,881.5	1,873.5	71.5	70.9
American Indian or Alaska Native total[2,3]	45,991	44,928	10.3	9.9	46.4	44.8	1,334.5	1,288.5	66.4	65.7
Asian or Pacific Islander total[2,3]	253,915	272,949	14.3	14.6	59.2	60.7	1,681.0	1,715.5	17.0	16.4
Hispanic[2]	901,033	914,065	16.7	16.5	72.9	72.1	2,149.0	2,130.5	53.3	52.9

1 Includes births to White Hispanic and Black Hispanic women and births with origin not stated, not shown separately.   2 Hispanic origin are reported separately on birth certificates. Persons of Hispanic origin may be of any race. Multiple-race data, when reported, were bridged to single-race categories in order to maintain comparability among all reported areas.   3 Includes persons of Hispanic origin, and origin not stated, according to the mother's reported race.

Table 1-2. Births and Birth Rates, by Race and Hispanic Origin of Mother, Final 2000–2014

(Number, rate per 100,000 population in specified group.)

Year and characteristic	All races and origins[1]	Non-Hispanic White[2]	Non-Hispanic Black[2]	American Indian or Alaska Native[2,3]	Asian or Pacific Islander[2,3]	Hispanic[2]
Number						
2000	4,058,814	2,362,968	604,346	41,668	200,543	815,868
2001	4,025,933	2,326,578	589,917	41,872	200,279	851,851
2002	4,021,726	2,298,156	578,335	42,368	210,907	876,642
2003	4,089,950	2,321,904	576,033	43,052	221,203	912,329
2004	4,112,052	2,296,683	578,772	43,927	229,123	946,349
2005	4,138,349	2,279,768	583,759	44,813	231,108	985,505
2006	4,265,555	2,308,640	617,247	47,721	241,045	1,039,077
2007	4,316,233	2,310,333	627,191	49,443	254,488	1,062,779
2008	4,247,694	2,267,817	623,029	49,537	253,185	1,041,239
2009	4,130,665	2,212,552	609,584	48,665	251,089	999,548
2010	3,999,386	2,162,406	589,808	46,760	246,886	945,180
2011	3,953,590	2,146,566	582,345	46,419	253,915	918,129
2012	3,952,841	2,134,044	583,489	46,093	272,802	907,677
2013	3,932,181	2,129,196	583,834	45,991	265,673	901,033
2014	3,988,076	2,149,302	588,891	44,928	282,723	914,065
Birth Rate						
2000	14.4	12.2	17.3	14.0	17.1	23.1
2001	14.1	11.9	16.6	13.5	16.1	22.9
2002	14.0	11.7	16.1	13.2	16.3	22.7
2003	14.1	11.8	15.9	13.0	16.4	22.8
2004	14.0	11.7	15.8	12.8	16.4	22.8
2005	14.0	11.6	15.8	12.6	15.9	22.9
2006	14.3	11.7	16.5	12.9	16.0	23.3
2007	14.3	11.7	16.6	12.9	16.4	23.0
2008	14.0	11.5	16.3	12.4	15.7	21.8
2009	13.5	11.2	15.7	11.8	15.1	20.3
2010	13.0	10.9	15.1	11.0	14.5	18.7
2011	12.7	10.8	14.7	10.7	14.5	17.6
2012	12.1	10.7	14.6	10.5	15.1	17.1
2013	12.0	10.7	14.4	10.3	14.3	16.7
2014	12.0	10.8	14.4	9.9	14.6	16.5
Fertility Rate						
2000	65.9	58.5	71.4	58.7	65.8	95.9
2001	65.1	57.7	69.1	57.0	62.5	95.4
2002	65.0	57.6	67.5	55.8	63.4	94.7
2003	66.1	58.9	67.1	55.0	64.2	95.2
2004	66.4	58.9	67.1	54.3	64.5	95.7
2005	66.7	59.0	67.2	53.6	63.0	96.4
2006	68.6	60.3	70.7	55.4	63.6	98.3
2007	69.3	61.0	71.4	55.6	65.3	97.4
2008	68.1	60.5	70.8	54.1	63.3	92.7
2009	66.2	59.6	68.9	51.7	61.3	86.5
2010	64.1	58.7	66.6	48.6	59.2	80.2
2011	63.2	58.7	65.4	47.7	59.9	76.2
2012	63.0	58.6	65.0	47.0	62.2	74.4
2013	62.5	58.7	64.6	46.4	59.2	72.9
2014	62.9	59.5	64.5	44.8	60.7	72.1

1 Includes births to White Hispanic and Black Hispanic women and births with origin not stated, not shown separately.   2 Hispanic origin are reported separately on birth certificates. Persons of Hispanic origin may be of any race. Multiple-race data, when reported, were bridged to single-race categories in order to maintain comparability among all reported areas.   3 Includes persons of Hispanic origin, and origin not stated, according to the mother's reported race.

Table 1-3. Births and Birth Rates, by Age, Race, and Hispanic Origin of Mother, 2013 and 2014

(Number, rates per 1,000 women in specified age group.)

Age, race, and Hispanic origin of mother	2013		2014	
	Number	Rate	Number	Rate
All Races and Origins [1]				
Total[2]	3,932,181	62.5	3,988,076	62.9
10 to 14 years	3,098	0.3	2,769	0.3
15 to 19 years	273,105	26.5	249,078	24.2
20 to 24 years	896,745	80.7	882,567	79.0
25 to 29 years	1,120,777	105.5	1,145,392	105.8
30 to 34 years	1,036,927	98.0	1,081,058	100.8
35 to 39 years	483,873	49.3	508,748	51.0
40 to 44 years	109,484	10.4	110,021	10.6
45 to 49 years[3]	7,495	0.8	7,700	0.8
50 to 54 years	677	NA	743	NA
Non-Hispanic White [4]				
Total[2]	2,129,196	58.7	2,149,302	59.5
10 to 14 years	717	0.1	679	0.1
15 to 19 years	107,886	18.6	99,220	17.3
20 to 24 years	431,540	68.3	420,224	67.1
25 to 29 years	637,710	103.5	646,907	103.9
30 to 34 years	620,788	101.9	642,219	104.7
35 to 39 years	269,221	48.0	280,788	49.6
40 to 44 years	56,896	9.1	55,609	9.1
45 to 49 years[3]	4,085	0.7	4,123	0.7
50 to 54 years	353	NA	343	NA
Non-Hispanic Black [4]				
Total[2]	583,834	64.6	588,891	64.5
10 to 14 years	1,043	0.7	955	0.6
15 to 19 years	62,066	39.0	54,819	34.9
20 to 24 years	185,662	105.6	182,435	102.8
25 to 29 years	153,903	102.7	160,935	103.3
30 to 34 years	112,650	77.3	116,939	79.6
35 to 39 years	53,546	40.3	57,647	42.5
40 to 44 years	13,851	9.9	14,000	10.1
45 to 49 years[3]	1,010	0.8	1,043	0.9
50 to 54 years	103	NA	118	NA
American Indian or Alaska Native Total [4,5]				
Total[2]	45,991	46.4	44,928	47.0
10 to 14 years	70	0.4	55	0.5
15 to 19 years	5,718	31.1	5,001	34.9
20 to 24 years	14,970	78.9	14,099	81.7
25 to 29 years	12,673	75.6	12,784	73.9
30 to 34 years	8,142	50.4	8,592	49.7
35 to 39 years	3,591	24.7	3,576	22.3
40 to 44 years	781	5.5	784	5.5
45 to 49 years[3]	39	0.3	35	0.5
50 to 54 years	7	NA	2	NA
Asian or Pacific Islander Total [4,5]				
Total[2]	265,673	59.2	282,723	44.8
10 to 14 years	58	0.1	40	0.3
15 to 19 years	5,083	8.7	4,637	27.3
20 to 24 years	27,250	39.1	27,003	37.5
25 to 29 years	70,886	89.5	74,950	90.0
30 to 34 years	95,865	114.6	105,442	121.3
35 to 39 years	52,872	66.6	56,449	68.9
40 to 44 years	12,648	16.1	13,157	16.1
45 to 49 years[3]	917	1.5	911	1.5
50 to 54 years	94	NA	134	NA
Hispanic [6]				
Total[2]	901,033	72.9	914,065	72.1
10 to 14 years	1,214	0.5	1,037	0.4
15 to 19 years	92,960	41.7	85,970	38.0
20 to 24 years	237,705	107.2	239,121	104.5
25 to 29 years	244,243	119.1	248,171	118.7
30 to 34 years	196,417	94.8	204,232	96.5
35 to 39 years	102,663	52.4	107,644	53.6
40 to 44 years	24,491	13.3	25,636	13.5
45 to 49 years[3]	1,274	0.8	1,374	0.9
50 to 54 years	66	NA	80	NA

1 Includes births to race and origin groups not shown separately, such as white Hispanic and black Hispanic women, and births with origin not stated.   2 Includes births to women of all ages. The rate shown for all ages is the fertility rate, which is defined as the total number of births (regardless of the age of the mother) per 1,000 women age 15 to 44 years.   3 The birth rate for women age 45 to 49 years is computed by relating the number of births to women age 45 and over to women age 45 to 49 years, as most of the births are to women age 45 to 49 years.   4 Race and Hispanic origin are reported separately on birth certificates. Persons of Hispanic origin may be of any race. Multiple-race data, when reported, were bridged to single-race categories in order to maintain comparability among all reported areas.   5 Includes persons of Hispanic origin, and origin not stated, according to the mother's reported race.   6 Includes all persons of Hispanic origin of any race.

Table 1-4. Birth Rates, by Age of Mother, Live-Birth Order, and Race and Hispanic Origin of Mother, 2014

(Rates per 1,000 women in specified age groups.)

Live-birth order and race and Hispanic origin of mother	15 to 44 years[1]	10 to 14 years	15 to 19 years	20 to 24 years	25 to 29 years	30 to 34 years	35 to 39 years	40 to 44 years	45 to 49 years[1]
All Races and Origins	62.9	0.3	24.2	79.0	105.8	100.8	51.0	10.6	0.8
1st child	24.6	0.3	20.1	40.1	39.8	30.6	11.6	2.3	0.2
2nd child	20.1	0.0	3.6	25.9	35.0	34.5	16.6	2.9	0.2
3rd child	10.6	*	0.5	9.6	19.2	20.0	11.3	2.2	0.1
4th child	4.5	*	0.1	2.6	7.7	9.2	5.9	1.4	0.1
5th child	1.8	*	0.0	0.6	2.7	3.7	2.7	0.7	0.1
6th and 7th child	1.1	*	0.0	0.2	1.2	2.3	2.0	0.6	0.1
8th child and over	0.3	*	*	0.0	0.2	0.6	0.9	0.4	0.0
Non-Hispanic White	59.5	0.1	17.3	67.1	103.9	104.7	49.6	9.1	0.7
1st child	24.5	0.1	14.8	36.3	43.7	34.7	12.5	2.3	0.2
2nd child	19.7	*	2.2	21.8	35.0	37.6	17.1	2.7	0.2
3rd child	9.4	*	0.2	7.0	16.7	19.4	10.6	1.8	0.1
4th child	3.6	*	0.0	1.6	5.9	7.8	4.8	1.0	0.1
5th child	1.3	*	0.0	0.3	1.8	2.9	2.1	0.5	0.0
6th and 7th child	0.8	*	*	0.1	0.7	1.8	1.6	0.4	0.0
8th child and over	0.3	*	*	0.0	0.1	0.4	0.8	0.4	0.0
Non-Hispanic Black	64.5	0.6	34.9	102.8	103.3	79.6	42.5	10.1	0.9
1st child	23.9	0.6	28.4	48.7	29.6	18.0	8.0	1.9	0.2
2nd child	18.6	*	5.5	32.7	32.3	23.3	11.4	2.4	0.2
3rd child	11.5	*	0.9	14.5	22.3	18.0	9.7	2.2	0.2
4th child	5.6	*	0.1	4.9	11.2	10.0	6.0	1.5	0.1
5th child	2.5	*	0.0	1.5	4.8	5.1	3.1	0.9	0.1
6th and 7th child	1.7	*	*	0.4	2.7	3.9	2.8	0.8	0.1
8th child and over	0.6	*	*	0.1	0.5	1.3	1.4	0.5	0.0
American Indian or Alaska Native	.44.8	0.3	27.3	73.2	74.7	52.3	24.1	5.5	0.3
1st child	14.8	0.0	22.3	30.6	16.3	8.6	3.3	0.7	*
2nd child	12.0	*	4.3	24.9	21.7	12.0	4.3	0.9	*
3rd child	8.5	*	0.6	12.1	18.4	12.3	5.1	1.0	*
4th child	4.8	*	*	4.2	10.5	8.7	4.4	1.0	*
5th child	2.4	*	*	1.1	4.8	5.1	2.7	0.7	*
6th and 7th child	1.8	*	*	0.3	2.7	4.3	3.0	0.9	*
8th child and over	0.5	*	*	*	0.3	1.3	1.0	0.4	*
Asian or Pacific Islander	60.7	0.1	7.7	37.5	90.0	121.3	68.9	16.1	1.5
1st child	27.2	0.0	6.4	23.0	50.3	50.9	19.8	4.3	0.5
2nd child	22.1	*	1.1	10.1	26.6	49.0	30.6	6.1	0.4
3rd child	7.4	*	0.1	3.1	8.5	13.9	12.1	3.3	0.3
4th child	2.5	*	*	0.9	2.9	4.5	3.9	1.3	0.1
5th child	0.9	*	*	0.2	1.0	1.6	1.4	0.6	0.1
6th and 7th child	0.5	*	*	0.1	0.5	1.0	0.9	0.4	0.1
8th child and over	0.2	*	*	*	0.1	0.3	0.3	0.2	0.0
Hispanic [2]	72.1	0.4	38.0	104.5	118.7	96.5	53.6	13.5	0.9
1st child	24.5	0.4	30.7	48.7	32.2	19.5	8.2	1.9	0.2
2nd child	21.6	*	6.3	36.3	40.5	27.9	13.2	2.8	0.2
3rd child	14.4	*	0.9	14.3	28.3	25.5	14.1	3.1	0.2
4th child	7.0	*	0.1	4.0	11.9	14.2	9.6	2.5	0.2
5th child	2.8	*	0.0	0.9	3.9	5.7	4.8	1.5	0.1
6th and 7th child	1.5	*	*	0.2	1.6	3.1	3.0	1.2	0.1
8th child and over	0.3	*	*	0.0	0.2	0.6	0.7	0.4	0.0

* = Figure does not meet standards of reliability or precision.   0.0 = Quantity more than zero but less than 0.05.   1 Birth rates computed by relating births to women aged 45 and over to women aged 45–49.
2 Includes all persons of Hispanic origin of any race.

Table 1-5. Birth Rates for Women Under 20 Years of Age, by Age and Race and Hispanic Origin of Mother, Selected Years, 1991–2014

(Rates per 1,000 women in specified group.)

Age, race, and Hispanic origin of mother	Year					Percent change		
	1991	2007	2010	2011	2014	1991–2014	2007–2014	2011–2014
10 to 14 Years								
All races and origins[1]	1.4	0.6	0.4	0.4	0.3	-78.6	-50.0	-25.0
Non-Hispanic White[2]	0.5	0.2	0.2	0.2	0.1	-80.0	-50.0	-50.0
Non-Hispanic Black[2]	4.9	1.4	1.0	0.9	0.6	-87.8	-57.1	-33.3
American Indian or Alaska Native total[2,3]	1.6	0.7	0.5	0.5	0.3	-81.3	-57.1	-40.0
Asian or Pacific Islander total[2,3]	0.8	0.2	0.1	0.1	0.1	-87.5	-50.0	†
Hispanic[4]	2.4	1.2	0.8	0.7	0.4	-83.3	-66.7	-42.9
15 to 19 Years								
All races and origins[1]	61.8	41.5	34.2	31.3	24.2	-60.8	-41.7	-22.7
Non-Hispanic White[2]	43.4	27.2	23.5	21.7	17.3	-60.1	-36.4	-20.3
Non-Hispanic Black[2]	118.2	62.0	51.5	47.3	34.9	-70.5	-43.7	-26.2
American Indian or Alaska Native total[2,3]	84.1	49.3	38.7	36.1	27.3	-67.5	-44.6	-24.4
Asian or Pacific Islander total[2,3]	27.3	14.8	10.9	10.2	7.7	-71.8	-48.0	-24.5
Hispanic[4]	104.6	75.3	55.7	49.6	38.0	-63.7	-49.5	-23.4
15 to 17 Years								
All races and origins[1]	38.6	21.7	17.3	15.4	10.9	-71.8	-49.8	-29.2
Non-Hispanic White[2]	23.6	11.9	10.0	9.0	6.7	-71.6	-43.7	-25.6
Non-Hispanic Black[2]	86.1	34.6	27.4	24.6	16.6	-80.7	-52.0	-32.5
American Indian or Alaska Native total[2,3]	51.9	26.1	20.1	18.2	13.2	-74.6	-49.4	-27.5
Asian or Pacific Islander total[2,3]	16.3	7.4	5.1	4.6	3.3	-79.8	-55.4	-28.3
Hispanic[4]	69.2	44.4	32.3	28.0	19.3	-72.1	-56.5	-31.1
18 to 19 Years								
All races and origins[1]	94.0	71.7	58.2	54.1	43.8	-53.4	-38.9	-19.0
Non-Hispanic White[2]	70.6	50.4	42.5	39.9	32.9	-53.4	-34.7	-17.5
Non-Hispanic Black[2]	162.2	105.2	85.6	78.8	61.5	-62.1	-41.5	-22.0
American Indian or Alaska Native total[2,3]	134.2	86.3	66.1	61.6	48.6	-63.8	-43.7	-21.1
Asian or Pacific Islander total[2,3]	42.2	24.9	18.7	18.1	13.9	-67.1	-44.2	-23.2
Hispanic[4]	155.5	124.7	90.7	81.5	66.1	-57.5	-47.0	-18.9

† = Difference not statistically significant.   1 Includes births to race and origin groups not shown separately, such as white Hispanic and black Hispanic women, and births with origin not stated.   2 Race and Hispanic origin are reported separately on birth certificates. Persons of Hispanic origin may be of any race. Multiple-race data, when reported, were bridged to single-race categories in order to maintain comparability among all reported areas.   3 Includes persons of Hispanic origin, and origin not stated, according to the mother's reported race.   4 Includes all persons of Hispanic origin of any race.

Table 1-6. Birth Rate for Teenagers Age 15 to 19 Years, by State and Territory, 2010 and 2014

(Rate per 1,000 female population age 15 to 19 years.)

State	2010	2014	Percent change
United States [1]	34.2	24.2	-29.2
Alabama	43.6	32.0	-26.6
Alaska	38.3	27.8	†
Arizona	41.9	29.9	-28.6
Arkansas	52.5	39.5	†
California	31.5	21.1	-33.0
Colorado	33.4	20.3	-39.2
Connecticut	18.7	11.5	-38.5
Delaware	30.5	20.7	†
District of Columbia	45.4	28.4	†
Florida	32.0	22.5	-29.7
Georgia	41.4	28.4	-31.4
Hawaii	32.5	23.1	-28.9
Idaho	33.0	23.2	-29.7
Illinois	33.0	22.8	-30.9
Indiana	37.3	28.0	-24.9
Iowa	28.6	19.8	-30.8
Kansas	39.3	27.6	-29.8
Kentucky	46.2	35.3	-23.6
Louisiana	47.7	35.8	-24.9
Maine	21.4	16.5	†
Maryland	27.3	17.8	-34.8
Massachusetts	17.2	10.6	-38.4
Michigan	30.1	21.1	-29.9
Minnesota	22.5	15.5	-31.1
Mississippi	55.0	38.0	-30.9
Missouri	37.1	27.2	-26.7
Montana	35.0	26.4	-24.6
Nebraska	31.1	22.2	-28.6
Nevada	38.6	28.5	-26.2
New Hampshire	15.7	11.0	-29.9
New Jersey	20.1	13.1	-34.8
New Mexico	53.0	37.8	-28.7
New York	22.7	16.1	-29.1
North Carolina	38.3	25.9	-32.4
North Dakota	28.8	23.9	†
Ohio	34.1	25.1	-26.4
Oklahoma	50.4	38.5	-23.6
Oregon	28.2	20.0	-29.1
Pennsylvania	27.0	19.3	-28.5
Rhode Island	22.3	15.8	†
South Carolina	42.6	28.5	-33.1
South Dakota	34.9	26.2	†
Tennessee	43.2	33.0	-23.6
Texas	52.2	37.8	-27.6
Utah	27.9	19.4	-30.5
Vermont	17.9	14.2	†
Virginia	27.4	18.4	-32.8
Washington	26.7	19.1	-28.5
West Virginia	44.4	36.6	†
Wisconsin	26.2	18.0	-31.3
Wyoming	39.0	30.1	-22.8
Puerto Rico	51.4	40.4	†
Virgin Islands	50.5	NA	†
Guam	60.1	48.4	†
American Samoa	34.1	46.8	†
Northern Marianas	53.4	38.6	†

† = Difference not statistically significant.   1 Excludes data for the territories.

Figure 1-2. Percent of Births, by Race and Hispanic Origin, 2014

Figure 1-3. Percent of Births to Unmarried Women by Race and Hispanic Origin

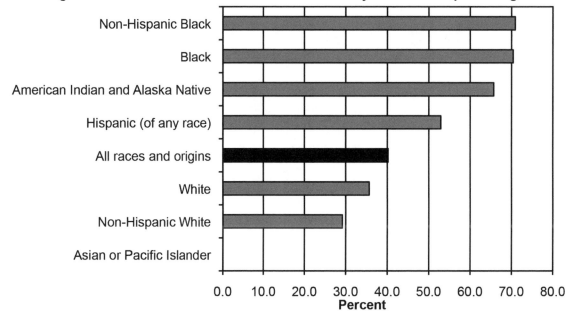

Table 1-7. Number, Percent, and Rate of Births to Unmarried Women, by Age, 2014

(Number, percent, rate per 1,000 unmarried women.)

Age of mother	Number	Percent	Rate
Total	1,604,870	40.2	43.9
Under 20 years	223,386	NA	NA
Under 15 years	2,752	99.4	NA
15 to 19 years	220,634	88.6	22
20 to 24 years	579,760	65.7	61.6
25 to 29 years	419,792	36.7	67.6
30 to 34 years	243,054	22.5	58.1
35 to 39 years	110,058	21.6	33.4
40 years and over	28,830	24.3	8.5

NA = Not available.

Table 1-8 Live Births, by Race and Hispanic Origin of Mother, and Birth and Fertility Rates, by State and Territory, 2014

(Birth rates are total births per 1,000 women; fertility rates are total births per 1,000 women age 15-44 years.)

State and territory	All races and origins[1]	Non-Hispanic White[2]	Non-Hispanic Black[2]	American Indian or Alaskan Native[2,3]	Asian or Pacific Islander[2,3]	Hispanic[4]	Birth rate for all races	Fertility rate for all races
United States [5]	3,988,076	2,149,302	588,891	44,928	282,723	914,065	12.5	62.9
Alabama	59,422	35,929	18,230	200	1,227	4,019	12.3	61.8
Alaska	11,392	6,541	446	2,450	1,106	841	15.5	77.3
Arizona	86,887	38,608	4,673	5,473	3,519	35,034	12.9	66.4
Arkansas	38,511	25,940	7,254	301	1,202	3,837	13.0	67.0
California	502,879	144,318	28,312	3,509	84,224	237,539	13.0	62.4
Colorado	65,830	40,629	3,355	777	3,010	17,655	12.3	60.7
Connecticut	36,285	20,933	4,615	308	2,280	8,129	10.1	53.0
Delaware	10,972	5,904	2,847	26	644	1,541	11.7	60.8
District of Columbia	9,509	2,966	4,775	16	482	1,282	14.4	53.6
Florida	219,991	100,837	49,313	406	7,402	61,849	11.1	59.7
Georgia	130,946	60,104	45,022	292	6,519	17,242	13.0	62.2
Hawaii	18,550	4,881	558	30	11,535	2,764	13.1	69.3
Idaho	22,876	18,188	207	429	501	3,651	14.0	72.7
Illinois	158,556	86,227	27,187	227	10,174	33,803	12.3	61.1
Indiana	84,080	64,076	10,344	125	2,322	7,239	12.7	64.9
Iowa	39,687	32,423	2,359	284	1,408	3,315	12.8	67.8
Kansas	39,223	28,504	2,938	347	1,359	6,132	13.5	70.0
Kentucky	56,170	46,701	5,352	76	1,275	2,819	12.7	65.8
Louisiana	64,497	34,264	24,222	373	1,537	4,249	13.9	68.4
Maine	12,698	11,654	442	158	248	200	9.5	54.3
Maryland	73,921	33,178	23,968	260	5,797	10,974	12.4	61.5
Massachusetts	71,908	44,542	7,165	151	6,599	12,722	10.7	52.5
Michigan	114,375	80,304	21,650	784	4,284	7,352	11.5	60.6
Minnesota	69,904	50,332	7,745	1,428	5,669	4,678	12.8	66.4
Mississippi	38,736	19,839	16,621	223	583	1,547	12.9	64.4
Missouri	75,360	57,150	11,453	423	2,186	3,959	12.4	64.1
Montana	12,432	10,153	90	1,585	169	494	12.1	67.0
Nebraska	26,794	19,471	1,852	553	1,048	4,143	14.2	73.6
Nevada	35,861	15,151	4,259	475	3,145	13,006	12.6	63.3
New Hampshire	12,302	10,917	189	21	528	591	9.3	50.5
New Jersey	103,305	48,196	15,528	193	11,977	27,267	11.6	59.9
New Mexico	26,052	7,222	468	3,581	578	14,449	12.5	65.5
New York	238,773	116,013	36,958	757	26,786	55,329	12.1	59.0
North Carolina	120,975	67,551	29,017	2,025	5,730	17,784	12.2	61.0
North Dakota	11,359	9,036	460	1,032	314	480	15.4	78.8
Ohio	139,467	104,102	23,663	301	4,232	6,884	12.0	63.1
Oklahoma	53,339	33,577	5,044	6,051	1,734	7,219	13.8	69.9
Oregon	45,556	32,338	1,219	778	2,811	8,524	11.5	58.7
Pennsylvania	142,268	99,306	20,169	368	7,067	14,496	11.1	59.1
Rhode Island	10,823	6,573	851	130	594	2,585	10.3	51.5
South Carolina	57,627	33,639	17,878	193	1,293	4,646	11.9	61.1
South Dakota	12,283	9,122	340	2,055	271	603	14.4	77.8
Tennessee	81,602	55,499	16,989	240	2,180	6,986	12.5	63.0
Texas	399,766	140,992	47,983	1,168	20,844	189,462	14.8	70.7
Utah	51,154	39,433	573	713	1,850	7,764	17.4	80.0
Vermont	6,130	5,724	116	16	163	92	9.8	52.9
Virginia	103,300	59,885	21,623	255	8,356	13,490	12.4	61.3
Washington	88,585	55,872	4,659	2,059	10,306	15,779	12.5	63.3
West Virginia	20,301	18,860	762	29	214	350	11.0	60.3
Wisconsin	67,161	49,440	7,063	980	3,333	6,375	11.7	61.8
Wyoming	7,696	6,258	85	294	108	895	13.2	69.4
Puerto Rico	34,434	30,246	4,171	- - -	NA	31,693	9.7	48.2
Virgin Islands	NA	NA	NA	NA	NA	NA	NA	NA
Guam	3,395	1	5	13	3,109	61	21.1	99.1
American Samoa	1,077	–	–	–	1,077	NA	19.8	85.2
Northern Marianas	517	8	2	–	509	3	10.0	39.6

NA = Not available.   - = Quantity zero   1 Includes births to race and origin groups not shown separately, such as white Hispanic and black Hispanic women, and births with origin not stated.   2 Race and Hispanic origin are reported separately on birth certificates.   3 Includes persons of Hispanic origin according to the mother's reported race.   4 Includes all persons of Hispanic origin of any race.   5 Excludes data for the territories.

Table 1-9. Selected Characteristics of Births, by Race and Hispanic Origin of Mother, 2011 and 2014

(Number, rate.)

Race and Hispanic origin of mother	Number Total[2]		Cesarean rate[1] Late[3]		Preterm Total[4]		Very low birthweight[5]			Low birthweight		
	2011	2014	2011	2014	2011	2014	2011	2014	2011	2014	2011	2014
All Races and Origins [6]	3,953,590	3,988,076	32.8	32.2	11.7	11.5	8.3	8.1	8.1	8.0	1.4	1.4
Non-Hispanic White[7]	2,146,566	2,149,302	32.4	31.4	10.5	8.9	7.6	6.5	7.1	7.0	1.1	1.1
Non-Hispanic Black[7]	582,345	588,891	35.5	35.6	16.8	13.2	10.7	6.5	13.3	13.2	3.0	2.9
American Indian or Alaska Native total[7,8]	46,419	44,928	28.4	28.5	13.5	10.2	9.6	2.7	7.6	7.6	1.3	1.3
Asian or Pacific Islander total[7,8]	253,915	272,949	33.2	33.2	10.4	8.5	7.6	2.2	8.4	8.1	1.2	1.2
Hispanic[9]	918,129	914,065	32.0	31.9	11.7	9.5	8.4	6.8	7.0	8.0	1.2	1.2

1 All births by cesarean delivery per 100 live births.   2 Born prior to 37 completed weeks of gestation.   3 Born between 34 and 36 completed weeks of gestation.   4 Birthweight of less than 2,500 grams (5 lb 8 oz).   5 Birthweight of less than 1,500 grams (3 lb 4 oz).   6 Includes births to White Hispanic and Black Hispanic women and births with origin not stated, not shown separately.   7 Race and Hispanic origin are reported separately on birth certificates. Persons of Hispanic origin may be of any race. Multiple-race data, when reported, were bridged to single-race categories in order to maintain comparability among all reported areas.   8 Includes persons of Hispanic and non-Hispanic origin and origin not stated, according to the mother's reported race.   9 Persons of Hispanic origin may be of any race.

Table 1-10. Preterm Births, 2007–2014

(Percent.)

Year	Total preterm[1]	Late preterm[2]	Early preterm (less than 34 weeks)		
			Total	32–33 weeks	Less than 32 weeks
2007	10.4	7.5	2.9	1.2	1.7
2008	10.4	7.5	2.9	1.2	1.7
2009	10.1	7.2	2.9	1.2	1.7
2010	10.0	7.2	2.8	1.2	1.7
2011	9.8	7.0	2.8	1.2	1.6
2012	9.8	7.0	2.8	1.2	1.6
2013	9.6	6.8	2.8	1.2	1.6
2014	9.6	6.8	2.8	1.2	1.6

1 Preterm is less than 37 completed weeks of gestation.   2 Late preterm is 34 to 36 completed weeks of gestation.

Table 1-11. Birth Rates, by Live-Birth Order and by Race and Hispanic Origin of Mother, 2000–2014

(Rates are live births per 1,000 women age 15 to 44 years.)

Year, race, and Hispanic origin of mother	Fertility rate	Live-birth order			
		1st child	2nd child	3rd child	4th child and over
All Races and Origins [1,2]					
2000	65.9	26.5	21.4	11.0	7.0
2001	65.1	25.9	21.3	11.0	7.0
2002	65.0	25.8	21.2	10.9	7.0
2003	66.1	26.5	21.4	11.1	7.1
2004	66.4	26.4	21.4	11.2	7.3
2005	66.7	26.5	21.5	11.3	7.4
2006	68.6	27.4	21.9	11.6	7.7
2007	69.3	27.8	22.0	11.7	7.8
2008	68.1	27.5	21.5	11.4	7.8
2009	66.2	26.8	20.8	11.0	7.6
2010	64.1	25.9	20.2	10.6	7.5
2011	63.2	25.4	20.0	10.4	7.4
2012	63.0	25.2	19.9	10.4	7.4
2013	62.5	24.7	19.9	10.4	7.4
2014	62.9	24.6	20.1	10.6	7.6
Non-Hispanic White [2,3]					
2000	58.5	24.2	19.8	9.4	5.1
2001	57.7	23.6	19.7	9.4	5.1
2002	57.6	23.6	19.6	9.3	5.1
2003	58.9	24.5	19.8	9.4	5.2
2004	58.9	24.4	19.8	9.5	5.3
2005	59.0	24.4	19.8	9.5	5.3
2006	60.3	25.1	20.0	9.6	5.5
2007	61.0	25.6	20.1	9.7	5.6
2008	60.5	25.5	19.8	9.5	5.6
2009	59.6	25.3	19.5	9.2	5.6
2010	58.7	25.0	19.2	9.1	5.5
2011	58.7	24.9	19.2	9.0	5.6
2012	58.6	24.7	19.2	9.1	5.6
2013	58.7	24.4	19.3	9.2	5.7
2014	59.5	24.5	19.7	9.4	5.9
Non-Hispanic Black [2,3]					
2000	71.4	26.7	21.2	12.8	10.8
2001	69.1	25.9	20.4	12.4	10.5
2002	67.5	25.4	19.7	12.1	10.4
2003	67.1	25.4	19.6	11.9	10.3
2004	67.1	25.5	19.4	11.9	10.3
2005	67.2	25.8	19.3	11.8	10.3
2006	70.7	27.5	20.3	12.3	10.6
2007	71.4	27.9	20.4	12.3	10.8
2008	70.8	28.1	20.0	12.1	10.7
2009	68.9	27.3	19.4	11.7	10.5
2010	66.6	26.3	18.9	11.3	10.1
2011	65.4	25.6	18.5	11.1	10.1
2012	65.0	25.1	18.6	11.2	10.1
2013	64.6	24.4	18.6	11.3	10.3
2014	64.5	23.9	18.6	11.5	10.4
Hispanic [4]					
2000	95.9	35.8	29.2	18.0	12.9
2001	95.4	35.2	29.3	18.0	12.9
2002	94.7	34.7	29.1	18.0	12.9
2003	95.2	34.5	29.4	18.3	13.0
2004	95.7	34.4	29.3	18.7	13.4
2005	96.4	34.4	29.6	19.0	13.5
2006	98.3	35.1	29.9	19.3	14.0
2007	97.4	34.7	29.4	19.3	14.1
2008	92.7	33.0	27.8	18.3	13.6
2009	86.5	30.6	25.9	17.0	13.0
2010	80.2	28.0	24.0	15.9	12.4
2011	76.2	26.3	22.9	15.2	11.8
2012	74.4	25.5	22.3	14.9	11.7
2013	72.9	24.9	21.8	14.6	11.6
2014	72.1	24.5	21.6	14.4	11.6

Year, race, and Hispanic origin of mother	Fertility rate	Live-birth order			
		1st child	2nd child	3rd child	4th child and over

1 Includes births to race and origin groups not shown separately, such as white Hispanic and black Hispanic women, and births with origin not stated.   2 Includes origin not stated.   3 Race and Hispanic origin are reported separately on birth certificates. Persons of Hispanic origin may be of any race. Multiple-race data, when reported, were bridged to single-race categories in order to maintain comparability among all reported areas.   4 Includes all persons of Hispanic origin of any race.

Table 1-12. Birth Rates for Teenagers Age 15 to 19 Years, by State and Territory of Residence, Selected Years, 1991–2014

(Birth rates per 1,000 estimated female population age 15 to 19 years in each area, percent.)

State and territory	1991	2005	2009	2010	2014	Percent change, 1991–2014	Percent change, 2005–2014	Percent change, 2009–2014	Percent change, 2010–2014
United States [1]	61.8	40.5	39.1	34.2	24.2	-60.8	-40.2	-38.1	-29.2
Alabama	73.6	49.7	50.7	43.6	32.0	-56.5	-35.6	-36.9	-26.6
Alaska	66.0	37.3	44.5	38.3	27.8	-57.9	-25.5	-37.5	-27.4
Arizona	79.7	58.2	50.6	41.9	29.9	-62.5	-48.6	-40.9	-28.6
Arkansas	79.5	59.1	59.2	52.5	39.5	-50.3	-33.2	-33.3	-24.8
California	73.8	38.8	36.6	31.5	21.1	-71.4	-45.6	-42.3	-33.0
Colorado	58.3	42.6	38.5	33.4	20.3	-65.2	-52.3	-47.3	-39.2
Connecticut	40.1	23.3	21.0	18.7	11.5	-71.3	-50.6	-45.2	-38.5
Delaware	60.4	44.0	35.3	30.5	20.7	-65.7	-53.0	-41.4	-32.1
District of Columbia	109.6	63.4	47.7	45.4	28.4	-74.1	-55.2	-40.5	-37.4
Florida	67.9	42.4	39.0	32.0	22.5	-66.9	-46.9	-42.3	-29.7
Georgia	76.0	52.7	47.7	41.4	28.4	-62.6	-46.1	-40.5	-31.4
Hawaii	59.2	36.2	40.9	32.5	23.1	-61.0	-36.2	-43.5	-28.9
Idaho	53.9	37.7	35.9	33.0	23.2	-57.0	-38.5	-35.4	-29.7
Illinois	64.5	38.6	36.1	33.0	22.8	-64.7	-40.9	-36.8	-30.9
Indiana	60.4	43.2	42.5	37.3	28.0	-53.6	-35.2	-34.1	-24.9
Iowa	42.5	32.6	32.1	28.6	19.8	-53.4	-39.3	-38.3	-30.8
Kansas	55.4	41.4	43.8	39.3	27.6	-50.2	-33.3	-37.0	-29.8
Kentucky	68.8	49.1	51.3	46.2	35.3	-48.7	-28.1	-31.2	-23.6
Louisiana	76.0	49.1	52.7	47.7	35.8	-52.9	-27.1	-32.1	-24.9
Maine	43.5	24.4	24.4	21.4	16.5	-62.1	-32.4	-32.4	-22.9
Maryland	54.1	31.8	31.3	27.3	17.8	-67.1	-44.0	-43.1	-34.8
Massachusetts	37.5	21.8	19.6	17.2	10.6	-71.7	-51.4	-45.9	-38.4
Michigan	58.9	32.5	32.7	30.1	21.1	-64.2	-35.1	-35.5	-29.9
Minnesota	37.3	26.1	24.3	22.5	15.5	-58.4	-40.6	-36.2	-31.1
Mississippi	85.3	60.5	64.2	55.0	38.0	-55.5	-37.2	-40.8	-30.9
Missouri	64.4	42.5	41.6	37.1	27.2	-57.8	-36.0	-34.6	-26.7
Montana	46.8	35.2	38.5	35.0	26.4	-43.6	-25.0	-31.4	-24.6
Nebraska	42.4	34.2	34.6	31.1	22.2	-47.6	-35.1	-35.8	-28.6
Nevada	74.5	50.1	47.4	38.6	28.5	-61.7	-43.1	-39.9	-26.2
New Hampshire	33.1	17.9	16.4	15.7	11.0	-66.8	-38.5	-32.9	-29.9
New Jersey	41.3	23.4	22.7	20.1	13.1	-68.3	-44.0	-42.3	-34.8
New Mexico	79.5	61.6	63.9	53.0	37.8	-52.5	-38.6	-40.8	-28.7
New York	45.5	26.5	24.4	22.7	16.1	-64.6	-39.2	-34.0	-29.1
North Carolina	70.0	48.5	44.9	38.3	25.9	-63.0	-46.6	-42.3	-32.4
North Dakota	35.5	29.7	27.9	28.8	23.9	-32.7	-19.5	-14.3	-17.0
Ohio	60.5	38.9	38.9	34.1	25.1	-58.5	-35.5	-35.5	-26.4
Oklahoma	72.1	54.2	60.1	50.4	38.5	-46.6	-29.0	-35.9	-23.6
Oregon	54.8	33.0	33.1	28.2	20.0	-63.5	-39.4	-39.6	-29.1
Pennsylvania	46.7	30.4	29.3	27.0	19.3	-58.7	-36.5	-34.1	-28.5
Rhode Island	44.7	31.4	26.8	22.3	15.8	-64.7	-49.7	-41.0	-29.1
South Carolina	72.5	51.0	49.1	42.6	28.5	-60.7	-44.1	-42.0	-33.1
South Dakota	47.6	37.5	38.4	34.9	26.2	-45.0	-30.1	-31.8	-24.9
Tennessee	74.8	54.9	50.6	43.2	33.0	-55.9	-39.9	-34.8	-23.6
Texas	78.4	61.6	60.7	52.2	37.8	-51.8	-38.6	-37.7	-27.6
Utah	48.0	33.4	30.7	27.9	19.4	-59.6	-41.9	-36.8	-30.5
Vermont	39.2	18.6	17.4	17.9	14.2	-63.8	-23.7	-18.4	-20.7
Virginia	53.4	34.4	31.0	27.4	18.4	-65.5	-46.5	-40.6	-32.8
Washington	53.7	31.1	31.9	26.7	19.1	-64.4	-38.6	-40.1	-28.5
West Virginia	58.0	43.4	49.8	44.8	36.6	-36.9	-15.7	-26.5	-18.3
Wisconsin	43.7	30.3	29.4	26.2	18.0	-58.8	-40.6	-38.8	-31.3
Wyoming	54.3	43.2	45.0	39.0	30.1	-44.6	-30.3	-33.1	-22.8
Puerto Rico	72.4	61.2	54.7	51.4	40.4	-44.2	-34.0	-26.1	-21.4
Virgin Islands	77.9	50.0	51.5	50.5	NA	NA	NA	NA	NA
Guam	95.7	59.2	50.8	60.1	48.4	-49.4	-18.2	-4.7	-19.5
America Samoa	NA	34.2	35.2	34.1	46.8	NA	36.8	33.0	37.2
Northern Marinas	NA	30.4	50.2	53.4	38.6	NA	27.0	-23.1	-27.7

NA = Not available.   1 Excludes data for the territories.

Figure 1-4. Birth Rates for Teenagers Age 15–19 by Race and Hispanic Origin, 1991 and 2014

Figure 1-5. Highest and Lowest Birth Rates for Teenagers (Age 15 to 19 Years) by State, 2014

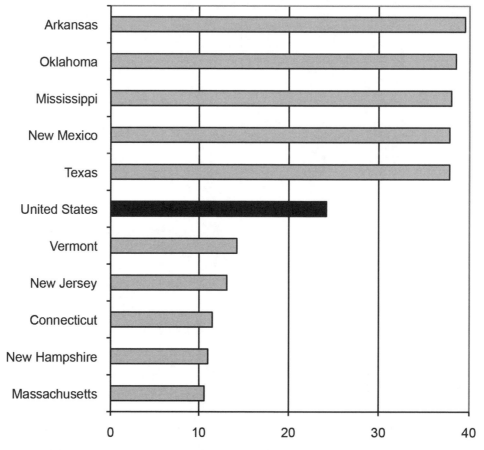

Table 1-13. Responses to the Statement, "If You Got Pregnant Now or Got a Female Pregnant Now, How Would You Feel?" for Never-Married Females and Males Age 15 to 19 Years, 2002 and 2006–2010

(Numbers in thousands, percent.)

Characteristic	Number of respondents	Percent surveyed[1]	Very upset		A little upset		A little pleased		Very pleased	
			Percent	Standard error	Percent	Standard error	Percent	Standard error	Percent	Standard error
2002, Total	9,598	100.0	60.2	1.8	26.7	1.6	8.0	0.9	4.7	0.8
2006–2010 [2], Total	10,361	100.0	57.5	1.5	29.1	1.3	8.2	0.8	4.8	0.7
2006–2010										
Hispanic Origin and Race										
Hispanic or Latina	1,849	100.0	47.7	3.0	32.5	3.0	13.2	2.5	6.0	1.3
Non-Hispanic white	6,150	100.0	63.1	2.0	28.2	1.9	5.4	1.0	3.2	0.8
Non-Hispanic black	1,691	100.0	48.9	3.0	30.6	2.4	9.9	1.6	9.5	1.7
Age										
15–17 years	5,820	100.0	63.3	1.9	28.6	1.6	5.7	1.0	2.2	0.5
18–19 years	4,541	100.0	50.0	2.3	29.7	2.1	11.5	1.1	8.3	1.4
Ever Had Sex										
Yes	4,417	100.0	44.2	2.1	33.9	1.9	12.7	1.4	8.6	1.4
No	5,944	100.0	67.3	2.0	25.5	1.8	4.9	0.9	2.1	0.6
Family Structure at Age 14										
Both biological or adoptive parents	6,317	100.0	63.7	2.0	25.2	1.8	7.1	1.0	3.8	0.8
Other[2]	4,044	100.0	47.7	2.1	35.2	1.8	10.1	1.3	6.6	1.1
Male										
Total 2002	10,139	100.0	51.4	2.0	33.4	1.8	11.0	1.4	3.7	0.6
Total 2006–2010[1]	10,766	100.0	46.4	1.8	34.0	1.5	14.3	1.2	4.3	0.5
Male, 2006–2010										
Hispanic origin and race:										
Hispanic or Latino	2,000	100.0	26.6	2.9	37.8	2.6	23.3	3.2	11.7	2.2
Non-Hispanic white	6,405	100.0	56.0	2.1	32.1	2.0	9.7	1.2	1.5	0.5
Non-Hispanic black	1,673	100.0	29.9	3.3	40.0	3.3	22.4	2.4	6.5	1.3
Age										
15–17 years	6,623	100.0	53.1	2.2	32.3	2.0	11.1	1.4	2.8	0.5
18–19 years	4,143	100.0	35.8	2.4	36.9	2.0	19.2	1.9	6.8	1.1
Ever Had Sex										
Yes	4,501	100.0	32.8	2.0	37.5	1.8	21.1	2.2	6.9	1.0
No	6,266	100.0	56.2	2.2	31.5	2.1	9.3	1.1	2.5	0.6
Family Structure at Age 14										
Both biological or adoptive parents	6,737	100.0	52.0	2.1	32.5	1.6	11.5	1.3	3.3	0.6
Other[3]	4,029	100.0	37.1	2.0	36.7	2.3	18.9	1.8	6.0	0.8

1 Percentages may not add to 100 because responses of "would not care" (coded only if respondent insisted) are not shown separately.   2 Includes persons of other or unknown origin and race groups, not shown separately.   3 Refers to anything other than two biological or adoptive parents or biological mother and stepfather, including one biological parent and no other parents(s)/parent figures or no parent(s)/parent figures.

Table 1-14. Birth Rates for Women Age 10 to 19 Years, by Age, Race, and Hispanic Origin of Mother, Selected Years, 1991–2014

(Rates per 1,000 women in specified age, race, and Hispanic origin groups.)

Age, race, and Hispanic origin of mother	1991	2007	2013	2014	Percent change, 1991–2014	Percent change, 2007–2014	Percent change, 2010–2014
10 to 14 Years							
All races and origins[1]	1.4	0.6	0.3	0.3	−79	−50	†
Non-Hispanic White[2]	0.5	0.2	0.1	0.1	−80	−50	†
Non-Hispanic Black[2]	4.9	1.4	0.7	0.6	−88	−57	−14
American Indian or Alaska Native total[2,3]	1.6	0.7	0.4	0.3	−81	−57	−25
Asian or Pacific Islander total[2,3]	0.8	0.2	0.1	0.1	−88	−50	†
Hispanic[4]	2.4	1.2	0.5	0.4	−83	−67	−20
15 to 19 Years							
All races and origins[1]	61.8	41.5	26.5	24.2	−61	−42	−9
Non-Hispanic White[2]	43.4	27.2	18.6	17.3	−60	−36	−7
Non-Hispanic Black[2]	118.2	62.0	39.0	34.9	−70	−44	−11
American Indian or Alaska Native total[2,3]	84.1	49.3	31.1	27.3	−68	−45	−12
Asian or Pacific Islander total[2,3]	27.3	14.8	8.7	7.7	−72	−48	−11
Hispanic[4]	104.6	75.3	41.7	38.0	−64	−50	−9
15 to 17 Years							
All races and origins[1]	38.6	21.7	12.3	10.9	−72	−50	−11
Non-Hispanic White[2]	23.6	11.9	7.4	6.7	−72	−44	−9
Non-Hispanic Black[2]	86.1	34.6	18.9	16.6	−81	−52	−12
American Indian or Alaska Native total[2,3]	51.9	26.1	15.9	13.2	−75	−49	−17
Asian or Pacific Islander total[2,3]	16.3	7.4	3.7	3.3	−80	−55	−11
Hispanic[4]	69.2	44.4	22.0	19.3	−72	−57	−12
18 to 19 Years							
All races and origins[1]	94.0	71.7	47.1	43.8	−53	−39	−7
Non-Hispanic White[2]	70.6	50.4	35.0	32.9	−53	−35	−6
Non-Hispanic Black[2]	162.2	105.2	67.0	61.5	−62	−42	−8
American Indian or Alaska Native total[2,3]	134.2	86.3	53.3	48.6	−64	−44	−9
Asian or Pacific Islander total[2,3]	42.2	24.9	16.1	13.9	−67	−44	−14
Hispanic[4]	155.5	124.7	70.8	66.1	−57	−47	−7

† = Difference not statistically significant.   1 Includes births to race and origin groups not shown separately, such as white Hispanic and black Hispanic women, and births with origin not stated.   2 Race and Hispanic origin are reported separately on birth certificates. Persons of Hispanic origin may be of any race. Multiple-race data, when reported, were bridged to single-race categories in order to maintain comparability among all reported areas.   3 Includes persons of Hispanic origin, and origin not stated, according to the mother's reported race.   4 Includes all persons of Hispanic origin of any race.

Table 1-15. Mean Age of Mother, by Live-Birth Order and Race and Hispanic Origin of Mother, Selected Years, 1980–2014

(Arithmetic average of the age of mothers at the times of births.)

Year, race, and Hispanic origin of mother	Total	Live-birth order							Unknown or not stated
		1	2	3	4	5	6 and 7	8 and over	
All Races [1]									
1980 [2]	25.0	22.7	25.4	27.3	29.0	30.6	32.7	36.0	23.9
1985	25.8	23.7	26.3	27.9	29.3	30.6	32.5	35.7	26.1
1990	26.4	24.2	26.9	28.3	29.4	30.6	32.1	35.1	27.4
1995	26.9	24.5	27.5	29.1	30.1	31.2	32.6	35.4	27.1
2000	27.2	24.9	27.7	29.2	30.3	31.4	32.9	35.8	27.4
2001	27.3	25.0	27.8	29.2	30.3	31.4	32.9	35.9	27.0
2002	27.3	25.1	27.9	29.2	30.3	31.4	32.9	35.9	27.7
2003	27.4	25.2	28.0	29.3	30.4	31.4	33.0	35.8	27.9
2004	27.5	25.2	28.0	29.4	30.4	31.4	32.9	35.9	27.6
2005	27.4	25.2	28.0	29.4	30.4	31.4	32.9	35.9	28.0
2006	27.4	25.0	27.9	29.3	30.4	31.4	33.0	35.8	28.0
2007	27.4	25.0	27.9	29.3	30.4	31.5	32.9	35.7	27.9
2008	27.4	25.1	27.9	29.4	30.5	31.5	32.9	35.7	27.7
2009	27.5	25.2	28.0	29.5	30.6	31.6	32.9	35.7	27.6
2010	27.7	25.4	28.2	29.6	30.7	31.7	33.0	35.7	27.7
2011	27.9	25.6	28.3	29.7	30.8	31.8	33.1	35.5	28.2
2012	28.0	25.8	28.4	29.8	30.9	31.9	33.2	35.7	27.9
2013	28.2	26.0	28.6	29.9	31.1	32.0	33.3	35.7	28.3
2014	28.3	26.3	28.7	30.0	31.0	32.0	33.4	35.7	28.7
Non-Hispanic White [3]									
1990 [4]	27.1	25.0	27.6	29.1	30.3	31.6	33.2	36.2	28.5
1995	27.6	25.4	28.3	29.9	31.2	32.4	33.9	36.7	28.5
2000	28.0	25.9	28.6	30.0	31.3	32.4	34.0	37.0	28.9
2001	28.1	26.0	28.6	30.1	31.3	32.4	33.9	37.0	28.2
2002	28.2	26.1	28.7	30.1	31.2	32.3	33.9	37.1	28.6
2003	28.2	26.2	28.8	30.1	31.2	32.3	33.9	37.0	28.8
2004	28.2	26.2	28.8	30.2	31.2	32.2	33.8	36.9	28.7
2005	28.2	26.2	28.8	30.1	31.2	32.2	33.8	36.9	29.1
2006	28.1	26.0	28.8	30.1	31.1	32.1	33.7	36.7	29.1
2007	28.1	26.0	28.7	30.0	31.1	32.1	33.7	36.7	28.8
2008	28.1	26.0	28.7	30.1	31.1	32.1	33.6	36.7	28.7
2009	28.1	26.1	28.8	30.1	31.1	32.1	33.6	36.7	28.6
2010	28.3	26.3	28.9	30.2	31.1	32.2	33.6	36.6	28.7
2011	28.4	26.5	29.0	30.2	31.2	32.2	33.7	36.4	29.0
2012	28.5	26.6	29.0	30.2	31.3	32.2	33.7	36.5	28.6
2013	28.6	26.8	29.1	30.3	31.3	32.3	33.7	36.6	29.0
2014	28.8	27.0	29.2	30.4		32.3	33.8	36.6	29.3
Non-Hispanic Black [3]									
1990 [4]	24.4	21.7	24.6	26.3	27.4	28.7	30.3	33.3	26.0
1995	24.8	21.9	25.3	27.0	28.0	29.3	30.8	33.2	25.4
2000	25.2	22.3	25.5	27.1	28.2	29.5	31.0	33.9	26.0
2001	25.3	22.4	25.7	27.2	28.3	29.6	31.2	34.1	26.4
2002	25.4	22.6	25.8	27.3	28.5	29.6	31.2	34.1	26.5
2003	25.6	22.7	25.9	27.5	28.6	29.7	31.3	34.0	26.3
2004	25.6	22.7	25.9	27.5	28.6	29.8	31.2	34.1	25.7
2005	25.6	22.7	26.0	27.6	28.8	29.8	31.3	34.2	25.8
2006	25.6	22.7	26.0	27.7	28.8	29.9	31.4	34.1	25.9
2007	25.6	22.7	26.0	27.7	28.9	30.0	31.4	34.2	26.1
2008	25.6	22.8	26.0	27.8	29.0	30.0	31.5	34.2	26.2
2009	25.7	22.9	26.1	27.9	29.1	30.2	31.5	34.3	26.2
2010	25.9	23.1	26.3	28.0	29.3	30.3	31.7	34.2	26.5
2011	26.1	23.4	26.4	28.2	29.4	30.5	31.8	34.2	26.6
2012	26.3	23.6	26.6	28.3	29.5	30.5	31.9	34.2	26.5
2013	26.6	23.9	26.8	28.5	29.6	30.6	31.9	34.4	27.1
2014	26.9	24.2	27.0	28.6	29.8	30.7	32.1	34.3	17.7
Hispanic [5]									
1990 [4]	25.3	22.4	25.2	27.4	29.1	30.6	32.3	35.3	26.1
1995	25.4	22.4	25.5	27.8	29.6	31.1	32.8	35.5	24.2
2000	25.7	22.7	25.8	28.1	29.8	31.3	33.0	35.5	24.2
2001	25.9	22.8	25.9	28.2	29.9	31.4	33.1	35.7	24.4
2002	26.0	23.0	26.0	28.3	29.9	31.4	33.1	35.7	25.7
2003	26.1	23.1	26.1	28.4	30.0	31.4	33.1	35.4	25.8
2004	26.2	23.1	26.2	28.5	30.1	31.5	33.1	35.5	25.8

Table 1-15. Mean Age of Mother, by Live-Birth Order and Race and Hispanic Origin of Mother, Selected Years, 1980–2014— continued

(Arithmetic average of the age of mothers at the times of births.)

Year, race, and Hispanic origin of mother	Total	Live-birth order							
		1	2	3	4	5	6 and 7	8 and over	Unknown or not stated
2005	26.2	23.1	26.2	28.5	30.1	31.4	33.2	35.6	26.5
2006	26.2	23.1	26.2	28.6	30.2	31.5	33.2	35.5	26.6
2007	26.3	23.1	26.3	28.6	30.3	31.6	33.1	35.3	26.7
2008	26.4	23.1	26.4	28.7	30.4	31.6	33.2	35.3	26.7
2009	26.5	23.3	26.5	28.9	30.5	31.8	33.1	35.3	26.8
2010	26.8	23.4	26.7	29.0	30.7	32.0	33.3	35.3	27.2
2011	27.0	23.7	26.9	29.2	30.9	32.1	33.3	35.0	28.0
2012	27.1	23.8	27.0	29.3	31.0	32.2	33.5	35.1	27.6
2013	27.3	24.0	27.2	29.4	31.1	32.3	33.6	35.2	27.9
2014	27.5	24.3	27.3	29.5	31.2	32.4	33.7	35.2	28.1

1 Includes races other than White and Black and origin not stated.   2 Based on 100 percent of births in selected states and on a 50-percent sample of births in all other states.   3 Race and Hispanic origin are reported separately on birth certificates. Persons of Hispanic origin may be of any race. Multiple-race data, when reported, were bridged to single-race categories in order to maintain comparability among all reported areas.   4 Excludes data for New Hampshire and Oklahoma, which did not report Hispanic origin.   5 Includes all persons of Hispanic origin of any race.

Table 1-16. Live Births, Birth Rates, and Fertility Rates, by Race, Selected Years, 1940–2014

(Number, rate per 1,000 population in specified group.)

Characteristic and year	Number					Birth rate				Fertility rate			
	All races[1]	White	Black	American Indian or Alaska Native	Asian or Pacific Islander	White	Black	American Indian or Alaska Native	Asian or Pacific Islander	White	Black	American Indian or Alaska Native	Asian or Pacific Islander
Race of Mother													
1980 [2]	3,612,258	2,936,351	568,080	29,389	74,355	15.1	21.3	20.7	19.9	65.6	84.7	82.7	73.2
1981 [2]	3,629,238	2,947,679	564,955	29,688	84,553	15.0	20.8	20.0	20.1	64.8	82.0	79.6	73.7
1982 [2]	3,680,537	2,984,817	568,506	32,436	93,193	15.1	20.7	21.1	20.3	64.8	80.9	83.6	74.8
1983 [2]	3,638,933	2,946,468	562,624	32,881	95,713	14.8	20.2	20.6	19.5	63.4	78.7	81.8	71.7
1984 [2]	3,669,141	2,967,100	568,138	33,256	98,926	14.8	20.1	20.1	18.8	63.2	78.2	79.8	69.2
1985	3,760,561	3,037,913	581,824	34,037	104,606	15.0	20.4	19.8	18.7	64.1	78.8	78.6	68.4
1986	3,756,547	3,019,175	592,910	34,169	107,797	14.8	20.5	19.2	18.0	63.1	78.9	75.9	66.0
1987	3,809,394	3,043,828	611,173	35,322	116,560	14.9	20.8	19.1	18.4	63.3	80.1	75.6	67.1
1988	3,909,510	3,102,083	638,562	37,088	129,035	15.0	21.5	19.3	19.2	64.5	82.6	76.8	70.2
1989	4,040,958	3,192,355	673,124	39,478	133,075	15.4	22.3	19.7	18.7	66.4	86.2	79.0	68.2
1990	4,158,212	3,290,273	684,336	39,051	141,635	15.8	22.4	18.9	19.0	68.3	86.8	76.2	69.6
1991	4,110,907	3,241,273	682,602	38,841	145,372	15.3	21.8	18.3	18.3	66.7	84.8	73.9	67.1
1992	4,065,014	3,201,678	673,633	39,453	150,250	15.0	21.1	17.9	17.9	66.1	82.4	73.1	66.1
1993	4,000,240	3,149,833	658,875	38,732	152,800	14.6	20.2	17.0	17.3	64.9	79.6	69.7	64.3
1994	3,952,767	3,121,004	636,391	37,740	157,632	14.3	19.1	16.0	17.1	64.2	75.9	65.8	63.9
1995	3,899,589	3,098,885	603,139	37,278	160,287	14.1	17.8	15.3	16.7	63.6	71.0	63.0	62.6
1996	3,891,494	3,093,057	594,781	37,880	165,776	13.9	17.3	14.9	16.5	63.3	69.2	61.8	62.3
1997	3,880,894	3,072,640	599,913	38,572	169,769	13.7	17.1	14.7	16.2	62.8	69.0	60.8	61.3
1998	3,941,553	3,118,727	609,902	40,272	172,652	13.8	17.1	14.8	15.9	63.6	69.4	61.3	60.1
1999	3,959,417	3,132,501	605,970	40,170	180,776	13.7	16.8	14.2	15.9	64.0	68.5	59.0	60.9
2000	4,058,814	3,194,005	622,598	41,668	200,543	13.9	17.0	14.0	17.1	65.3	70.0	58.7	65.8
2001	4,025,933	3,177,626	589,616*	41,872	200,279	13.7	16.3	13.5	16.1	65.0	67.5	56.8	62.5
2002	4,021,726	3,174,760	593,691	42,368	210,907	13.6	15.7	13.2	16.3	65.1	65.7	55.7	63.3
2003	4,089,950	3,225,848	599,847	43,052	221,203	13.7	15.7	13.0	16.4	66.4	66.0	54.8	64.2
2004	4,112,052	3,222,928	616,074	43,927	229,123	13.6	15.9	12.8	16.4	66.5	67.2	54.2	64.5
2005	4,138,349	3,229,294	633,134	44,813	231,108	13.6	16.1	12.6	15.9	66.8	68.5	53.6	63.0
2006	4,265,555	3,310,308	666,481	47,721	241,045	13.8	16.7	12.9	16.0	68.7	71.4	55.3	63.7
2007	4,316,233	3,336,626	675,676	49,443	254,488	13.8	16.7	12.9	16.4	69.4	71.7	55.5	65.3
2008	4,247,694	3,274,163	670,809	49,537	253,185	13.5	16.3	12.4	15.7	68.3	70.6	54.0	63.3
2009	4,130,665	3,173,293	657,618	48,665	251,089	13.0	15.8	11.8	15.1	66.4	68.8	51.6	61.3
2010	3,999,386	3,069,315	636,425	46,760	246,886	12.5	15.1	11.0	14.5	64.4	66.3	48.6	59.2
2011	3,953,590	3,020,355	632,901	46,419	253,915	12.2	14.8	10.7	14.5	63.4	65.5	47.7	59.9
2012	3,952,841	2,999,820	634,126	46,093	272,802	12.1	14.7	10.5	15.1	63.0	65.1	47.0	62.2
2013	3,932,181	2,985,757	634,760	45,991	265,673	12.0	14.5	10.3	14.3	62.7	64.7	46.4	59.2
2014	3,988,076	3,019,863	640,562	44,928	282,723	12.0	14.5	9.9	14.6	63.2	64.6	44.8	60.7
Race of Child													
1960 [3]	4,257,850	3,600,744	602,264	21,114	NA	22.7	31.9	NA	NA	113.2	153.5	NA	NA
1961 [3]	4,268,326	3,600,864	611,072	21,464	NA	22.2	NA	NA	NA	112.3	NA	NA	NA
1962 [3,5]	4,167,362	3,394,068	584,610	21,968	NA	21.4	NA	NA	NA	107.5	NA	NA	NA
1963 [3,5]	4,098,020	3,326,344	580,658	22,358	NA	20.7	NA	NA	NA	103.6	NA	NA	NA
1964 [3]	4,027,490	3,369,160	607,556	24,382	NA	20.0	29.5	NA	NA	99.8	142.6	NA	NA
1965 [3]	3,760,358	3,123,860	581,126	24,066	NA	18.3	27.7	NA	NA	91.3	133.2	NA	NA
1966 [3]	3,606,274	2,993,230	558,244	23,014	NA	17.4	26.2	NA	NA	86.2	124.7	NA	NA
1967 [4]	3,520,959	2,922,502	543,976	22,665	NA	16.8	25.1	NA	NA	82.8	118.5	NA	NA
1968 [3]	3,501,564	2,912,224	531,152	24,156	NA	16.6	24.2	NA	NA	81.3	112.7	NA	NA
1969 [3]	3,600,206	2,993,614	543,132	24,008	NA	16.9	24.4	NA	NA	82.2	112.1	NA	NA
1970 [3]	3,731,386	3,091,264	572,362	25,864	NA	17.4	25.3	NA	NA	84.1	115.4	NA	NA
1971 [3]	3,555,970	2,919,746	564,960	27,148	NA	16.1	24.4	NA	NA	77.3	109.7	NA	NA
1972 [2]	3,258,411	2,655,558	531,329	27,368	NA	14.5	22.5	NA	NA	68.9	99.9	NA	NA
1973 [2]	3,136,965	2,551,030	512,597	26,464	NA	13.8	21.4	NA	NA	64.9	93.6	NA	NA
1974 [2]	3,159,958	2,575,792	507,162	26,631	NA	13.9	20.8	NA	NA	64.2	89.7	NA	NA
1975 [2]	3,144,198	2,551,996	511,581	27,546	NA	13.6	20.7	NA	NA	62.5	87.9	NA	NA
1976 [2]	3,167,788	2,567,614	514,479	29,009	NA	13.6	20.5	NA	NA	61.5	85.8	NA	NA
1977 [2]	3,326,632	2,691,070	544,221	30,500	NA	14.1	21.4	NA	NA	63.2	88.1	NA	NA
1978 [2]	3,333,279	2,681,116	551,540	33,160	NA	14.0	21.3	NA	NA	61.7	86.7	NA	NA
1979 [2]	3,494,398	2,808,420	577,855	34,269	NA	14.5	22.0	NA	NA	63.4	88.3	NA	NA
1980 [2]	3,612,258	2,898,732	589,616	36,797	NA	14.9	22.1	NA	NA	64.7	88.1	NA	NA
Births adjusted for underregistration													
Race of Child													
1940	2,559,000	2,199,000	NA	NA	NA	18.6	NA	NA	NA	77.1	NA	NA	NA
1945	2,858,000	2,471,000	NA	NA	NA	19.7	NA	NA	NA	83.4	NA	NA	NA
1950	3,632,000	3,108,000	NA	NA	NA	23.0	NA	NA	NA	102.3	NA	NA	NA

Table 1-16. Live Births, Birth Rates, and Fertility Rates, by Race, Selected Years, 1940–2014— continued

(Number, rate per 1,000 population in specified group.)

Characteristic and year	Number					Birth rate				Fertility rate			
	All races[1]	White	Black	American Indian or Alaska Native	Asian or Pacific Islander	White	Black	American Indian or Alaska Native	Asian or Pacific Islander	White	Black	American Indian or Alaska Native	Asian or Pacific Islander
1955	4,097,000	3,485,000	NA	NA	NA	23.8	NA	NA	NA	113.7	NA	NA	NA

NA = Not available.   1 Data for 1960–1991 includes births to races not shown separately. For 1992 and later years, unknown race of mother is imputed.   2 Based on 100 percent of births in selected states and on a 50 percent sample of births in all other states.   3 Based on a 50 percent sample of births.   4 Based on a 20 to 50 percent sample of births.   5 Figures by race exclude New Jersey.

Table 1-17. Births and Birth Rates, by Hispanic Origin of Mother and by Race for Mothers of Non-Hispanic Origin, 1989–2014

(Birth rates are live births per 1,000 population in specified group; fertility rates are live births per 1,000 women age 15 to 44 years in specified group.)

Measure and year	All origins[1]	Hispanic (may be of any race)						Non-Hispanic		
		Total	Mexican	Puerto Rican	Cuban	Central and South American	Other and unknown Hispanic	Total[2]	White	Black
Number										
1989[3]	3,903,012	532,249	327,233	56,229	10,842	72,443	65,502	3,297,493	2,526,367	611,269
1990[4]	4,092,994	595,073	385,640	58,807	11,311	83,008	56,307	3,457,417	2,626,500	661,701
1991[5]	4,094,566	623,085	411,233	59,833	11,058	86,908	54,053	3,434,464	2,589,878	666,758
1992[5]	4,049,024	643,271	432,047	59,569	11,472	89,031	51,152	3,365,862	2,527,207	657,450
1993	4,000,240	654,418	443,733	58,102	11,916	92,371	48,296	3,295,345	2,472,031	641,273
1994	3,952,767	665,026	454,536	57,240	11,889	93,485	47,876	3,245,115	2,438,855	619,198
1995	3,899,589	679,768	469,615	54,824	12,473	94,996	47,860	3,160,495	2,382,638	587,781
1996	3,891,494	701,339	489,666	54,863	12,613	97,888	46,309	3,133,484	2,358,989	578,099
1997	3,880,894	709,767	499,024	55,450	12,887	97,405	45,001	3,115,174	2,333,363	581,431
1998	3,941,553	734,661	516,011	57,349	13,226	98,226	49,849	3,158,975	2,361,462	593,127
1999	3,959,417	764,339	540,674	57,138	13,088	103,307	50,132	3,147,580	2,346,450	588,981
2000	4,058,814	815,868	581,915	58,124	13,429	113,344	49,056	3,199,994	2,362,968	604,346
2001	4,025,933	851,851	611,000	57,568	14,017	121,365	47,901	3,149,572	2,326,578	589,917
2002	4,021,726	876,642	627,505	57,465	14,232	125,981	51,459	3,119,944	2,298,156	578,335
2003	4,089,950	912,329	654,504	58,400	14,867	135,586	48,972	3,149,034	2,321,904	576,033
2004	4,112,052	946,349	677,621	61,221	14,943	143,520	49,044	3,133,125	2,296,683	578,772
2005	4,138,349	985,505	693,197	63,340	16,064	151,201	61,703	3,123,005	2,279,768	583,759
2006	4,265,555	1,039,077	718,146	66,932	16,936	165,321	71,742	3,196,082	2,308,640	617,247
2007	4,316,233	1,062,779	722,055	68,488	16,981	169,851	85,404	3,222,460	2,310,333	627,191
2008	4,247,694	1,041,239	684,883	69,015	16,718	155,578	115,045	3,173,629	2,267,817	623,029
2009	4,130,665	999,548	645,297	68,486	16,641	148,647	120,477	3,101,330	2,212,552	609,584
2010	3,999,396	945,180	598,317	66,368	16,882	142,692	120,921	3,026,314	2,162,406	589,808
2011	3,953,590	918,129	566,699	67,018	17,131	136,221	131,060	3,008,200	2,146,566	582,345
2012	3,952,841	907,677	555,823	67,182	17,396	131,794	135,482	3,014,304	2,134,044	583,489
2013	3,932,181	901,033	545,303	68,302	18,854	131,305	137,370	3,003,556	2,129,196	583,834
2014	3,988,076	914,065	545,977	69,879	20,163	136,656	141,390	3,043,519	2,149,302	588,891
Birth Rate										
1989[3,6]	16.3	26.2	25.7	23.7	10.0	28.3	[6]	15.4	14.2	22.8
1990[4,6]	16.7	26.7	28.7	21.6	10.9	27.5	[6]	15.7	14.4	23.0
1991[5,6]	16.2	26.5	27.6	23.3	9.8	28.3	[6]	15.2	13.9	22.4
1992[5,6]	15.8	26.1	27.4	22.9	10.1	27.5	[6]	14.8	13.4	21.6
1993[6]	15.4	25.4	26.8	21.5	10.5	26.3	[6]	14.3	13.1	20.7
1994[6]	15.0	24.7	26.1	20.8	10.7	24.9	[6]	13.9	12.8	19.5
1995[6]	14.6	24.1	25.8	19.0	10.8	24.2	[6]	13.5	12.5	18.2
1996[6]	14.4	23.8	26.2	17.2	10.6	22.5	[6]	13.3	12.3	17.6
1997[6]	14.2	23.0	25.3	17.2	10.0	21.3	[6]	13.1	12.2	17.4
1998[6]	14.3	22.7	24.6	17.9	9.7	21.7	[6]	13.2	12.2	17.5
1999[6]	14.2	22.5	24.2	18.0	9.4	21.7	[6]	13.0	12.1	17.1
2000[6]	14.4	23.1	25.0	18.1	9.7	21.8	[6]	13.2	12.2	17.3
2001[6]	14.1	22.9	24.7	17.7	10.3	21.7	[6]	12.8	11.9	16.6
2002[6]	14.0	22.7	24.3	16.5	10.1	22.5	[6]	12.6	11.7	16.1
2003[6]	14.1	22.8	24.6	15.0	10.0	23.0	[6]	12.7	11.8	15.9
2004[6]	14.0	22.8	24.8	16.0	9.3	22.1	[6]	12.6	11.7	15.8
2005[6]	14.0	22.9	24.5	17.0	10.2	22.7	[6]	12.5	11.6	15.8
2006[6]	14.3	23.3	24.6	17.5	10.4	23.8	[6]	12.7	11.7	16.5
2007[6]	14.3	23.0	23.9	17.1	10.2	24.6	[6]	12.8	11.7	16.6
2008[6]	14.0	21.8	21.7	16.4	10.1	26.1	[6]	12.5	11.5	16.3
2009[6]	13.5	20.3	19.8	15.5	9.5	25.5	[6]	12.2	11.2	15.7
2010[6]	13.0	18,7	18.2	14.1	9.0	23.4	[6]	11.8	10.9	15.1
2011[6]	12.7	17.6	16.9	13.7	9.1	23.0	[6]	11.7	10.8	14.7
2012[6]	12.6	17.1	16.3	16.3	13.5	8.9	[6]	11.7	10.7	14.6
2013[6]	12.4	16.7	15.8	15.8	13.3	9.4	[6]	11.6	10.7	14.4
2014[6]	12.5	16.5	NA	NA	NA	NA	[6]	11.7	10.8	14.4
Fertility Rate										
1989[3,6]	69.2	104.9	106.6	86.6	49.8	95.8	[6]	65.7	60.5	84.8
1990[4,6]	71.0	107.7	118.9	82.9	52.6	102.7	[6]	67.1	62.8	89.0
1991[5,6]	69.3	106.9	114.9	87.9	47.6	105.5	[6]	65.2	60.9	87.0
1992[5,6]	68.4	106.1	113.3	87.9	49.4	104.7	[6]	64.2	60.0	84.5
1993[6]	67.0	103.3	110.9	79.8	53.9	101.5	[6]	62.7	58.9	81.5
1994[6]	65.9	100.7	109.9	78.2	53.6	93.2	[6]	61.6	58.2	77.5
1995[6]	64.6	98.8	109.9	71.3	52.2	89.1	[6]	60.2	57.5	72.8
1996[6]	64.1	97.5	110.7	66.5	55.1	84.2	[6]	59.6	57.1	70.7
1997[6]	63.6	94.2	106.6	65.8	53.1	80.6	[6]	59.3	56.8	70.3
1998[6]	64.3	93.2	103.2	69.7	46.5	83.5		60.0	57.6	70.9

Table 1-17. Births and Birth Rates, by Hispanic Origin of Mother and by Race for Mothers of Non-Hispanic Origin, 1989–2014—continued

(Birth rates are live births per 1,000 population in specified group; fertility rates are live births per 1,000 women age 15 to 44 years in specified group.)

Measure and year	All origins[1]	Hispanic (may be of any race)						Non-Hispanic		
		Total	Mexican	Puerto Rican	Cuban	Central and South American	Other and unknown Hispanic	Total[2]	White	Black
1999[6]	64.4	93.0	101.5	71.1	47.0	84.8	[6]	60.0	57.7	69.9
2000[6]	65.9	95.9	105.1	73.5	49.3	85.1	[6]	61.1	58.5	71.4
2001[6]	65.1	95.4	105.0	71,7	56.4	82.2	[6]	60.0	57.7	69.1
2002[6]	65.0	94.7	103.0	65.6	59.3	86.5	[6]	59.8	57.6	67.5
2003[6]	66.1	95.2	103.7	60.6	60.8	89.7	[6]	60.7	58.9	67.1
2004[6]	66.4	95.7	104.5	66.8	52.2	87.4	[6]	60.8	58.9	67.1
2005[6]	66.7	96.4	104.5	69.8	49.1	90.5	[6]	60.8	59.0	67.2
2006[6]	68.6	98.3	105.6	71.6	47.9	95.6	[6]	62.5	60.3	70.7
2007[6]	69.3	97.4	102.8	70.3	47.6	100.1	[6]	63.3	61.0	71.4
2008[6]	68.1	92.7	92.6	67.0	50.1	109.1	[6]	62.7	60.5	70.8
2009[6]	66.2	86.5	84.8	63.7	46.0	107.5	[6]	61.6	59.6	68.9
2010[6]	64.1	80.2	78.2	59.7	46.4	97.1	[6]	60.4	58.7	66.6
2011[6]	63.2	76.2	73.0	59.6	46.1	96.3	[6]	60.1	58.7	65.4
2012[6]	63.0	74.4	70.7	58.2	45.4	94.9	[6]	60.3	58.5	65.0
2013[6]	62.5	72.9	68.4	57.8	48.0	94.4	[6]	59.9	58.7	64.6
2014[6]	62.9	72.1	NA	NA	NA	NA	[6]	60.7	59.5	64.5

1 Includes origin not stated.   2 Includes races other than White and Black.   3 Excludes data for Louisiana, New Hampshire, and Oklahoma, which did not report Hispanic origin.   4 Excludes data for New Hampshire and Oklahoma, which did not report Hispanic origin.   5 Excludes data for New Hampshire, which did not report Hispanic origin.   6 Rates for the Central and South American population includes other and unknown Hispanic.

Table 1-18. Live Births, by Age of Mother, Live-Birth Order, and Race of Mother, 1989–2014

(Number of children born alive to mother.)

Measure and year	All origins[1]	Hispanic (may be of any race)						Non-Hispanic		
		Total	Mexican	Puerto Rican	Cuban	Central and South American	Other and unknown Hispanic	Total[2]	White	Black
Number										
1989[3]	3,903,012	532,249	327,233	56,229	10,842	72,443	65,502	3,297,493	2,526,367	611,269
1990[4]	4,092,994	595,073	385,640	58,807	11,311	83,008	56,307	3,457,417	2,626,500	661,701
1991[5]	4,094,566	623,085	411,233	59,833	11,058	86,908	54,053	3,434,464	2,589,878	666,758
1992[5]	4,049,024	643,271	432,047	59,569	11,472	89,031	51,152	3,365,862	2,527,207	657,450
1993	4,000,240	654,418	443,733	58,102	11,916	92,371	48,296	3,295,345	2,472,031	641,273
1994	3,952,767	665,026	454,536	57,240	11,889	93,485	47,876	3,245,115	2,438,855	619,198
1995	3,899,589	679,768	469,615	54,824	12,473	94,996	47,860	3,160,495	2,382,638	587,781
1996	3,891,494	701,339	489,666	54,863	12,613	97,888	46,309	3,133,484	2,358,989	578,099
1997	3,880,894	709,767	499,024	55,450	12,887	97,405	45,001	3,115,174	2,333,363	581,431
1998	3,941,553	734,661	516,011	57,349	13,226	98,226	49,849	3,158,975	2,361,462	593,127
1999	3,959,417	764,339	540,674	57,138	13,088	103,307	50,132	3,147,580	2,346,450	588,981
2000	4,058,814	815,868	581,915	58,124	13,429	113,344	49,056	3,199,994	2,362,968	604,346
2001	4,025,933	851,851	611,000	57,568	14,017	121,365	47,901	3,149,572	2,326,578	589,917
2002	4,021,726	876,642	627,505	57,465	14,232	125,981	51,459	3,119,944	2,298,156	578,335
2003	4,089,950	912,329	654,504	58,400	14,867	135,586	48,972	3,149,034	2,321,904	576,033
2004	4,112,052	946,349	677,621	61,221	14,943	143,520	49,044	3,133,125	2,296,683	578,772
2005	4,138,349	985,505	693,197	63,340	16,064	151,201	61,703	3,123,005	2,279,768	583,759
2006	4,265,555	1,039,077	718,146	66,932	16,936	165,321	71,742	3,196,082	2,308,640	617,247
2007	4,316,233	1,062,779	722,055	68,488	16,981	169,851	85,404	3,222,460	2,310,333	627,191
2008	4,247,694	1,041,239	684,883	69,015	16,718	155,578	115,045	3,173,629	2,267,817	623,029
2009	4,130,665	999,548	645,297	68,486	16,641	148,647	120,477	3,101,330	2,212,552	609,584
2010	3,999,396	945,180	598,317	66,368	16,882	142,692	120,921	3,026,314	2,162,406	589,808
2011	3,953,590	918,129	566,699	67,018	17,131	136,221	131,060	3,008,200	2,146,566	582,345
2012	3,952,841	907,677	555,823	67,182	17,396	131,794	135,482	3,014,304	2,134,044	583,489
2013	3,932,181	901,033	545,303	68,302	18,854	131,305	137,370	3,003,556	2,129,196	583,834
2014	3,988,076	914,065	545,977	69,879	20,163	136,656	141,390	3,043,519	2,149,302	588,891
Birth Rate										
1989[3,6]	16.3	26.2	25.7	23.7	10.0	28.3	[6]	15.4	14.2	22.8
1990[4,6]	16.7	26.7	28.7	21.6	10.9	27.5	[6]	15.7	14.4	23.0
1991[5,6]	16.2	26.5	27.6	23.3	9.8	28.3	[6]	15.2	13.9	22.4
1992[5,6]	15.8	26.1	27.4	22.9	10.1	27.5	[6]	14.8	13.4	21.6
1993[6]	15.4	25.4	26.8	21.5	10.5	26.3	[6]	14.3	13.1	20.7
1994[6]	15.0	24.7	26.1	20.8	10.7	24.9	[6]	13.9	12.8	19.5
1995[6]	14.6	24.1	25.8	19.0	10.8	24.2	[6]	13.5	12.5	18.2
1996[6]	14.4	23.8	26.2	17.2	10.6	22.5	[6]	13.3	12.3	17.6
1997[6]	14.2	23.0	25.3	17.2	10.0	21.3	[6]	13.1	12.2	17.4
1998[6]	14.3	22.7	24.6	17.9	9.7	21.7	[6]	13.2	12.2	17.5
1999[6]	14.2	22.5	24.2	18.0	9.4	21.7	[6]	13.0	12.1	17.1
2000[6]	14.4	23.1	25.0	18.1	9.7	21.8	[6]	13.2	12.2	17.3
2001[6]	14.1	22.9	24.7	17.7	10.3	21.7	[6]	12.8	11.9	16.6
2002[6]	14.0	22.7	24.3	16.5	10.1	22.5	[6]	12.6	11.7	16.1
2003[6]	14.1	22.8	24.6	15.0	10.0	23.0	[6]	12.7	11.8	15.9
2004[6]	14.0	22.8	24.8	16.0	9.3	22.1	[6]	12.6	11.7	15.8
2005[6]	14.0	22.9	24.5	17.0	10.2	22.7	[6]	12.5	11.6	15.8
2006[6]	14.3	23.3	24.6	17.5	10.4	23.8	[6]	12.7	11.7	16.5
2007[6]	14.3	23.0	23.9	17.1	10.2	24.6	[6]	12.8	11.7	16.6
2008[6]	14.0	21.8	21.7	16.4	10.1	26.1	[6]	12.5	11.5	16.3
2009[6]	13.5	20.3	19.8	15.5	9.5	25.5	[6]	12.2	11.2	15.7
2010[6]	13.0	18.7	18.2	14.1	9.0	23.4	[6]	11.8	10.9	15.1
2011[6]	12.7	17.6	16.9	13.7	9.1	23.0	[6]	11.7	10.8	14.7
2012[6]	12.6	17.1	16.3	16.3	13.5	8.9	[6]	11.7	10.7	14.6
2013[6]	12.4	16.7	15.8	15.8	13.3	9.4	[6]	11.6	10.7	14.4
2014[6]	12.5	16.5	NA	NA	NA	NA	[6]	11.7	10.8	14.4
Fertility Rate										
1989[3,6]	69.2	104.9	106.6	86.6	49.8	95.8	[6]	65.7	60.5	84.8
1990[4,6]	71.0	107.7	118.9	82.9	52.6	102.7	[6]	67.1	62.8	89.0
1991[5,6]	69.3	106.9	114.9	87.9	47.6	105.5	[6]	65.2	60.9	87.0
1992[5,6]	68.4	106.1	113.3	87.9	49.4	104.7	[6]	64.2	60.0	84.5
1993[6]	67.0	103.3	110.9	79.8	53.9	101.5	[6]	62.7	58.9	81.5
1994[6]	65.9	100.7	109.9	78.2	53.6	93.2	[6]	61.6	58.2	77.5
1995[6]	64.6	98.8	109.9	71.3	52.2	89.1	[6]	60.2	57.5	72.8
1996[6]	64.1	97.5	110.7	66.5	55.1	84.2	[6]	59.6	57.1	70.7
1997[6]	63.6	94.2	106.6	65.8	53.1	80.6	[6]	59.3	56.8	70.3
1998[6]	64.3	93.2	103.2	69.7	46.5	83.5		60.0	57.6	70.9

Table 1-18. Live Births, by Age of Mother, Live-Birth Order, and Race of Mother, 1989–2014— continued

(Number of children born alive to mother.)

Measure and year	All origins[1]	Hispanic (may be of any race)						Non-Hispanic		
		Total	Mexican	Puerto Rican	Cuban	Central and South American	Other and unknown Hispanic	Total[2]	White	Black
1999[6]	64.4	93.0	101.5	71.1	47.0	84.8	(6)	60.0	57.7	69.9
2000[6]	65.9	95.9	105.1	73.5	49.3	85.1	(6)	61.1	58.5	71.4
2001[6]	65.1	95.4	105.0	71,7	56.4	82.2	(6)	60.0	57.7	69.1
2002[6]	65.0	94.7	103.0	65.6	59.3	86.5	(6)	59.8	57.6	67.5
2003[6]	66.1	95.2	103.7	60.6	60.8	89.7	(6)	60.7	58.9	67.1
2004[6]	66.4	95.7	104.5	66.8	52.2	87.4	(6)	60.8	58.9	67.1
2005[6]	66.7	96.4	104.5	69.8	49.1	90.5	(6)	60.8	59.0	67.2
2006[6]	68.6	98.3	105.6	71.6	47.9	95.6	(6)	62.5	60.3	70.7
2007[6]	69.3	97.4	102.8	70.3	47.6	100.1	(6)	63.3	61.0	71.4
2008[6]	68.1	92.7	92.6	67.0	50.1	109.1	(6)	62.7	60.5	70.8
2009[6]	66.2	86.5	84.8	63.7	46.0	107.5	(6)	61.6	59.6	68.9
2010[6]	64.1	80.2	78.2	59.7	46.4	97.1	(6)	60.4	58.7	66.6
2011[6]	63.2	76.2	73.0	59.6	46.1	96.3	(6)	60.1	58.7	65.4
2012[6]	63.0	74.4	70.7	58.2	45.4	94.9	(6)	60.3	58.5	65.0
2013[6]	62.5	72.9	68.4	57.8	48.0	94.4	(6)	59.9	58.7	64.6
2014[6]	62.9	72.1	NA	NA	NA	NA	(6)	60.7	59.5	64.5

– = Quantity zero.   1 Includes origin not stated.   2 Includes races other than white and black.   3 Excludes data for Louisiana, New Hampshire, and Oklahoma, which did not report Hispanic origin.   4 Excludes data for New Hampshire and Oklahoma, which did not report Hispanic origin.   5 Excludes data for New Hampshire, which did not report Hispanic origin.   6 Rates for the Central and South American population include other and unknown Hispanic origin.

Table 1-19. Live Births, by Age of Mother, Live-Birth Order, and Hispanic Origin, 2014

(Number of children born alive to mother; includes births with stated origin of mother only.)

Live-birth order and origin of mother	15 years	16 years	17 years	18 years	19 years	20 to 24 years	25 to 29 years	30 to 34 years	35 to 39 years	40 to 44 years	45 to 49 years	50 to 54 years
Hispanic[1] , Total	3,309	8,210	14,776	24,085	35,590	239,121	248,971	204,232	107,644	25,636	1,374	80
1st child	3,194	7,670	12,885	19,343	26,083	110,928	67,331	41,018	16,340	3,577	254	21
2nd child	101	487	1,689	4,115	7,876	82,829	84,524	58,859	26,486	5,254	267	16
3rd child	6	28	126	472	1,300	32,702	59,140	53,629	28,097	5,947	244	15
4th child	–	6	8	54	166	9,053	24,832	29,935	19,200	4,824	242	8
5th child	–	1	4	4	20	2,143	8,207	11,959	9,548	2,838	137	7
6th child	–	1	2	1	3	436	2,601	4,765	4,202	1,556	110	7
7th child	–	1	–	–	3	89	833	1,828	1,781	757	57	1
8th child and over	–	–	–	2	1	61	431	1,299	1,486	758	57	3
Not stated	8	16	62	94	138	880	1,072	940	504	125	6	2
Mexican	2,079	5,281	9,475	15,369	22,481	146,071	148,067	118,730	62,002	15,030	719	28
1st child	2,005	4,928	8,268	12,233	16,294	64,972	35,410	19,752	7,347	1,592	100	8
2nd child	67	319	1,076	2,732	5,117	51,712	49,086	30,857	12,486	2,398	107	5
3rd child	5	18	83	317	858	21,189	38,326	34,016	17,049	3,514	121	3
4th child	–	4	6	32	108	5,920	16,707	20,281	13,118	3,235	141	3
5th child	–	1	3	4	16	1,418	5,393	8,141	6,668	2,038	92	3
6th child	–	1	1	1	1	284	1,730	3,157	2,892	1,155	69	3
7th child	–	1	–	–	3	58	561	1,204	1,172	529	45	–
8th child and over	–	–	–	–	1	33	283	809	984	494	41	1
Not stated	2	9	38	50	83	485	571	513	286	75	3	2
Puerto Rican	251	618	1,145	2,037	3,149	21,349	19,148	13,829	6,737	1,437	81	7
1st child	242	578	983	1,657	2,363	9,984	5,432	3,245	1,349	283	16	2
2nd child	6	35	144	316	649	7,412	6,591	4,313	2,050	375	26	1
3rd child	–	–	9	40	105	2,767	4,186	3,107	1,539	324	11	1
4th child	–	–	–	3	13	829	1,757	1,646	855	220	11	1
5th child	–	–	1	–	1	182	701	761	438	107	5	2
6th child	–	–	–	–	1	40	227	373	226	47	10	–
7th child	–	–	–	–	–	9	80	158	121	25	–	–
8th child and over	–	–	–	–	–	8	43	112	107	48	1	–
Not stated	3	5	8	21	17	118	131	114	52	8	1	–
Cuban	15	48	120	229	434	4,132	6,430	5,267	2,706	719	49	6
1st child	15	45	110	202	358	2,655	3,044	1,953	777	169	19	3
2nd child	–	3	8	22	63	1,121	2,302	2,126	1,126	293	16	1
3rd child	–	–	1	3	10	269	767	815	530	150	8	1
4th child	–	–	–	1	–	63	196	226	164	62	3	1
5th child	–	–	–	–	–	10	79	73	54	22	1	–
6th child	–	–	–	–	–	4	15	26	23	7	1	–
7th child	–	–	–	–	–	–	7	14	11	4	1	–
8th child and over	–	–	–	–	–	2	4	12	12	6	–	–
Not stated	–	–	1	1	3	8	16	22	9	6	–	–
Central and South American	334	742	1,401	2,142	3,268	25,763	37,094	37,579	22,351	5,500	347	19
1st child	327	696	1,242	1,785	2,467	13,480	12,102	9,532	4,445	1,008	79	5
2nd child	4	42	144	309	677	8,533	13,342	12,529	6,932	1,438	71	6
3rd child	1	3	6	30	93	2,891	7,702	8,766	5,449	1,308	74	2
4th child	–	–	1	3	7	617	2,688	4,166	2,943	820	58	–
5th child	–	–	–	–	2	103	778	1,526	1,410	433	25	2
6th child	–	–	1	–	–	15	209	565	618	219	20	3
7th child	–	–	–	–	–	2	50	195	274	128	6	–
8th child and over	–	–	–	2	–	7	27	134	178	126	13	1
Not stated	2	1	7	13	22	115	196	166	102	20	1	–
Other and Unknown Hispanic	630	1,521	2,635	4,308	6,258	41,806	38,232	28,827	13,848	2,950	178	20
1st child	605	1,423	2,282	3,466	4,601	19,837	11,343	6,536	2,422	525	40	3
2nd child	24	88	317	736	1,370	14,051	13,203	9,034	3,892	750	47	3
3rd child	–	7	27	82	234	5,586	8,159	6,925	3,530	651	30	8
4th child	–	2	1	15	38	1,624	3,484	3,616	2,120	487	29	3
5th child	–	–	–	–	1	430	1,256	1,458	978	238	14	–
6th child	–	–	–	–	1	93	420	644	443	128	10	1
7th child	–	–	–	–	–	20	135	257	203	71	5	1
8th child and over	–	–	–	–	–	11	74	232	205	84	2	1
Not stated	1	1	8	9	13	154	158	125	55	16	1	–

– = Quantity zero.   1 Includes all persons of Hispanic origin of any race.

Table 1-20. Live Births, by Race of Mother, by State and Territory, 2014

(Number.)

State and territory	All races	White	Black	American Indian or Alaska Native	Asian or Pacific Islander
United States [1]	3,988,076	3,019,863	640,562	44,928	282,723
Alabama	59,422	39,578	18,417	200	1,227
Alaska	11,392	7,288	548	2,450	1,106
Arizona	86,887	72,687	5,208	5,473	3,519
Arkansas	38,511	29,632	7,376	301	1,202
California	502,879	383,492	31,654	3,509	84,224
Colorado	65,830	58,117	3,926	777	3,010
Connecticut	36,285	28,543	5,154	308	2,280
Delaware	10,972	7,314	2,988	26	644
District of Columbia	9,509	3,985	5,026	16	482
Florida	219,991	159,035	53,148	406	7,402
Georgia	130,946	76,226	47,909	292	6,519
Hawaii	18,550	6,368	617	30	11,535
Idaho	22,876	21,696	250	429	501
Illinois	158,556	119,995	28,160	227	10,174
Indiana	84,080	70,967	10,666	125	2,322
Iowa	39,687	35,528	2,467	284	1,408
Kansas	39,223	34,420	3,097	347	1,359
Kentucky	56,170	49,248	5,571	76	1,275
Louisiana	64,497	37,562	25,025	373	1,537
Maine	12,698	11,842	450	158	248
Maryland	73,921	42,525	25,339	260	5,797
Massachusetts	71,908	55,882	9,276	151	6,599
Michigan	114,375	87,070	22,237	784	4,284
Minnesota	69,904	54,774	8,033	1,428	5,669
Mississippi	38,736	20,894	17,036	223	583
Missouri	75,360	60,968	11,783	423	2,186
Montana	12,432	10,572	106	1,585	169
Nebraska	26,794	23,178	2,015	553	1,048
Nevada	35,861	27,638	4,603	475	3,145
New Hampshire	12,302	11,494	259	21	528
New Jersey	103,305	71,033	20,102	193	11,977
New Mexico	26,052	21,161	732	3,581	578
New York	238,773	164,486	46,744	757	26,786
North Carolina	120,975	81,257	31,963	2,025	5,730
North Dakota	11,359	9,509	504	1,032	314
Ohio	139,467	110,003	24,931	301	4,232
Oklahoma	53,339	40,258	5,296	6,051	1,734
Oregon	45,556	40,634	1,333	778	2,811
Pennsylvania	142,268	110,809	24,024	368	7,067
Rhode Island	10,823	8,734	1,365	130	594
South Carolina	57,627	37,543	18,598	193	1,293
South Dakota	12,283	9,601	356	2,055	271
Tennessee	81,602	61,391	17,791	240	2,180
Texas	399,766	326,480	51,274	1,168	20,844
Utah	51,154	47,851	740	713	1,850
Vermont	6,130	5,825	126	16	163
Virginia	103,300	71,861	22,828	255	8,356
Washington	88,585	70,966	5,254	2,059	10,306
West Virginia	20,301	19,245	813	29	214
Wisconsin	67,161	55,520	7,328	980	3,333
Wyoming	7,696	7,178	116	294	108
Puerto Rico	34,434	30,246	4,171	- - -	NA
Virgin Islands	NA	NA	NA	NA	NA
Guam	3,395	236	37	13	3,109
American Samoa	1,077	–	–	–	1,077
Northern Marianas	517	8	–	–	509

NA = Not available.   - = Quantity zero.   1 Excludes data for the territories.

Table 1-21. Live Births, by Hispanic Origin of Mother and by Race for Mothers of Non-Hispanic Origin, by State and Territory, 2014

(Number.)

State and territory	All origins	Hispanic (may be of any race)						Non-Hispanic			Not stated
		Total	Mexican	Puerto Rican	Cuban	Central and South American	Other and unknown Hispanic	Total[1]	White	Black	
United States [2]	3,988,076	914,065	545,977	69,879	20,163	136,656	141,390	3,043,519	2,149,302	588,891	30,492
Alabama	59,422	4,019	2,585	210	39	1,059	126	55,391	35,929	18,230	12
Alaska	11,392	841	461	104	14	106	156	10,375	6,541	446	176
Arizona	86,887	35,034	31,480	495	189	1,193	1,677	51,553	38,608	4,673	300
Arkansas	38,511	3,837	2,898	69	18	634	218	34,592	25,940	7,254	82
California	502,879	237,539	178,810	2,200	757	18,689	37,083	254,458	144,318	28,312	10,882
Colorado	65,830	17,655	11,329	419	108	1,064	4,735	47,294	40,629	3,355	881
Connecticut	36,285	8,129	887	4,240	91	2,691	220	28,072	20,933	4,615	84
Delaware	10,972	1,541	657	341	23	411	109	9,411	5,904	2,847	20
District of Columbia	9,509	1,282	158	45	25	891	163	8,170	2,966	4,775	57
Florida	219,991	61,849	12,126	12,673	13,376	19,766	3,908	157,461	100,837	49,313	681
Georgia	130,946	17,242	10,400	1,189	293	3,759	1,601	111,241	60,104	45,022	2,463
Hawaii	18,550	2,764	773	914	26	143	908	15,782	4,881	558	4
Idaho	22,876	3,651	2,955	51	12	159	474	19,172	18,188	207	53
Illinois	158,556	33,803	27,681	2,471	217	2,432	1,002	123,552	86,227	27,187	1,201
Indiana	84,080	7,239	5,360	362	42	769	706	76,779	64,076	10,344	62
Iowa	39,687	3,315	2,457	98	27	543	190	36,361	32,423	2,359	11
Kansas	39,223	6,132	4,680	159	50	541	702	33,048	28,504	2,938	43
Kentucky	56,170	2,819	1,636	207	194	518	264	53,284	46,701	5,352	67
Louisiana	64,497	4,249	1,581	189	113	1,830	536	60,176	34,264	24,222	72
Maine	12,698	200	60	58	12	38	32	12,492	11,654	442	6
Maryland	73,921	10,974	1,821	689	126	7,130	1,208	62,760	33,178	23,968	187
Massachusetts	71,908	12,722	519	4,437	139	3,737	3,890	58,234	44,542	7,165	952
Michigan	114,375	7,352	4,683	528	104	705	1,332	106,883	80,304	21,650	140
Minnesota	69,904	4,678	3,192	176	50	909	351	64,867	50,332	7,745	359
Mississippi	38,736	1,547	901	89	26	387	144	37,179	19,839	16,621	10
Missouri	75,360	3,959	2,457	202	71	662	567	71,045	57,150	11,453	356
Montana	12,432	494	300	22	5	37	130	11,892	10,153	90	46
Nebraska	26,794	4,143	2,986	64	88	739	266	22,628	19,471	1,852	23
Nevada	35,861	13,006	10,381	307	259	1,305	754	22,757	15,151	4,259	98
New Hampshire	12,302	591	85	159	13	115	219	11,625	10,917	189	86
New Jersey	103,305	27,267	4,801	6,346	743	13,639	1,738	75,570	48,196	15,528	468
New Mexico	26,052	14,449	5,108	123	57	143	9,018	11,148	7,222	468	455
New York	238,773	55,329	8,942	13,003	582	17,212	15,590	179,561	116,013	36,958	3,883
North Carolina	120,975	17,784	10,462	1,399	267	4,429	1,227	103,123	67,551	29,017	68
North Dakota	11,359	480	329	40	6	18	87	10,735	9,036	460	144
Ohio	139,467	6,884	3,174	1,650	105	1,199	756	132,068	104,102	23,663	515
Oklahoma	53,339	7,219	5,416	213	49	691	850	46,026	33,577	5,044	94
Oregon	45,556	8,524	7,365	140	80	530	409	36,849	32,338	1,219	183
Pennsylvania	142,268	14,496	2,433	7,193	253	1,887	2,730	126,042	99,306	20,169	1,730
Rhode Island	10,823	2,585	158	747	25	813	842	8,038	6,573	851	200
South Carolina	57,627	4,646	2,570	460	63	1,105	448	52,769	33,639	17,878	212
South Dakota	12,283	603	337	41	7	154	64	11,656	9,122	340	24
Tennessee	81,602	6,986	4,305	392	110	1,562	617	74,538	55,499	16,989	78
Texas	399,766	189,462	138,579	2,175	852	13,111	34,745	209,955	140,992	47,983	349
Utah	51,154	7,764	5,381	138	46	1,215	984	42,204	39,433	573	1,186
Vermont	6,130	92	23	17	2	25	25	6,015	5,724	116	23
Virginia	103,300	13,490	3,135	1,167	225	4,198	4,765	89,665	59,885	21,623	145
Washington	88,585	15,779	11,873	479	121	1,225	2,081	71,868	55,872	4,659	938
West Virginia	20,301	350	149	72	10	44	75	19,845	18,860	762	106
Wisconsin	67,161	6,375	4,537	890	49	440	459	60,608	49,440	7,063	178
Wyoming	7,696	895	601	27	4	54	209	6,702	6,258	85	99
Puerto Rico	3,434	31,691	44	30,626	27	192	804	2,731	30,246	4171	10
Virgin Islands	NA	NA	NA	NA	NA	NA	NA	NA	NA	NA	NA
Guam	3,395	61	29	9	3	5	15	3,287	1	5	47
American Samoa	1,077	NA	NA	NA	NA	NA	NA	-	-	-	1,077
Northern Marianas	517	3	1	1	-	1	-	509	8	-	5

NA = Not available.   - = Quantity zero.   1 Includes races other than White and Black.   2 Excludes data for the territories.

Table 1-22. Birth Rates, by Age of Mother, State, and Territory, 2014

(Fertility rates are births per 1,000 women age 15 to 44 years estimated in each area; total fertility rates are sums of birth rates for 5-year age groups multiplied by 5; birth rates by age are births per 1,000 women in specified age group estimated in each area.)

State and territory	Birth rate	Fertility rate	Total fertility rate	10 to 14 years	15 to 19 years Total	15 to 17 years	18 to 19 years	20 to 24 years	25 to 29 years	30 to 34 years	35 to 39 years	40 to 44 years	45 to 49 years [1]
United States [2]	12.5	62.9	1,862.5	0.3	24.2	10.9	43.8	79.0	105.8	100.8	51.0	10.6	0.8
Alabama	12.3	61.8	1,825.5	0.4	32.0	14.5	58.4	97.1	113.1	83.5	33.0	5.7	0.3
Alaska	15.5	77.3	2,188.5	*	27.8	9.5	59.5	113.1	124.5	108.3	51.4	11.5	*
Arizona	12.9	66.4	1,971.0	0.2	29.9	13.4	55.0	90.9	115.7	97.8	49.0	10.0	0.7
Arkansas	13	67.0	1,971.0	0.4	39.5	16.2	75.7	115.2	118.1	81.8	32.6	6.2	0.4
California	13	62.4	1,841.0	0.2	21.1	9.6	38.0	66.8	93.9	106.1	63.8	15.0	1.3
Colorado	12.3	60.7	1,772.5	0.2	20.3	8.9	37.2	71.9	97.0	99.7	53.1	11.5	0.8
Connecticut	10.1	53.0	1,634.5	*	11.5	5.5	19.7	47.3	88.3	108.4	58.4	11.9	1.0
Delaware	11.7	60.8	1,791.0	*	20.7	10.1	34.5	73.5	101.5	103.1	47.7	10.7	*
District of Columbia	14.4	53.6	1,517.0	*	28.4	22.3	32.4	55.6	46.2	78.3	71.7	20.0	2.6
Florida	11.1	59.7	1,769.5	0.3	22.5	9.3	42.8	77.4	100.8	93.4	48.5	10.3	0.7
Georgia	13	62.2	1,866.0	0.3	28.4	12.5	52.3	89.7	107.1	91.9	45.5	9.6	0.7
Hawaii	13.1	69.3	1,998.5	*	23.1	9.6	43.9	84.1	104.6	105.4	63.7	17.1	1.6
Idaho	14	72.7	2,154.5	*	23.2	9.0	45.8	114.7	135.6	102.4	45.1	9.2	0.6
Illinois	12.3	61.1	1,809.5	0.2	22.8	10.4	41.7	69.3	98.3	105.4	54.2	10.9	0.8
Indiana	12.7	64.9	1,932.5	0.3	28.0	11.9	52.1	92.0	124.0	95.5	39.0	7.3	0.4
Iowa	12.8	67.8	2,019.0	0.2	19.8	8.6	34.9	79.2	142.7	110.7	43.6	7.2	0.4
Kansas	13.5	70.0	2,053.0	0.2	27.6	11.9	50.7	89.8	132.8	106.9	44.8	8.0	0.5
Kentucky	12.7	65.8	1,957.0	0.3	35.3	14.7	66.6	104.9	121.8	87.3	35.5	6.0	0.3
Louisiana	13.9	68.4	1,956.0	0.7	35.8	15.7	67.4	107.0	116.9	86.5	37.3	6.6	0.4
Maine	9.5	54.3	1,655.5	*	16.5	6.7	30.6	72.4	100.6	91.5	41.9	7.6	*
Maryland	12.4	61.5	1,818.5	0.3	17.8	8.5	31.4	65.1	96.2	109.5	61.0	12.7	1.1
Massachusetts	10.7	52.5	1,576.5	*	10.6	4.9	17.2	39.2	73.6	111.7	65.6	13.5	1.0
Michigan	11.5	60.6	1,832.0	0.2	21.1	8.9	39.3	75.5	115.8	101.5	43.6	8.1	0.6
Minnesota	12.8	66.4	1,943.0	0.1	15.5	6.8	28.4	64.0	121.0	121.5	55.4	10.2	0.9
Mississippi	12.9	64.4	1,886.5	0.7	38.0	17.6	67.3	112.6	115.5	75.3	29.5	5.2	0.5
Missouri	12.4	64.1	1,874.0	0.3	27.2	11.8	50.4	88.7	115.9	95.0	39.8	7.5	0.4
Montana	12.1	67.0	1,953.5	*	26.4	13.0	46.2	82.3	126.5	101.2	44.0	9.6	*
Nebraska	14.2	73.6	2,162.0	0.3	22.2	9.7	39.8	82.8	144.4	121.9	50.8	9.4	0.6
Nevada	12.6	63.3	1,870.0	0.3	28.5	12.2	56.6	90.7	103.2	92.8	47.0	10.5	1.0
New Hampshire	9.3	50.5	1,578.5	*	11.0	4.4	19.6	49.4	97.6	103.3	46.7	7.0	0.6
New Jersey	11.6	59.9	1,811.0	0.2	13.1	5.8	25.0	55.0	94.7	119.2	65.2	13.8	1.0
New Mexico	12.5	65.5	1,907.0	0.5	37.8	19.0	66.0	101.7	110.2	82.3	39.8	8.6	0.5
New York	12.1	59.0	1,727.5	0.2	16.1	7.2	28.1	58.5	86.5	103.8	64.0	15.1	1.3
North Carolina	12.2	61.0	1,832.0	0.3	25.9	12.2	45.5	86.5	106.4	93.8	44.3	8.6	0.6
North Dakota	15.4	78.8	2,236.0	*	23.9	8.6	42.1	80.4	156.6	126.2	51.0	8.3	*
Ohio	12	63.1	1,880.5	0.3	25.1	10.6	46.9	87.0	113.5	99.4	42.8	7.5	0.5
Oklahoma	13.8	69.9	2,025.5	0.5	38.5	16.9	71.8	109.3	126.4	87.3	35.9	6.9	0.3
Oregon	11.5	58.7	1,723.0	0.2	20.0	8.5	37.6	70.1	100.0	94.2	48.7	10.6	0.8
Pennsylvania	11.1	59.1	1,762.5	0.3	19.3	9.0	32.7	68.5	100.1	104.9	49.5	9.2	0.7
Rhode Island	10.3	51.5	1,559.0	*	15.8	7.6	24.3	50.9	83.9	100.0	50.9	9.6	*
South Carolina	11.9	61.1	1,800.5	0.3	28.5	13.4	50.1	90.0	106.1	88.3	38.9	7.5	0.5
South Dakota	14.4	77.8	2,268.0	*	26.2	13.2	44.6	94.1	155.9	119.7	48.6	8.5	*
Tennessee	12.5	63.0	1,866.5	0.4	33.0	13.6	62.7	97.2	110.7	87.6	36.9	7.1	0.4
Texas	14.8	70.7	2,092.0	0.5	37.8	18.8	67.7	103.0	117.2	100.3	48.6	10.3	0.7
Utah	17.4	80.0	2,328.5	*	19.4	7.9	37.9	92.9	162.8	123.1	55.4	11.1	0.9
Vermont	9.8	52.9	1,634.0	*	14.2	5.5	23.6	54.2	99.0	100.5	48.5	9.5	*
Virginia	12.4	61.3	1,810.5	0.2	18.4	7.7	33.2	69.1	100.8	105.2	56.0	11.5	0.9
Washington	12.5	63.3	1,847.5	0.2	19.1	8.3	36.2	72.6	105.6	104.7	55.1	11.4	0.8
West Virginia	11	60.3	1,813.5	0.5	36.6	15.8	66.9	101.8	113.9	73.7	31.1	4.6	0.5
Wisconsin	11.7	61.8	1,846.0	0.2	18.0	7.5	33.0	67.2	120.7	107.9	46.6	8.2	0.4
Wyoming	13.2	69.4	1,991.0	*	30.1	11.8	58.7	103.7	128.6	90.0	38.1	7.4	*
Puerto Rico	9.7	48.2	1,432.0	0.5	40.4	21.4	67.8	90.0	76.8	50.7	22.9	4.8	0.3
Virgin Islands	NA	NA	NA	NA	NA	NA	NA	NA	NA	NA	NA	NA	NA
Guam	21.1	99.1	2,960.5	*	48.4	22.2	86.7	152.8	149.7	137.7	82.9	19.6	*
American Samoa	19.8	85.2	2,601.5	*	46.8	23.4	71.0	94.3	149.5	124.5	80.5	23.7	*
Northern Marianas	10	39.6	1,244.0	*	38.6	*	66.6	88.0	51.5	26.8	30.5	11.7	*

* = Figure does not meet standards of reliability or percision; birth rates based on fewer than 20 births.   1 Birth rates computed by relating births to women age 45 years and over to women age 45 to 49 years.   2 Excludes data for the territories.

Figure 1-6. Birth Rates, by Age of Mother, 1980–2014

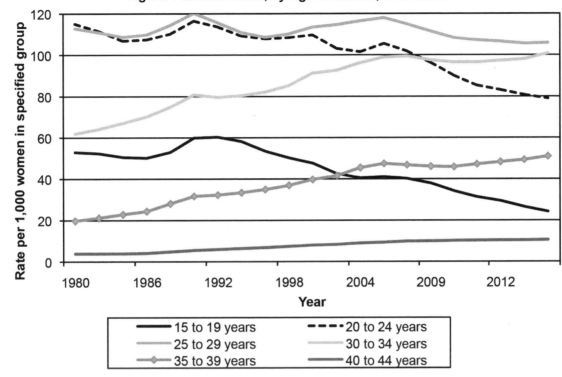

Table 1-23. Birth Rates, by Age of Mother, Live-Birth Order, and Race of Mother, 2011

(Live births per 1,000 women in specified age and racial group.)

Live-birth order and race of mother	15 to 44 years	10 to 14 years	15 to 19 years Total	15 to 17 years	18 to 19 years	20 to 24 years	25 to 29 years	30 to 34 years	35 to 39 years	40 to 44 years	45 to 49 years[1]
All Races	62.9	0.3	24.2	10.9	43.8	79.0	105.8	100.8	51.0	10.6	0.8
1st child	24.6	0.3	20.1	10.1	34.8	40.1	39.8	30.6	11.6	2.3	0.2
2nd child	20.1	0.0	3.6	0.8	7.7	25.9	35.0	34.5	16.6	2.9	0.2
3rd child	10.6	*	0.5	0.1	1.1	9.6	19.2	20.0	11.3	2.2	0.1
4th child	4.5	*	0.1	0.0	0.1	2.6	7.7	9.2	5.9	1.4	0.1
5th child	1.8	*	0.0	*	0.0	0.6	2.7	3.7	2.7	0.7	0.1
6th and 7th child	1.1	*	0.0	*	*	0.2	1.2	2.3	2.0	0.6	0.1
8th child and over	0.3	*	*	*	*	0.0	0.2	0.6	0.9	0.4	0.0
White	63.2	0.2	23.0	10.2	42.0	77.3	108.6	103.9	51.2	10.2	0.7
1st child	24.7	0.2	19.2	9.4	33.7	39.7	41.4	31.4	11.6	2.2	0.2
2nd child	20.4	*	3.3	0.7	7.2	25.7	36.7	35.6	16.3	2.8	0.2
3rd child	10.8	*	0.4	0.0	0.9	8.9	19.7	21.1	11.6	2.1	0.1
4th child	4.5	*	0.0	0.0	0.1	2.2	7.4	9.5	6.1	1.3	0.1
5th child	1.7	*	0.0	*	0.0	0.5	2.4	3.6	2.8	0.7	0.0
6th and 7th child	1.0	*	*	*	*	0.1	1.0	2.1	2.0	0.6	0.1
8th child and over	0.3	*	*	*	*	0.0	0.1	0.5	0.8	0.4	0.0
Black	64.6	0.6	35.1	16.7	61.9	102.6	103.1	79.4	42.6	10.2	0.8
1st child	23.9	0.6	28.6	15.4	48.0	48.9	29.5	17.8	7.9	1.9	0.2
2nd child	18.7	*	5.5	1.3	11.7	32.7	32.5	23.4	11.5	2.4	0.2
3rd child	11.5	*	0.9	0.1	2.0	14.4	22.3	18.2	9.9	2.2	0.2
4th child	5.6	*	0.1	*	0.2	4.8	11.1	10.0	6.1	1.5	0.1
5th child	2.5	*	0.0	*	0.0	1.4	4.7	5.0	3.2	0.9	0.1
6th and 7th child	1.7	*	*	*	*	0.4	2.6	3.8	2.8	0.8	0.1
8th child and over	0.6	*	*	*	*	0.1	0.4	1.2	1.4	0.5	0.0
American Indian or Alaska Native	.44.8	0.3	27.3	13.2	48.6	73.2	74.7	52.3	24.1	5.5	0.3
1st child	14.8	0.0	22.3	12.0	37.7	30.6	16.3	8.6	3.3	0.7	*
2nd child	12.0	*	4.3	1.0	9.2	24.9	21.7	12.0	4.3	0.9	*
3rd child	8.5	*	0.6	*	1.5	12.1	18.4	12.3	5.1	1.0	*
4th child	4.8	*	*	*	*	4.2	10.5	8.7	4.4	1.0	*
5th child	2.4	*	*	*	*	1.1	4.8	5.1	2.7	0.7	*
6th and 7th child	1.8	*	*	*	*	0.3	2.7	4.3	3.0	0.9	*
8th child and over	0.5	*	*	*	*	*	0.3	1.3	1.0	0.4	*
Asian or Pacific Islander	60.7	0.1	7.7	3.3	13.9	37.5	90.0	121.3	68.9	16.1	1.5
1st child	27.2	0.0	6.4	3.0	11.2	23.0	50.3	50.9	19.8	4.3	0.5
2nd child	22.1	*	1.1	0.2	2.3	10.1	26.6	49.0	30.6	6.1	0.4
3rd child	7.4	*	0.1	*	0.3	3.1	8.5	13.9	12.1	3.3	0.3
4th child	2.5	*	*	*	*	0.9	2.9	4.5	3.9	1.3	0.1
5th child	0.9	*	*	*	*	0.2	1.0	1.6	1.4	0.6	0.1
6th and 7th child	0.5	*	*	*	*	0.1	0.5	1.0	0.9	0.4	0.1
8th child and over	0.2	*	*	*	*	*	0.1	0.3	0.3	0.2	0.0

* = Figure does not meet standards of reliability or precision; based on fewer than 20 births in the numerator.   0.0 = Quantity more than zero but less than 0.05.   1 Birth rates computed by relating births to women age 45 years and over to women age 45 to 49 years.

Table 1-24. Birth Rates, by Age and Selected Race of Father, 1980–2014

(Rates are births per 1,000 men in specified group.)

Year and race of father	Total, 15 to 54 years[1]	Age of father								
		15 to 19 years[2]	20 to 24 years	25 to 29 years	30 to 34 years	35 to 39 years	40 to 44 years	45 to 49 years	50 to 54 years	55 years and over
All Races [3]										
1980[4]	57.0	18.8	92.0	123.1	91.0	42.8	17.1	6.1	2.2	0.3
1981[4]	56.3	18.4	88.4	119.1	88.7	43.3	17.0	6.2	2.3	0.4
1982[4]	56.4	18.6	86.5	117.3	90.3	44.5	17.5	6.4	2.3	0.4
1983[4]	55.1	18.2	82.6	113.0	89.1	45.2	17.4	6.4	2.3	0.4
1984[4]	55.0	17.8	80.7	111.4	89.9	46.0	17.8	6.3	2.4	0.4
1985	55.6	18.0	81.2	112.3	91.1	47.3	18.1	6.6	2.5	0.4
1986	54.8	17.9	80.3	109.6	90.3	46.8	18.3	6.7	2.6	0.4
1987	55.0	18.3	80.5	109.9	91.2	48.6	19.0	6.9	2.6	0.4
1988	55.8	19.6	82.4	111.6	93.2	49.9	19.9	7.1	2.7	0.4
1989	57.2	21.9	85.4	114.3	94.8	51.3	20.4	7.4	2.7	0.6
1990	58.4	23.5	88.0	116.4	97.8	53.0	21.0	7.5	2.8	0.4
1991	56.8	24.7	87.9	113.5	94.3	51.6	20.2	7.4	2.7	0.4
1992	55.3	24.4	87.1	111.1	93.0	51.1	20.4	7.3	2.7	0.4
1993	53.7	24.4	86.0	108.1	91.7	50.7	20.2	7.3	2.7	0.4
1994	52.4	24.6	85.6	105.3	91.1	50.5	20.3	7.2	2.6	0.3
1995	51.0	23.9	83.9	103.2	90.7	50.4	20.3	7.0	2.5	0.3
1996	50.2	22.7	83.4	102.8	91.3	51.1	20.5	6.9	2.5	0.3
1997	49.4	21.9	82.1	102.6	92.0	51.5	20.7	7.0	2.5	0.3
1998	49.6	21.3	82.3	104.4	94.4	53.1	21.0	7.1	2.5	0.3
1999	49.2	20.6	81.1	105.3	95.9	53.9	21.1	7.0	2.4	0.3
2000	50.0	19.8	82.1	106.5	99.5	56.3	22.2	7.3	2.5	0.3
2001	48.9	18.3	78.3	106.7	99.9	57.1	22.3	7.3	2.4	0.3
2002	48.7	17.2	75.7	107.1	100.7	58.3	22.7	7.4	2.4	0.3
2003	49.3	16.6	74.7	109.1	104.0	60.9	23.6	7.6	2.5	0.3
2004	49.3	16.6	73.4	108.9	104.7	62.5	24.1	7.7	2.4	0.3
2005	49.3	16.4	72.7	109.4	105.9	63.4	24.5	7.9	2.5	0.2
2006	50.4	17.3	75.3	111.4	108.6	65.2	25.3	8.1	2.6	0.2
2007	50.8	18.2	75.6	110.4	110.3	65.6	25.7	8.2	2.6	0.3
2008	49.8	18.4	73.2	106.4	108.3	64.8	25.8	8.3	2.6	0.3
2009	48.3	17.7	69.5	101.5	105.5	63.8	25.9	8.2	2.6	0.3
2010	46.8	16.1	64.6	97.1	103.6	63.4	25.9	8.2	2.6	0.3
2011	46.1	14.7	60.5	94.4	102.2	64.6	26.4	8.3	2.6	0.3
2012	46.1	13.8	58.3	92.5	102.0	65.9	26.8	8.6	2.6	0.3
2013	45.8	12.3	55.7	90.6	101.8	66.6	27.0	8.8	2.7	0.3
2014	46.3	11.3	53.9	89.7	103.9	68.8	27.9	9.3	2.8	0.4
White										
1980[4]	53.4	15.4	84.9	119.4	87.8	39.7	15.0	5.1	1.8	0.3
1981[4]	52.9	15.0	81.7	115.8	85.8	40.3	15.0	5.2	1.8	0.3
1982[4]	53.1	14.9	80.1	114.2	87.5	41.7	15.6	5.3	1.9	0.3
1983[4]	52.0	14.4	76.3	110.2	86.8	42.6	15.5	5.3	1.8	0.3
1984[4]	51.8	14.0	74.3	108.8	87.9	43.5	16.0	5.3	1.9	0.3
1985	52.6	14.0	74.7	109.9	89.5	44.8	16.3	5.6	1.9	0.3
1986	51.7	13.8	73.3	107.0	88.7	44.4	16.6	5.7	2.0	0.3
1987	51.6	13.9	72.8	107.0	89.5	46.2	17.3	5.9	2.0	0.3
1988	52.2	14.8	73.7	108.3	91.2	47.6	18.1	6.1	2.1	0.3
1989	53.3	16.7	75.9	110.8	93.0	49.1	18.7	6.3	2.1	0.4
1990	54.6	18.1	78.3	113.2	96.1	50.9	19.2	6.5	2.2	0.3
1991	53.1	19.0	78.4	110.2	92.8	49.6	18.5	6.5	2.2	0.3
1992	51.8	18.8	77.8	108.2	91.9	49.1	18.8	6.4	2.2	0.3
1993	50.3	18.9	77.2	105.5	90.7	48.9	18.7	6.4	2.2	0.2
1994	49.3	19.5	77.4	103.1	90.4	48.9	18.9	6.3	2.2	0.3
1995	48.4	19.4	77.0	101.7	90.4	49.1	19.1	6.2	2.1	0.2
1996	47.7	18.7	76.7	101.4	91.1	49.9	19.2	6.1	2.1	0.2
1997	46.8	18.0	75.3	100.9	91.7	50.2	19.3	6.2	2.1	0.3
1998	47.1	17.7	75.6	102.7	94.3	51.9	19.6	6.3	2.1	0.3
1999	46.9	17.3	74.7	104.1	96.2	52.7	19.8	6.3	2.1	0.3
2000	47.6	16.6	75.8	105.4	99.5	54.7	20.7	6.5	2.1	0.3
2001	46.9	15.4	73.1	106.6	100.3	55.8	20.8	6.5	2.0	0.3
2002	46.8	14.7	71.4	107.5	101.2	57.0	21.2	6.6	2.1	0.3
2003	47.5	14.1	70.7	109.9	104.5	59.6	22.0	6.8	2.1	0.3
2004	47.4	14.1	69.1	109.6	105.0	61.1	22.5	6.9	2.0	0.2
2005	47.3	14.0	68.2	110.0	106.2	61.9	22.8	6.9	2.1	0.2
2006	48.3	14.6	70.5	112.0	108.8	63.4	23.5	7.1	2.1	0.1
2007	48.6	15.5	70.6	111.1	110.5	63.5	23.8	7.1	2.1	0.3

Table 1-24. Birth Rates, by Age and Selected Race of Father, 1980–2014— continued

(Rates are births per 1,000 men in specified group.)

Year and race of father	Total, 15 to 54 years[1]	Age of father								
		15 to 19 years[2]	20 to 24 years	25 to 29 years	30 to 34 years	35 to 39 years	40 to 44 years	45 to 49 years	50 to 54 years	55 years and over
2008	47.7	15.7	68.1	107.0	108.8	62.6	23.9	7.2	2.1	0.3
2009	46.3	15.2	64.3	102.0	106.2	61.7	24.0	7.1	2.1	0.3
2010	44.8	13.9	59.6	97.5	104.6	61.3	24.0	7.1	2.0	0.2
2011	44.1	12.8	55.5	94.5	103.0	62.5	24.3	7.1	2.0	0.2
2012	44.0	12.1	53.7	92.3	102.5	63.4	24.4	7.3	2.1	0.2
2013	43.8	10.9	51.3	90.4	102.5	64.6	24.6	7.4	2.1	0.2
2014		10.1	50.1	89.8	104.4	66.5	25.3	7.9	2.2	0.2
Black										
1980[4]	83.0	40.1	145.3	152.8	109.6	62.0	31.2	13.6	5.9	1.1
1981[4]	80.4	38.9	138.4	145.6	104.3	61.3	29.7	13.3	5.7	1.2
1982[4]	79.5	40.3	133.4	141.2	103.6	61.1	29.6	13.9	6.0	1.2
1983[4]	77.2	40.7	129.1	134.4	99.0	59.6	29.6	13.5	6.0	1.2
1984[4]	76.7	40.9	128.0	132.2	98.3	58.4	29.3	13.3	6.1	1.2
1985	77.2	41.8	129.5	132.7	97.3	59.4	29.5	13.3	6.5	1.2
1986	77.2	42.6	131.4	131.6	97.4	58.0	29.1	13.5	6.7	1.3
1987	78.3	44.6	136.1	133.9	97.4	58.0	30.0	13.8	6.6	1.3
1988	80.7	48.1	144.1	137.9	100.0	58.0	30.6	14.3	6.9	1.4
1989	84.1	52.9	153.4	143.5	101.4	59.9	31.1	14.9	6.9	2.7
1990	84.9	55.2	158.2	144.9	103.2	60.4	31.1	15.0	7.1	1.4
1991	83.0	57.8	158.5	142.0	99.2	58.5	29.4	14.1	6.7	1.4
1992	80.4	57.0	157.1	138.6	95.8	56.7	28.4	13.7	6.1	1.4
1993	77.6	56.2	152.7	134.2	94.0	56.3	27.7	13.4	6.3	1.3
1994	74.0	54.1	149.1	129.6	91.4	53.8	26.4	12.8	5.8	1.1
1995	69.1	49.9	139.2	123.9	87.7	52.0	25.7	11.9	5.4	1.1
1996	67.2	46.7	137.6	123.9	87.0	51.8	25.7	11.3	5.3	1.1
1997	66.7	45.1	136.3	126.3	88.8	52.6	26.1	11.4	5.2	1.0
1998	66.8	42.8	137.0	130.3	90.9	54.0	26.7	11.6	5.0	1.0
1999	65.4	41.0	133.8	129.6	91.6	54.3	26.5	11.2	4.9	1.0
2000	66.2	39.6	135.5	131.0	95.2	56.9	28.4	11.7	5.0	1.0
2001	63.3	36.2	124.9	127.6	96.1	57.1	28.2	11.8	4.6	1.0
2002	61.2	32.8	117.3	126.4	95.1	58.0	28.4	11.9	4.7	0.9
2003	61.2	31.8	114.4	127.7	97.6	60.1	29.3	12.3	4.7	0.9
2004	61.7	31.8	113.9	129.0	100.2	62.0	30.2	12.5	4.8	0.7
2005	62.5	31.1	114.7	131.5	102.8	64.2	31.2	13.3	5.0	0.7
2006	64.8	32.9	119.8	135.1	107.1	67.5	32.4	13.7	5.3	0.6
2007	63.8	33.9	118.5	128.1	105.1	67.7	33.2	13.9	5.4	1.0
2008	64.4	35.8	115.8	119.0	103.5	68.3	34.0	14.4	5.7	1.0
2009	61.9	32.2	114.4	122.3	102.1	66.0	33.3	13.9	5.5	1.0
2010	59.6	29.0	107.0	117.0	98.9	65.7	33.9	13.8	5.8	1.0
2011	58.7	26.6	99.4	114.6	98.3	66.7	34.5	14.2	5.7	1.0
2012	58.2	24.6	93.8	112.7	98.0	68.2	35.1	14.6	5.7	1.0
2013	58.0	21.5	88.7	111.5	99.3	69.2	36.1	15.5	6.0	1.0
2014	57.8	19.1	84.4	108.4		71.2	37.0	15.9	6.1	1.1

1 Rates computed by relating total births, regardless of age of father, to men age 15 to 54 years.   2 Rates computed by relating births to fathers under 20 years of age to men age 15 to 19 years.   3 Includes races other than White and Black.   4 Based on 100 percent of births in selected states and on a 50-percent sample of births in all other states.   NOTE: Race and Hispanic origin are reported separately on birth certificates.

Table 1-25. Total Fertility Rates and Birth Rates by Age of Mother, 1970–2014, and by Age and Race of Mother, 1980–2014

(Live births per 1,000 women in specified group.)

Year and race	Total fertility rate	10 to 14 years	15 to 19 years			20 to 24 years	25 to 29 years	30 to 34 years	35 to 39 years	40 to 44 years	45 to 49 years[1]
			Total	15 to 17 years	18 to 19 years						
All Races [2]											
1980[3]	1,839.5	1.1	53.0	32.5	82.1	115.1	112.9	61.9	19.8	3.9	0.2
1981[3]	1,812.0	1.1	52.2	32.0	80.0	112.2	111.5	61.4	20.0	3.8	0.2
1982[3]	1,827.5	1.1	52.4	32.3	79.4	111.6	111.0	64.1	21.2	3.9	0.2
1983[3]	1,799.0	1.1	51.4	31.8	77.4	107.8	108.5	64.9	22.0	3.9	0.2
1984[3]	1,806.5	1.2	50.6	31.0	77.4	106.8	108.7	67.0	22.9	3.9	0.2
1985	1,844.0	1.2	51.0	31.0	79.6	108.3	111.0	69.1	24.0	4.0	0.2
1986	1,837.5	1.3	50.2	30.5	79.6	107.4	109.8	70.1	24.4	4.1	0.2
1987	1,872.0	1.3	50.6	31.7	78.5	107.9	111.6	72.1	26.3	4.4	0.2
1988	1,934.0	1.3	53.0	33.6	79.9	110.2	114.4	74.8	28.1	4.8	0.2
1989	2,014.0	1.4	57.3	36.4	84.2	113.8	117.6	77.4	29.9	5.2	0.2
1990	2,081.0	1.4	59.9	37.5	88.6	116.5	120.2	80.8	31.7	5.5	0.2
1991	2,062.5	1.4	61.8	38.6	94.0	115.3	117.2	79.2	31.9	5.5	0.2
1992	2,046.0	1.4	60.3	37.6	93.6	113.7	115.7	79.6	32.3	5.9	0.3
1993	2,019.5	1.4	59.0	37.5	91.1	111.3	113.2	79.9	32.7	6.1	0.3
1994	2,001.5	1.4	58.2	37.2	90.2	109.2	111.0	80.4	33.4	6.4	0.3
1995	1,978.0	1.3	56.0	35.5	87.7	107.5	108.8	81.1	34.0	6.6	0.3
1996	1,976.0	1.2	53.5	33.3	84.7	107.8	108.6	82.1	34.9	6.8	0.3
1997	1,971.0	1.1	51.3	31.4	82.1	107.3	108.3	83.0	35.7	7.1	0.4
1998	1,999.0	1.0	50.3	29.9	80.9	108.4	110.2	85.2	36.9	7.4	0.4
1999	2,007.5	0.9	48.8	28.2	79.1	107.9	111.2	87.1	37.8	7.4	0.4
2000	2,056.0	0.9	47.7	26.9	78.1	109.7	113.5	91.2	39.7	8.0	0.5
2001	2,030.5	0.8	45.0	24.5	75.5	105.6	113.8	91.8	40.5	8.1	0.5
2002	2,020.5	0.7	42.6	23.1	72.2	103.1	114.7	92.6	41.6	8.3	0.5
2003	2,047.5	0.6	41.1	22.2	69.6	102.3	116.7	95.7	43.9	8.7	0.5
2004	2,051.5	0.6	40.5	21.8	68.7	101.5	116.5	96.2	45.5	9.0	0.5
2005	2,057.0	0.6	39.7	21.1	68.4	101.8	116.5	96.7	46.4	9.1	0.6
2006	2,108.0	0.6	41.1	21.6	71.2	105.5	118.0	98.9	47.5	9.4	0.6
2007	2,120.0	0.6	41.5	21.7	71.7	105.4	118.1	100.6	47.6	9.6	0.6
2008	2,072.0	0.6	40.2	21.1	68.2	101.8	115.0	99.4	46.8	9.9	0.7
2009	2,002.0	0.5	37.9	19.6	64.0	96.2	111.5	97.5	46.1	10.0	0.7
2010	1,931.0	0.4	34.2	17.3	58.2	90.0	108.3	96.5	45.9	10.2	0.7
2011	1,894.5	0.4	31.3	15.4	54.1	85.3	107.2	96.5	47.2	10.3	0.7
2012	1,880.5	0.4	29.4	14.1	51.4	83.1	106.5	97.3	48.3	10.4	0.8
2013	1,857.5	0.3	26.5	12.3	47.1	80.7	105.5	98.0	49.3	10.4	0.8
2014	1,862.5	0.3	24.2	10.9	43.8	79.0	106.5	100.8	51.0	10.0	0.7
White											
1980[3]	1,773.0	0.6	45.4	25.5	73.2	111.1	113.8	61.2	18.8	3.5	0.2
1981[3]	1,748.0	0.5	44.9	25.4	71.5	108.3	112.3	61.0	19.0	3.4	0.2
1982[3]	1,767.0	0.6	45.0	25.5	70.8	107.7	111.9	64.0	20.4	3.6	0.2
1983[3]	1,740.5	0.6	43.9	25.0	68.8	103.8	109.4	65.3	21.3	3.6	0.2
1984[3]	1,748.5	0.6	42.9	24.3	68.4	102.7	109.8	67.7	22.2	3.6	0.2
1985	1,787.0	0.6	43.3	24.4	70.4	104.1	112.3	69.9	23.3	3.7	0.2
1986	1,776.0	0.6	42.3	23.8	70.1	102.7	110.8	70.9	23.9	3.8	0.2
1987	1,804.5	0.6	42.5	24.6	68.9	102.3	112.3	73.0	25.9	4.1	0.2
1988	1,856.5	0.6	44.4	26.0	69.6	103.7	114.8	75.4	27.7	4.5	0.2
1989	1,931.0	0.7	47.9	28.1	72.9	106.9	117.8	78.1	29.7	4.9	0.2
1990	2,003.0	0.7	50.8	29.5	78.0	109.8	120.7	81.7	31.5	5.2	0.2
1991	1,988.0	0.8	52.6	30.5	83.3	108.8	118.0	80.2	31.8	5.2	0.2
1992	1,978.0	0.8	51.4	29.9	83.2	107.7	116.9	80.8	32.1	5.7	0.2
1993	1,961.5	0.8	50.6	30.0	81.5	106.1	114.7	81.3	32.6	5.9	0.3
1994	1,957.5	0.8	50.5	30.4	81.2	105.0	113.0	82.2	33.5	6.2	0.3
1995	1,954.5	0.8	49.5	29.6	80.2	104.7	111.7	83.3	34.2	6.4	0.3
1996	1,960.5	0.7	47.5	28.0	77.6	105.3	111.7	84.6	35.3	6.7	0.3
1997	1,955.0	0.7	45.5	26.6	75.0	104.5	111.3	85.7	36.1	6.9	0.3
1998	1,991.0	0.6	44.9	25.6	74.1	105.4	113.6	88.5	37.5	7.3	0.4
1999	2,007.5	0.6	44.0	24.4	73.0	105.0	114.9	90.7	38.5	7.4	0.4
2000	2,051.0	0.6	43.2	23.3	72.3	106.6	116.7	94.6	40.2	7.9	0.4
2001	2,042.5	0.5	41.0	21.4	70.4	103.4	117.8	95.9	41.4	8.0	0.5
2002	2,041.5	0.5	39.2	20.4	67.7	101.6	119.0	96.7	42.6	8.2	0.5
2003	2,075.0	0.5	38.0	19.6	65.6	100.9	121.3	100.1	45.0	8.7	0.5
2004	2,074.5	0.5	37.4	19.4	64.4	99.8	120.8	100.3	46.7	8.9	0.5
2005	2,078.5	0.5	36.7	18.8	64.0	99.9	120.7	100.7	47.6	9.0	0.6

Table 1-25. Total Fertility Rates and Birth Rates by Age of Mother, 1970–2014, and by Age and Race of Mother, 1980–2014— continued

(Live births per 1,000 women in specified group.)

Year and race	Total fertility rate	10 to 14 years	15 to 19 years Total	15 to 17 years	18 to 19 years	20 to 24 years	25 to 29 years	30 to 34 years	35 to 39 years	40 to 44 years	45 to 49 years[1]
2006	2,125.0	0.5	37.9	19.2	66.7	103.4	122.0	102.7	48.6	9.3	0.6
2007	2,137.0	0.5	38.4	19.5	67.2	103.5	122.0	104.4	48.5	9.5	0.6
2008	2,087.0	0.4	37.3	19.1	64.0	99.8	118.8	103.3	47.5	9.7	0.6
2009	2,016.5	0.4	35.3	17.8	60.2	94.1	114.9	101.3	46.7	9.9	0.7
2010	1,947.5	0.3	31.9	15.8	54.8	87.9	111.9	100.5	46.4	10.0	0.6
2011	1,905.0	0.3	29.1	14.1	50.8	83.0	110.2	100.1	47.6	10.1	0.6
2012	1,885.5	0.3	27.4	13.0	48.3	80.8	109.2	100.2	48.5	10.0	0.7
2013	1,868.0	0.2	24.9	11.3	44.7	78.5	108.3	101.3	49.6	10.1	0.7
2014	1,875.5	0.2	23.0	10.2	42.0	77.3	108.6	103.9	51.2	10.2	0.7
Black											
1980[3]	2,176.5	4.3	97.8	72.5	135.1	140.0	103.9	59.9	23.5	5.6	0.3
1981[3]	2,117.5	4.0	94.5	69.3	131.0	136.5	102.3	57.4	23.1	5.4	0.3
1982[3]	2,106.5	4.0	94.3	69.7	128.9	135.4	101.3	57.5	23.3	5.1	0.4
1983[3]	2,066.0	4.1	93.9	69.6	127.1	131.9	98.4	56.2	23.3	5.1	0.3
1984[3]	2,070.5	4.4	94.1	69.2	128.1	132.2	98.4	56.7	23.3	4.8	0.2
1985	2,109.0	4.5	95.4	69.3	132.4	135.0	100.2	57.9	23.9	4.6	0.3
1986	2,135.5	4.7	95.8	69.3	135.1	137.3	101.1	59.3	23.8	4.8	0.3
1987	2,198.0	4.8	97.6	72.1	135.8	142.7	104.3	60.6	24.6	4.8	0.2
1988	2,298.0	4.9	102.7	75.7	142.7	149.7	108.2	63.1	25.6	5.1	0.3
1989	2,432.5	5.1	111.5	81.9	151.9	156.8	114.4	66.3	26.7	5.4	0.3
1990	2,480.0	4.9	112.8	82.3	152.9	160.2	115.5	68.7	28.1	5.5	0.3
1991	2,462.0	4.7	114.8	83.5	157.6	159.7	112.0	67.3	28.2	5.5	0.2
1992	2,416.0	4.6	111.3	80.5	156.3	156.2	109.7	67.0	28.6	5.6	0.2
1993	2,351.0	4.5	107.3	78.9	150.2	150.2	106.4	66.6	29.0	5.9	0.3
1994	2,258.5	4.5	102.9	75.1	146.2	142.9	101.5	65.0	28.7	5.9	0.3
1995	2,127.5	4.1	94.4	68.5	135.0	133.7	95.6	63.0	28.4	6.0	0.3
1996	2,088.5	3.5	89.6	63.3	130.5	133.2	94.3	62.0	28.7	6.1	0.3
1997	2,091.5	3.1	86.3	59.3	127.7	135.2	95.0	62.6	29.3	6.5	0.3
1998	2,111.5	2.8	83.5	55.4	124.8	138.4	97.5	63.2	30.0	6.6	0.3
1999	2,082.5	2.5	79.1	50.5	120.6	137.9	97.3	62.7	30.2	6.5	0.3
2000	2,129.0	2.3	77.4	49.0	118.8	141.3	100.3	65.4	31.5	7.2	0.4
2001	2,049.5	2.0	71.3	43.7	112.9	132.9	99.6	64.9	31.6	7.2	0.4
2002	1,990.0	1.8	65.8	39.5	106.3	126.9	99.4	64.7	31.6	7.4	0.4
2003	1,994.5	1.5	62.5	37.5	101.3	125.9	101.4	66.4	33.1	7.6	0.5
2004	2,026.0	1.6	61.7	36.3	101.3	127.5	104.4	67.8	33.8	7.9	0.5
2005	2,062.0	1.6	60.1	34.5	101.2	129.5	107.0	70.2	35.1	8.4	0.5
2006	2,143.0	1.5	62.2	35.3	105.6	135.2	110.6	73.8	36.3	8.5	0.5
2007	2,145.5	1.4	62.1	34.7	105.2	134.6	110.4	74.9	36.4	8.7	0.6
2008	2,102.5	1.3	60.1	33.5	99.5	130.6	107.9	74.8	36.4	8.8	0.6
2009	2,036.0	1.1	56.5	30.9	92.9	125.1	105.3	73.5	36.2	8.9	0.6
2010	1,957.0	1.0	51.1	27.3	84.8	118.1	101.8	73.0	36.4	9.3	0.7
2011	1,920.0	0.9	47.3	24.7	78.8	111.9	101.7	74.1	38.0	9.4	0.7
2012	1,899.5	0.8	44.0	22.0	74.4	106.7	101.7	75.1	39.2	9.7	0.7
2013	1,882.5	0.7	39.1	19.0	67.3	105.5	102.6	77.3	40.5	10.0	0.8
2014	1,872.0	0.6	35.1	16.7	61.9	102.6	103.1	79.4	42.6	10.2	0.8
American Indian or Alaska Native											
1980[3]	2,165.0	1.9	82.2	51.5	129.5	143.7	106.6	61.8	28.1	8.2	*
1981[3]	2,092.5	2.1	78.4	49.7	121.5	141.2	105.6	58.9	25.2	6.6	*
1982[3]	2,215.0	1.4	83.5	52.6	127.6	148.1	115.8	60.9	26.9	6.0	*
1983[3]	2,182.0	1.9	84.2	55.2	121.4	145.5	113.7	58.9	25.5	6.4	*
1984[3]	2,137.5	1.7	81.5	50.7	124.7	142.4	109.2	60.5	26.3	5.6	*
1985	2,129.5	1.7	79.2	47.7	124.1	139.1	109.6	62.6	27.4	6.0	*
1986	2,083.0	1.8	78.1	48.7	125.3	138.8	107.9	60.7	23.8	5.3	*
1987	2,100.5	1.7	77.2	48.8	122.2	140.0	107.9	63.0	24.4	5.6	*
1988	2,155.0	1.7	77.5	49.7	121.1	145.2	110.9	64.5	25.6	5.3	*
1989	2,248.5	1.5	82.7	51.6	128.9	152.4	114.2	64.8	27.4	6.4	*
1990	2,184.5	1.6	81.1	48.5	129.3	148.7	110.3	61.5	27.5	5.9	*
1991	2,142.5	1.6	84.1	51.9	134.2	143.8	105.6	60.8	26.4	5.8	0.4
1992	2,135.5	1.6	82.4	52.3	130.5	142.3	107.0	61.0	26.7	5.9	*
1993	2,048.5	1.4	79.8	51.5	126.3	134.2	103.5	59.5	25.5	5.6	*
1994	1,950.0	1.8	76.4	48.4	123.7	126.5	98.2	56.6	24.8	5.4	0.3
1995	1,878.5	1.6	72.9	44.6	122.2	123.1	91.6	56.5	24.3	5.5	*
1996	1,855.0	1.6	68.2	42.7	113.3	123.5	91.1	56.5	24.4	5.5	*

Table 1-25. Total Fertility Rates and Birth Rates by Age of Mother, 1970–2014, and by Age and Race of Mother, 1980–2014— continued

(Live births per 1,000 women in specified group.)

| Year and race | Total fertility rate | 10 to 14 years | 15 to 19 years | | | 20 to 24 years | 25 to 29 years | 30 to 34 years | 35 to 39 years | 40 to 44 years | 45 to 49 years[1] |
			Total	15 to 17 years	18 to 19 years						
1997	1,834.5	1.5	65.2	41.0	107.1	122.5	91.6	56.0	24.4	5.4	0.3
1998	1,851.0	1.5	64.7	39.7	106.9	125.1	92.0	56.8	24.6	5.3	*
1999	1,783.5	1.4	59.9	36.5	98.0	120.7	90.6	53.8	24.3	5.7	0.3
2000	1,772.5	1.1	58.3	34.1	97.1	117.2	91.8	55.5	24.6	5.7	0.3
2001	1,675.5	0.8	50.9	28.8	85.3	110.7	88.9	53.7	24.1	5.7	0.3
2002	1,639.5	0.9	49.0	27.9	82.1	107.0	89.3	52.8	23.3	5.2	0.4
2003	1,610.5	0.8	47.2	26.7	79.9	105.4	87.1	51.9	23.9	5.6	0.2
2004	1,584.0	0.8	46.0	26.3	78.0	102.9	86.3	51.8	23.3	5.4	0.3
2005	1,625.0	0.7	46.9	25.9	80.8	106.8	89.0	52.0	23.9	5.4	0.3
2006	1,621.5	0.7	49.3	26.1	86.3	105.8	86.2	52.5	24.3	5.2	0.3
2007	1,569.0	0.7	47.3	25.8	80.2	102.7	83.2	51.2	23.1	5.3	0.3
2008	1,569.0	0.7	47.3	25.8	80.2	102.7	83.2	51.2	23.1	5.3	0.3
2009	1,494.0	0.6	43.7	23.6	73.5	96.3	79.3	50.7	22.6	5.3	0.3
2010	1,404.0	0.5	38.7	20.1	66.1	91.0	74.4	48.4	22.3	5.2	0.3
2011	1,373.5	0.5	36.1	18.2	61.6	86.6	75.4	47.3	23.1	5.5	0.2
2012	1,350.0	0.5	34.9	17.0	60.5	81.7	73.9	49.7	23.3	5.5	0.5
2013	1,334.5	0.4	31.1	15.9	53.3	78.9	75.6	50.4	24.7	5.5	0.3
2014	1,288.5	0.3	27.3	13.2	48.6	73.2	74.7	52.3	24.1	5.5	0.3
Asian or Other Pacific Islander											
1980[3]	1,953.5	0.3	26.2	12.0	46.2	93.3	127.4	96.0	38.3	8.5	0.7
1981[3]	1,976.0	0.3	28.5	13.4	49.5	96.4	129.1	93.4	38.0	8.6	0.9
1982[3]	2,015.5	0.4	29.4	14.0	50.8	98.9	130.9	94.4	39.2	8.8	1.1
1983[3]	1,943.5	0.5	26.1	12.9	44.5	94.0	126.2	93.3	39.4	8.2	1.0
1984[3]	1,892.0	0.5	24.2	12.6	40.7	86.7	124.3	92.4	40.6	8.7	1.0
1985	1,885.0	0.4	23.8	12.5	40.8	83.6	123.0	93.6	42.7	8.7	1.2
1986	1,836.0	0.5	22.8	12.1	38.8	79.2	119.9	92.6	41.9	9.3	1.0
1987	1,886.0	0.6	22.4	12.6	37.0	79.7	122.7	97.0	44.2	9.5	1.1
1988	1,983.5	0.6	24.2	13.6	39.6	80.7	128.0	104.4	47.5	10.3	1.0
1989	1,947.5	0.6	25.6	15.0	40.4	78.8	124.0	102.3	47.0	10.2	1.0
1990	2,002.5	0.7	26.4	16.0	40.2	79.2	126.3	106.5	49.6	10.7	1.1
1991	1,928.0	0.8	27.3	16.3	42.2	73.8	118.9	103.3	49.2	11.2	1.1
1992	1,894.5	0.7	26.5	15.4	41.9	71.7	114.6	102.7	50.7	11.1	0.9
1993	1,841.5	0.7	26.5	16.1	41.2	68.1	110.3	101.2	49.4	11.2	0.9
1994	1,834.0	0.7	26.6	16.3	41.3	66.4	108.0	102.2	50.4	11.5	1.0
1995	1,795.5	0.7	25.5	15.6	40.1	64.2	103.7	102.3	50.1	11.8	0.8
1996	1,787.0	0.6	23.5	14.7	36.8	63.5	102.8	104.1	50.2	11.9	0.8
1997	1,757.5	0.5	22.3	14.0	34.9	61.2	101.6	102.5	51.0	11.5	0.9
1998	1,731.5	0.5	22.2	13.8	34.5	59.2	98.7	101.6	51.4	11.8	0.9
1999	1,754.5	0.4	21.4	12.4	33.9	58.9	100.8	104.3	52.9	11.3	0.9
2000	1,892.0	0.3	20.5	11.6	32.6	60.3	108.4	116.5	59.0	12.6	0.8
2001	1,785.0	0.2	19.3	10.1	32.0	56.0	102.3	109.9	56.2	12.2	0.9
2002	1,798.5	0.3	17.7	8.8	29.9	55.5	102.4	112.5	57.8	12.6	0.9
2003	1,819.0	0.2	16.4	8.5	27.3	54.3	102.7	115.9	60.0	13.4	0.9
2004	1,825.0	0.2	16.0	8.4	26.6	53.3	100.4	118.3	62.2	13.6	1.0
2005	1,784.5	0.2	15.4	7.7	26.4	52.9	96.6	115.3	61.8	13.7	1.0
2006	1,803.0	0.1	15.3	8.2	25.4	53.8	95.7	117.3	63.4	14.0	1.0
2007	1,850.5	0.2	14.8	7.4	24.9	53.2	99.2	121.6	65.8	14.2	1.1
2008	1,797.5	0.2	13.8	7.0	23.0	50.4	96.6	117.7	64.9	14.7	1.2
2009	1,743.0	0.1	12.6	6.3	20.9	46.4	94.6	115.1	63.8	14.9	1.1
2010	1,689.0	0.1	10.9	5.1	18.7	42.6	91.5	113.6	62.8	15.1	1.2
2011	1,706.5	0.1	10.2	4.6	18.1	41.9	93.7	114.9	64.1	15.2	1.2
2012	1,769.5	0.1	9.7	4.1	17.7	41.4	95.8	121.3	68.1	16.1	1.4
2013	1,681.0	0.1	8.7	3.7	16.1	39.1	89.5	114.6	66.6	16.1	1.5
2014	1,715.5	0.1	7.7	3.3	13.9	37.5	90.0	121.3	68.9	16.1	1.5

* = Figure does not meet standards of reliability or precision.　　1 Beginning in 1997, rates computed by relating births to women age 45 years and over to women age 45 to 49 years.　　2 For 1970 to 1991 includes births to races not shown separately. For 1992 and later years, unknown race of mother is imputed.　　3 Based on 100-percent of births in selected states and on a 50-percent sample of births in all other states.

Table 1-26. Fertility Rates and Birth Rates, by Age, Live-Birth Order, Specified Hispanic Origin, and Race of Mother, 2014

(Live births per 1,000 women in specified age and race groups.)

Live-birth order and race of mother	15 to 44 years[1]	10 to 14 years	15 to 19 years			20 to 24 years	25 to 29 years	30 to 34 years	35 to 39 years	40 to 44 years	45 to 49 years[2]
			Total	15 to 17 years	18 to 19 years						
HISPANIC[3]											
Total	72.1	0.4	38.0	19.3	66.1	104.5	118.7	96.5	53.6	13.5	0.9
1st child	24.5	0.4	30.7	17.5	50.5	48.7	32.2	19.5	8.2	1.9	0.2
2nd child	21.6	*	6.3	1.7	13.3	36.3	40.5	27.9	13.2	2.8	0.2
3rd child	14.4	*	0.9	0.1	2.0	14.3	28.3	25.5	14.1	3.1	0.2
4th child	7.0	*	0.1	*	0.2	4.0	11.9	14.2	9.6	2.5	0.2
5th child	2.8	*	0.0	*	0.0	0.9	3.9	5.7	4.8	1.5	0.1
6th and 7th child	1.5	*	*	*	*	0.2	1.6	3.1	3.0	1.2	0.1
8th child and over	0.3	*	*	*	*	0.0	0.2	0.6	0.7	0.4	0.0
NON-HISPANIC[4]											
Total[5]	60.7	0.2	20.3	8.5	37.6	72.4	102.7	101.9	50.3	10.0	0.8
1st child	24.6	0.2	17.1	7.9	30.5	37.9	41.6	33.3	12.4	2.4	0.2
2nd child	19.7	*	2.8	0.5	6.1	23.2	33.7	36.1	17.4	3.0	0.2
3rd child	9.6	*	0.4	0.0	0.8	8.3	17.0	18.6	10.6	2.0	0.1
4th child	3.9	*	0.0	0.0	0.1	2.3	6.7	7.9	5.0	1.1	0.1
5th child	1.5	*	0.0	*	0.0	0.6	2.4	3.2	2.2	0.6	0.0
6th and 7th child	0.9	*	*	*	*	0.2	1.1	2.1	1.8	0.5	0.0
8th child and over	0.3	*	*	*	*	0.0	0.2	0.6	0.9	0.4	0.0
White	59.5	0.1	17.3	6.7	32.9	67.1	103.9	104.7	49.6	9.1	0.7
1st child	24.5	0.1	14.8	6.3	27.4	36.3	43.7	34.7	12.5	2.3	0.2
2nd child	19.7	*	2.2	0.4	4.9	21.8	35.0	37.6	17.1	2.7	0.2
3rd child	9.4	*	0.2	0.0	0.6	7.0	16.7	19.4	10.6	1.8	0.1
4th child	3.6	*	0.0	*	0.0	1.6	5.9	7.8	4.8	1.0	0.1
5th child	1.3	*	0.0	*	*	0.3	1.8	2.9	2.1	0.5	0.0
6th and 7th child	0.8	*	*	*	*	0.1	0.7	1.8	1.6	0.4	0.0
8th child and over	0.3	*	*	*	*	0.0	0.1	0.4	0.8	0.4	0.0
Black	64.5	0.6	34.9	16.6	61.5	102.8	103.3	79.6	42.5	10.1	0.9
1st child	23.9	0.6	28.4	15.2	47.6	48.7	29.6	18.0	8.0	1.9	0.2
2nd child	18.6	*	5.5	1.3	11.6	32.7	32.3	23.3	11.4	2.4	0.2
3rd child	11.5	*	0.9	0.1	2.0	14.5	22.3	18.0	9.7	2.2	0.2
4th child	5.6	*	0.1	*	0.2	4.9	11.2	10.0	6.0	1.5	0.1
5th child	2.5	*	0.0	*	0.0	1.5	4.8	5.1	3.1	0.9	0.1
6th and 7th child	1.7	*	*	*	*	0.4	2.7	3.9	2.8	0.8	0.1
8th child and over	0.6	*	*	*	*	0.1	0.5	1.3	1.4	0.5	0.0

* = Figure does not meet standards of reliability or precision.   0.0 = Quantity more than zero but less than 0.05.   1 Fertility rates computed by relating total births, regardless of age of mother, to women age 15 to 44 years.   2 Birth rates computed by relating births to women age 45 years and over to women age 45 to 49 years.   3 Includes Central and South American and other and unknown Hispanic. Includes all persons of Hispanic origin of any race.   4 Includes origin not stated.   5 Includes races other than White and Black.

Table 1-27. Fertility Rates and Birth Rates, by Live-Birth Order and by Race and Hispanic Origin of Mother, 1989–2014

(Births per 1,000 women age 15 to 44 years.)

Year, origin, and race of mother	Total fertility rate	Fertility rate[1]	10–14 years	15–19 years			20–24 years	25–29 years	30–34 years	35–39 years	40–44 years	45–49 years[2]
				Total	15–17 years	18–19 years						
ALL ORIGINS												
1989	2,014.0	69.2	1.4	57.3	36.4	84.2	113.8	117.6	77.4	29.9	5.2	0.2
1990	2,081.0	70.9	1.4	59.9	37.5	88.6	116.5	120.2	80.8	31.7	5.5	0.2
1991	2,062.5	69.3	1.4	61.8	38.6	94.0	115.3	117.2	79.2	31.9	5.5	0.2
1992	2,046.0	68.4	1.4	60.3	37.6	93.6	113.7	115.7	79.6	32.3	5.9	0.3
1993	2,019.5	67.0	1.4	59.0	37.5	91.1	111.3	113.2	79.9	32.7	6.1	0.3
1994	2,001.5	65.9	1.4	58.2	37.2	90.2	109.2	111.0	80.4	33.4	6.4	0.3
1995	1,978.0	64.6	1.3	56.0	35.5	87.7	107.5	108.8	81.1	34.0	6.6	0.3
1996	1,976.0	64.1	1.2	53.5	33.3	84.7	107.8	108.6	82.1	34.9	6.8	0.3
1997	1,971.0	63.6	1.1	51.3	31.4	82.1	107.3	108.3	83.0	35.7	7.1	0.4
1998	1,999.0	64.3	1.0	50.3	29.9	80.9	108.4	110.2	85.2	36.9	7.4	0.4
1999	2,007.5	64.4	0.9	48.8	28.2	79.1	107.9	111.2	87.1	37.8	7.4	0.4
2000	2,056.0	65.9	0.9	47.7	26.9	78.1	109.7	113.5	91.2	39.7	8.0	0.5
2001	2,030.5	65.1	0.8	45.0	24.5	75.5	105.6	113.8	91.8	40.5	8.1	0.5
2002	2,020.5	65.0	0.7	42.6	23.1	72.2	103.1	114.7	92.6	41.6	8.3	0.5
2003	2,047.5	66.1	0.6	41.1	22.2	69.6	102.3	116.7	95.7	43.9	8.7	0.5
2004	2,051.5	66.4	0.6	40.5	21.8	68.7	101.5	116.5	96.2	45.5	9.0	0.5
2005	2,057.0	66.7	0.6	39.7	21.1	68.4	101.8	116.5	96.7	46.4	9.1	0.6
2006	2,108.0	68.6	0.6	41.1	21.6	71.2	105.5	118.0	98.9	47.5	9.4	0.6
2007	2,120.0	69.3	0.6	41.5	21.7	71.7	105.4	118.1	100.6	47.6	9.6	0.6
2008	2,072.0	68.1	0.6	40.2	21.1	68.2	101.8	115.0	99.4	46.8	9.9	0.7
2009	2,002.0	66.2	0.5	37.9	19.6	64.0	96.2	111.5	97.5	46.1	10.0	0.7
2010	1,931.0	64.1	0.4	34.2	17.3	58.2	90.0	108.3	96.5	45.9	10.2	0.7
2011	1,894.5	63.2	0.4	31.3	15.4	54.1	85.3	107.2	96.5	47.2	10.3	0.7
2012	1,880.5	63.0	0.4	29.4	14.1	51.4	83.1	106.5	97.3	48.3	10.4	0.8
2013	1,857.5	62.5	0.3	26.5	12.3	47.1	80.7	105.5	98.0	49.3	10.4	0.8
2014	1,862.5	62.9	0.3	24.2	10.9	43.8	79.0	106.5	100.8	51.0	10.0	0.7
HISPANIC[3]												
Total												
1989 [4]	2,903.5	104.9	2.3	100.8	NA	NA	184.4	146.6	92.1	43.5	10.4	0.6
1990 [5]	2,959.5	107.7	2.4	100.3	65.9	147.7	181.0	153.0	98.3	45.3	10.9	0.7
1991 [6]	2,963.5	106.9	2.4	104.6	69.2	155.5	184.6	150.0	95.1	44.7	10.7	0.6
1992 [6]	2,957.5	106.1	2.5	103.3	68.9	153.9	185.2	148.8	94.8	45.3	11.0	0.6
1993	2,894.5	103.3	2.6	101.8	68.5	151.1	180.0	146.0	93.2	44.1	10.6	0.6
1994	2,839.0	100.7	2.6	101.3	69.9	147.5	175.7	142.4	91.1	43.4	10.7	0.6
1995	2,798.5	98.8	2.6	99.3	68.3	145.4	171.9	140.4	90.5	43.7	10.7	0.6
1996	2,772.0	97.5	2.4	94.6	64.2	140.0	170.2	140.7	91.3	43.9	10.7	0.6
1997	2,680.5	94.2	2.1	89.6	61.1	132.4	162.6	137.5	89.6	43.4	10.7	0.6
1998	2,652.5	93.2	1.9	87.9	58.5	131.5	159.3	136.1	90.5	43.4	10.8	0.6
1999	2,649.0	93.0	1.9	86.8	56.9	129.5	157.3	135.8	92.3	44.5	10.6	0.6
2000	2,730.0	95.9	1.7	87.3	55.5	132.6	161.3	139.9	97.1	46.6	11.5	0.6
2001	2,030.5	65.1	0.8	45.0	24.5	75.5	105.6	113.8	91.8	40.5	8.1	0.5
2002	2,020.5	65.0	0.7	42.6	23.1	72.2	103.1	114.7	92.6	41.6	8.3	0.5
2003	2,047.5	66.1	0.6	41.1	22.2	69.6	102.3	116.7	95.7	43.9	8.7	0.5
2004	2,051.5	66.4	0.6	40.5	21.8	68.7	101.5	116.5	96.2	45.5	9.0	0.5
2005	2,057.0	66.7	0.6	39.7	21.1	68.4	101.8	116.5	96.7	46.4	9.1	0.6
2006	2,108.0	68.6	0.6	41.1	21.6	71.2	105.5	118.0	98.9	47.5	9.4	0.6
2007	2,120.0	69.3	0.6	41.5	21.7	71.7	105.4	118.1	100.6	47.6	9.6	0.6
2008	2,072.0	68.1	0.6	40.2	21.1	68.2	101.8	115.0	99.4	46.8	9.9	0.7
2009	2,002.0	66.2	0.5	37.9	19.6	64.0	96.2	111.5	97.5	46.1	10.0	0.7
2010	1,931.0	64.1	0.4	34.2	17.3	58.2	90.0	108.3	96.5	45.9	10.2	0.7
2011	1,894.5	63.2	0.4	31.3	15.4	54.1	85.3	107.2	96.5	47.2	10.3	0.7
2012	2,189.5	74.4	0.6	46.3	22.5	77.2	111.5	119.6	94.3	51.6	13.2	0.8
2013	2,149.5	72.9	0.5	41.7	22.0	70.8	107.2	119.1	94.8	52.4	13.3	0.8
2014	2,130.5	72.1	0.4	38.0	19.3	66.1	104.5	118.7	96.5	53.6	13.5	0.9
Mexican												
1989 [4]	2,916.5	106.6	2.0	94.5	NA	NA	184.3	153.7	96.1	41.0	11.1	0.6
1990 [5]	3,214.0	118.9	2.5	108.0	69.7	162.2	200.3	165.3	104.4	49.1	12.4	0.8
1991 [6]	3,103.5	114.9	2.5	108.3	70.0	164.7	192.4	156.1	99.7	49.1	11.9	0.7
1992 [6]	3,107.0	113.3	2.4	105.1	NA	NA	196.6	160.2	97.1	47.4	11.8	0.8
1993	3,041.5	110.9	2.5	103.6	68.4	156.6	187.9	159.5	97.2	45.5	11.3	0.8
1994	3,024.0	109.9	2.7	109.2	73.6	163.3	189.1	153.6	92.5	45.3	11.7	0.7
1995	3,033.5	109.9	2.7	115.9	79.1	170.7	190.4	146.6	93.0	45.5	11.9	0.7
1996	3,052.0	110.7	2.6	112.2	77.7	161.6	185.3	154.7	96.5	46.4	12.0	0.7
1997	2,957.0	106.6	2.3	103.4	71.3	151.6	180.9	150.0	95.3	47.4	11.5	0.6
1998	2,878.0	103.2	2.1	96.4	62.9	149.2	176.5	147.4	94.9	46.9	10.8	0.6
1999	2,823.0	101.5	2.1	94.3	60.8	145.6	170.8	141.4	97.4	47.2	10.7	0.7
2000	2,906.5	105.1	1.9	95.4	60.6	146.7	174.9	144.7	102.3	49.2	12.2	0.7
2001	2,905.0	105.0	1.7	93.2	58.2	142.5	173.8	146.8	102.1	50.1	12.6	0.7
2002	2,869.0	103.0	1.5	91.4	57.0	141.0	171.2	146.8	101.1	48.5	12.5	0.8

Table 1-27. Fertility Rates and Birth Rates, by Live-Birth Order and by Race and Hispanic Origin of Mother, 1989–2014— continued

(Births per 1,000 women age 15 to 44 years.)

Year, origin, and race of mother	Total fertility rate	Fertility rate[1]	10–14 years	15–19 years Total	15–17 years	18–19 years	20–24 years	25–29 years	30–34 years	35–39 years	40–44 years	45–49 years[2]
2003	2,903.0	103.7	1.4	88.8	54.4	140.7	172.2	151.0	104.2	49.6	12.7	0.7
2004	2,948.5	104.5	1.4	90.3	55.6	142.5	173.4	152.5	105.5	53.5	12.4	0.7
2005	2,954.5	104.5	1.4	87.5	52.3	144.5	173.5	152.1	107.1	55.3	13.2	0.8
2006	2,997.0	105.6	1.3	86.6	50.7	145.4	180.3	152.3	109.0	55.5	13.6	0.8
2007	2,944.5	102.8	1.2	81.7	49.9	130.6	176.0	150.2	110.1	55.4	13.5	0.8
2008	2,663.5	92.6	1.1	71.4	44.4	111.7	154.3	138.4	101.9	51.4	13.4	0.8
2009	2,442.0	84.8	1.0	62.9	37.8	100.5	135.2	129.0	96.0	50.6	13.0	0.7
2010	2,276.5	78.2	0.8	55.3	32.6	89.9	123.3	122.9	91.5	48.1	12.7	0.7
2011	2,143.0	73.0	0.6	47.9	27.7	77.6	111.6	118.2	89.3	47.9	12.4	0.7
2012	2,082.5	70.7	0.6	44.5	24.8	74.2	106.0	113.5	88.3	48.1	12.5	0.8
2013	2,018.5	68.4	0.5	39.5	21.2	66.5	101.6	115.7	87.4	47.7	12.7	0.8
2014	NA	NA	NA	NA	NA	NA	NA	NA	NA	NA	NA	NA
Puerto Rican												
1989[4]	2,421.0	86.6	3.8	112.7	NA	NA	171.0	98.0	65.2	26.9	6.3	*
1990[5]	2,301.0	82.9	2.9	101.6	71.6	141.6	150.1	109.9	62.8	26.2	6.2	0.5
1991[6]	2,573.5	87.9	2.7	111.0	*	*	193.3	108.9	68.1	23.9	6.5	*
1992[6]	2,568.5	87.9	3.4	106.5	NA	NA	199.1	102.6	65.3	29.9	6.6	*
1993	2,416.0	79.8	3.1	104.9	70.1	*	184.6	102.8	54.4	26.7	6.2	*
1994	2,341.5	78.2	3.1	99.6	68.8	*	169.0	103.8	59.5	27.5	5.6	0.2
1995	2,078.0	71.3	2.9	82.8	57.3	*	138.1	97.9	61.2	26.9	5.5	0.3
1996	1,965.0	66.5	1.9	76.5	48.6	*	133.7	95.6	54.3	25.2	5.6	*
1997	1,931.5	65.8	1.7	68.9	45.0	*	136.0	92.9	54.1	26.1	6.2	0.4
1998	2,043.5	69.7	1.8	76.2	51.7	*	146.7	88.7	61.9	25.8	7.2	0.4
1999	2,104.5	71.1	1.6	74.0	49.4	*	146.0	106.5	58.0	27.3	7.2	0.3
2000	2,178.5	73.5	1.7	82.9	54.7	120.4	149.5	101.6	61.1	32.0	6.6	0.3
2001	2,144.5	71.7	1.7	80.3	*	*	144.5	93.9	70.6	30.8	6.7	0.4
2002	1,937.0	65.6	1.3	59.3	38.6	*	132.2	92.1	63.6	32.0	6.4	0.5
2003	1,805.0	60.6	1.0	57.9	34.4	*	124.5	86.3	55.4	29.2	6.3	0.4
2004	2,005.0	66.8	0.9	59.1	37.0	*	133.9	101.5	66.0	32.4	6.7	0.5
2005	2,065.5	69.8	0.9	59.2	35.1	*	124.1	108.8	76.6	35.3	7.8	0.4
2006	2,088.5	71.6	1.0	64.7	35.8	*	130.7	100.7	72.3	39.2	8.5	0.6
2007	2,101.0	70.3	0.8	61.8	32.8	*	139.2	105.9	65.0	39.8	7.3	0.4
2008	2,004.0	67.0	0.7	56.0	28.8	*	119.3	114.3	65.9	37.3	6.9	0.4
2009	1,922.5	63.7	0.7	50.8	28.2	82.4	118.9	106.6	66.9	32.6	7.4	0.6
2010	1,747.5	59.7	0.6	45.4	25.0	73.4	105.7	90.7	66.0	32.6	7.9	0.6
2011	1,747.5	59.6	0.5	42.8	22.9	69.5	106.0	93.8	64.9	33.2	7.8	0.5
2012	1,688.5	58.2	0.4	40.6	22.0	64.8	96.4	91.3	66.0	34.0	8.4	0.7
2013	1,684.0	57.8	0.5	36.3	18.2	61.8	94.8	91.5	70.6	34.5	8.0	0.5
2014	NA	NA	NA	NA	NA	NA	NA	NA	NA	NA	NA	NA
Cuban												
1989[4]	1,479.0	49.8	*	*	NA	NA	*	*	*	*	*	*
1990[5]	1,459.5	52.6	*	30.3	18.2	46.1	64.6	95.4	67.6	28.2	4.9	*
1991[6]	1,352.5	47.6	*	*	*	*	*	*	*	*	*	*
1992[6]	1,453.5	49.4	*	*	NA	NA	*	*	*	*	*	*
1993	1,570.0	53.9	*	*	*	*	*	*	*	*	*	*
1994	1,587.0	53.6	*	*	*	*	*	*	*	*	*	*
1995	1,584.0	52.2	*	*	*	*	*	*	*	*	*	*
1996	1,617.0	55.1	*	*	*	*	*	*	*	*	*	*
1997	1,619.5	53.1	*	*	*	*	*	*	*	*	*	*
1998	1,402.5	46.5	*	*	*	*	*	*	*	*	*	*
1999	1,388.5	47.0	*	*	*	*	*	*	*	*	*	*
2000	1,528.0	49.3	*	23.5	14.2	43.4	64.2	104.0	68.1	37.3	7.9	*
2001	1,786.0	56.4	*	*	*	*	*	*	*	*	*	*
2002	1,958.5	59.3	*	*	*	*	*	*	*	*	*	*
2003	2,032.5	60.8	*	*	*	*	*	*	*	*	*	*
2004	1,699.5	52.2	*	*	*	*	*	*	*	*	*	*
2005	1,540.5	49.1	*	*	*	*	*	*	*	*	*	*
2006	1,556.5	47.9	*	*	*	*	*	*	*	*	6.8	*
2007	1,542.5	47.6	*	*	*	*	*	*	*	*	6.4	*
2008	1,536.5	50.1	*	*	*	*	*	*	*	*	*	*
2009	1,352.0	46.0	*	*	*	*	*	*	*	*	*	*
2010	1,452.5	46.4	*	17.8	8.0	29.7	61.6	80.6	82.8	39.1	8.0	0.5
2011	1,433.5	46.1	*	15.8	6.7	29.0	54.7	86.1	78.4	42.0	9.1	0.5
2012	1,370.5	45.4	*	15.0	6.6	24.9	57.3	78.7	72.9	40.7	8.8	0.6
2013	1,449.0	48.0	*	14.9	6.0	26.2	58.4	85.2	78.2	44.0	8.5	0.5
2014	NA	NA	NA	NA	NA	NA	NA	NA	NA	NA	NA	NA
Other Hispanic[7]												
1989[4]	2,683.0	95.8	1.7	66.4	NA	NA	159.2	150.4	85.1	60.3	12.7	0.8
1990[5]	2,877.0	102.7	2.1	86.0	57.2	123.8	162.9	155.8	106.9	49.4	11.6	0.7
1991[6]	3,064.5	105.5	2.2	100.7	67.3	145.6	184.1	164.5	100.2	49.2	11.4	0.6
1992[6]	2,989.0	104.7	2.4	108.2	NA	NA	168.0	151.9	104.4	49.9	12.5	0.5
1993	2,914.5	101.5	2.6	102.0	74.7	134.6	167.5	139.4	106.7	51.7	12.5	0.5

Table 1-27. Fertility Rates and Birth Rates, by Live-Birth Order and by Race and Hispanic Origin of Mother, 1989–2014— continued

(Births per 1,000 women age 15 to 44 years.)

Year, origin, and race of mother	Total fertility rate	Fertility rate[1]	10–14 years	15–19 years Total	15–17 years	18–19 years	20–24 years	25–29 years	30–34 years	35–39 years	40–44 years	45–49 years[2]
1994	2,693.0	93.2	2.5	82.6	62.7	105.0	151.2	137.0	104.4	48.4	11.9	0.6
1995	2,629.5	89.1	2.3	72.1	51.3	99.4	144.3	147.7	97.9	49.4	11.6	0.6
1996	2,516.5	84.2	2.2	64.8	43.4	95.6	149.6	127.9	98.0	49.1	11.0	0.7
1997	2,376.5	80.6	1.8	66.4	44.5	98.0	129.3	125.8	95.6	43.9	11.8	0.7
1998	2,448.5	83.5	1.8	75.0	53.3	100.3	122.7	133.6	97.8	45.4	12.8	0.6
1999	2,517.0	84.8	1.5	75.5	53.1	100.5	130.2	138.4	98.3	46.5	12.3	0.7
2000	2,563.5	85.1	1.2	69.9	44.4	102.0	133.2	143.9	103.6	47.7	12.5	0.7
2001	2,503.5	82.2	1.1	63.8	35.0	111.6	133.6	143.7	95.6	50.4	11.6	0.9
2002	2,612.0	86.5	1.1	60.9	33.7	105.4	138.8	149.5	101.7	57.3	12.3	0.8
2003	2,690.0	89.7	1.0	57.5	34.9	88.0	138.4	152.3	111.8	62.4	13.8	0.8
2004	2,594.0	87.4	1.1	54.6	31.1	90.2	131.1	143.5	113.5	59.2	15.0	0.8
2005	2,737.0	90.5	1.1	58.2	35.0	90.2	148.1	152.3	115.0	57.6	14.3	0.8
2006	2,918.0	95.6	1.1	62.5	36.3	99.7	154.3	172.7	118.0	59.3	14.7	1.0
2007	2,995.0	100.1	1.2	68.1	38.8	113.4	154.5	173.4	124.1	60.7	15.9	1.1
2008	3,278.0	109.1	1.4	80.5	47.9	129.3	180.5	171.1	135.9	69.1	16.0	1.1
2009	3,248.5	107.5	1.3	78.4	44.2	131.3	181.3	169.4	133.5	68.3	16.3	1.2
2010	2,870.0	97.1	1.0	67.4	39.6	105.2	146.6	154.2	120.5	67.0	16.2	1.1
2011	2,847.5	96.3	1.1	62.1	35.1	99.9	142.3	150.3	127.3	68.6	16.7	1.1
2012	2,812.5	94.9	0.9	58.9	33.2	93.4	140.7	153.6	122.3	68.0	17.7	1.1
2013	2,799.5	94.4	0.7	52.2	28.6	84.7	136.3	154.2	125.5	72.2	17.0	1.1
2014	NA	NA	NA	NA	NA	NA	NA	NA	NA	NA	NA	NA
NON-HISPANIC [8]												
Total [9]												
1989 [4]	1,921.0	65.7	1.3	53.4	---	---	107.8	113.4	74.7	28.6	4.8	0.2
1990 [5]	1,979.5	67.1	1.3	54.8	33.8	81.4	108.1	116.5	79.2	30.7	5.1	0.2
1991 [6]	1,953.0	65.2	1.3	56.1	34.4	86.1	106.5	113.1	77.5	30.8	5.1	0.2
1992 [6]	1,929.0	64.2	1.2	54.3	33.2	85.3	104.3	111.4	77.9	31.1	5.4	0.2
1993	1,901.5	62.7	1.2	52.7	32.9	82.3	101.7	108.7	78.4	31.6	5.7	0.3
1994	1,883.5	61.6	1.2	51.7	32.3	81.4	99.5	106.5	79.1	32.4	6.0	0.3
1995	1,856.5	60.2	1.1	49.3	30.5	78.6	97.4	104.1	79.9	33.0	6.2	0.3
1996	1,852.0	59.6	1.0	47.0	28.4	75.8	97.3	103.6	80.8	33.9	6.5	0.3
1997	1,853.0	59.3	0.9	45.0	26.7	73.7	97.4	103.5	82.0	34.8	6.7	0.3
1998	1,887.5	60.0	0.8	44.0	25.2	72.4	98.9	105.8	84.4	36.2	7.0	0.4
1999	1,894.0	60.0	0.8	42.2	23.3	70.2	98.4	106.7	86.2	37.0	7.1	0.4
2000	1,931.5	61.1	0.7	40.7	21.9	68.2	99.5	108.4	90.2	38.8	7.6	0.4
2001	1,898.0	60.0	0.6	37.8	19.6	65.0	94.6	108.1	90.8	39.5	7.7	0.5
2002	1,885.0	59.8	0.6	35.4	18.2	61.6	91.8	108.7	91.6	40.5	7.9	0.5
2003	1,909.0	60.7	0.5	33.9	17.2	58.9	90.6	110.6	94.6	42.8	8.3	0.5
2004	1,906.0	60.8	0.5	33.1	16.7	57.6	89.5	110.1	94.7	44.3	8.5	0.5
2005	1,902.0	60.8	0.5	32.1	15.9	56.9	89.2	109.5	94.7	45.2	8.6	0.6
2006	1,946.0	62.5	0.5	33.2	16.5	59.0	92.3	110.7	96.9	46.2	8.8	0.6
2007	1,959.5	63.3	0.5	33.8	16.4	60.1	92.3	110.9	98.7	46.1	9.0	0.6
2008	1,926.0	62.7	0.4	33.1	16.0	57.8	90.0	108.6	97.9	45.3	9.3	0.6
2009	1,877.5	61.6	0.4	31.6	15.1	54.7	86.0	106.0	96.7	44.7	9.4	0.7
2010	1,831.0	60.4	0.3	28.8	13.4	50.3	81.5	104.2	96.5	44.5	9.7	0.7
2011	1,810.5	60.1	0.3	26.5	12.0	47.0	78.0	103.8	96.8	46.2	9.8	0.7
2012	1,803.0	60.3	0.3	24.8	10.9	44.5	76.2	103.3	98.0	47.5	9.8	0.8
2013	1,784.0	59.9	0.2	22.3	9.5	40.6	74.1	102.3	98.8	48.5	9.8	0.8
2014	1,793.0	60.7	0.2	20.3	8.5	37.6	72.4	102.7	101.9	50.3	10.0	0.7
White												
1989 [3]	1,770.0	60.5	0.4	39.9	NA	NA	94.7	111.7	75.0	27.8	4.3	0.2
1990 [4]	1,850.5	62.8	0.5	42.5	23.2	66.6	97.5	115.3	79.4	30.0	4.7	0.2
1991 [5]	1,822.5	60.9	0.5	43.4	23.6	70.6	95.7	112.1	77.7	30.2	4.7	0.2
1992 [5]	1,803.5	60.0	0.5	41.7	22.7	69.8	93.9	110.6	78.3	30.4	5.1	0.2
1993	1,786.0	58.9	0.5	40.7	22.7	67.7	92.2	108.2	79.0	31.0	5.4	0.2
1994	1,782.5	58.2	0.5	40.4	22.7	67.6	90.9	106.6	80.2	32.0	5.7	0.2
1995	1,777.5	57.5	0.4	39.3	22.0	66.2	90.2	105.1	81.5	32.8	5.9	0.3
1996	1,781.0	57.1	0.4	37.6	20.6	64.0	90.1	104.9	82.8	33.9	6.2	0.3
1997	1,785.5	56.8	0.4	36.0	19.3	62.1	90.0	104.8	84.3	34.8	6.5	0.3
1998	1,825.0	57.6	0.3	35.3	18.3	60.9	91.2	107.4	87.2	36.4	6.8	0.4
1999	1,838.5	57.7	0.3	34.1	17.1	59.4	90.6	108.6	89.5	37.3	6.9	0.4
2000	1,866.0	58.5	0.3	32.6	15.8	57.5	91.2	109.4	93.2	38.8	7.3	0.4
2001	1,846.0	57.7	0.3	30.3	14.0	54.7	87.0	109.6	94.3	39.8	7.5	0.4
2002	1,840.0	57.6	0.2	28.6	13.1	52.0	84.7	110.4	95.0	40.9	7.7	0.5
2003	1,874.5	58.9	0.2	27.4	12.4	50.0	84.1	112.7	98.4	43.5	8.1	0.5
2004	1,871.0	58.9	0.2	26.7	12.0	48.6	83.0	112.1	98.3	45.1	8.3	0.5
2005	1,869.0	59.0	0.2	26.0	11.5	48.0	82.7	111.7	98.4	46.0	8.3	0.5
2006	1,900.5	60.3	0.2	26.7	11.8	49.4	85.1	112.2	100.0	46.8	8.5	0.6
2007	1,908.0	61.0	0.2	27.2	11.9	50.4	85.1	112.0	101.5	46.3	8.7	0.6
2008	1,874.5	60.5	0.2	26.7	11.6	48.6	82.8	109.7	100.8	45.2	8.9	0.6
2009	1,830.0	59.6	0.2	25.7	11.0	46.2	79.2	107.1	99.7	44.4	9.1	0.6

Table 1-27. Fertility Rates and Birth Rates, by Live-Birth Order and by Race and Hispanic Origin of Mother, 1989–2014— continued

(Births per 1,000 women age 15 to 44 years.)

Year, origin, and race of mother	Total fertility rate [1]	Fertility rate [2]	10–14 years	15–19 years			20–24 years	25–29 years	30–34 years	35–39 years	40–44 years	45–49 years [2]
				Total	15–17 years	18–19 years						
2010	1,791.0	58.7	0.2	23.5	10.0	42.5	74.9	105.8	99.9	44.1	9.2	0.6
2011	1,773.5	58.7	0.2	21.7	9.0	39.9	71.8	105.2	100.1	45.8	9.3	0.6
2012	1,761.5	58.6	0.2	20.5	8.4	37.9	70.2	104.4	104.7	46.8	9.1	0.6
2013	1,751.0	58.7	0.1	18.6	7.4	35.0	68.3	103.5	101.9	48.0	9.1	0.7
2014	1,762.5	59.5	0.1	17.3	6.7	32.9	67.1	103.9	100.5	49.6	9.1	0.7
Black												
1989 [4]	2,424.0	84.8	5.2	111.9	NA	NA	156.3	113.8	65.7	26.3	5.3	0.3
1990 [5]	2,547.5	89.0	5.0	116.2	84.9	157.5	165.1	118.4	70.2	28.7	5.6	0.3
1991 [6]	2,532.0	87.0	4.9	118.2	86.1	162.2	164.8	115.1	68.9	28.7	5.6	0.2
1992 [6]	2,482.5	84.5	4.8	114.7	82.9	161.1	160.8	112.8	68.4	29.1	5.7	0.2
1993	2,412.5	81.5	4.6	110.5	81.1	154.6	154.5	109.2	68.1	29.4	5.9	0.3
1994	2,314.5	77.5	4.6	105.7	77.0	150.4	146.8	104.1	66.3	29.1	6.0	0.3
1995	2,186.5	72.8	4.2	97.2	70.4	139.2	137.8	98.5	64.4	28.8	6.1	0.3
1996	2,140.0	70.7	3.6	91.9	64.8	134.1	137.0	96.7	63.2	29.1	6.2	0.3
1997	2,137.5	70.3	3.2	88.3	60.7	131.0	138.8	97.2	63.6	29.6	6.5	0.3
1998	2,164.0	70.9	2.9	85.7	56.8	128.2	142.5	99.9	64.4	30.4	6.7	0.3
1999	2,134.0	69.9	2.6	81.0	51.7	123.9	142.1	99.8	63.9	30.6	6.5	0.3
2000	2,178.5	71.4	2.4	79.2	50.1	121.9	145.4	102.8	66.5	31.8	7.2	0.4
2001	2,107.0	69.1	2.1	73.1	44.8	115.9	137.3	102.8	66.4	32.0	7.3	0.4
2002	2,053.0	67.5	1.9	67.7	40.6	109.5	131.4	103.1	66.5	32.1	7.5	0.4
2003	2,037.5	67.1	1.6	63.8	38.2	103.4	128.8	104.0	67.7	33.4	7.7	0.5
2004	2,030.5	67.1	1.6	61.9	36.4	101.6	127.9	105.0	67.8	33.6	7.8	0.5
2005	2,030.5	67.2	1.6	59.4	34.1	100.2	127.9	105.5	68.8	34.2	8.2	0.5
2006	2,128.5	70.7	1.5	61.9	35.2	105.1	134.4	110.0	73.2	35.9	8.3	0.5
2007	2,142.0	71.4	1.4	62.0	34.6	105.2	134.5	110.5	74.7	36.2	8.5	0.6
2008	2,115.5	70.8	1.4	60.4	33.6	100.0	131.6	108.8	75.3	36.3	8.7	0.6
2009	2,046.5	68.9	1.1	56.8	31.0	93.5	125.9	106.0	73.9	36.1	8.9	0.6
2010	1,971.5	66.6	1.0	51.5	27.4	85.6	119.4	102.5	73.6	36.4	9.2	0.7
2011	1,919.5	65.4	0.9	47.3	24.6	78.8	112.3	101.7	73.9	37.8	9.3	0.7
2012	1,898.5	65.0	0.8	43.9	21.9	74.1	109.0	101.7	75.1	38.9	9.6	0.7
2013	1,881.5	64.6	0.7	39.0	18.9	67.0	105.6	102.7	77.3	40.3	9.9	0.8
2014	1,873.5	64.5	0.6	34.9	16.6	61.5	102.8	103.3	79.6	42.5	10.1	0.9

1 Fertility rates computed by relating total births.   2 Beginning in 1997, rates computed by relating births to women age 45 to 54 years to women 45 to 49 years.   3 Includes all persons of Hispanic origin of any race.   4 Excludes data for Louisiana, New Hampshire, and Oklahoma, which did not report Hispanic origin.   5 Excludes data for New Hampshire and Oklahoma, which did not report Hispanic origin.   6 Excludes data for New Hampshire, which did not report Hispanic origin.   7 Includes Central and South American and other unknown Hispanic origin.   8 Includes origin not stated.   9 Includes races other than black and white.

Table 1-28. Fertility Rates and Birth Rates, by Live-Birth Order and by Race and Hispanic Origin of Mother, 1980–2014

(Births per 1,000 women age 15 to 44 years.)

Year, race, and Hispanic origin of mother	Fertility rate	Live-birth order						
		1	2	3	4	5	6 and 7	8 and over
All Races [1,2]								
1980 [3]	68.4	29.5	21.8	10.3	3.9	1.5	1.0	0.4
1981 [3]	67.3	29.0	21.6	10.1	3.8	1.5	0.9	0.4
1982 [3]	67.3	28.6	22.0	10.2	3.8	1.4	0.9	0.3
1983 [3]	65.7	27.8	21.5	10.1	3.7	1.4	0.9	0.3
1984 [3]	65.5	27.4	21.7	10.1	3.7	1.4	0.9	0.3
1985	66.3	27.6	22.0	10.4	3.8	1.4	0.8	0.3
1986	65.4	27.2	21.6	10.3	3.8	1.4	0.8	0.3
1987	65.8	27.2	21.6	10.5	3.9	1.4	0.8	0.3
1988	67.3	27.6	22.0	10.9	4.1	1.5	0.9	0.3
1989	69.2	28.4	22.4	11.3	4.3	1.6	0.9	0.3
1990	70.9	29.0	22.8	11.7	4.5	1.7	1.0	0.3
1991	69.3	28.2	22.3	11.4	4.4	1.7	1.0	0.3
1992	68.4	27.6	22.2	11.2	4.4	1.7	1.0	0.3
1993	67.0	27.3	21.7	10.9	4.3	1.6	1.0	0.3
1994	65.9	27.1	21.2	10.6	4.1	1.6	0.9	0.3
1995	64.6	26.9	20.7	10.3	4.0	1.5	0.9	0.3
1996	64.1	26.3	20.7	10.4	4.0	1.5	0.9	0.3
1997	63.6	25.9	20.7	10.4	4.0	1.5	0.9	0.3
1998	64.3	25.9	21.0	10.6	4.1	1.5	0.9	0.3
1999	64.4	26.0	21.0	10.7	4.1	1.5	0.9	0.3
2000	65.9	26.5	21.4	11.0	4.2	1.6	0.9	0.3
2001	65.1	25.9	21.3	11.0	4.3	1.6	0.9	0.3
2002	65.0	25.8	21.2	10.9	4.3	1.6	0.9	0.3
2003	66.1	26.5	21.4	11.1	4.3	1.6	0.9	0.3
2004								
	66.4	26.4	21.4	11.2	4.4	1.6	0.9	0.3
2005	66.7	26.5	21.5	11.3	4.5	1.6	0.9	0.3
2006	68.6	27.4	21.9	11.6	4.7	1.7	1.0	0.3
2007	69.3	27.8	22.0	11.7	4.7	1.8	1.0	0.3
2008	68.1	27.5	21.5	11.4	4.7	1.7	1.0	0.3
2009	66.2	26.8	20.8	11.0	4.6	1.7	1.0	0.3
2010	64.1	25.9	20.2	10.6	4.4	1.7	1.0	0.3
2011	63.2	25.4	20.0	10.4	4.4	1.7	1.0	0.3
2012	63.0	25.2	19.9	10.4	4.4	1.7	1.0	0.3
2013	62.5	24.7	19.9	10.4	4.4	1.7	1.0	0.3
2014	62.9	24.6	20.1	10.6	4.5	1.8	1.1	0.3
Non-Hispanic White [2,4]								
1990 [5]	62.8	26.7	21.2	9.9	3.3	1.1	0.5	0.2
1991 [6]	60.9	25.8	20.6	9.6	3.2	1.0	0.5	0.2
1992 [6]	60.0	25.1	20.5	9.5	3.2	1.0	0.5	0.2
1993	58.9	24.8	20.1	9.2	3.1	1.0	0.5	0.2
1994	58.2	24.6	19.7	9.1	3.1	1.0	0.5	0.2
1995	57.5	24.5	19.3	8.9	3.0	1.0	0.5	0.2
1996	57.1	24.1	19.3	8.9	3.0	1.0	0.5	0.2
1997	56.8	23.8	19.3	8.9	3.0	1.0	0.5	0.2
1998	57.6	23.8	19.7	9.2	3.1	1.0	0.6	0.2
1999	57.7	24.0	19.6	9.2	3.2	1.0	0.6	0.2
2000	58.5	24.2	19.8	9.4	3.3	1.1	0.6	0.2
2001	57.7	23.6	19.7	9.4	3.3	1.1	0.6	0.2
2002	57.6	23.6	19.6	9.3	3.3	1.1	0.6	0.2
2003	58.9	24.5	19.8	9.4	3.3	1.1	0.6	0.2
2004								
	58.9	24.4	19.8	9.5	3.3	1.1	0.6	0.2
2005	59.0	24.4	19.8	9.5	3.4	1.1	0.6	0.2
2006	60.3	25.1	20.0	9.6	3.5	1.1	0.6	0.2
2007	61.0	25.6	20.1	9.7	3.5	1.2	0.7	0.2
2008	60.5	25.5	19.8	9.5	3.5	1.2	0.7	0.2
2009	59.6	25.3	19.5	9.2	3.4	1.2	0.7	0.3
2010	58.7	25.0	19.2	9.1	3.4	1.2	0.7	0.3
2011	58.7	24.9	19.2	9.0	3.4	1.2	0.7	0.3
2012	58.6	24.7	19.2	9.1	3.4	1.2	0.7	0.3
2013	58.7	24.4	19.3	9.2	3.5	1.2	0.7	0.3
2014	59.5	24.5	19.7	9.4	3.6	1.3	0.8	0.3

Table 1-28. Fertility Rates and Birth Rates, by Live-Birth Order and by Race and Hispanic Origin of Mother, 1980–2014— continued

(Births per 1,000 women age 15 to 44 years.)

Year, race, and Hispanic origin of mother	Fertility rate	Live-birth order						
		1	2	3	4	5	6 and 7	8 and over
Non-Hispanic Black [2,4]								
1990 [5]	89.0	33.2	26.3	16.0	7.6	3.3	2.0	0.6
1991 [6]	87.0	32.1	25.5	15.7	7.5	3.4	2.2	0.6
1992 [6]	84.5	31.1	24.8	15.2	7.3	3.4	2.2	0.6
1993	81.5	30.5	23.6	14.3	7.0	3.2	2.2	0.7
1994	77.5	30.0	22.4	13.2	6.3	2.9	2.0	0.6
1995	72.8	28.9	20.9	12.1	5.8	2.7	1.9	0.6
1996	70.7	27.6	20.5	12.0	5.6	2.6	1.8	0.6
1997	70.3	27.2	20.6	12.0	5.7	2.5	1.8	0.6
1998	70.9	27.0	21.0	12.3	5.7	2.6	1.8	0.6
1999	69.9	26.4	20.8	12.3	5.7	2.5	1.7	0.6
2000	71.4	26.7	21.2	12.8	5.9	2.6	1.8	0.6
2001	69.1	25.9	20.4	12.4	5.8	2.5	1.7	0.6
2002	67.5	25.4	19.7	12.1	5.7	2.5	1.7	0.6
2003	67.1	25.4	19.6	11.9	5.6	2.5	1.6	0.5
2004								
	67.1	25.5	19.4	11.9	5.6	2.5	1.7	0.5
2005	67.2	25.8	19.3	11.8	5.6	2.5	1.7	0.5
2006	70.7	27.5	20.3	12.3	5.8	2.5	1.7	0.5
2007	71.4	27.9	20.4	12.3	5.9	2.6	1.7	0.5
2008	70.8	28.1	20.0	12.1	5.8	2.6	1.7	0.5
2009								
	68.9	27.3	19.4	11.7	5.7	2.5	1.7	0.6
2010	66.6	26.3	18.9	11.3	5.4	2.5	1.7	0.5
2011	65.4	25.6	18.5	11.1	5.4	2.4	1.7	0.6
2012	65.0	25.1	18.6	11.2	5.5	2.4	1.7	0.5
2013	64.6	24.4	18.6	11.3	5.5	2.5	1.7	0.6
2014	64.5	23.9	18.6	11.5	5.6	2.5	1.7	0.6
Hispanic [7]								
1990 [5]	107.7	40.7	30.9	19.5	9.3	4.0	2.6	0.8
1991 [6]	106.9	40.8	30.6	19.2	9.2	3.9	2.5	0.7
1992 [6]	106.1	40.1	30.9	19.0	9.1	3.9	2.5	0.7
1993	103.3	39.3	30.4	18.3	8.6	3.7	2.3	0.6
1994	100.7	39.0	29.7	17.6	8.2	3.4	2.1	0.6
1995	98.8	38.4	29.3	17.4	7.8	3.3	2.0	0.6
1996	97.5	37.2	29.4	17.4	7.8	3.2	1.9	0.5
1997	94.2	35.6	28.6	17.1	7.6	3.0	1.8	0.5
1998	93.2	34.8	28.5	17.2	7.6	3.0	1.7	0.4
1999	93.0	34.6	28.5	17.3	7.5	2.9	1.7	0.4
2000	95.9	35.8	29.2	18.0	7.7	3.0	1.7	0.4
2001	95.4	35.2	29.3	18.0	7.9	3.0	1.7	0.4
2002	94.7	34.7	29.1	18.0	7.9	3.0	1.6	0.4
2003	95.2	34.5	29.4	18.3	8.0	3.0	1.6	0.4
2004								
	95.7	34.4	29.3	18.7	8.2	3.1	1.6	0.4
2005	96.4	34.4	29.6	19.0	8.4	3.1	1.6	0.4
2006	98.3	35.1	29.9	19.3	8.7	3.3	1.7	0.4
2007	97.4	34.7	29.4	19.3	8.7	3.3	1.7	0.4
2008	92.7	33.0	27.8	18.3	8.4	3.2	1.7	0.3
2009	86.5	30.6	25.9	17.0	8.0	3.0	1.6	0.3
2010	80.2	28.0	24.0	15.9	7.5	2.9	1.5	0.3
2011	76.2	26.3	22.9	15.2	7.2	2.8	1.5	0.3
2012	74.4	25.5	22.3	14.9	7.1	2.8	1.5	0.3
2013	72.9	24.9	21.8	14.6	7.0	2.8	1.5	0.3
2014	72.1	24.5	21.6	14.4	7.0	2.8	1.5	0.3

1 Includes races other than White and Black.   2 Includes origin not stated.   3 Based on 100 percent of births in selected states and on a 50 percent sample of births in all other states.   4 Race and Hispanic origin are reported separately on birth certificates. Persons of Hispanic origin may be of any race. Multiple-race data, when reported, were bridged to single-race categories in order to maintain comparability among all reported areas. Persons of Hispanic origin may be of any race.   5 Excludes data for New Hampshire and Oklahoma, which did not report Hispanic origin.   6 Excludes data for New Hampshire, which did not report Hispanic origin.   7 Includes all persons of Hispanic origin of any race.

Table 1-29. Selected Demographic Characteristics of Births, by Race of Mother, 2014

(Number; rates are live births per 1,000 population; percent.)

Characteristic	All races	White	Black	American Indian or Alaska Native	Asian or Pacific Islander
Number					
Births	3,988,076	3,019,863	640,562	44,928	282,723
Rate					
Birth rate	12.5	12.0	14.5	9.9	14.6
Fertility rate	1862.5	1875.5	1872.0	1288.5	1715.5
Total fertility rate	1,894.5	1,905.0	1,920.0	1,373.5	1,706.5
Sex ratio[1]	1,048	1,051	1,029	1,031	1,063
Percent, All Births					
Births to mothers under 20 years	6.3	6.0	9.5	11.3	1.7
4th and higher-order births[2]	12.2	11.7	16.1	21.2	6.6
Births to unmarried mothers	40.2	35.7	70.4	65.7	16.4
Mothers born in the 50 states and DC	78.1	81.8	83.4	94.2	23.3
Mean					
Age of mother at first birth	26.3	26.4	24.2	23.1	29.5

1 Male live births per 1,000 female live births.   2 Based on live-birth order.

Table 1-30. Births, by Day of Week and Index of Occurrence, by Method of Delivery, 2014

(Number, ratio.)

Day of the week	Average number of births	Index of occurrence[1]		
		Total[2]	Method of delivery	
			Vaginal	Cesarean
Total, All Days	10,926	100.0	100.0	100.0
Sunday	7,371	67.5	76.6	48.3
Monday	11,805	108.0	101.9	121.1
Tuesday	12,630	115.6	112.0	123.3
Wednesday	12,155	111.2	109.4	115.2
Thursday	12,112	110.9	109.0	114.7
Friday	12,042	110.2	105.6	119.9
Saturday	8,344	76.4	85.5	57.2

1 Index is the ratio of the average number of births by a specified method of delivery on a given day of the week to the average daily number of births by a specified method of delivery for the year, multiplied by 100.   2 Includes method of delivery not stated.

Table 1-31. Births and Observed and Seasonally Adjusted Birth and Fertility Rates, by Month, 2014

(Rates on an annual basis per 1,000 population for specified month; birth rates are live births per 1,000 total population; fertility rates are births per 1,000 women age 15 to 44 years.)

Month	Number	Observed		Seasonally adjusted [1]	
		Birth rate	Fertility rate	Birth rate	Fertility rate
Total, All Months	3,988,076	12.5	62.9	X	X
January	326,366	12.1	60.8	13.6	66.1
February	298,404	12.2	61.5	13.5	66.0
March	323,572	12.0	60.2	13.5	65.8
April	318,990	12.2	61.3	13.4	65.8
May	334,613	12.4	62.2	13.5	66.0
June	325,981	12.4	62.6	13.5	66.1
July	355,524	13.1	66.1	13.5	66.0
August	354,257	13.1	65.8	13.4	65.7
September	348,424	13.3	66.9	13.4	65.6
October	343,356	12.7	63.8	13.4	65.7
November	317,998	12.1	61.0	13.4	65.4
December	340,591	12.5	63.2	13.4	65.6

X = Not applicable.   1 Method of seasonal adjustment developed by the U.S. Census Bureau. For more information, see: http://www.census.gov/ts/papers/ShiskinYoungMusgrave1967.pdf

Table 1-32. Number, Rate, and Percent of Births to Unmarried Women and Birth Rate for Married Women, Selected Years, 1980–2014

(Number, rate per 1,000 women age 15 to 44 years; percent.)

Year	Births to unmarried women			Birth rate for married women[3]
	Number	Rate[1]	Percent[2]	
1980	665,747	29.4	18.4	97.0
1985	828,174	32.8	22.0	93.3
1990	1,165,384	43.8	28.0	93.2
1995	1,253,976	44.3	32.2	82.6
2000	1,347,043	44.1	33.2	87.4
2001	1,349,249	43.7	33.5	86.6
2002	1,365,966	43.6	34.0	86.9
2003	1,415,995	44.7	34.6	88.4
2004	1,470,189	46.0	35.8	88.1
2005	1,527,034	47.2	36.9	87.9
2006	1,641,946	50.3	38.5	88.7
2007	1,715,047	51.8	39.7	89.1
2008	1,726,566	51.8	40.6	86.9
2009	1,693,658	49.9	41.0	85.6
2010	1,633,471	47.5	40.8	84.3
2011	1,607,773	46.0	40.7	85.1
2012	1,609,619	45.3	40.7	86.0
2013	1,595,873	44.4	40.6	86.9
2014	1,604,870	43.9	40.2	88.9

Note: Rates for 2001 to 2009 have been revised using revised intercensal populations based on the 2010 census.   1 Births to unmarried women per 1,000 unmarried women age 15 to 44 years.   2 Percentage of all births to unmarried women.   3 Births to married women per 1,000 married women age 15 to 44 years.

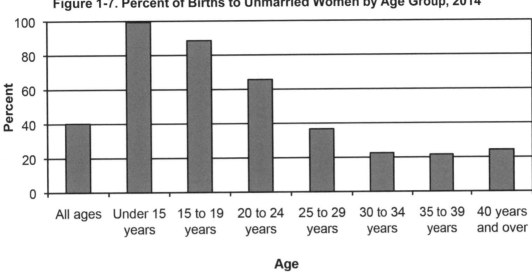

Figure 1-7. Percent of Births to Unmarried Women by Age Group, 2014

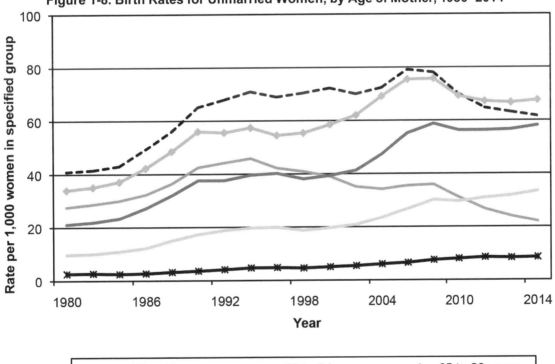

Figure 1-8. Birth Rates for Unmarried Women, by Age of Mother, 1980–2014

Table 1-33. Birth Rates for Unmarried Women, by Age of Mother, Selected Years, 1970–2014, and by Age, Race, and Hispanic Origin of Mother, Selected Years, 1970–2014

(Births to unmarried women per 1,000 unmarried women.)

Characteristic	Age of mother								
	15 to 44 years[1]	15 to 19 years			20 to 24 years	25 to 29 years	30 to 34 years	35 to 39 years	40 to 44 years[2]
		Total	15 to 17 years	18 to 19 years					
All Races [3]									
1970 [4,5]	26.4	22.4	17.1	32.9	38.4	37.0	27.1	13.6	3.5
1975 [5,6]	24.5	23.9	19.3	32.5	31.2	27.5	17.9	9.1	2.6
1980 [5,6]	29.4	27.6	20.6	39.0	40.9	34.0	21.1	9.7	2.6
1980 [6,7]	28.4	27.5	20.7	38.7	39.7	31.4	18.5	8.4	2.3
1981 [6,7]	29.5	27.9	20.9	39.0	41.1	34.5	20.8	9.8	2.6
1982 [6,7]	30.0	28.7	21.5	39.6	41.5	35.1	21.9	10.0	2.7
1983 [6,7]	30.3	29.5	22.0	40.7	41.8	35.5	22.4	10.2	2.6
1984 [6,7]	31.0	30.0	21.9	42.5	43.0	37.1	23.3	10.9	2.5
1985 [7]	32.8	31.4	22.4	45.9	46.5	39.9	25.2	11.6	2.5
1986 [7]	34.2	32.3	22.8	48.0	49.3	42.2	27.2	12.2	2.7
1987 [7]	36.0	33.8	24.5	48.9	52.6	44.5	29.6	13.5	2.9
1988 [7]	38.5	36.4	26.4	51.5	56.0	48.5	32.0	15.0	3.2
1989 [7]	41.6	40.1	28.7	56.0	61.2	52.8	34.9	16.0	3.4
1990 [7]	43.8	42.5	29.6	60.7	65.1	56.0	37.6	17.3	3.6
1991 [7]	45.0	44.6	30.8	65.4	67.8	56.0	37.9	17.9	3.8
1992 [7]	44.9	44.2	30.2	66.7	67.9	55.6	37.6	18.8	4.1
1993 [7]	44.8	44.0	30.3	66.2	68.5	55.9	38.0	18.9	4.4
1994 [7]	46.2	45.8	31.7	69.1	70.9	57.4	39.6	19.7	4.7
1995 [7]	44.3	43.8	30.1	66.5	68.7	54.3	38.9	19.3	4.7
1996 [7]	43.8	42.2	28.5	64.9	68.9	54.5	40.2	19.9	4.8
1997 [7]	42.9	41.4	27.7	63.9	68.9	53.4	37.9	18.7	4.6
1998 [7]	43.3	40.9	26.5	63.6	70.4	55.4	38.1	18.7	4.6
1999 [7]	43.3	39.7	25.0	62.3	70.8	56.9	38.1	19.0	4.6
2000 [7]	44.1	39.0	23.9	62.2	72.2	58.5	39.3	19.7	5.0
2001 [7]	43.7	36.8	21.8	60.2	70.8	59.6	40.3	20.4	5.3
2002 [7]	43.6	35.1	20.7	58.1	70.0	62.0	41.3	20.9	5.4
2003 [7]	44.7	34.3	20.1	56.6	71.0	66.2	44.2	22.3	5.8
2004 [7]	46.0	34.2	19.9	56.6	72.3	69.1	47.3	23.5	6.0
2005 [7]	47.2	33.9	19.4	57.0	74.5	71.5	50.4	24.5	6.2
2006 [7]	50.3	35.5	20.1	60.3	79.1	75.4	55.3	26.8	6.5
2007 [7]	51.8	36.5	20.4	61.9	79.8	76.9	58.0	28.7	6.8
2008 [7]	51.8	35.9	20.1	59.7	78.1	75.7	58.8	30.2	7.5
2009 [7]	49.9	34.0	18.8	56.3	74.4	73.0	57.1	29.7	7.8
2010 [7]	47.5	31.1	16.8	52.0	70.0	69.2	56.3	29.6	8.0
2011 [7]	46.0	28.4	14.9	48.2	66.7	67.8	56.2	29.9	8.2
White									
1980 [6,7]	18.1	16.5	12.0	24.1	25.1	21.5	14.1	7.1	1.8
1981 [6,7]	18.6	17.2	12.6	24.6	25.8	22.3	14.2	7.2	1.9
1982 [6,7]	19.3	18.0	13.1	25.3	26.5	23.1	15.3	7.4	2.1
1983 [6,7]	19.8	18.7	13.6	26.4	27.1	23.8	15.9	7.8	2.0
1984 [6,7]	20.6	19.3	13.7	27.9	28.5	25.5	16.8	8.4	2.0
1985 [7]	22.5	20.8	14.5	31.2	31.7	28.5	18.4	9.0	2.0
1986 [7]	23.9	21.8	14.9	33.5	34.2	30.5	20.1	9.7	2.2
1987 [7]	25.3	23.2	16.2	34.5	36.6	32.0	22.3	10.7	2.4
1988 [7]	27.4	25.3	17.6	36.8	39.2	35.4	24.2	12.1	2.7
1989 [7]	30.2	28.0	19.3	40.2	43.8	39.1	26.8	13.1	2.9
1990 [7]	32.9	30.6	20.4	44.9	48.2	43.0	29.9	14.5	3.2
1991 [7]	34.5	32.7	21.7	49.4	51.4	44.3	30.9	15.2	3.2
1992 [7]	35.0	32.7	21.4	51.2	52.4	44.8	31.3	16.1	3.6
1993 [7]	35.6	33.3	21.9	52.0	53.8	46.0	31.9	16.3	3.9
1994 [7]	37.8	35.8	23.9	55.8	57.5	48.6	33.8	17.2	4.3
1995 [7]	37.0	35.0	23.3	54.7	57.2	47.4	33.7	16.8	4.2
1996 [7]	37.0	34.0	22.3	53.5	57.9	48.1	35.4	17.7	4.3
1997 [7]	36.3	33.6	22.0	52.9	57.9	47.0	33.6	16.6	3.9
1998 [7]	36.9	33.6	21.5	53.1	59.5	48.6	34.1	16.9	4.1
1999 [7]	37.4	33.2	20.6	52.9	60.2	50.8	34.9	17.4	4.1
2000 [7]	38.2	32.7	19.7	53.1	61.7	52.9	35.9	17.9	4.5
2001 [7]	38.4	31.2	18.1	51.9	61.5	54.9	37.2	18.6	4.9
2002 [7]	39.0	30.3	17.5	50.8	61.6	57.5	38.8	19.5	5.1
2003 [7]	40.5	29.9	17.1	50.0	63.2	61.7	42.3	21.3	5.5
2004 [7]	41.8	29.9	17.0	49.9	64.5	65.0	46.2	22.8	5.6

Table 1-33. Birth Rates for Unmarried Women, by Age of Mother, Selected Years, 1970–2014, and by Age, Race, and Hispanic Origin of Mother, Selected Years, 1970–2014— continued

(Births to unmarried women per 1,000 unmarried women.)

| Characteristic | 15 to 44 years[1] | Age of mother | | | 20 to 24 years | 25 to 29 years | 30 to 34 years | 35 to 39 years | 40 to 44 years[2] |
| | | 15 to 19 years | | | | | | | |
		Total	15 to 17 years	18 to 19 years					
2005 [7]	43.2	29.7	16.7	50.3	67.0	67.7	49.8	23.9	5.9
2006 [7]	46.4	31.1	17.3	53.3	71.7	72.4	55.5	26.6	6.3
2007 [7]	48.3	32.3	17.9	55.1	72.6	74.3	59.5	29.1	6.5
2008 [7]	48.4	31.9	17.8	53.3	70.9	73.1	60.0	31.1	7.3
2009 [7]	46.6	30.4	16.7	50.5	67.3	69.7	57.7	30.6	7.8
2010 [7]	44.5	27.9	15.1	46.9	63.4	65.8	56.8	30.7	8.1
2011 [7]	42.7	25.5	13.4	43.4	60.1	63.8	56.2	30.6	8.3
2012 [7]	45.3	26.7	13.7	45.8	64.7	67.2	56.3	30.9	8.5
2013 [7]	44.3	24.0	11.9	42.1	63.1	66.7	56.6	31.8	8.3
2014 [7]	43.9	22.0	10.6	39.4	61.6	67.6	58.1	33.4	8.5
White									
1990 [7,8]	24.4	25.0	16.2	37.0	36.4	30.3	20.5	6.1	NA
1991 [7]	NA	NA	NA	NA	NA	NA	NA	NA	NA
1992 [7]	NA	NA	NA	NA	NA	NA	NA	NA	NA
1993 [7]	NA	NA	NA	NA	NA	NA	NA	NA	NA
1994 [7]	28.4	28.1	17.9	45.0	43.8	34.7	24.6	12.8	3.1
1995 [7]	28.1	27.7	17.6	44.6	43.9	34.4	25.1	12.9	3.2
1996 [7]	28.2	27.0	16.9	43.9	44.5	35.0	26.4	13.8	3.3
1997 [7]	27.5	26.4	16.2	43.3	44.8	34.4	24.9	12.7	2.9
1998 [7]	27.9	26.2	15.5	43.1	46.3	35.4	25.0	13.1	3.1
1999 [7]	27.9	25.6	14.6	42.7	46.3	36.2	24.8	13.0	3.1
2000 [7]	28.0	24.7	13.6	42.1	47.0	36.9	24.8	12.9	3.3
2001 [7]	27.8	23.1	12.1	40.3	46.4	37.8	25.4	13.2	3.6
2002 [7]	27.9	22.1	11.4	38.8	46.3	38.9	26.2	13.6	3.7
2003 [7]	28.8	21.5	11.0	37.8	47.6	41.5	28.0	14.8	4.1
2004 [7]	29.6	21.3	10.7	37.4	48.6	44.2	30.0	15.7	4.2
2005 [7]	30.4	20.9	10.3	37.4	49.9	46.0	31.7	16.2	4.3
2006 [7]	32.4	21.6	10.7	38.9	52.6	49.1	35.1	17.9	4.5
2007 [7]	33.8	22.6	10.9	40.7	53.4	50.7	37.2	19.2	4.6
2008 [7]	34.3	22.5	10.8	39.7	52.9	50.8	38.4	20.4	5.2
2009 [7]	33.6	21.8	10.4	38.1	51.4	49.3	37.9	20.0	5.5
2010 [7]	32.9	20.3	9.5	36.0	49.5	48.0	38.7	20.2	5.8
2011 [7]	32.3	18.8	8.6	33.6	47.8	47.8	39.2	20.7	6.0
2012 [7]	42.1	24.1	12.4	41.4	58.3	63.2	56.3	31.5	8.5
2013 [7]	40.8	21.9	10.8	38.6	56.9	62.5	56.2	32.3	7.7
2014 [7]	40.6	20.3	9.7	36.4	55.9	63.5	57.7	34.0	7.6
Black									
1980 [6,7]	81.1	87.9	68.8	118.2	112.3	81.4	46.7	19.0	5.5
1981 [6,7]	79.4	85.0	65.9	114.2	110.7	83.1	45.5	19.6	5.6
1982 [6,7]	77.9	85.1	66.3	112.7	109.3	82.7	44.1	19.5	5.2
1983 [6,7]	76.2	85.5	66.8	111.9	107.2	79.7	43.8	19.4	4.8
1984 [6,7]	75.2	86.1	66.5	113.6	107.9	77.8	43.8	19.4	4.3
1985 [7]	77.0	87.6	66.8	117.9	113.1	79.3	47.5	20.4	4.3
1986 [7]	79.0	88.5	67.0	121.1	118.0	84.6	50.0	20.6	4.4
1987 [7]	82.6	90.9	69.9	123.0	126.1	91.6	53.1	22.4	4.7
1988 [7]	86.5	96.1	73.5	130.5	133.6	97.2	57.4	24.1	5.0
1989 [7]	90.7	104.5	78.9	140.9	142.4	102.9	60.5	24.9	5.0
1990 [7]	90.5	106.0	78.8	143.7	144.8	105.3	61.5	25.5	5.1
1991 [7]	89.0	107.8	79.9	147.7	146.4	100.0	59.8	25.5	5.4
1992 [7]	85.7	104.8	77.2	146.4	142.6	96.8	57.3	25.6	5.4
1993 [7]	83.0	101.2	75.9	140.0	139.9	92.8	56.7	25.7	5.8
1994 [7]	80.8	99.3	73.9	139.6	135.2	91.3	56.5	26.0	5.9
1995 [7]	74.5	91.2	67.4	129.2	124.6	82.3	53.3	25.3	6.0
1996 [7]	72.8	87.5	62.6	127.2	122.6	81.2	53.4	25.2	6.1
1997 [7]	71.5	84.5	59.0	124.8	124.2	81.4	51.0	24.3	6.5
1998 [7]	71.6	81.5	55.0	121.5	127.8	86.5	50.5	24.3	6.0
1999 [7]	69.7	76.5	50.0	115.8	126.8	85.5	49.0	24.2	5.8
2000 [7]	70.5	75.0	48.3	115.0	129.0	85.9	50.2	25.4	6.3
2001 [7]	68.0	69.4	43.5	109.1	122.5	84.4	51.2	25.4	6.3
2002 [7]	66.1	64.0	39.4	102.8	119.0	86.3	50.2	24.9	6.3
2003 [7]	65.9	61.0	37.4	98.0	117.8	91.3	51.2	25.2	6.5
2004 [7]	66.8	60.1	36.1	98.0	119.6	92.5	52.0	25.7	6.8

Table 1-33. Birth Rates for Unmarried Women, by Age of Mother, Selected Years, 1970–2014, and by Age, Race, and Hispanic Origin of Mother, Selected Years, 1970–2014— continued

(Births to unmarried women per 1,000 unmarried women.)

| Characteristic | 15 to 44 years[1] | 15 to 19 years | | | 20 to 24 years | 25 to 29 years | 30 to 34 years | 35 to 39 years | 40 to 44 years[2] |
		Total	15 to 17 years	18 to 19 years					
2005[7]	67.2	58.7	34.4	97.9	120.4	94.7	53.9	25.9	7.1
2006[7]	70.7	61.1	35.4	103.3	125.5	98.0	58.4	27.3	7.2
2007[7]	71.4	61.3	34.8	103.6	125.3	99.1	59.9	28.0	7.4
2008[7]	71.0	59.7	33.9	98.4	124.0	97.0	61.1	28.5	7.6
2009[7]	68.7	55.9	31.1	91.3	119.5	95.6	60.3	28.4	7.6
2010[7]	65.3	50.8	27.6	83.6	112.6	92.5	58.6	27.8	7.8
2011[7]	63.7	46.7	24.7	77.4	106.9	92.4	59.1	28.9	7.8
2012[7]	62.6	43.4	22.0	73.2	103.5	91.2	59.6	29.7	8.1
2013[7]	61.7	38.5	19.0	66.2	100.7	92.3	60.6	31.1	8.4
2014[7]	61.5	34.4	16.7	60.9	97.4	93.3	67.0	32.0	8.8
Asian or Pacific Islander									
2000[7]	20.9	15.2	9.6	23.2	24.2	25.4	29.7	18.4	6.9
2001[7]	20.5	14.2	8.5	22.4	23.9	25.7	28.7	19.5	6.3
2002[7]	20.6	13.0	7.3	21.0	24.4	26.7	29.4	19.1	6.9
2003[7]	21.1	12.3	7.1	19.6	24.2	29.0	31.8	19.8	7.9
2004[7]	22.1	12.3	7.3	19.4	24.8	30.7	35.8	20.7	8.6
2005[7]	22.8	11.9	6.8	19.3	25.8	31.4	36.8	24.6	9.3
2006[7]	23.4	12.0	7.3	18.9	26.8	30.5	37.6	29.7	9.4
2007[7]	23.9	11.9	6.7	19.2	27.1	32.3	36.9	28.8	9.9
2008[7]	23.9	11.4	6.3	18.4	26.4	33.5	37.9	30.3	10.8
2009[7]	23.6	10.6	5.9	17.1	25.3	36.2	39.2	27.3	9.9
2010[7]	22.3	9.2	4.8	15.4	23.2	35.0	40.0	26.6	9.9
2011[7]	22.4	8.6	4.4	14.8	22.3	35.1	42.3	27.0	9.9
2012[7]	22.9	8.1	3.9	14.2	22.0	35.2	43.6	30.1	12.1
2013[7]	21.8	7.2	3.5	12.6	20.7	31.5	44.1	31.5	12.6
2014[7]	21.7	6.2	3.0	10.6	19.4	31.4	47.0	36.0	12.6
Hispanic[9]									
1990[7,8]	89.6	65.9	45.9	98.9	129.8	131.7	88.1	50.8	13.7
1991[7]	92.5	71.0	49.5	107.5	134.2	135.1	88.2	47.6	14.1
1992[7]	92.8	70.3	49.2	106.6	138.2	133.4	89.9	47.8	14.6
1993[7]	91.4	71.1	49.6	108.8	134.3	130.4	87.8	47.1	14.1
1994[7]	95.8	77.7	55.7	115.4	144.5	131.7	91.2	47.4	13.9
1995[7]	88.8	73.2	52.8	108.6	135.8	122.3	84.1	42.2	12.1
1996[7]	86.2	69.3	49.7	102.3	131.6	122.0	84.6	41.2	12.3
1997[7]	83.2	69.2	50.7	100.6	122.8	114.8	78.8	40.5	12.1
1998[7]	82.8	69.3	49.8	101.2	120.6	115.9	78.2	38.8	12.0
1999[7]	84.9	68.6	48.7	99.9	126.1	119.6	84.2	42.4	11.2
2000[7]	87.2	68.5	47.0	102.2	130.5	121.6	89.4	46.1	12.2
2001[7]	86.8	65.5	43.4	101.1	129.8	121.0	91.4	49.6	12.2
2002[7]	87.0	63.9	41.9	100.7	127.2	125.1	91.0	52.4	12.8
2003[7]	89.9	63.5	41.1	101.2	130.2	135.6	98.7	54.0	13.2
2004[7]	92.7	64.2	41.2	102.9	133.4	142.5	108.8	56.0	13.7
2005[7]	96.2	63.7	40.3	103.9	142.5	151.2	116.7	58.1	14.1
2006[7]	101.5	65.9	40.5	110.2	155.1	160.7	122.9	61.3	14.8
2007[7]	102.1	65.4	40.6	109.2	153.8	161.1	127.0	64.9	14.9
2008[7]	97.3	62.4	39.4	101.1	141.0	151.1	121.6	66.9	16.2
2009[7]	89.4	56.7	35.3	90.9	125.4	139.4	112.4	63.7	17.1
2010[7]	80.6	50.0	30.8	79.8	110.5	123.9	105.8	61.7	16.3
2011[7]	75.1	44.7	27.0	71.7	100.6	116.2	106.0	58.0	16.2
2012[7]	72.6	41.8	24.5	68.5	96.5	113.2	103.9	57.6	16.5
2013[7]	69.9	37.6	21.1	63.0	93.1	112.0	100.1	56.8	16.8
2014[7]	68.5	34.4	18.6	59.5	92.3	111.2	97.3	58.2	16.8

NA = Not available.   1 Rates computed by relating total births to unmarried mothers, regardless of age of mother, to unmarried women age 15 to 44 years.   2 Beginning in 1997, birth rates computed by relating births to unmarried mothers age 40 years and over to unmarried women age 40 to 44 years.   3 Includes races other than White, Black, and Asian or Other Pacific Islander.   4 Births to unmarried women are estimated for the United States from data for registration areas in which marital status of mother was reported.   5 Based on a 50 percent sample of births.   6 Based on 100 percent of births in selected states and on a 50 percent sample of births in all other states.   7 Data for states in which marital status was not reported have been inferred and included with data from the remaining states.   8 Rates based on data for 48 states and the District of Columbia that reported Hispanic origin on the birth certificate. Rate for age group 35–39 years are based on births to unmarried women aged 35–44 years.   9 Persons of Hispanic origin may be of any race.

Table 1-34. Births and Birth Rates for Unmarried Women, by Age, Race, and Hispanic Origin of Mother, 2014

(Number, rate, percent.)

Measure and age of mother	All races[1]	White Total[2]	White Non-Hispanic	Black Total[2]	Black Non-Hispanic	American Indian or Alaska Native[2]	Asian or Pacific Islander[2]	Hispanic[3]
Number								
All ages	1,604,870	1,078,215	628,078	450,784	417,518	29,529	46,342	483,807
Under 15 years	2,752	1,631	672	1,026	953	55	40	1,030
15 to 19 years	220,634	154,190	84,148	58,176	53,416	4,644	3,624	75,307
15 years	7,998	5,292	2,245	2,405	2,205	179	122	3,263
16 years	19,463	13,512	6,137	5,219	4,746	428	304	7,875
17 years	36,443	25,769	12,854	9,242	8,446	815	617	13,835
18 years	62,078	43,834	24,190	15,895	14,536	1,323	1,026	21,152
19 years	94,652	65,783	38,722	25,415	23,483	1,899	1,555	29,182
20 to 24 years	579,760	383,980	235,014	172,845	161,345	10,814	12,121	161,047
25 to 29 years	419,792	279,270	167,132	119,396	110,795	7,755	13,371	120,669
30 to 34 years	243,054	163,763	91,192	64,825	59,622	4,260	10,206	77,634
35 to 39 years	110,058	75,204	39,124	27,973	25,418	1,634	5,247	38,357
40 years and over	28,820	20,177	10,796	6,543	5,969	367	1,733	9,763
Rate per 1,000 Unmarried Women in Specified Group								
15 to 44 years[4]	43.9	40.6	31.8	61.5	NA	NA	21.7	68.5
15 to 19 years	22.0	20.3	15.0	34.4	NA	NA	6.2	34.4
15 to 17 years	10.6	9.7	6.3	16.7	NA	NA	3.0	18.6
18 to 19 years	39.4	36.4	28.1	60.9	NA	NA	10.6	59.5
20 to 24 years	61.6	55.9	44.4	97.4	NA	NA	19.4	92.3
25 to 29 years	67.6	63.5	49.1	93.3	NA	NA	31.4	111.2
30 to 34 years	58.1	57.7	43.1	67.0	NA	NA	47.0	97.3
35 to 39 years	33.4	34.0	24.2	32.0	NA	NA	36.0	58.2
40 to 44 years[5]	8.5	7.6	6.5	8.8	NA	NA	12.6	16.8
Percent of Births to Unmarried Women								
All ages	40.2	35.7	29.2	70.4	70.9	65.7	16.4	52.9
Under 15 years	99.4	99.1	99.0	99.8	99.8	100.0	100.0	99.3
15 to 19 years	88.6	85.9	84.8	97.0	97.4	92.9	78.2	87.6
15 years	98.9	98.6	98.6	99.8	99.8	99.4	94.6	98.6
16 years	96.6	95.5	95.2	99.5	99.6	97.7	90.7	95.9
17 years	94.5	93.1	92.8	98.9	99.2	97.5	87.8	93.6
18 years	89.5	87.1	86.8	97.3	97.6	93.8	79.7	87.8
19 years	83.8	80.2	79.4	95.5	96.1	88.9	71.3	82.0
20 to 24 years	65.7	59.6	55.9	87.7	88.4	76.7	44.9	67.3
25 to 29 years	36.7	31.6	25.9	68.2	68.8	60.7	17.8	48.5
30 to 34 years	22.5	19.5	14.2	50.8	51.0	49.6	9.7	38.0
35 to 39 years	21.6	19.5	13.9	44.2	44.1	45.7	9.3	35.6
40 years and over	24.3	23.2	18.0	39.7	39.4	44.7	12.2	36.0

NA = Not available.   1 Includes races other than White and Black and origin not stated.   2 Race and Hispanic origin are reported separately on birth certificates. Persons of Hispanic origin may be of any race. Multiple-race data, when reported, were bridged to single-race categories in order to maintain comparability among all reported areas.   3 Persons of Hispanic origin may be of any race.   4 Birth rates computed by relating total births to unmarried mothers, regardless of age of mother, to unmarried women age 15 to 44 years.   5 Birth rates computed by relating births to unmarried mothers age 40 years and over to unmarried women age 40 to 44 years.

Table 1-35. Selected Demographic Characteristics of Births, by Hispanic Origin of Mother and by Race for Mothers of Non-Hispanic Origin, 2014

(Birth rates are births per 1,000 population; fertility rates are computed by relating total births, regardless of age of mother, to women age 15 to 44 years; total fertility rates are sums of birth rates for 5-year age groups multiplied by 5.)

Characteristic	All origins[1]	Hispanic[2]						Non-Hispanic		
		Total	Mexican	PuertoRican	Cuban	Central and South American	Other and unknown Hispanic	Total[3]	White	Black
Number										
Births	3,988,076	914,065	545,977	68,879	20,163	136,656	141,390	3,043,519	2,149,302	588,891
Rate										
Birth rate[4]	12.5	16.5	NA	NA	NA	(4)	NA	11.7	10.8	14.4
Fertility rate[4]	62.9	72.1	NA	NA	NA	(4)	NA	60.7	59.5	64.5
Total fertility rate[4]	1,862.5	2,130.5	NA	NA	NA	(4)	NA	1793.0	1,762.5	1,873.5
Sex ratio[5]	1,048	1,041	1,042	1,047	1,047	1,038	1,050	1,050	1,055	1,027
Percent										
Births to mothers under 20 years	6.3	9.5	10.1	14.0	4.2	5.9	11.0	5.4	4.6	9.5
4th and higher-order births[6]	12.2	16.1	18.2	12.6	5.5	13.5	13.4	11.0	9.9	16.2
Births to unmarried mothers	40.2	52.9	51.6	65.0	49.8	50.4	55.5	36.5	29.2	70.9
Mothers born in the 50 states and D.C.	78.1	52.4	50.2	72.9	48.9	17.4	72.0	85.8	93.7	85.4
Mean										
Age of mother at first birth	26.3	24.3	23.7	24.1	27.0	26.5	24.0	26.7	27.0	24.2

1 Includes origin not stated.   2 Persons of Hispanic origin may be of any race.   3 Includes races other than White and Black.   4 Rates for Central and South American include other and unknown Hispanic.
5 Male births per 1,000 female births.   6Based on live-birth order.

Table 1-36. Percent of Births with Selected Medical or Health Characteristics, by Race of Mother, 2011

(Percent, rate.)

Characteristic	All races	White	Black	American or Alaska Indian Native	Asian or Pacific Islander
ALL BIRTHS					
Mother					
Diabetes during pregnancy	5.5	5.3	5.0	7.5	9.2
Weight gain of less than 11 lbs	8.5	7.7	12.9	11.9	6.0
Weight gain of more than 40 lbs	21.2	21.7	21.1	21.4	15.2
Induction of labor	23.2	24.1	21.9	21.9	17.2
CNM delivery[1]	7.8	7.9	7.4	16.7	6.5
Cesarean delivery	32.8	32.3	35.2	28.4	33.2
Infant					
Gestational age					
Preterm[2]	11.7	10.8	16.5	13.5	10.4
Early preterm[3]	3.4	3.0	5.9	3.9	2.8
Late preterm[4]	8.3	7.8	10.6	9.6	7.6
Birthweight					
Very low birthweight[5]	1.4	1.2	2.9	1.3	1.2
Low birthweight[6]	8.1	7.1	13.0	7.5	8.4
4,000 grams or more[7]	7.8	8.7	4.4	9.8	4.8
Low 5-minute Apgar[8]	1.9	1.6	3.1	2.3	1.2
Twin birth[9] (rate)	33.2	32.8	36.4	23.4	31.2
Triplet or higher-order multiple birth[10] (rate)	137.0	145.5	110.3	43.1	119.7

1 Births delivered by certified nurse midwives.   2 Born prior to 37 completed weeks of gestation.   3 Born prior to 34 completed weeks of gestation.   4 Born between 34 and 36 completed weeks of gestation.   5 Birthweight of less than 1,500 grams (3 lb 4 oz).   6 Birthweight of less than 2,500 grams (5 lb 8 oz).   7 Equivalent to 8 lb 14 oz.   8 Score of less than 7 on a 10-point scale.   9 Live births in twin deliveries per 1,000 live births.   10 Live births in triplet and other higher-order multiple deliveries per 100,000 live births.

Table 1-37. Percent of Births with Selected Medical or Health Characteristics, by Hispanic Origin of Mother and by Race for Mothers of Non-Hispanic Origin, 2011

(Percent, rate.)

Characteristic	All origins[1]	Origin of mother								
		Hispanic						Non-Hispanic		
		Total	Mexican	Puerto Rican	Cuban	Central and South American	Other and unknown Hispanic	Total[2]	White	Black
ALL BIRTHS										
Mother										
Diabetes during pregnancy	5.5	5.8	6.2	6.1	5.1	5.5	4.6	5.4	5.1	4.9
Weight gain of less than 11 lbs	8.5	9.4	9.8	8.8	5.1	8.7	8.8	8.2	7.1	13.1
Weight gain of more than 40 lbs	21.2	16.7	15.5	22.7	27.1	15.3	19.3	22.6	23.8	21.2
Induction of labor	23.2	18.0	17.4	21.2	20.5	16.5	19.7	24.9	26.6	22.0
CNM delivery[3]	7.8	8.0	7.5	10.3	4.6	9.4	7.8	7.8	7.9	7.1
Cesarean delivery	32.8	32.0	30.8	34.5	47.9	32.8	33.5	33.0	32.4	35.5
Infant										
Gestational age										
Preterm[4]	11.7	11.7	11.3	13.2	12.4	11.8	12.3	11.7	10.5	16.8
Early preterm[5]	3.4	3.3	3.1	4.0	3.4	3.3	3.5	3.5	2.9	6.0
Late preterm[6]	8.3	8.4	8.2	9.2	9.0	8.5	8.8	8.2	7.6	10.7
Birthweight										
Very low birthweight[7]	1.4	1.2	1.1	1.8	1.3	1.2	1.4	1.5	1.1	3.0
Low birthweight[8]	8.1	7.0	6.5	9.7	7.1	6.7	8.0	8.4	7.1	13.3
4,000 grams or more[9]	7.8	7.2	7.6	5.8	7.3	7.0	6.1	8.0	9.3	4.2
Low 5-minute Apgar[10]	1.9	1.4	1.3	1.7	1.4	1.3	1.6	2.0	1.8	3.2
Twin birth[11] (rate)	33.2	23.1	20.9	32.0	29.4	25.2	25.3	36.1	36.6	37.2
Triplet or higher-order multiple birth[12] (rate)	137.0	78.7	60.7	114.9	181.0	105.7	96.9	153.2	171.0	108.9

1 Includes origin not stated.   2 Includes races other than White and Black.   3 Births delivered by certified nurse midwives.   4 Born prior to 37 completed weeks of gestation.   5 Born prior to 34 completed weeks of gestation.   6 Born between 34 and 36 completed weeks of gestation.   7 Birthweight of less than 1,500 grams (3 lb 4 oz).   8 Birthweight of less than 2,500 grams (5 lb 8 oz).   9 Equivalent to 8 lb 14 oz.   10 Score of less than 7 on a 10 point scale.   11 Live births in twin deliveries per 1,000 live births.   12 Live births in triplet and other higher-order multiple deliveries per 100,000 live births.

Table 1-38. Births to Unmarried Women, by Race and Hispanic Origin of Mother, by State and Territory of Residence, 2011

(Number, percent.)

State and territory	Births to unmarried women				Percent unmarried			
	All races[1]	Non-Hispanic		Hispanic[3]	All races[1]	Non-Hispanic		Hispanic[3]
		White[2]	Black[2]			White[2]	Black[2]	
United States [4]	1,604,870	628,078	417,518	483,807	40.2	29.2	70.9	52.9
Alabama	25,721	10,456	13,848	1,196	43.3	29.1	76.0	29.8
Alaska	4,061	1,532	187	287	35.6	23.4	41.9	34.1
Arizona	39,224	11,926	2,913	19,807	45.1	30.9	62.3	56.5
Arkansas	16,925	8,809	5,735	1,881	43.9	34.0	79.1	49.0
California	194,960	34,263	18,899	125,459	38.8	23.7	66.8	52.8
Colorado	14,748	6,825	1,321	5,885	22.4	16.8	39.4	33.3
Connecticut	13,477	4,955	3,068	5,203	37.1	23.7	66.5	64.0
Delaware	5,116	2,122	1,985	937	46.6	35.9	69.7	60.8
District of Columbia	4,771	186	3,748	770	50.2	6.3	78.5	60.1
Florida	105,422	38,084	34,116	31,620	47.9	37.8	69.2	51.1
Georgia	59,415	17,183	31,646	8,773	45.4	28.6	70.3	50.9
Hawaii	6,886	1,122	129	1,291	37.1	23.0	23.1	46.7
Idaho	6,367	4,379	66	1,624	27.8	24.1	31.9	44.5
Illinois	63,555	22,757	21,599	17,775	40.1	26.4	79.4	52.6
Indiana	36,409	23,821	8,217	4,041	43.3	37.2	79.4	55.8
Iowa	13,949	10,127	1,650	1,742	35.1	31.2	69.9	52.5
Kansas	14,298	8,651	2,081	3,156	36.5	30.4	70.8	51.5
Kentucky	23,545	17,795	4,009	1,514	41.9	38.1	74.9	53.7
Louisiana	34,006	11,915	19,194	2,389	52.7	34.8	79.2	56.2
Maine	5,236	4,805	157	89	41.2	41.2	35.5	44.5
Maryland	29,372	8,337	14,591	5,930	39.7	25.1	60.9	54.0
Massachusetts	23,872	11,259	3,873	7,628	33.2	25.3	54.1	60.0
Michigan	47,817	25,909	17,301	3,726	41.8	32.3	79.9	50.7
Minnesota	22,610	12,615	4,269	2,505	32.3	25.1	55.1	53.5
Mississippi	20,935	6,469	13,369	841	54.0	32.6	80.4	54.4
Missouri	30,292	18,748	8,795	2,022	40.2	32.8	76.8	51.1
Montana	4,586	3,089	50	238	36.9	30.4	55.6	48.2
Nebraska	8,840	5,126	1,227	2,032	33.0	26.3	66.3	49.0
Nevada	16,431	5,216	3,078	7,018	45.8	34.4	72.3	54.0
New Hampshire	4,147	3,706	87	268	33.7	33.9	46.0	45.3
New Jersey	36,646	9,231	10,493	16,181	35.5	19.2	67.6	59.3
New Mexico	13,358	2,077	251	8,411	51.3	28.8	53.6	58.2
New York	94,658	29,497	25,026	35,238	39.6	25.4	67.7	63.7
North Carolina	49,574	18,143	20,645	9,080	41.0	26.9	71.1	51.1
North Dakota	3,680	2,392	191	223	32.4	26.5	41.5	46.5
Ohio	60,620	37,108	18,508	4,185	43.5	35.6	78.2	60.8
Oklahoma	22,512	11,765	3,746	3,535	42.2	35.0	74.3	49.0
Oregon	16,459	10,488	687	4,318	36.1	32.4	56.4	50.7
Pennsylvania	58,383	31,583	15,536	9,487	41.0	31.8	77.0	65.4
Rhode Island	4,918	2,419	529	1,657	45.4	36.8	62.2	64.1
South Carolina	27,261	10,571	13,860	2,438	47.3	31.4	77.5	52.5
South Dakota	4,632	2,441	169	331	37.7	26.8	49.7	54.9
Tennessee	35,911	18,818	13,252	3,492	44.0	33.9	78.0	50.0
Texas	166,754	38,063	30,463	95,943	41.7	27.0	63.5	50.6
Utah	9,497	5,313	217	3,166	18.6	13.5	37.9	40.8
Vermont	2,421	2,303	45	36	39.5	40.2	38.8	39.1
Virginia	35,066	13,963	13,910	6,499	33.9	23.3	64.3	48.2
Washington	28,450	15,202	2,232	7,806	32.1	27.2	47.9	49.5
West Virginia	9,111	8,280	572	168	44.9	43.9	75.1	48.0
Wisconsin	25,411	14,401	5,943	3,526	37.8	29.1	84.1	55.3
Wyoming	2,555	1,833	35	440	33.2	29.3	41.2	49.2
Puerto Rico	23,142	1,595	189	21,345	67.2	64.8	75.0	67.3
Virgin Islands	NA	NA	NA	NA	NA	NA	NA	NA
Guam	2,068	30	5	14	60.9	14.6	*	*
American Samoa	372	NA	NA	NA	34.5	NA	NA	NA
Northern Marianas	373	–	–	1	72.1	*	*	*

NA = Not available.   - = Quantity zero.   * = Figure does not meet standards of reliability or precision.   1 Includes races other than White and Black and origin not stated.   2 Race and Hispanic origin are reported separately on birth certificates. Persons of Hispanic origin may be of any race. Multiple-race data, when reported, were bridged to single-race categories in order to maintain comparability among all reported areas.   3 Includes all persons of Hispanic origin of any race.   4 Excludes data for the territories.

Table 1-39. Births, by Weight Gain of Mother During Pregnancy, by Plurality, Gestational Age, and Race and Hispanic Origin of Mother, 2014

(Number, percent distribution.)

Period of gestation[1], race, and Hispanic origin of mother	All births	Less than 11 pounds	11 to 20 pounds	21 to 30 pounds	31 to 40 pounds	41 to 98 pounds	Not stated
NUMBER							
All Pluralities							
All Gestational Ages [2]							
All races[3]	3,988,076	333,525	625,309	1,077,724	953,971	821,542	176,005
Non-Hispanic White[4]	2,149,302	148,782	282,206	570,534	562,523	502,600	82,657
Non-Hispanic Black[4]	588,891	72,375	103,321	139,224	114,805	121,221	37,945
Hispanic[5]	914,065	88,445	182,651	263,932	194,444	147,424	37,169
Under 37 Weeks							
All races[3]	381,321	48,893	77,458	97,012	69,557	65,093	23,308
Non-Hispanic White[4]	191,311	20,025	34,315	49,068	38,916	38,666	10,321
Non-Hispanic Black[4]	77,860	13,436	16,758	17,363	11,707	12,092	6,504
Hispanic[5]	82,459	12,046	19,892	21,995	13,597	10,558	4,371
37 Weeks and Over							
All races[3]	3,603,509	284,236	547,555	980,319	884,171	756,212	151,016
Non-Hispanic White[4]	1,956,803	128,592	247,760	521,295	523,490	463,817	71,849
Non-Hispanic Black[4]	510,519	58,844	86,510	121,796	103,065	109,088	31,216
Hispanic[5]	830,970	76,309	162,681	241,821	180,783	136,807	32,569
Live Births in Singleton Deliveries							
All Gestational Ages [2]							
All races[3]	3,848,214	324,953	610,703	1,051,621	921,931	770,206	168,800
Non-Hispanic White[4]	2,067,486	144,896	275,196	556,471	543,151	468,844	78,928
Non-Hispanic Black[4]	564,817	69,788	99,979	134,577	110,248	114,031	36,194
Hispanic[5]	891,426	86,874	179,618	258,955	189,163	140,651	36,165
Under 37 Weeks							
All races[3]	297,460	42,734	67,099	79,839	50,635	38,578	18,575
Non-Hispanic White[4]	142,627	17,235	29,282	39,706	27,442	21,089	7,873
Non-Hispanic Black[4]	62,741	11,583	14,339	14,292	8,905	8,302	5,320
Hispanic[5]	68,806	10,877	17,799	18,801	10,475	7,136	3,718
37 Weeks and Over							
All races[3]	3,547,586	42,734	67,099	79,839	50,635	38,578	18,575
Non-Hispanic White[4]	1,923,697	17,235	29,282	39,706	27,442	21,089	7,873
Non-Hispanic Black[4]	501,584	11,583	14,339	14,292	8,905	8,302	5,320
Hispanic[5]	822,002	10,877	17,799	18,801	10,475	7,136	3,718
PERCENT DISTRIBUTION							
All Pluralities							
All Gestational Ages [2]							
All races[3]	100.0	8.7	16.4	28.3	25.0	21.6	X
Non-Hispanic White[4]	100.0	7.2	13.7	27.6	27.2	24.3	X
Non-Hispanic Black[4]	100.0	13.1	18.8	25.3	20.8	22.0	X
Hispanic[5]	100.0	10.1	20.8	30.1	22.2	16.8	X
Under 37 Weeks							
All races[3]	100.0	13.7	21.6	27.1	19.4	18.2	X
Non-Hispanic White[4]	100.0	11.1	19.0	27.1	21.5	21.4	X
Non-Hispanic Black[4]	100.0	18.8	23.5	24.3	16.4	16.9	X
Hispanic[5]	100.0	15.4	25.5	28.2	17.4	13.5	X
37 Weeks and Over							
All races[3]	100.0	8.2	15.9	28.4	25.6	21.9	X
Non-Hispanic White[4]	100.0	6.8	13.1	27.7	27.8	24.6	X
Non-Hispanic Black[4]	100.0	12.3	18.0	25.4	21.5	22.8	X
Hispanic[5]	100.0	9.6	20.4	30.3	22.6	17.1	X
Live Births in Singleton Deliveries							
All Gestational Ages [2]							
All races[3]	100.0	8.8	16.6	28.6	25.1	20.9	X
Non-Hispanic White[4]	100.0	7.3	13.8	28.0	27.3	23.6	X
Non-Hispanic Black[4]	100.0	13.2	18.9	25.5	20.9	21.6	X
Hispanic[5]	100.0	10.2	21.0	30.3	22.1	16.4	X

Table 1-39. Births, by Weight Gain of Mother During Pregnancy, by Plurality, Gestational Age, and Race and Hispanic Origin of Mother, 2014— continued

(Number, percent distribution.)

Period of gestation[1], race, and Hispanic origin of mother	All births	Less than 11 pounds	11 to 20 pounds	21 to 30 pounds	31 to 40 pounds	41 to 98 pounds	Not stated
Under 37 Weeks							
All races[3]	100.0	15.3	24.1	28.6	18.2	13.8	X
Non-Hispanic White[4]	100.0	11.4	20.0	29.7	22.1	16.8	X
Non-Hispanic Black[4]	100.0	18.5	23.9	25.9	16.8	14.9	X
Hispanic[5]	100.0	14.0	25.8	29.8	18.2	12.2	X
37 Weeks and Over							
All races[3]	100.0	8.3	16.0	28.6	25.5	21.5	X
Non-Hispanic White[4]	100.0	6.9	13.3	27.9	27.8	24.2	X
Non-Hispanic Black[4]	100.0	12.3	18.2	25.5	21.5	22.4	X
Hispanic[5]	100.0	9.6	20.5	30.4	22.6	16.9	X

X = Not applicable.   1Expressed in completed weeks.   2Includes births with period of gestation not stated.   3Includes races other than White and Black and origin not stated.   4Race and Hispanic origin are reported separately on birth certificates. Persons of Hispanic origin may be of any race. Multiple-race data, when reported, were bridged to single-race categories in order to maintain comparability among all reported areas.   5Includes all persons of Hispanic origin of any race.

Table 1-40. Selected Risk Factors, Obstetric Procedures, Characteristics of Labor and Delivery, and Congenital Anomalies, by Age, Race, and Hispanic Origin of Mother, 2011

(Rates are number of live births with specified risk factors, procedures, or anomaly per 1,000 live births in specified group; congenital anomalies are per 100,000 live births.)

Risk factor, procedure, characteristic, and anomaly	All births[1]	Factor reported	Under 20 years	20 to 24 years	25 to 29 years	30 to 34 years	35 to 39 years	40 to 54 years	Not stated[2]
ALL RACES [3]									
Risk factors in This Pregnancy									
Diabetes	3,988,076	249,506	22.2	34.9	54.5	75.4	104.7	137.8	7,385
Hypertension, pregnancy-associated	3,988,076	201,994	54.2	49.1	49.1	49.1	54.7	70.0	7,385
Hypertension, chronic	3,988,076	63,044	5.6	9.0	13.2	18.4	27.1	42.0	7,385
Obstetric Procedures and Characteristics of Labor or Delivery									
Induction of labor	3,988,076	926,070	269.7	252.0	236.6	217.0	207.0	217.7	4,091
Breech/malpresentation	3,988,076	222,044	45.0	47.4	53.0	61.4	71.6	88.9	89,680
Congenital Anomalies									
Anencephaly	3,988,076	441	13.9	13.1	9.9	9.9	11.0	*	12,159
Meningomyelocele/Spina Bifida	3,988,076	554	13.5	14.5	14.8	14.0	10.8	*	12,159
Omphalocele/Gastroschisis	3,988,076	1,495	106.3	70.4	28.3	17.3	17.0	*	12,159
Cleft lip/palate	3,988,076	2,888	75.7	82.1	70.5	66.5	68.8	89.0	12,159
Down syndrome	3,988,076	1,978	28.3	27.6	24.6	37.8	114.2	336.5	12,159
NON-HISPANIC WHITE [4]									
Risk factors in This Pregnancy									
Diabetes									
Hypertension, pregnancy-associated	2,149,302	120,379	25.6	36.1	49.3	63.1	84.5	112.2	3,032
Hypertension, chronic	2,149,302	116,924	60.1	54.2	54.4	51.8	55.8	70.0	3,032
	2,149,302	32,105	6.0	8.9	12.8	16.8	23.6	36.0	3,032
Obstetric Procedures and Characteristics of Labor or Delivery									
Induction of labor									
Breech/malpresentation	2,149,302	562,932	333.0	297.6	267.2	238.9	228.8	244.8	1,531
	2,149,302	116,954	42.0	44.9	51.7	60.0	68.9	85.5	43,882
Congenital Anomalies									
Anencephaly									
Meningomyelocele/Spina Bifida	2,149,302	243	*	11.4	11.0	10.1	13.6	*	5,044
Omphalocele/Gastroschisis	2,149,302	362	*	19.8	18.1	15.6	11.8	*	5,044
Cleft lip/palate	2,149,302	898	123.4	89.0	34.9	18.1	17.9	*	5,044
Down syndrome	2,149,302	1,858	100.3	105.4	83.1	78.2	78.9	96.8	5,044
	2,149,302	1,208	29.1	32.4	28.4	43.1	123.5	397.4	5,044
NON-HISPANIC BLACK [4]									
Risk factors in This Pregnancy									
Diabetes	588,891	32,581	18.0	29.4	52.5	80.6	108.9	142.0	1,859
Hypertension, pregnancy-associated	588,891	36,335	62.5	56.6	58.5	65.7	72.8	88.5	1,859
Hypertension, chronic	588,891	18,631	8.9	15.4	28.0	45.8	70.0	97.5	1,859
Obstetric Procedures and Characteristics of Labor or Delivery									
Induction of labor	588,891	131,483	258.3	230.7	219.3	211.6	208.3	212.6	1,255
Breech/malpresentation	588,891	33,326	45.0	50.3	56.1	65.1	79.0	94.6	16,580
Congenital Anomalies									
Anencephaly	588,891	62	*	12.7	*	*	*	*	3,318
Meningomyelocele/Spina Bifida	588,891	60	*	*	*	*	*	*	3,318
Omphalocele/Gastroschisis	588,891	182	77.5	38.0	18.7	22.4	*	*	3,318
Cleft lip/palate	588,891	241	43.3	44.6	36.2	38.7	47.1	*	3,318
Down syndrome	588,891	202	*	24.2	17.5	31.0	75.1	219.1	3,318
HISPANIC [5]									
Risk factors in This Pregnancy									
Diabetes	914,065	62,970	19.9	34.4	59.6	93.1	135.1	175.0	1,581
Hypertension, pregnancy-associated	914,065	37,164	42.7	36.7	36.5	41.3	50.4	66.4	1,581
Hypertension, chronic	914,065	9,034	3.2	5.0	7.6	13.0	20.0	33.0	1,581
Obstetric Procedures and Characteristics of Labor or Delivery									
Induction of labor	914,065	170,312	210.2	196.9	182.7	175.2	174.4	186.0	792
Breech/malpresentation	914,065	51,294	48.1	49.1	54.0	63.2	73.2	86.7	21,232
Congenital Anomalies									
Anencephaly	914,065	105	*	14.7	9.3	10.3	*	*	2,329
Meningomyelocele/Spina Bifida	914,065	107	*	9.2	12.9	11.3	*	*	2,329
Omphalocele/Gastroschisis	914,065	322	101.4	57.0	20.5	14.2	*	*	2,329
Cleft lip/palate	914,065	547	68.0	67.5	56.0	45.7	60.6	111.1	2,329
Down syndrome	914,065	455	26.5	23.5	22.5	32.9	138.9	385.3	2,329

* = Figure does not meet standards of reliability or precision; precision; based on fewer than 20 births in the numerator.   1 Total number of births to residents of areas reporting risk factors, procedure or anomaly.   2 No response reported for specific item.   3 Includes races not shown.   4 Race and Hispanic origin are reported separately on birth certificates. Multiple-race data, when reported, were bridged to single-race categories in order to maintain comparability among all reported areas.   5 Includes all persons of Hispanic origin of any race.

Table 1-41. Births Delivered by Forceps or Vacuum Extraction, Selected Years, 1990–2014

(Percent.)

Year and type of birth	Forceps	Vacuum extraction	Forceps or vacuum
All Births			
1990 [1]	5.1	3.9	9.0
1995	3.5	5.9	9.4
2000	2.1	4.9	7.0
1005	0.9	3.9	4.8
2007	0.8	3.5	4.2
2008	0.7	3.2	3.9
2009	0.7	3.0	3.7
2010	0.7	3.0	3.6
2011	0.7	2.9	3.5
2012	0.6	2.8	3.4
2013	0.6	2.7	3.2
2014	0.6	2.6	3.2

1 Excludes data for Oklahoma, which did not require reporting method of delivery.

Table 1-42. Births, by Method of Delivery and Race and Hispanic Origin of Mother, 1989–2014

(Number, rate.)

Year	All births	Vaginal — Number				Cesarean — Number				Cesarean — Percentage of all live births by cesarean delivery			
		Total[1]	Non-Hispanic White[2]	Non-Hispanic Black[2]	Hispanic[3]	Total[1]	Non-Hispanic White[2]	Non-Hispanic Black[2]	Hispanic[3]	Total[1]	Non-Hispanic White[2]	Non-Hispanic Black[2]	Hispanic[3]
1989[4]	3,798,734	2,793,463	1,806,753	440,310	385,462	826,955	556,585	125,290	105,268	22.8	23.6	22.2	21.5
1990[5]	4,110,563	3,111,421	1,972,754	503,720	458,242	914,096	603,467	142,838	122,969	22.7	23.4	22.1	21.2
1991[6]	4,110,907	3,100,891	1,941,726	507,522	472,126	905,077	587,802	142,417	129,752	22.6	23.2	21.9	21.6
1992[6]	4,065,014	3,100,710	1,916,414	502,669	494,338	888,622	566,788	143,153	133,369	22.3	22.8	22.2	21.2
1993	4,000,240	3,098,796	1,902,433	496,333	514,493	861,987	542,013	139,702	136,279	21.8	22.2	22.0	20.9
1994	3,952,767	3,087,576	1,896,609	480,551	525,928	830,517	518,021	134,526	135,569	21.2	21.5	21.9	20.5
1995	3,899,589	3,063,724	1,867,024	457,104	539,731	806,722	496,103	127,171	136,640	20.8	21.0	21.8	20.2
1996	3,891,494	3,061,092	1,851,058	449,544	558,105	797,119	485,530	124,836	139,554	20.7	20.8	21.7	20.0
1997	3,880,894	3,046,621	1,829,213	451,744	563,114	799,033	481,982	126,138	142,907	20.8	20.9	21.8	20.2
1998	3,941,553	3,078,537	1,842,420	457,186	580,143	825,870	495,550	131,999	150,317	21.2	21.2	22.4	20.6
1999	3,959,417	3,063,870	1,810,682	449,580	599,118	862,086	514,051	135,508	161,035	22.0	22.1	23.2	21.2
2000	4,058,814	3,108,188	1,804,550	454,736	633,220	923,991	540,794	146,042	179,583	22.9	23.1	24.3	22.1
2001	4,025,933	3,027,993	1,746,551	435,455	648,821	978,411	567,488	151,908	199,874	24.4	24.5	25.9	23.6
2002	4,021,726	2,958,423	1,687,144	416,516	653,516	1,043,846	598,682	159,297	219,777	26.1	26.2	27.7	25.2
2003	4,089,950	2,949,853	1,671,414	405,671	667,656	1,119,388	637,482	167,506	241,159	27.5	27.6	29.2	26.5
2004	4,112,052	2,903,341	1,617,994	397,877	679,118	1,190,210	667,836	178,461	263,454	29.1	29.2	31.0	28.0
2005	4,138,349	2,873,918	1,579,613	392,064	698,089	1,248,815	690,260	189,287	285,376	30.3	30.4	32.6	29.0
2006	4,265,555	2,929,590	1,580,794	411,097	728,854	1,321,054	718,960	203,723	307,981	31.1	31.3	33.1	29.7
2007	4,316,233	2,933,056	1,565,555	413,088	737,478	1,367,340	735,744	211,615	322,554	31.8	32.0	33.9	30.4
2008	4,247,694	2,864,343	1,527,340	406,379	716,811	1,369,273	732,641	214,416	321,859	32.3	32.4	34.5	31.0
2009	4,130,665	2,764,285	1,481,660	392,715	682,512	1,353,572	723,687	214,810	315,025	32.9	32.8	35.4	31.6
2010	3,999,386	2,680,947	1,454,861	379,617	643,682	1,309,182	702,548	208,520	300,138	32.8	32.6	35.5	31.8
2011	3,953,590	2,651,428	1,447,969	374,978	623,010	1,293,267	693,591	206,009	293,816	32.8	32.4	35.5	32.0
2012	3,952,841	2,650,744	1,441,894	374,035	615,095	1,296,070	688,932	208,562	291,637	32.8	32.3	35.8	32.2
2013	3,932,181	2,642,892	1,446,270	374,054	610,196	1,284,339	680,521	209,015	290,016	32.7	32.0	35.8	32.2
2014	3,988,076	2,699,951	1,473,298	379,055	622,033	1,284,551	674,254	209,361	291,520	32.2	31.4	35.6	31.9

1 Includes races other than White and Black and origin not stated.   2 Race and Hispanic origin are reported separately on birth certificates. Persons of Hispanic origin may be of any race. Multiple-race data, when reported, were bridged to single-race categories in order to maintain comparability among all reported areas.   3 Includes all persons of Hispanic origin of any race.   4 Excludes data for Louisiana, Maryland, Nebraska, Nevada, and Oklahoma, which did not report method of delivery on the birth certificate; data by Hispanic origin also excludes New Hampshire, which did not report Hispanic origin.   5 Excludes data for New Hampshire and Oklahoma, which did not report data by Hispanic origin. Oklahoma did not report method of delivery.   6 Excludes data for New Hampshire, which did not report Hispanic origin.

Table 1-43. Births, by Method of Delivery and Age, Race, and Hispanic Origin of Mother, 2014

(Number; rate of cesarean delivery.)

Age, race, and Hispanic origin of mother	Number				Cesarean delivery rate[1]
	All births	Vaginal	Cesarean	Not stated	
All Races [2]	3,988,076	2,699,951	1,284,551	3,574	32.2
Under 20 years	251,847	198,899	52,825	123	21.0
20 to 24 years	882,567	644,568	237,279	720	26.9
25 to 29 years	1,145,392	793,120	351,313	959	30.7
30 to 34 years	1,081,058	703,447	376,574	1,037	34.9
35 to 39 years	508,748	299,641	208,551	556	41.0
40 years and over	118,464	60,276	58,009	179	49.0
Non-Hispanic White [3]	2,149,302	1,473,298	674,254	1,750	31.4
Under 20 years	99,899	78,808	21,047	44	21.1
20 to 24 years	420,224	310,106	109,781	337	26.1
25 to 29 years	646,097	456,308	189,334	455	29.3
30 to 34 years	642,219	426,603	215,061	555	33.5
35 to 39 years	280,788	170,052	110,460	276	39.4
40 years and over	60,075	31,421	28,571	83	47.6
Non-Hispanic Black [3]	588,891	379,055	209,361	475	35.6
Under 20 years	55,774	42,793	12,952	29	23.2
20 to 24 years	182,435	126,866	55,459	110	30.4
25 to 29 years	160,935	102,923	57,883	129	36.0
30 to 34 years	116,939	69,123	47,696	120	40.8
35 to 39 years	57,647	30,465	27,115	67	47.1
40 years and over	15,161	6,885	8,256	20	54.5
Hispanic [4]	914,065	622,033	291,520	512	31.9
Under 20 years	87,007	69,739	17,229	39	19.8
20 to 24 years	239,121	175,971	63,056	94	26.4
25 to 29 years	248,971	169,931	78,898	142	31.7
30 to 34 years	204,232	130,095	74,001	136	36.3
35 to 39 years	107,644	62,341	45,225	78	42.0
40 years and over	27,090	13,956	13,111	23	48.4

1 Percentage of all live births by cesarean delivery.   2 Includes races other than White and Black and origin not stated.   3 Race and Hispanic origin are reported separately on birth certificates. Persons of Hispanic origin may be of any race. Multiple-race data, when reported, were bridged to single-race categories in order to maintain comparability among all reported areas.   4 Includes all persons of Hispanic origin of any race.

Table 1-44. Cesarean Deliveries, by Race and Hispanic Origin of Mother, by State and Territory of Residence, 2014

(Percent.)

State and territory	Total cesarean delivery rate[1]				Low-risk cesarean delivery rate[2]			
	All races[3]	Non-Hispanic		Hispanic[5]	All races[3]	Non-Hispanic		Hispanic[5]
		White[4]	Black[4]			White[4]	Black[4]	
United States [6]	32.2	31.4	35.6	31.9	26.0	25.0	29.9	25.8
Alabama	35.4	35.4	37.0	28.3	29.7	29.1	32.4	23.7
Alaska	23.7	25.3	33.3	28.7	20.8	21.9	31.3	26.2
Arizona	27.8	28.9	33.1	26.2	22.1	22.7	28.1	20.7
Arkansas	32.0	32.0	33.4	29.9	24.2	24.0	24.9	23.7
California	32.7	31.5	37.8	32.2	25.5	25.0	29.8	24.8
Colorado	25.6	26.1	27.7	23.5	20.4	20.5	23.6	18.5
Connecticut	34.2	34.3	36.8	32.3	28.2	28.0	30.4	26.0
Delaware	31.5	31.6	32.7	28.7	25.5	24.8	28.0	22.4
District of Columbia	32.8	31.3	34.7	28.9	27.9	26.2	29.8	24.9
Florida	37.2	34.2	38.3	41.0	31.0	27.7	31.9	36.1
Georgia	33.8	33.9	35.7	29.0	27.4	26.9	29.2	24.5
Hawaii	24.6	22.6	30.9	25.5	17.9	16.4	23.2	19.3
Idaho	24.2	23.7	27.5	25.9	19.3	18.8	*	22.1
Illinois	31.2	31.7	31.9	28.6	24.6	24.5	25.5	23.1
Indiana	30.3	30.1	32.4	28.7	24.0	23.6	25.8	23.4
Iowa	30.0	29.7	32.0	31.1	23.7	23.2	26.7	24.2
Kansas	29.8	30.0	31.8	27.6	23.5	23.5	25.4	22.3
Kentucky	35.1	35.0	37.3	32.2	28.8	28.4	31.9	27.1
Louisiana	38.3	39.1	38.0	34.5	30.9	31.2	30.7	29.2
Maine	29.8	29.8	29.6	28.0	22.4	22.1	28.7	*
Maryland	34.9	32.8	39.3	31.3	29.8	27.4	34.2	27.5
Massachusetts	31.6	31.8	34.7	30.0	23.8	23.9	28.5	20.8
Michigan	32.8	32.7	33.2	31.1	27.0	26.4	28.5	27.0
Minnesota	26.5	27.2	26.8	24.5	21.1	20.9	24.3	19.2
Mississippi	37.7	37.9	38.3	30.6	31.5	31.2	32.3	26.2
Missouri	30.1	29.8	31.3	29.6	23.6	22.8	27.0	23.5
Montana	31.4	30.8	24.4	32.2	26.4	25.8	*	27.0
Nebraska	30.8	31.4	29.9	28.7	23.6	23.4	25.6	22.7
Nevada	34.4	34.1	41.4	32.1	28.7	27.9	37.1	25.8
New Hampshire	29.9	29.8	25.4	31.3	23.5	23.2	*	23.4
New Jersey	37.4	36.0	39.9	37.4	31.6	30.5	33.9	31.6
New Mexico	23.8	23.9	30.6	24.1	17.0	18.2	21.7	16.3
New York	33.9	32.2	38.4	34.5	28.4	27.0	33.4	28.3
North Carolina	29.5	30.0	32.0	23.8	22.7	22.0	26.2	18.9
North Dakota	27.6	27.1	26.5	28.3	21.2	20.3	28.7	23.4
Ohio	30.5	30.3	32.1	29.4	24.3	23.6	27.3	25.0
Oklahoma	33.1	33.7	35.1	30.1	25.1	25.5	28.8	22.6
Oregon	27.4	27.2	33.0	26.6	21.9	21.6	23.8	21.4
Pennsylvania	30.4	30.3	31.2	30.5	25.1	24.7	27.7	24.5
Rhode Island	30.7	31.6	30.6	29.5	25.8	27.0	27.9	22.4
South Carolina	34.3	33.8	36.8	28.6	27.7	26.7	30.6	24.0
South Dakota	24.8	24.0	27.4	26.5	19.3	18.9	*	22.0
Tennessee	33.7	33.6	35.5	29.5	28.2	27.5	31.1	24.2
Texas	34.9	34.7	38.6	34.0	28.0	27.6	32.4	27.0
Utah	22.3	21.6	25.5	23.3	17.6	16.9	25.3	18.2
Vermont	25.8	25.6	28.4	27.2	20.1	19.8	*	*
Virginia	33.1	31.8	36.0	31.4	25.9	23.4	30.1	26.9
Washington	27.6	26.6	32.2	26.7	22.7	21.3	27.6	22.0
West Virginia	35.4	35.5	34.5	32.1	25.4	25.4	27.5	20.5
Wisconsin	26.1	26.6	25.6	25.7	21.2	21.0	23.2	20.4
Wyoming	27.8	26.8	35.3	32.8	21.4	21.0	*	25.3
Puerto Rico	48.0	46.7	42.1	48.2	42.2	40.3	35.2	42.4
Virgin Islands	NA	NA	NA	NA	NA	NA	NA	NA
Guam	23.2	17.7	*	*	*	*	*	*
American Samoa	NA	NA	NA	NA	NA	NA	NA	NA
Northern Marianas	23.0	*	*	*	*	*	*	*

NA = Not available.   * = Figure does not meet standards of reliability or precision; based on fewer than 20 births in the numerator.   1 Percent of all live births by cesarean delivery.   2 Low-risk cesarean is defined as singleton, term (37 or more weeks of gestation), vertex (not breech) cesarean deliveries to women having a first birth per 100 women delivering singleton, term, vertex first births.   3 Includes races other than White and Black and origin not stated.   4 Race and Hispanic origin are reported separately on birth certificates. Persons of Hispanic origin may be of any race. Multiple-race data, when reported, were bridged to single-race categories in order to maintain comparability among all reported areas.   5 Includes all persons of Hispanic origin of any race.   6Excludes data for the territories.

Table 1-45. Births, by Birthweight, Gestational Age, and Race and Hispanic Origin of Mother, 2014

(Number, percent.)

Birthweight[1], race, and Hispanic origin of mother	All births	Period of gestation[2]										Not stated
		Preterm					Term				Post-term	
		Total under 37 weeks	Under 28 weeks	28 to 31 weeks	32 to 33 weeks	34 to 36 weeks	Total, 37 to 41 weeks	37 to 38 weeks	39 weeks	40 to 41 weeks	42 weeks and over	
ALL RACES [3]												
Total	3,988,076	381,321	27,320	36,245	45,909	271,847	3,586,933	986,745	2,339,796	260,392	16,576	3,246
Less than 500 grams	5,936	5,881	5,804	69	2	6	5	4	1	–	–	50
500 to 999 grams	20,721	20,612	16,415	3,868	262	67	74	26	44	4	–	35
1,000 to 1,499 grams	29,290	28,522	3,769	17,896	4,798	2,059	736	364	345	27	5	27
1,500 to 1,999 grams	61,992	56,045	155	11,689	21,194	23,007	5,867	4,807	985	75	20	60
2,000 to 2,499 grams	200,908	109,032	88	1,514	15,748	91,682	91,583	69,154	21,655	774	85	208
2,500 to 2,999 grams	727,987	106,432	87	453	2,765	103,127	620,079	306,171	299,305	14,603	896	580
3,000 to 3,499 grams	1,546,274	41,800	–	413	746	40,641	1,499,005	406,977	1,005,253	86,775	4,580	889
3,500 to 3,999 grams	1,071,007	9,187	–	218	228	8,741	1,054,510	162,733	781,822	109,955	6,772	538
4,000 to 4,499 grams	276,592	1,841	–	–	48	1,793	271,277	30,065	200,368	40,844	3,345	129
4,500 to 4,999 grams	39,353	432	–	–	9	423	38,160	5,011	26,536	6,613	742	19
5,000 grams or more	4,746	126	–	–	8	118	4,496	1,117	2,777	602	114	10
Not stated	3,270	1,411	1,002	125	101	183	1,141	316	705	120	17	701
Percent												
Very low birthweight[4]	1.4	14.5	98.7	60.4	11.1	0.8	0.0	0.0	0.0	0.0	0.0	4.4
Low birthweight[5]	8.0	57.9	99.7	97.0	91.7	43.0	2.7	7.5	1.0	0.3	0.7	14.9
NON-HISPANIC WHITE [6]												
Total	2,149,302	191,311	10,646	16,974	22,996	140,695	1,946,215	495,474	1,293,001	157,740	10,588	1,188
Less than 500 grams	2,118	2,100	2,063	31	2	4	2	2	–	–	–	16
500 to 999 grams	8,206	8,154	6,376	1,621	120	37	43	15	26	2	–	9
1,000 to 1,499 grams	13,308	12,919	1,690	8,042	2,195	992	374	179	178	17	3	12
1,500 to 1,999 grams	29,947	27,111	64	5,938	10,380	10,729	2,806	2,322	446	38	7	23
2,000 to 2,499 grams	95,995	54,679	40	776	8,365	45,498	41,180	31,301	9,498	381	39	97
2,500 to 2,999 grams	340,534	56,306	37	186	1,391	54,692	283,547	140,662	135,757	7,128	450	231
3,000 to 3,499 grams	807,151	23,152	–	191	349	22,612	781,037	207,707	525,483	47,847	2,603	359
3,500 to 3,999 grams	641,453	4,988	–	112	97	4,779	631,776	92,358	470,421	68,997	4,438	251
4,000 to 4,499 grams	180,378	987	–	–	24	963	176,947	17,423	131,428	28,096	2,377	67
4,500 to 4,999 grams	25,897	217	–	–	4	213	25,097	2,762	17,622	4,713	569	14
5,000 grams or more	2,859	69	–	–	3	66	2,696	555	1,697	444	90	4
Not stated	1,456	629	376	77	66	110	710	188	445	77	12	105
Percent												
Very low birthweight[4]	1.1	12.2	98.6	57.4	10.1	0.7	0.0	0.0	0.0	0.0	0.0	3.4
Low birthweight[5]	7.0	55.0	99.6	97.1	91.9	40.7	2.3	6.8	0.8	0.3	0.5	14.5
NON-HISPANIC BLACK [6]												
Total	588,891	77,860	9,045	9,105	9,882	49,828	508,502	160,090	317,267	31,145	2,017	512
Less than 500 grams	2,187	2,172	2,150	20	–	2	3	2	1	–	–	12
500 to 999 grams	6,837	6,813	5,447	1,277	72	17	11	4	7	–	–	13
1,000 to 1,499 grams	7,845	7,677	956	4,915	1,320	486	159	87	67	5	–	9
1,500 to 1,999 grams	14,742	13,265	47	2,389	5,110	5,719	1,457	1,197	246	14	3	17
2,000 to 2,499 grams	45,844	22,935	25	277	2,743	19,890	22,842	17,101	5,566	175	23	44
2,500 to 2,999 grams	145,566	17,601	20	103	442	17,036	127,690	61,467	63,349	2,874	156	119
3,000 to 3,499 grams	227,376	5,511	–	76	121	5,314	221,002	58,656	149,549	12,797	699	164
3,500 to 3,999 grams	111,315	1,122	–	22	41	1,059	109,360	17,672	80,185	11,503	776	57
4,000 to 4,499 grams	22,778	217	–	–	6	211	22,251	3,099	15,869	3,283	301	9
4,500 to 4,999 grams	3,209	48	–	–	2	46	3,111	611	2,052	448	50	–
5,000 grams or more	465	13	–	–	3	10	442	135	270	37	9	1
Not stated	727	486	400	26	22	38	174	59	106	9	–	67
Percent												
Very low birthweight[4]	2.9	21.5	98.9	68.4	14.1	1.0	0.0	0.1	0.0	0.0	0.0	7.6
Low birthweight[5]	13.2	68.3	99.8	97.8	93.8	52.4	4.8	11.5	1.9	0.6	1.3	21.3
HISPANIC [7]												
Total	914,065	82,459	5,722	7,491	9,636	59,610	828,013	241,191	534,789	52,033	2,957	636
Less than 500 grams	1,152	1,134	1,121	13	–	–	–	–	–	–	–	18
500 to 999 grams	4,311	4,287	3,537	690	51	9	16	6	10	–	–	8
1,000 to 1,499 grams	5,774	5,614	830	3,536	869	379	155	76	74	5	2	3
1,500 to 1,999 grams	12,332	11,212	41	2,561	4,156	4,454	1,103	859	225	19	6	11
2,000 to 2,499 grams	40,855	22,574	17	376	3,513	18,668	18,229	13,705	4,375	149	15	37
2,500 to 2,999 grams	167,417	24,125	23	127	728	23,247	142,955	72,135	67,793	3,027	216	121
3,000 to 3,499 grams	373,521	10,140	–	111	222	9,807	362,206	104,398	239,239	18,569	946	229
3,500 to 3,999 grams	242,122	2,489	–	68	76	2,345	238,338	40,732	175,709	21,897	1,170	125
4,000 to 4,499 grams	57,020	516	–	–	10	506	55,970	7,581	41,253	7,136	502	32

Table 1-45. Births, by Birthweight, Gestational Age, and Race and Hispanic Origin of Mother, 2014— continued

(Number, percent.)

Birthweight[1], race, and Hispanic origin of mother	All births	Period of gestation[2]										Not stated
		Preterm					Term				Post-term	
		Total under 37 weeks	Under 28 weeks	28 to 31 weeks	32 to 33 weeks	34 to 36 weeks	Total, 37 to 41 weeks	37 to 38 weeks	39 weeks	40 to 41 weeks	42 weeks and over	
4,500 to 4,999 grams	8,058	140	–	–	3	137	7,826	1,317	5,398	1,111	89	3
5,000 grams or more	1,097	34	–	–	1	33	1,050	335	620	95	10	3
Not stated	406	194	153	9	7	25	165	47	93	25	1	46
Percent												
Very low birthweight[4]	1.2	13.4	98.5	56.7	9.6	0.7	0.0	0.0	0.0	0.0	0.1	4.9
Low birthweight[5]	7.1	54.5	99.6	95.9	89.2	39.5	2.4	6.1	0.9	0.3	0.8	13.1

– = Quantity zero.   0.0 = Quantity more than zero but less than 0.05.   1 Equivalents of the gram weights in pounds and ounces are shown in Notes.   2 Expressed in completed weeks.   3 Includes races other than White and Black and origin not stated.   4 Birthweight of less than 1,500 grams (3 lb 4 oz).   5 Birthweight of less than 2,500 grams (5 lb 8 oz).   6 Race and Hispanic origin are reported separately on birth certificates. Persons of Hispanic origin may be of any race. Multiple-race data, when reported, were bridged to single-race categories in order to maintain comparability among all reported areas.   7 Includes all persons of Hispanic origin of any race.

Figure 1-9. Cesarean Deliveries, by Age of Mother, 2014

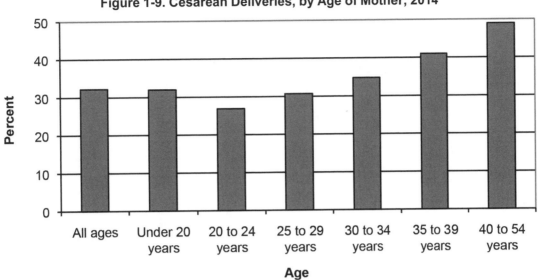

Figure 1-10. Percent of Birth with Low and Very Low Birth Weights, Selected Years, 1986–2011

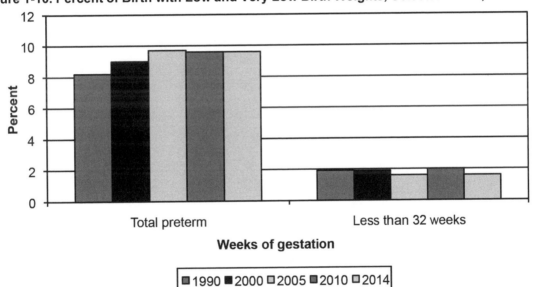

Table 1-46A. Very Preterm and Preterm Births and Very Low Birthweight and Low Birthweight Births, by Race and Hispanic Origin of Mother, 2007–2014

(Percent.)

Year	Very preterm[1]				Preterm[2]			
	All races[3]	Non-Hispanic		Hispanic[5]	All races[3]	Non-Hispanic		Hispanic[5]
		White[4]	Black[4]			White[4]	Black[4]	
2007	1.71	1.39	3.48	1.46	10.44	9.90	14.71	9.35
2008	1.67	1.37	3.26	1.43	10.36	9.81	14.38	9.38
2009	1.65	1.35	3.28	1.41	10.07	9.50	14.05	9.12
2010	1.65	1.36	3.20	1.41	9.98	9.41	13.81	9.09
2011	1.64	1.33	3.20	1.42	9.81	9.21	13.54	9.02
2012	1.63	1.32	3.19	1.45	9.76	9.13	13.48	9.09
2013	1.62	1.31	3.16	1.44	9.62	8.94	13.25	9.08
2014	1.60	1.29	3.08	1.45	9.57	8.91	13.23	9.03

Table 1-46B. Very Preterm and Preterm Births and Very Low Birthweight and Low Birthweight Births, by Race and Hispanic Origin of Mother, 1989–2014

(Percent.)

Year	Very low birthweight[6]				Low birthweight[7]			
	All races[3]	Non-Hispanic		Hispanic[5]	All races[3]	Non-Hispanic		Hispanic[5]
		White[4]	Black[4]			White[4]	Black[4]	
1989 [8]	1.28	0.93	2.97	1.05	7.05	5.62	13.61	6.18
1990 [9]	1.27	0.93	2.93	1.03	6.97	5.61	13.32	6.06
1991 [10]	1.29	0.94	2.97	1.02	7.12	5.72	13.62	6.15
1992 [10]	1.29	0.94	2.97	1.04	7.08	5.73	13.40	6.10
1993	1.33	1.00	2.99	1.06	7.22	5.92	13.43	6.24
1994	1.33	1.01	2.99	1.08	7.28	6.06	13.34	6.25
1995	1.35	1.04	2.98	1.11	7.32	6.20	13.21	6.29
1996	1.37	1.08	3.02	1.12	7.39	6.36	13.12	6.28
1997	1.42	1.12	3.05	1.13	7.51	6.47	13.11	6.42
1998	1.45	1.15	3.11	1.15	7.57	6.55	13.17	6.44
1999	1.45	1.15	3.18	1.14	7.62	6.64	13.23	6.38
2000	1.43	1.14	3.10	1.14	7.57	6.60	13.13	6.41
2001	1.44	1.17	3.08	1.14	7.68	6.76	13.07	6.47
2002	1.46	1.17	3.15	1.17	7.82	6.91	13.39	6.55
2003	1.45	1.18	3.12	1.16	7.93	7.04	13.55	6.69
2004	1.48	1.20	3.15	1.20	8.08	7.20	13.74	6.79
2005	1.49	1.21	3.27	1.20	8.19	7.29	14.02	6.88
2006	1.49	1.20	3.15	1.19	8.26	7.32	13.97	6.99
2007	1.49	1.19	3.20	1.21	8.22	7.28	13.90	6.93
2008	1.46	1.18	3.01	1.20	8.18	7.22	13.71	6.96
2009	1.45	1.16	3.06	1.19	8.16	7.19	13.61	6.94
2010	1.45	1.16	2.98	1.20	8.15	7.14	13.53	6.97
2011	1.44	1.14	2.99	1.20	8.10	7.09	13.33	7.02
2012	1.42	1.13	2.94	1.22	7.99	6.97	13.18	6.97
2013	1.41	1.11	2.90	1.21	8.02	6.98	13.08	7.09
2014	1.40	1.10	2.86	1.23	8.00	6.96	13.15	7.05

NA = Not available.   1Births of less than 32 completed weeks of gestation.   2Births of less than 37 completed weeks of gestation.   3Includes races other than White and Black and origin not stated.   4Race and Hispanic origin are reported separately on birth certificates. Persons of Hispanic origin may be of any race. Multiple-race data, when reported, were bridged to single-race categories in order to maintain comparability among all reported areas.   5Includes all persons of Hispanic origin of any race.   6Less than 1,500 grams (3 lb. 4 oz.).   7Less than 2,500 grams (5 lb. 8 oz.).   8Data by Hispanic origin exclude New Hampshire, Oklahoma, and Louisiana, which did not report Hispanic origin.   9Data by Hispanic origin exclude New Hampshire and Oklahoma, which did not report Hispanic origin.   10Data by Hispanic origin exclude New Hampshire, which did not report Hispanic origin.

Table 1-47. Birthweight Distribution in 500-Gram Intervals, Selected Years, 1990–2014

(Percent.)

Weight	All births					Percent change		
	1990	2006	2008	2009	2014	1990–2009	1990–2014	2009–2014
Less than 1,000 grams	0.63	0.72	0.70	0.70	0.67	11.1	6.1	-4.5
1,000–1,499 grams	0.65	0.76	0.75	0.75	0.73	15.4	13.0	-2.1
1,500–1,999 grams	1.33	1.63	1.58	1.59	1.55	19.5	16.9	-2.2
2,000–2,499 grams	4.37	5.15	5.14	5.12	5.04	17.2	15.3	-1.6
2,500–2,999 grams	16.03	18.44	18.57	18.59	18.25	16.0	13.9	-1.8
3,000–3,499 grams	36.71	38.87	39.20	39.22	38.77	6.8	5.6	-1.1
3,500–3,999 grams	29.40	26.61	26.41	26.43	26.86	-10.1	-8.7	1.6
4,000–4,499 grams	9.10	6.75	6.60	6.57	6.94	-27.8	-23.8	5.6
4,500–4,999 grams	1.59	0.96	0.92	0.92	0.99	-42.1	-37.9	7.3
5,000 grams or more	0.19	0.11	0.10	0.10	0.12	-47.4	-37.4	19.0

Note: Totals do not sum to 100 due to rounding.

Table 1-48. Preterm and Low Birthweight Births, by Age and Race and Hispanic Origin of Mother, 2014

(Percent, number.)

Age, race, and Hispanic origin of mother	Preterm[1] Percent			Preterm[1] Number				Low birthweight[2] Percent			Low birthweight[2] Number			
	Total	Early[3]	Late[4]	Total	Early[3]	Late[4]	Unknown	Total	Very[5]	Moderately[6]	Total	Very[5]	Moderately[6]	Unknown
All Races[7]														
All ages	9.57	2.75	6.82	381,321	109,474	271,847	5,469	8.00	1.40	6.60	318,847	55,947	262,900	3,270
Under 15 years	14.04	4.75	9.29	387	131	256	11	11.16	2.93	8.24	309	81	228	1
15 to 19 years	9.82	3.00	6.82	24,431	7,471	16,960	384	9.30	1.66	7.64	23,146	4,138	19,008	190
15 years	11.78	4.15	7.63	951	335	616	27	10.70	2.18	8.52	864	176	688	10
16 years	10.18	3.29	6.88	2,048	663	1,385	38	9.54	1.82	7.73	1,922	366	1,556	21
17 years	9.91	3.02	6.89	3,815	1,162	2,653	53	9.40	1.71	7.70	3,622	657	2,965	24
18 years	9.95	3.05	6.91	6,900	2,113	4,787	106	9.31	1.72	7.60	6,455	1,189	5,266	53
19 years	9.50	2.83	6.66	10,717	3,198	7,519	160	9.11	1.55	7.56	10,283	1,750	8,533	82
20 to 24 years	9.17	2.64	6.52	80,817	23,289	57,528	1,179	8.25	1.39	6.86	72,780	12,272	60,508	719
25 to 29 years	8.90	2.50	6.40	101,883	28,624	73,259	1,409	7.36	1.27	6.09	84,262	14,524	69,738	931
30 to 34 years	9.36	2.64	6.71	101,074	28,566	72,508	1,475	7.45	1.30	6.15	80,524	14,089	66,435	858
35 to 39 years	11.01	3.18	7.82	55,949	16,188	39,761	772	8.67	1.61	7.06	44,086	8,180	35,906	438
40 to 44 years	13.41	4.11	9.30	14,737	4,515	10,222	216	10.94	2.13	8.81	12,021	2,342	9,679	124
45 to 54 years	24.23	8.19	16.05	2,043	690	1,353	23	20.38	3.81	16.58	1,719	321	1,398	9
Non-Hispanic White[8]														
All ages	8.91	2.36	6.55	191,311	50,616	140,695	2,318	6.96	1.10	5.86	149,574	23,632	125,942	1,456
Under 15 years	12.83	5.01	7.82	87	34	53	6	10.16	2.95	7.22	69	20	49	–
15 to 19 years	9.55	2.81	6.75	9,469	2,781	6,688	135	8.18	1.48	6.70	8,112	1,467	6,645	69
15 years	11.77	4.10	7.67	267	93	174	9	9.07	1.98	7.09	206	45	161	6
16 years	10.08	3.26	6.82	649	210	439	14	8.45	1.59	6.87	544	102	442	10
17 years	9.81	2.81	7.00	1,357	389	968	14	8.02	1.54	6.48	1,110	213	897	10
18 years	9.67	2.91	6.76	2,693	810	1,883	37	8.35	1.59	6.76	2,326	444	1,882	17
19 years	9.24	2.62	6.61	4,503	1,279	3,224	61	8.05	1.36	6.69	3,926	663	3,263	26
20 to 24 years	8.57	2.27	6.31	36,006	9,513	26,493	437	7.11	1.09	6.02	29,855	4,587	25,268	265
25 to 29 years	8.29	2.15	6.15	53,557	13,872	39,685	644	6.46	1.00	5.45	41,701	6,485	35,216	423
30 to 34 years	8.71	2.29	6.42	55,901	14,677	41,224	677	6.57	1.02	5.55	42,169	6,559	35,610	478
35 to 39 years	10.09	2.67	7.43	28,323	7,488	20,841	326	7.60	1.22	6.38	21,337	3,428	17,909	175
40 to 44 years	12.46	3.46	8.99	6,922	1,925	4,997	84	9.84	1.71	8.13	5,467	948	4,519	39
45 to 54 years	23.33	7.31	16.02	1,040	326	714	9	19.38	3.09	16.28	864	138	726	7
Non-Hispanic Black[8]														
All ages	13.23	4.76	8.47	77,860	28,032	49,828	1,596	13.17	2.87	10.30	77,455	16,869	60,586	727
Under 15 years	14.75	4.74	10.01	140	45	95	4	12.88	3.04	9.84	123	29	94	–
15 to 19 years	11.92	4.34	7.59	6,528	2,374	4,154	121	13.62	2.67	10.95	7,457	1,462	5,995	71
15 years	13.91	5.62	8.29	307	124	183	9	14.92	3.17	11.75	329	70	259	4
16 years	11.59	4.52	7.07	551	215	336	8	12.92	2.67	10.25	615	127	488	3
17 years	11.80	4.44	7.36	1,004	378	626	19	13.81	2.89	10.92	1,175	246	929	5
18 years	12.12	4.28	7.83	1,802	637	1,165	34	13.60	2.67	10.93	2,023	397	1,626	21
19 years	11.73	4.18	7.55	2,864	1,020	1,844	51	13.58	2.55	11.04	3,315	622	2,693	38
20 to 24 years	12.28	4.26	8.01	22,376	7,774	14,602	437	13.04	2.57	10.47	23,769	4,690	19,079	199
25 to 29 years	12.79	4.54	8.25	20,561	7,294	13,267	419	12.39	2.69	9.70	19,913	4,325	15,588	200
30 to 34 years	13.80	5.09	8.71	16,128	5,949	10,179	363	13.00	3.09	9.91	15,185	3,608	11,577	133
35 to 39 years	16.21	6.08	10.13	9,339	3,504	5,835	188	14.64	3.70	10.94	8,426	2,132	6,294	102
40 to 44 years	17.98	6.97	11.01	2,515	975	1,540	59	16.63	3.98	12.65	2,325	556	1,769	21
45 to 54 years	23.55	10.09	13.46	273	117	156	5	22.16	5.78	16.38	257	67	190	1
Hispanic[9]														
All ages	9.03	2.50	6.53	82,459	22,849	59,610	636	7.05	1.23	5.82	64,424	11,237	53,187	406
Under 15 years	13.94	4.16	9.78	144	43	101	4	10.33	1.72	7.46	107	26	81	1
15 to 19 years	8.72	2.37	6.35	7,489	2,032	5,457	83	7.85	1.24	6.61	6,745	1,066	5,679	30
15 years	10.31	3.30	7.02	341	109	232	3	9.19	1.72	7.46	304	57	247	–
16 years	9.32	2.64	6.69	764	216	548	14	8.26	1.52	6.74	678	125	553	6
17 years	8.78	2.34	6.44	1,295	345	950	21	8.08	1.18	6.90	1,193	174	1,019	8
18 years	8.96	2.43	6.52	2,156	586	1,570	19	7.85	1.28	6.57	1,891	309	1,582	8
19 years	8.25	2.18	6.07	2,933	776	2,157	26	7.53	1.13	6.40	2,679	401	2,278	8
20 to 24 years	7.94	2.14	5.81	18,974	5,102	13,872	159	6.68	1.06	5.62	15,975	2,534	13,441	118
25 to 29 years	8.39	2.28	6.11	20,869	5,674	15,195	184	6.44	1.11	5.33	16,033	2,758	13,275	94
30 to 34 years	9.42	2.64	6.78	19,229	5,390	13,839	118	6.87	1.26	5.61	14,027	2,574	11,453	85
35 to 39 years	11.21	3.21	7.99	12,055	3,458	8,597	69	8.13	1.58	6.55	8,752	1,703	7,049	54
40 to 44 years	13.11	4.05	9.06	3,358	1,037	2,321	16	9.77	2.05	7.72	2,502	524	1,978	23
45 to 54 years	23.50	7.79	15.71	341	113	228	3	19.48	3.58	15.90	283	52	231	1

- = Quantity zero.   1 Less than 37 completed weeks of gestation.   2 Less than 2,500 grams.   3 Less than 34 completed weeks of gestation.   4 Includes 34 to 36 completed weeks of gestation.   5 Less than 1,500 grams.   6 Includes 1,500–2,499 grams.   7 Includes races other than White and Black and origin not stated.   8 Race and Hispanic origin are reported separately on birth certificates. Persons of Hispanic origin may be of any race. Multiple-race data, when reported, were bridged to single-race categories in order to maintain comparability among all reported areas.   9 Includes all persons of Hispanic origin of any race.

Table 1-49. Births of Very Low Birthweight, by Race and Hispanic Origin of Mother and by State and Territory of Residence, 2014

(Number, percent.)

State and territory	Number All races[1]	Number Non-Hispanic White[2]	Number Non-Hispanic Black[2]	Number Hispanic[3]	Percent All races[1]	Percent Non-Hispanic White[2]	Percent Non-Hispanic Black[2]	Percent Hispanic[3]
United States *	55,947	23,632	16,869	11,237	1.4	1.1	2.9	1.2
Alabama	1,135	441	647	34	1.9	1.2	3.6	0.8
Alaska	101	55	11	7	0.9	0.8	*	*
Arizona	1,004	420	116	373	1.2	1.1	2.5	1.1
Arkansas	558	291	201	45	1.4	1.1	2.8	1.2
California	5,727	1,274	749	2,598	1.1	0.9	2.6	1.1
Colorado	799	426	84	228	1.2	1.0	2.5	1.3
Connecticut	499	195	136	134	1.4	0.0	2.9	1.6
Delaware	194	69	90	24	1.8	1.2	3.2	1.5
District of Columbia	198	26	144	20	2.1	0.9	3.0	1.6
Florida	3,501	1,092	1,448	843	1.6	1.1	2.9	1.4
Georgia	2,321	657	1,337	210	1.8	1.1	3.0	1.2
Hawaii	243	37	12	36	1.3	0.8	*	1.3
Idaho	227	175	1	41	1.0	1.0	*	1.1
Illinois	2,409	1,052	808	401	1.5	1.2	3.0	1.2
Indiana	1,146	745	287	86	1.4	1.2	2.8	1.2
Iowa	460	342	52	42	1.2	1.1	2.2	1.3
Kansas	493	320	75	80	1.3	1.1	2.6	1.3
Kentucky	819	598	162	42	1.5	1.3	3.0	1.5
Louisiana	1,230	419	742	52	1.9	1.2	3.1	1.2
Maine	157	140	8	3	1.2	1.2	*	*
Maryland	1,186	351	634	139	1.6	1.1	2.6	1.3
Massachusetts	860	459	145	178	1.2	1.0	2.0	1.4
Michigan	1,688	906	622	93	1.5	1.1	2.9	1.3
Minnesota	790	498	143	62	1.1	1.0	1.8	1.3
Mississippi	804	256	522	18	2.1	1.3	3.1	*
Missouri	1,022	627	318	48	1.4	1.1	2.8	1.2
Montana	152	115	2	8	1.2	1.1	*	*
Nebraska	312	208	33	52	1.2	1.1	1.8	1.3
Nevada	509	171	129	158	1.4	1.1	3.0	1.2
New Hampshire	130	109	4	8	1.1	1.0	*	*
New Jersey	1,519	524	466	382	1.5	1.1	3.0	1.4
New Mexico	349	75	17	199	1.3	1.0	*	1.4
New York	3,298	1,156	1,010	796	1.4	1.0	2.7	1.4
North Carolina	1,997	826	882	211	1.7	1.2	3.0	1.2
North Dakota	116	90	8	2	1.0	1.0	*	*
Ohio	2,185	1,287	722	98	1.6	1.2	3.1	1.4
Oklahoma	766	461	139	76	1.4	1.4	2.8	1.1
Oregon	455	306	17	101	1.0	0.9	*	1.2
Pennsylvania	2,006	1,072	559	242	1.4	1.1	2.8	1.7
Rhode Island	150	81	16	36	1.4	1.2	*	1.4
South Carolina	1,016	382	549	61	1.8	1.1	3.1	1.3
South Dakota	125	84	8	8	1.0	0.9	*	*
Tennessee	1,260	681	474	80	1.5	1.2	2.8	1.1
Texas	5,722	1,662	1,385	2,376	1.4	1.2	2.9	1.3
Utah	552	406	9	90	1.1	1.0	*	1.2
Vermont	65	60	3	–	1.1	1.0	*	-
Virginia	1,547	660	625	147	1.5	1.1	2.9	1.1
Washington	888	469	94	178	1.0	0.8	2.0	1.1
West Virginia	278	243	25	6	1.4	1.3	3.3	*
Wisconsin	876	556	195	75	1.3	1.1	2.8	1.2
Wyoming	103	77	3	10	1.3	1.2	*	*
Puerto Rico	502	41	10	451	1.5	1.7	*	1.4
Virgin Islands	NA	NA	NA	NA	NA	NA	NA	NA
Guam	33	1	-	-	1.0	*	*	*
American Samoa	8	NA	NA	NA	*	NA	NA	NA
Northern Marianas	7	–	–	–	*	*	*	*

NA = Not available.   – = Quantity zero.   * = Figure does not meet standards of reliability or precision; based on fewer than 20 births in the numerator.   1 Includes races other than White and Black and origin not stated.   2 Race and Hispanic origin are reported separately on birth certificates. Persons of Hispanic origin may be of any race. Multiple-race data, when reported, were bridged to single-race categories in order to maintain comparability among all reported areas.   3 Includes all persons of Hispanic origin of any race.   4 Excludes data for the territories.

Table 1-50. Preterm Births (Less Than 37 Completed Weeks of Gestation), by Race and Hispanic Origin of Mother, by State and Territory of Residence, 2014

(Number, percent.)

State and territory	Number				Percent			
	All races[1]	Non-Hispanic		Hispanic[3]	All races[1]	Non-Hispanic		Hispanic[3]
		White[2]	Black[2]			White[2]	Black[2]	
United States [4]	381,321	191,311	77,860	82,459	9.57	8.91	13.23	9.03
Alabama	6,926	3,705	2,764	349	11.66	10.31	15.17	8.69
Alaska	967	485	36	62	8.51	7.43	8.09	7.40
Arizona	7,819	3,293	564	3,239	9.01	8.54	12.08	9.25
Arkansas	3,845	2,401	960	325	9.99	9.26	13.25	8.47
California	41,594	10,837	3,411	19,724	8.28	7.52	12.07	8.31
Colorado	5,517	3,223	360	1,536	8.38	7.93	10.74	8.70
Connecticut	3,347	1,779	561	807	9.23	8.50	12.16	9.93
Delaware	1,019	508	329	117	9.29	8.61	11.57	7.60
District of Columbia	915	202	563	111	9.63	6.81	11.80	8.66
Florida	21,846	9,014	6,546	5,545	9.93	8.94	13.28	8.97
Georgia	14,058	5,587	6,081	1,587	10.75	9.31	13.53	9.22
Hawaii	1,862	403	73	273	10.04	8.26	13.08	9.88
Idaho	1,863	1,471	14	309	8.15	8.09	*	8.47
Illinois	16,016	8,162	3,801	2,993	10.11	9.47	13.99	8.86
Indiana	8,142	5,914	1,389	630	9.69	9.23	13.43	8.71
Iowa	3,677	2,956	274	288	9.27	9.12	11.63	8.69
Kansas	3,423	2,398	373	500	8.73	8.42	12.70	8.16
Kentucky	6,033	4,990	682	236	10.74	10.69	12.75	8.38
Louisiana	7,925	3,642	3,734	374	12.29	10.63	15.43	8.80
Maine	1,060	973	30	15	8.35	8.35	6.80	*
Maryland	7,455	2,895	3,011	1,052	10.09	8.73	12.57	9.59
Massachusetts	6,177	3,748	717	1,134	8.61	8.42	10.01	8.92
Michigan	11,154	7,079	2,951	659	9.76	8.82	13.64	8.97
Minnesota	6,054	4,304	688	385	8.67	8.56	8.89	8.23
Mississippi	5,000	2,239	2,548	130	12.91	11.29	15.33	8.41
Missouri	7,346	5,111	1,612	347	9.76	8.95	14.09	8.77
Montana	1,157	873	12	40	9.31	8.60	*	8.10
Nebraska	2,439	1,710	231	363	9.11	8.79	12.48	8.77
Nevada	3,623	1,385	609	1,261	10.11	9.14	14.30	9.70
New Hampshire	1,013	908	12	45	8.24	8.32	*	7.64
New Jersey	9,885	4,222	2,064	2,563	9.57	8.76	13.30	9.40
New Mexico	2,387	668	59	1,331	9.17	9.25	12.63	9.23
New York	21,114	9,194	4,503	4,980	8.85	7.93	12.19	9.00
North Carolina	11,781	5,947	3,843	1,435	9.74	8.81	13.25	8.07
North Dakota	948	733	39	33	8.35	8.11	8.48	6.88
Ohio	14,302	9,910	3,251	699	10.26	9.53	13.75	10.16
Oklahoma	5,492	3,369	675	706	10.31	10.04	13.39	9.79
Oregon	3,510	2,467	117	652	7.71	7.63	9.60	7.65
Pennsylvania	13,291	8,587	2,567	1,431	9.36	8.66	12.74	9.88
Rhode Island	932	529	81	238	8.62	8.05	9.52	9.21
South Carolina	6,212	3,189	2,476	413	10.78	9.48	13.85	8.89
South Dakota	1,040	706	31	48	8.48	7.74	9.12	7.96
Tennessee	8,780	5,634	2,342	624	10.77	10.16	13.80	8.94
Texas	41,345	13,638	6,631	19,057	10.35	9.68	13.83	10.06
Utah	4,678	3,503	62	720	9.14	8.88	10.82	9.27
Vermont	486	456	12	3	7.93	7.97	*	*
Virginia	9,517	5,007	2,714	1,128	9.22	8.36	12.56	8.36
Washington	7,125	4,272	440	1,287	8.05	7.65	9.45	8.17
West Virginia	2,198	2,035	95	37	10.83	10.79	12.48	10.57
Wisconsin	6,163	4,373	913	519	9.19	8.85	12.99	8.18
Wyoming	863	677	9	119	11.22	10.82	*	13.30
Puerto Rico	4,066	302	38	3,724	11.8	12.3	15.1	11.8
Virgin Islands	NA	NA	NA	NA	NA	NA	NA	NA
Guam	326	8	1	2	9.7	*	*	*
American Samoa	NA	NA	NA	NA	NA	NA	NA	NA
Northern Marianas	48	–	–	–	9.3	*	*	*

NA = Not available.   – = Quantity zero.   * = Figure does not meet standards of reliability or precision; based on fewer than 20 births in the numerator.   1 Includes races other than White and Black and origin not stated.   2 Race and Hispanic origin are reported separately on birth certificates. Persons of Hispanic origin may be of any race. Multiple-race data, when reported, were bridged to single-race categories in order to maintain comparability among all reported areas.   3 Includes all persons of Hispanic origin of any race.   4 Excludes data for the territories.

Table 1-51. Low Birthweight Births (Less Than 2,500 Grams or 5 Lbs 8 Oz), by Race and Hispanic Origin of Mother, by State and Territory of Residence, 2014

(Number, percent.)

State and territory	Number				Percent			
	All races[1]	Non-Hispanic		Hispanic[3]	All races[1]	Non-Hispanic		Hispanic[3]
		White[2]	Black[2]			White[2]	Black[2]	
United States [4]	318,847	149,574	77,455	64,424	8.0	7.0	13.2	7.1
Alabama	5,989	2,851	2,740	292	10.1	7.9	15.0	7.3
Alaska	672	350	41	37	5.9	5.4	9.2	4.4
Arizona	6,086	2,577	555	2,345	7.0	6.7	11.9	6.7
Arkansas	3,432	1,998	1,041	261	8.9	7.7	14.4	6.8
California	33,586	8,338	3,250	15,008	6.7	5.8	11.5	6.3
Colorado	5,769	3,363	426	1,511	8.8	8.3	12.7	8.6
Connecticut	2,763	1,384	544	649	7.6	6.6	11.8	8.0
Delaware	908	395	349	105	8.3	6.7	12.3	6.8
District of Columbia	934	173	617	103	9.8	5.8	12.9	8.0
Florida	19,065	7,224	6,546	4,585	8.7	7.2	13.3	7.4
Georgia	12,385	4,228	6,206	1,180	9.5	7.0	13.8	6.9
Hawaii	1,462	293	57	199	7.9	6.0	10.2	7.2
Idaho	1,471	1,140	18	260	6.4	6.3	*	7.1
Illinois	12,929	6,004	3,726	2,204	8.2	7.0	13.7	6.5
Indiana	6,715	4,688	1,382	459	8.0	7.3	13.4	6.3
Iowa	2,675	2,032	275	226	6.7	6.3	11.7	6.8
Kansas	2,759	1,837	381	396	7.0	6.4	13.0	6.5
Kentucky	4,922	3,916	708	178	8.8	8.4	13.2	6.3
Louisiana	6,786	2,737	3,626	276	10.5	8.0	15.0	6.5
Maine	960	849	49	19	7.6	7.3	11.1	*
Maryland	6,345	2,182	2,887	800	8.6	6.6	12.1	7.3
Massachusetts	5,351	3,018	719	1,035	7.5	6.8	10.1	8.2
Michigan	9,545	5,602	2,992	488	8.4	7.0	13.8	6.6
Minnesota	4,595	3,072	685	299	6.6	6.1	8.9	6.4
Mississippi	4,374	1,623	2,590	106	11.3	8.2	15.6	6.9
Missouri	6,163	4,038	1,624	267	8.2	7.1	14.2	6.7
Montana	920	701	14	45	7.4	6.9	*	9.1
Nebraska	1,775	1,191	203	261	6.6	6.1	11.0	6.3
Nevada	2,972	1,140	579	943	8.3	7.5	13.6	7.3
New Hampshire	852	752	13	43	6.9	6.9	*	7.3
New Jersey	8,315	3,298	1,932	2,005	8.1	6.8	12.5	7.4
New Mexico	2,282	584	77	1,277	8.8	8.1	16.5	8.9
New York	18,722	7,621	4,397	4,244	7.9	6.6	11.9	7.7
North Carolina	10,720	5,022	3,950	1,165	8.9	7.4	13.6	6.6
North Dakota	704	549	39	19	6.2	6.1	8.5	*
Ohio	11,800	7,609	3,204	537	8.5	7.3	13.6	7.8
Oklahoma	4,238	2,506	665	515	8.0	7.5	13.2	7.1
Oregon	2,842	1,949	120	522	6.2	6.0	9.8	6.1
Pennsylvania	11,713	7,080	2,598	1,323	8.3	7.2	13.0	9.1
Rhode Island	765	410	77	203	7.1	6.2	9.1	7.9
South Carolina	5,435	2,432	2,563	319	9.4	7.2	14.3	6.9
South Dakota	804	570	35	44	6.5	6.2	10.3	7.3
Tennessee	7,297	4,344	2,351	428	9.0	7.8	13.9	6.1
Texas	32,744	10,172	6,360	14,268	8.2	7.2	13.3	7.5
Utah	3,572	2,641	59	568	7.0	6.7	10.3	7.3
Vermont	432	398	12	7	7.1	7.0	*	*
Virginia	8,130	3,874	2,665	892	7.9	6.5	12.3	6.6
Washington	5,705	3,341	450	955	6.4	6.0	9.7	6.1
West Virginia	1,852	1,702	90	36	9.1	9.0	11.8	10.3
Wisconsin	4,911	3,223	959	423	7.3	6.5	13.6	6.6
Wyoming	704	553	9	94	9.2	8.8	*	10.5
Puerto Rico	3,713	246	36	3,431	10.8	10.0	14.3	10.8
Virgin Islands	NA	NA	NA	NA	NA	NA	NA	NA
Guam	261	4	1	-	7.8	*	*	*
American Samoa	49	NA	NA	NA	4.5	NA	NA	NA
Northern Marianas	75	-	-	NA	7.6	*	*	NA

NA = Not available.   – = Quantity zero.   * = Figure does not meet standards of reliability or precision; based on fewer than 20 births in the numerator.   1 Includes races other than White and Black and origin not stated.   2 Race and Hispanic origin are reported separately on birth certificates. Persons of Hispanic origin may be of any race. Multiple-race data, when reported, were bridged to single-race categories in order to maintain comparability among all reported areas.   3 Includes all persons of Hispanic origin of any race.   4 Excludes data for the territories.

Table 1-52. Births, by Plurality, Age, and Race and Hispanic Origin of Mother, 2014

(Number, rate as stated.)

Plurality, race, and Hispanic origin of mother	All ages	Under 15 years	Age of mother								
			15 to 19 years			20 to 24 years	25 to 29 years	30 to 34 years	35 to 39 years	40 to 44 years	45 to 54 years
			Total	15 to 17 years	18 to 19 years						
					Number						
All Live Births											
All races[1]	3,988,076	2,769	249,078	66,791	182,287	882,567	1,145,392	1,081,058	508,748	110,021	8,443
Non-Hispanic White[2]	2,149,302	679	99,220	22,570	76,650	420,224	646,097	642,219	280,788	55,609	4,466
Non-Hispanic Black[2]	588,891	955	54,819	15,485	39,334	182,435	160,935	116,939	57,647	14,000	1,161
Hispanic[3]	914,065	1,037	85,970	26,295	59,675	239,121	248,971	204,232	107,644	25,636	1,454
Live Births in Single Deliveries											
All races[1]	3,848,214	2,741	245,030	65,856	179,174	861,890	1,109,520	1,035,762	482,936	103,578	6,757
Non-Hispanic White[2]	2,067,486	671	97,726	22,289	75,437	411,132	625,101	612,859	264,742	51,729	3,526
Non-Hispanic Black[2]	564,817	947	53,591	15,197	38,394	176,030	154,109	111,181	54,669	13,302	988
Hispanic[3]	891,426	1,027	84,761	25,960	58,801	234,742	243,143	198,008	103,765	24,723	1,257
Live Births in Twin Deliveries											
All races[1]	135,336	28	3,994	920	3,074	20,298	34,886	43,585	24,728	6,196	1,621
Non-Hispanic White[2]	78,788	8	1,471	278	1,193	8,907	20,335	28,122	15,297	3,723	925
Non-Hispanic Black[2]	23,546	8	1,207	279	928	6,304	6,710	5,588	2,904	673	152
Hispanic[3]	22,051	10	1,200	332	868	4,301	5,693	6,048	3,734	878	187
Live Births in Triplet and Higher-Order Multiple Births[4]											
All races[1]	4,526	–	54	15	39	379	986	1,711	1,084	247	65
Non-Hispanic White[2]	3,028	–	23	3	20	185	661	1,238	749	157	15
Non-Hispanic Black[2]	528	–	21	9	12	101	116	170	74	25	21
Hispanic[3]	588	–	9	3	6	78	135	176	145	35	10
Rate per 1,000 live births											
All Multiple Births											
All races[1]	35.1	10.1	16.3	14.0	17.1	23.4	31.3	41.9	50.7	58.6	199.7
Non-Hispanic White[2]	38.1	*	15.1	12.5	15.8	21.6	32.5	45.7	57.1	69.8	210.5
Non-Hispanic Black[2]	40.9	*	22.4	18.6	23.9	35.1	42.4	49.2	51.7	49.9	149.0
Hispanic[3]	24.8	*	14.1	12.7	14.6	18.3	23.4	30.5	36.0	35.6	135.5
Twin Births											
All races[1]	33.9	10.1	16.0	13.8	16.9	23.0	30.5	40.3	48.6	56.3	192.0
Non-Hispanic White[2]	36.7	*	14.8	12.3	15.6	21.2	31.5	43.8	54.5	66.9	207.1
Non-Hispanic Black[2]	40.0	*	22.0	18.0	23.6	34.6	41.7	47.8	50.4	48.1	130.9
Hispanic[3]	24.1	*	14.0	12.6	14.5	18.0	22.9	29.6	34.7	34.2	128.6
Triplet and Higher-Order Multiple Births[4]											
All races[1]	113.5	*	21.7	*	21.4	42.9	86.1	158.3	213.1	224.5	769.9
Non-Hispanic White[2]	140.9	*	23.2	*	26.1	44.0	102.3	192.8	266.7	282.3	*
Non-Hispanic Black[2]	89.7	*	38.3	*	*	55.4	72.1	145.4	128.4	178.6	1808.8
Hispanic[3]	64.3	*	*	*	*	32.6	54.2	86.2	134.7	136.5	*

– = Quantity zero.   * = Figure does not meet standards of reliability or precision; based on fewer than 20 births in the numerator.   1 Includes races other than White and Black and origin not stated.   2 Race and Hispanic origin are reported separately on birth certificates. Persons of Hispanic origin may be of any race. Multiple-race data, when reported, were bridged to single-race categories in order to maintain comparability among all reported areas.   3 Includes all persons of Hispanic origin of any race.   4 Triplet, quadruplet, quintuplet, and higher-order multiple deliveries.

Table 1-53. Numbers and Rates of Twin and Triplet and Higher-Order Multiple Births, by Race and Hispanic Origin of Mother, 1980–2014

(Number, rate per 1,000 live births; rate per 100,000 live births, as stated.)

Year, race, and Hispanic origin of mother	Total births	Twin births	Triplet and higher-order births	Multiple birth rate[1]	Twin birth rate[2]	Triplet or higher-order birth rate[3]
All Races [4]						
1980	3,612,258	68,339	1,337	19.3	18.9	37.0
1981	3,629,238	70,049	1,385	19.7	19.3	38.2
1982	3,680,537	71,631	1,484	19.9	19.5	40.3
1983	3,638,933	72,287	1,575	20.3	19.9	43.3
1984	3,669,141	72,949	1,653	20.3	19.9	45.1
1985	3,760,561	77,102	1,925	21.0	20.5	51.2
1986	3,756,547	79,485	1,814	21.6	21.2	48.3
1987	3,809,394	81,778	2,139	22.0	21.5	56.2
1988	3,909,510	85,315	2,385	22.4	21.8	61.0
1989	4,040,958	90,118	2,798	23.0	22.3	69.2
1990	4,158,212	93,865	3,028	23.3	22.6	72.8
1991	4,110,907	94,779	3,346	23.9	23.1	81.4
1992	4,065,014	95,372	3,883	24.4	23.5	95.5
1993	4,000,240	96,445	4,168	25.2	24.1	104.2
1994	3,952,767	97,064	4,594	25.7	24.6	116.2
1995	3,899,589	96,736	4,973	26.1	24.8	127.5
1996	3,891,494	100,750	5,939	27.4	25.9	152.6
1997	3,880,894	104,137	6,737	28.6	26.8	173.6
1998	3,941,553	110,670	7,625	30.0	28.1	193.5
1999	3,959,417	114,307	7,321	30.7	28.9	184.9
2000	4,058,814	118,916	7,325	31.1	29.3	180.5
2001	4,025,933	121,246	7,471	32.0	30.1	185.6
2002	4,021,726	125,134	7,401	33.0	31.1	184.0
2003	4,089,950	128,665	7,663	33.3	31.5	187.4
2004	4,112,052	132,219	7,275	33.9	32.2	176.9
2005	4,138,349	133,122	6,694	33.8	32.2	161.8
2006	4,265,555	137,085	6,540	33.7	32.1	153.3
2007	4,316,233	138,961	6,427	33.7	32.2	148.9
2008	4,247,694	138,660	6,268	34.1	32.6	147.6
2009	4,130,665	137,217	6,340	34.8	33.2	153.5
2010	3,999,386	132,562	5,503	34.5	33.1	137.6
2011	3,953,590	131,269	5,417	34.6	33.2	137.0
2012	3,952,841	131,024	4,919	34.4	33.1	124.4
2013	3,932,181	135,336	4,700	34.8	33.7	119.5
2014	3,988,076		4,526	35.1	33.9	113.5
Non-Hispanic White [5]						
1990 [6]	2,626,500	60,210	2,358	23.8	22.9	89.8
1991 [7]	2,589,878	60,904	2,612	24.5	23.5	100.9
1992 [7]	2,527,207	60,640	3,115	25.2	24.0	123.3
1993	2,472,031	61,525	3,360	26.2	24.9	135.9
1994	2,438,855	62,476	3,721	27.1	25.6	152.6
1995	2,382,638	62,370	4,050	27.9	26.2	170.0
1996	2,358,989	65,523	4,885	29.8	27.8	207.1
1997	2,333,363	67,191	5,386	31.1	28.8	230.8
1998	2,283,986	71,270	6,206	32.8	30.2	262.8
1999	2,346,450	73,964	5,909	34.0	31.5	251.8
2000	2,362,968	76,018	5,821	34.6	32.2	246.3
2001	2,326,578	77,882	5,894	36.0	33.5	253.3
2002	2,298,156	79,949	5,754	37.3	34.8	250.4
2003	2,321,904	81,691	5,922	37.7	35.2	255.0
2004	2,296,683	83,346	5,590	38.7	36.3	243.4
2005	2,279,768	82,223	4,966	38.2	36.1	217.8
2006	2,308,640	83,108	4,805	38.1	36.0	208.1
2007	2,310,333	83,632	4,559	38.2	36.2	197.3
2008	2,267,817	82,903	4,493	38.5	36.6	198.1
2009	2,212,552	81,954	4,457	39.1	37.0	201.4
2010	2,162,406	79,728	3,842	38.6	36.9	177.7
2011	2,146,566	78,638	3,670	38.3	36.6	171.0
2012	2,134,196	78,449	3,264	38.3	36.8	152.9
2013	2,129,196	78,072	3,134	38.1	36.7	147.2
2014	2,149,302	78,788	3,028	38.1	36.7	140.9

Table 1-53. Numbers and Rates of Twin and Triplet and Higher-Order Multiple Births, by Race and Hispanic Origin of Mother, 1980–2014— continued

(Number, rate per 1,000 live births; rate per 100,000 live births, as stated.)

Year, race, and Hispanic origin of mother	Total births	Twin births	Triplet and higher-order births	Multiple birth rate[1]	Twin birth rate[2]	Triplet or higher-order birth rate[3]
Non-Hispanic Black [5]						
1990 [6]	661,701	17,646	306	27.1	26.7	46.2
1991 [7]	666,758	18,243	367	27.9	27.4	55.0
1992 [7]	657,450	18,294	346	28.4	27.8	52.6
1993	641,273	18,115	314	28.7	28.2	49.0
1994	619,198	17,934	357	29.5	29.0	57.7
1995	587,781	16,622	340	28.9	28.3	57.8
1996	578,099	16,873	425	29.9	29.2	73.5
1997	581,431	17,472	523	30.9	30.0	90.0
1998	593,127	18,589	518	32.2	31.3	87.3
1999	588,981	18,920	561	33.1	32.1	95.2
2000	604,346	20,173	506	34.2	33.4	83.7
2001	589,917	19,974	531	34.8	33.9	90.0
2002	578,335	20,064	591	35.7	34.7	102.2
2003	576,033	20,010	631	35.8	34.7	109.5
2004	578,772	20,605	577	36.6	35.6	99.7
2005	583,759	21,254	616	37.5	36.4	105.5
2006	617,247	22,702	580	37.7	36.8	94.0
2007	627,191	23,101	612	37.8	36.8	97.6
2008	623,029	22,924	569	37.7	36.8	91.3
2009	609,584	23,159	644	39.0	38.0	105.6
2010	589,808	21,804	574	37.9	37.0	97.3
2011	582,345	21,681	634	38.3	37.2	108.9
2012	583,489	21,545	629	38.0	36.9	107.8
2013	583,834	22,346	623	39.3	38.3	106.7
2014	588,891	23,546	528	40.9	40.0	89.7
Hispanic [8]						
1990 [6]	595,073	10,713	235	18.4	18.0	39.5
1991 [7]	623,085	11,356	235	18.6	18.2	37.7
1992 [7]	643,271	11,932	239	18.9	18.5	37.2
1993	654,418	12,294	321	19.3	18.8	49.1
1994	665,026	12,206	348	18.9	18.4	52.3
1995	679,768	12,685	355	19.2	18.7	52.2
1996	701,339	13,014	409	19.1	18.6	58.3
1997	709,767	13,821	516	20.2	19.5	72.7
1998	734,661	15,015	553	21.2	20.4	75.3
1999	764,339	15,388	583	20.9	20.1	76.3
2000	815,868	16,470	659	21.0	20.2	80.8
2001	851,851	17,257	710	21.1	20.3	83.3
2002	876,642	18,128	737	21.5	20.7	84.1
2003	912,329	19,472	784	22.2	21.3	85.9
2004	946,349	20,351	723	22.3	21.5	76.4
2005	985,505	21,723	761	22.8	22.0	77.2
2006	1,039,077	22,698	787	22.6	21.8	75.7
2007	1,062,779	23,405	857	22.8	22.0	80.6
2008	1,041,239	23,266	834	23.1	22.3	80.1
2009	999,548	22,481	835	23.3	22.5	83.5
2010	945,180	21,359	721	23.4	22.6	76.3
2011	918,129	21,236	723	23.9	23.1	78.7
2012	907,677	20,505	636	23.3	22.6	46.2
2013	901,033	21,511	643	24.6	23.9	64.3
2014	914,065	22,051	588	24.8	24.1	70.1

1 The number of live births in all multiple deliveries per 1,000 live births.   2 The number of live births in twin deliveries per 1,000 live births.   3 The number of live births in triplet and other higher-order deliveries per 100,000 live births.   4 Includes races other than White and Black and origin not stated.   5 Race and Hispanic origin are reported separately on birth certificates. Persons of Hispanic origin may be of any race. Multiple-race data, when reported, were bridged to single-race categories in order to maintain comparability among all reported areas.   6 Excludes data for New Hampshire and Oklahoma, which did not report Hispanic origin.   7 Excludes data for New Hampshire, which did not report Hispanic origin.   8 Includes all persons of Hispanic origin of any race.

Table 1-54. Twin, Triplet, and Higher-Order Multiple Births, by State, 2012–2014

(Number, rate per 1,000 births.)

State	Twin		Triplet or higher order[1]	
	Number	Rate per 1,000 live births	Number	Rate per 100,000 live births
United States	398,684	33.6	14,145	119.1
Alabama	5,867	33.3	243	138.0
Alaska	1,004	29.5	6	*
Arizona	7,370	28.5	252	97.3
Arkansas	3,299	28.8	84	95.9
California	46,559	31.0	1,489	99.2
Colorado	6,277	32.0	177	90.3
Connecticut	4,410	40.5	162	148.7
Delaware	983	29.9	17	*
District of Columbia	990	35.1	28	99.3
Florida	20,693	31.9	713	109.9
Georgia	12,913	33.1	459	117.7
Hawaii	1,784	31.6	69	122.1
Idaho	2,079	30.5	68	99.7
Illinois	18,027	38.0	612	128.9
Indiana	8,194	32.7	311	124.2
Iowa	3,994	34.0	153	130.2
Kansas	3,822	32.3	162	136.8
Kentucky	5,370	32.0	222	132.4
Louisiana	6,629	34.8	269	141.3
Maine	1,321	34.5	45	117.6
Maryland	8,091	37.0	251	114.7
Massachusetts	9,249	42.8	267	123.5
Michigan	12,124	35.6	471	138.1
Minnesota	7,358	35.4	197	94.8
Mississippi	3,862	33.3	100	86.2
Missouri	7,765	34.3	248	109.7
Montana	1,158	31.4	36	97.5
Nebraska	2,615	33.2	154	191.5
Nevada	3,229	30.5	101	98.3
New Hampshire	1,427	38.5	30	81.0
New Jersey	13,364	43.1	456	147.0
New Mexico	1,911	24.0	68	85.6
New York	26,996	37.7	1,042	145.4
North Carolina	12,211	33.9	352	97.8
North Dakota	984	30.7	50	155.9
Ohio	14,405	34.6	707	169.6
Oklahoma	4,741	29.7	195	122.3
Oregon	4,505	33.2	103	75.9
Pennsylvania	14,900	35.0	500	117.5
Rhode Island	1,154	35.4	42	129.0
South Carolina	5,956	34.7	179	104.3
South Dakota	1,088	29.7	37	101.0
Tennessee	7,492	31.0	257	106.2
Texas	36,543	31.2	1,488	127.2
Utah	5,043	32.8	222	144.6
Vermont	599	33.1	14	*
Virginia	10,958	35.5	441	143.0
Washington	8,059	30.7	276	105.1
West Virginia	1,832	29.6	64	103.3
Wisconsin	6,758	33.6	218	108.4
Wyoming	722	31.5	12	*

* = Figure does not meet standards of reliability or precision.   1 Includes triplet, quadruplet, and other higher-order multiple births.

Table 1-55. Gestational Age and Birthweight Characteristics, by Plurality, 2014

(Number, percent.)

Characteristic	All births	Singletons	Twins	Triplets	Quadruplets	Quintuplets and higher-order multiples[1]
Number of Births	3,988,076	3,848,214	135,336	4,233	246	47
Percent, very preterm[2]	1.6	1.2	10.6	39.3	72.0	100.0
Percent, preterm[3]	9.6	7.7	58.7	98.3	98.0	100.0
Percent, very low birth-weight[4]	1.4	1.1	9.6	37.0	65.4	90.9
Percent, low birthweight[5]	8.0	6.2	55.3	95.1	97.5	100.0

1 Quintuplets, sextuplets, and higher-order multiple births are not differentiated in the national data set.   2 Very preterm is less than 32 completed weeks of gestation.   3 Preterm is less than 37 completed weeks of gestation.   4 Very low birthweight is less than 1,500 grams.   5 Low birthweight is less than 2,500 grams.

Table 1-56. Distribution of Births, by Selected Gestational Age, Selected Years, 1990–2014

(Percent.)

Gestational age	Obstetric estimate					
	1990	2000	2005	2006	2010	2014
Under 28 weeks	0.7	0.7	0.8	0.8	0.7	NA
28 to 31 weeks	1.2	1.2	1.3	1.3	1.2	0.9
32 to 33 weeks	1.4	1.5	1.6	1.6	1.5	1.2
Total under 34 weeks	3.3	3.4	3.6	3.7	3.5	NA
34 to 36 weeks	7.3	8.2	9.1	9.2	8.5	6.8
Total under 37 weeks	10.6	11.6	12.7	12.8	12.0	9.6
37 to 38 weeks	19.7	24.5	28.3	28.9	26.9	24.8
39 weeks [1]	21.7	24.3	25.3	25.4	28.3	NA
40 weeks [1]	22.6	21.3	19.2	18.9	19.1	NA
41 weeks	14.1	11.0	8.7	8.3	8.2	6.5
42 weeks or more	11.3	7.3	5.8	5.7	5.5	0.4

1 The value for 39 and 40 weeks combined is 58.7 percent.

Figure 1-11. Percent of Preterm Births by Completed Weeks of Gestation, Selected Years, 1990–2014

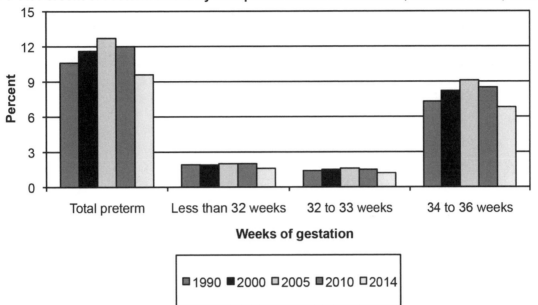

Figure 1-12. Twin, Triplet, and Higher Order Birth Rates, Selected Years, 1980–2014

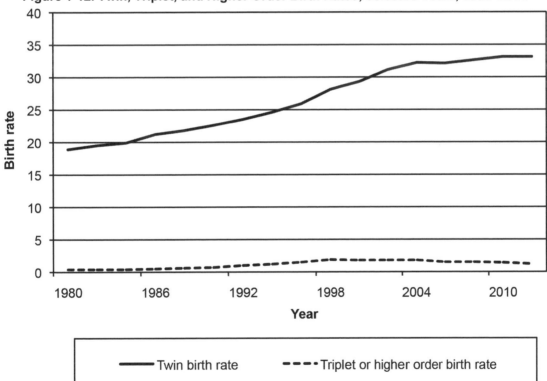

Table 1-57. Use of Contraception Among Sexually Experienced Males and Females Age 15 to 19 Years, by Method of Contraception, Selected Years, 1995–2010

(Number in thousands, percent.)

Method	Females		
	1995	2002	2006–2010
Percent Who Ever Used Method of Birth Control			
Any method	96.2	97.7	98.9
Pill	51.6	61.4	55.6
Injectable	9.7	20.7	20.3
Emergency contraception	*	8.1	13.7
Contraceptive patch	NA	1.5	10.3
Contraceptive ring	NA	NA	5.2
Condom	93.5	93.7	95.9
Female condom	1.1	1.7	1.5
Periodic abstinence-calendar	13.2	10.8	15
Withdrawal	42.3	55.0	57.3
Other methods	14.5	9.9	7.1

NA = Not available.   * = Figure does not meet standards of reliability or precision.

Table 1-58. Use of Contraception at First Sex Among Females and Males Age 15 to 19 Years, by Method Used, Selected Years, 1988–2010

(Number in thousands, percent.)

Characteristic	Number	Any method	No method	Pill (at all)[1]	Other hormonal[1,2]	Condom(at all)[1]	All other methods[3]	Dual methods (hormonal and condom)
Females								
1988	4,410	66.9	33.1	8.0	X	50.4	10.0	1.8
2002	4,598	74.5	25.5	16.5	2.1	66.4	2.6	13.1
2006–2010[4]	4,532	78.3	21.7	15.7	6.1	68.0	3.4	14.8
Females, 2006–2010								
Hispanic Origin and Race	833	74.0	26.0	7.2	5.8	65.4	1.3	5.7
Hispanic or Latina								
Non-Hispanic White	2,633	82.3	17.7	21.8	6.3	70.7	4.3	20.8
Non-Hispanic Black	785	71.1	28.9	8.9	6.6	64.1	*	9.5
Age at First Sex								
14 years or under	1,244	59.1	40.9	7.1	2.4	53.5	2.3	6.3
15 to 16 years	2,108	83.1	16.9	16.7	9.0	69.6	3.6	15.8
17 to 19 years	1,180	90.1	9.9	22.8	4.7	80.5	4.2	22.0
Age Difference Between Female and First Male Partner								
Male partner same age or younger	1,252	82.9	17.1	17.3	7.6	71.8	1.0	14.7
Male partner 1 year older	1,222	78.7	21.3	14.4	6.5	71.0	4.5	17.6
Male partner 2 to 3 years older	1,326	81.7	18.3	16.6	5.3	68.3	5.6	14.0
Male partner 4 or more years older	732	63.7	36.3	13.4	4.2	56.3	1.7	11.7
Males	5,379	71.4	28.6	9.5	X	55.0	10.6	2.6
1988								
1995	4,989	75.7	24.3	10.3	0.4	69.3	4.4	6.8
2002	4,697	82.0	18.0	14.9	2.1	70.9	4.7	10.4
2006–2010[4]	4,551	85.4	14.6	17.9	1.4	79.6	2.7	16.2
Males, 2006–2010								
Hispanic Origin and Race								
Hispanic or Latino	931	84.1	15.9	9.1	*	78.5	4.5	8.3
Non-Hispanic White	2,387	88.5	11.5	24.8	2.4	80.9	2.6	22.3
Non-Hispanic Black	977	81.7	18.3	11.7	*	79.6	*	11.1
Age at First Sex								
14 years or under	1,513	74.9	25.1	8.0	*	71.0	3.3	9.0
15 to 16 years	1,994	89.3	10.7	19.8	1.8	82.2	3.5	18.0
17 to 19 years	1,044	93.3	6.7	28.7	*	86.9	*	23.2
Age Difference Between Male and First Female Partner								
Female partner younger	723	88.3	11.7	14.5	*	79.6	5.0	15.1
Female partner same age	2,034	89.4	10.6	16.1	1.3	85.2	1.9	15.1
Female partner 1 year older	1,011	83.2	16.8	22.4	*	78.5	*	19.1
Female partner 2 or more years older	783	75.4	24.6	20.1	-	66.4	5.1	16.2

NOTE: Statistics not available for females in 1995 because of differences in the universe of respondents asked the questions.   X = Category not applicable.   - = Quantity zero.   * = Figure does not meet standards of reliability or precision.   1 Statistics for condom "at all," pill "at all," and other hormonal reflect use of that method regardless of whether it was used alone or in combination with another method. 2 Includes Lunelle injectable, emergency contraception, and contraceptive patch in 2002; adds contraceptive ring (Nuva-Ring) and Implanon implant in 2006–2010.   3 Excludes condom and hormonal methods. Thus, if other method was combined with condom or hormonal method, it is not counted. Other methods include withdrawal, sterilization, IUD, female condom, diaphragm, cervical cap, spermicidal foam, jelly, cream or suppository, sponge, calendar rhythm method, and "other" methods.   4 Includes persons of other or unknown origin and race groups.

Table 1-59. Use of Contraception at Last Sex in the Prior 3 Months Among Never-Married Females and Males Age 15 to 19 Years, by Method Used, Selected Years, 1988–2010

(Number in thousands, percent.)

Characteristic	Number	Any method	No method	Pill (at all)	Other hormonal[1]	Condom (at all)	All other methods[2]	Dual methods (hormonal and condom)
FEMALE								
1988	3,521	79.9	20.1	42.7	X	31.3	9.3	3.3
1995	3,225	70.7	29.3	25.0	7.0	38.2	9.6	8.4
2002	3,304	83.2	16.8	34.2	9.1	54.3	5.1	19.5
Total, 2006–2010[3]	3,175	85.6	14.4	30.5	12.2	52.0	11.0	20.1
Female, 2006–2010								
Hispanic Origin and Race								
Hispanic or Latina	539	79.5	20.5	17.2	18.0	47.7	10.6	14.0
Non-Hispanic White	1,873	89.3	10.7	38.6	10.5	52.4	12.3	24.4
Non-Hispanic Black	564	81.1	18.9	14.4	16.2	57.6	5.7	12.8
Age at First Sex								
14 years or under	835	73.0	27.0	18.0	11.6	38.3	16.7	11.7
15 to 16 years	1,528	88.7	11.3	33.5	12.9	50.1	10.9	18.7
17 to 19 years	812	92.8	7.2	37.9	11.3	69.6	5.5	31.4
MALE								
1988	3,847	84.2	15.8	37.4	...	53.3	13.6	15.2
1995	3,416	81.8	18.2	28.2	2.8	63.9	10.0	16.5
2002	3,165	90.7	9.3	31.0	6.3	70.7	2.0	23.9
Total, 2006–2010[3]	2,970	92.5	7.5	39.0	9.3	74.7	3.4	33.9
Male, 2006–2010								
Hispanic Origin and Race								
Hispanic or Latino	593	86.2	13.8	29.4	6.8	65.5	4.3	19.6
Non-Hispanic White	1,567	96.8	3.2	49.6	11.0	76.8	2.9	43.4
Non-Hispanic Black	638	91.6	8.4	25.6	9.8	79.0	4.1	26.9
Age at First Sex								
14 years or under	1,009	85.3	14.7	31.1	11.1	68.0	5.0	29.7
15 to 16 years	1,363	95.3	4.7	41.3	10.1	74.4	3.6	34.2
17 to 19 years	598	98.1	*	47.2	4.5	86.3	*	40.2

NOTE: Statistics for condom "at all," pill "at all," and other hormonal reflect use of that method regardless of whether it was used alone or in combination with another method.   X = Not applicable.   * = Figure does not meet standards of reliability or precision.   1 Includes Depo-Provera injectable and Norplant implants in 1995; adds Lunelle injectable, emergency contraception, and contraceptive patch in 2002; adds contraceptive ring (Nuva-Ring) and Implanon implant in 2006–2010.   2 Excludes condom and hormonal methods. Thus, if other method was combined with condom or hormonal method, it is not counted. Other methods include withdrawal, sterilization, IUD, female condom, diaphragm, cervical cap, spermicidal foam, jelly, cream or suppository, sponge, calendar rhythm method, and "other" methods. 3 Includes persons of other or unknown origin and race groups.

Table 1-60. Number of Live Births by Attendant, Place of Delivery, Race, and Hispanic Origin of Mother, 2014

(Number.)

Place of delivery and race and Hispanic origin of mother	All births	Physician			Midwife			Other	Unspecified
		Total	Doctor of medicine	Doctor of osteopathy	Total	Certified nurse midwife	Other midwife		
ALL RACES [1]									
Total	3,988,076	3,594,759	3,331,630	263,129	363,808	332,107	31,701	27,542	1,967
In hospital [2]	3,928,272	3,592,121	3,329,379	262,742	320,148	312,777	7,371	15,099	904
Not in hospital	59,674	2,584	2,203	381	43,647	19,324	24,323	12,402	1,041
Freestanding birthing center	18,219	561	432	129	16,848	9,825	7,023	779	31
Clinic or doctor's office	404	192	148	44	189	172	17	19	4
Residence	38,094	1,365	1,197	168	25,892	9,102	16,790	10,023	814
Other	2,957	466	426	40	718	225	493	1,581	192
Not specified	130	54	48	6	13	6	7	41	22
NON-HISPANIC WHITE [3]									
Total	2,149,302	1,917,811	1,751,589	166,222	214,908	189,583	25,325	15,580	1,003
In hospital [2]	2,100,900	1,916,178	1,750,278	165,900	177,684	173,269	4,415	6,593	445
Not in hospital	48,333	1,606	1,287	319	37,213	16,308	20,905	8,962	552
Freestanding birthing center	14,986	506	378	128	13,794	8,068	5,726	666	20
Clinic or doctor's office	322	131	93	38	179	163	16	10	2
Residence	31,299	722	596	126	22,610	7,893	14,717	7,512	455
Other	1,726	247	220	27	630	184	446	774	75
Not specified	69	27	24	3	11	6	5	25	6
NON-HISPANIC BLACK [3]									
Total	588,891	541,062	512,921	28,141	43,537	41,802	1,735	3,992	300
In hospital [2]	585,699	540,529	512,412	28,117	42,312	41,172	1,140	2,729	129
Not in hospital	3,166	519	495	24	1,225	630	595	1,254	168
Freestanding birthing center	745	25	25	–	684	391	293	27	9
Clinic or doctor's office	25	21	19	2	–	–	–	4	–
Residence	2,033	371	355	16	518	226	292	1,011	133
Other	363	102	96	6	23	13	10	212	26
Not specified	26	14	14	–	–	–	–	9	3
HISPANIC [4]									
Total	914,065	831,250	777,780	53,470	76,725	73,446	3,279	5,762	328
In hospital [2]	909,040	830,957	777,515	53,442	73,383	71,981	1,402	4,557	143
Not in hospital	5,016	287	259	28	3,341	1,465	1,876	1,203	185
Freestanding birthing center	1,758	25	24	1	1,671	915	756	60	2
Clinic or doctor's office	22	13	13	–	7	6	1	1	1
Residence	2,810	188	166	22	1,620	526	1,094	869	133
Other	426	61	56	5	43	18	25	273	49
Not specified	9	6	6	–	1	–	1	2	–

– = Quantity zero.   1 Includes races other than White and Black and origin not stated.   2 Includes births occurring en route to or on arrival at hospital.   3 Race and Hispanic origin are reported separately on birth certificates. Persons of Hispanic origin may be of any race. Multiple-race data, when reported, were bridged to single-race categories in order to maintain comparability among all reported areas. 4 Includes all persons of Hispanic origin of any race.

NOTES AND DEFINITIONS

SOURCES OF DATA

The tables in Part 1 are from the National Center for Health Statistics (NCHS), a component of the Centers for Disease Control and Prevention (CDC). Several different publications were used to obtain the data.

Most of the tables found in Part 1 were obtained from Hamilton BE, Martin JA, Osterman MJK, et al. *Births: Final Data for 2014*. National Vital Statistics Reports, Vol 64, No 12. Hyattsville, MD: National Center for Health Statistics. 2015.

Some data for the year 2013 was derived from Martin JA, Hamilton BE, Osterman MJK, et al. *Births: Final Data for 2013*. National Vital Statistics Reports: Vol 64, No 1. Hyattsville, MD: National Center for Health Statistics. 2015.

Data for Tables 1-13 and 1-57 through 1-59 were derived from Martinez G, Copen, CE, Abma, JC. *Teenagers in the United States: Sexual Activity, Contraceptive Use, and Childbearing, 2006–2010 National Survey of Family Growth*. National Center for Health Statistics. Vital Health Stat 23 (31). 2011.

NOTES ON THE DATA

Race and Hispanic origin are noted separately on birth certificates. Some rates for 2001 through 2009 have been revised using new population estimates that are based on the 2010 census; thus, these rates may differ from those previously published. Population estimates are generally for July 1 of the year shown.

CONCEPTS AND DEFINITIONS

Anencephaly—A congenital anomaly that consists of a partial or complete absence of the brain and skull.

Apgar score—This has been employed for over 50 years to assess the physical condition and short term prognosis of newborns. Historically, the score has been measured at 1 minute, 5 minutes, and if needed, at additional 5-minute intervals after delivery. Information on the 5 minute score is included in national birth certificate data. The Apgar score measures five easily identifiable characteristics of newborns. A 5-minute score of 0 to 3 indicates an infant in immediate need of resuscitation; 4 to 6 is considered intermediate, and 7 to 10 is considered normal. The Apgar score is a useful clinical indicator for reporting overall status of the neonate and need for, and response to resuscitation efforts.

Birth cohort—Consists of all persons born within a given period of time, such as a calendar year.

Birthweight—The first weight of the newborn obtained after birth. Low birthweight is defined as less than 2,500 grams or 5 pounds 8 ounces. Very low birthweight is defined as less than 1,500 grams or 3 pounds 4 ounces. Before 1979, low birthweight was defined as weighing 2,500 grams or less, and very low birthweight was defined as 1,500 grams or less. Equivalents of the gram weights in terms of pounds and ounces are as follows:

Less than 500 grams = 1 lb 1 oz or less

500–999 grams = 1 lb 2 oz–2 lb 3 oz

3 oz 1,000–1,499 grams = 2 lb 4 oz–3 lb 4 oz

1,500–1,999 grams = 3 lb 5 oz–4 lb 6 oz

2,000–2,499 grams = 4 lb 7 oz–5 lb 8 oz

2,500–2,999 grams = 5 lb 9 oz–6 lb 9 oz

3,000–3,499 grams = 6 lb 10 oz–7 lb 11 oz

3,500–3,999 grams = 7 lb 12 oz–8 lb 13 oz

4,000–4,499 grams = 8 lb 14 oz–9 lb 14 oz

4,500–4,999 grams = 9 lb 15 oz–11 lb 0 oz

5,000 grams or more = 11 lb 1oz or more

Birth rate—Calculated by dividing the number of live births in a population in a year by the midyear resident population. Birth rates are expressed as the number of live births per 1,000 population. The rate may be restricted to births to women of specific age, race, marital status, or geographic location (specific rate), or it may be related to the entire population (crude rate).

Breech/malpresentation—Presenting part of the fetus listed as breech, complete breech, frank breech, footling breech.

Cervical cerclage—Circumferential banding or suture of the cervix to prevent or treat early dilation of the cervix (e.g., incompetent cervix) in an attempt to avoid premature delivery.

Cleft lip/palate—Incomplete closure of the lip. May be unilateral, bilateral, or median. Cleft palate is incomplete fusion of the palatal shelves. May be limited to the soft palate, or may extend into the hard palate.

Contraception—The National Survey of Family Growth collects information on contraceptive use reported by women 15–44 years old. For current contraceptive use, women were asked about contraceptive use during the month of interview.

Women were classified by whether they reported using any of the 19 methods of contraception at any time in the month of interview.

Cyanotic heart disease—Congenital heart defects resulting in lack of oxygen that cause cyanosis.

Down syndrome—The most common chromosomal defect (trisomy 21).

Fertility rate—Total number of live births per 1,000 women of reproductive age (defined as women age 15 to 44 years).

Gestation—The time period between the first day of the last normal menstrual period and the day of birth or day of termination of pregnancy according to the National Vital Statistics System and the CDC's Abortion Surveillance.

Hispanic origin—Includes persons of Mexican, Puerto Rican, Cuban, Central and South American, and other or unknown Latin American or Spanish origins. Persons of Hispanic origin may be of any race.

Hypertension, chronic—Diagnosis prior to the onset of this pregnancy of elevated blood pressure above normal for age, gender, and physiological condition.

Hypertension, pregnancy-associated—Diagnosis in pregnancy of elevated blood pressure above normal for age, gender, and physiological condition.

Induction of labor—Initiation of uterine contractions by medical and/or surgical means for the purpose of delivery before the spontaneous onset of labor.

Maternal morbidities—Information on six maternal morbidities is collected on the 2003 revised birth certificate: maternal transfusion, third-or fourth-degree perineal laceration, ruptured uterus, unplanned hysterectomy, admission to intensive care unit, and unplanned operating room procedure. More than one morbidity may be reported. Maternal morbidity data are not available for Delaware for 2011 because of concerns with data quality.

Meconium, moderate/heavy—Staining of the amniotic fluid caused by passage of fetal bowel contents during labor and/or at delivery that is more than enough to cause a greenish color change of an otherwise clear fluid.

Meningomyecele/Spina bifida—Meningomyelocele is herniation of meninges and spinal cord tissue. Meningocele (herniation of meninges without spinal cord tissue) should also be included in this category. Both open and closed (covered with skin) lesions should be included. Spina bifida is herniation of the meninges and/or spinal cord tissue through a bony defect of spine closure.

Nonvertex presentation—Includes any nonvertex fetal presentation, that is, presentation of a part of the infant's body other than the upper and back part of the infant's head.

Omphalocele/Gastroschisis—Omphalocele is a defect in the anterior abdominal wall, accompanied by herniation of some abdominal organs through a widened umbilical ring into the umbilical stalk. Gastroschisis is an abnormality of the anterior abdominal wall, lateral to the umbilicus, resulting in herniation of the abdominal contents directly into the amniotic cavity.

Precipitous labor—Labor lasting less than 3 hours.

Prenatal care—Medical care provided to a pregnant woman to prevent complications and decrease the incidence of maternal and prenatal mortality. Information on when pregnancy care began is recorded on the birth certificate. Between 1970 and 1980, the reporting area for prenatal care expanded. In 1970, 39 states and the District of Columbia (D.C.) reported prenatal care on the birth certificate. Data were not available from Alabama, Alaska, Arkansas, Connecticut, Delaware, Georgia, Idaho, Massachusetts, New Mexico, Pennsylvania, and Virginia. In 1975, these data were available from three additional states—Connecticut, Delaware, and Georgia—increasing the number of states reporting prenatal care to 42 and D.C. During 1980–2002, prenatal care information was available for the entire United States.

Prepregnancy BMI—The 2003 Standard Certificate of Live Birth includes the components needed to compute both prepregnancy BMI and maternal weight gain (i.e., maternal height, prepregnancy weight, and weight at delivery). BMI is calculated as weight in kilograms divided by height in meters squared $(kg/m^2)(4)$.

Suspected chromosomal disorder—Includes any constellation of congenital malformations resulting from, or compatible with, known syndromes caused by detectable defects in chromosome structure.

Tocolysis—Administration of any agent with the intent to inhibit preterm uterine contractions to extend the length of the pregnancy.

WIC Program—The WIC program is run by the U.S. Department of Agriculture. It is intended to help low-income pregnant women, infants, and children through age 5 years receive proper nutrition by providing vouchers for food, nutrition counseling, health care screenings, and referrals.

PART 2

MORTALITY

PART 2: MORTALITY

Figure 2-1. Age-Adjusted Death Rates, 1940–2013

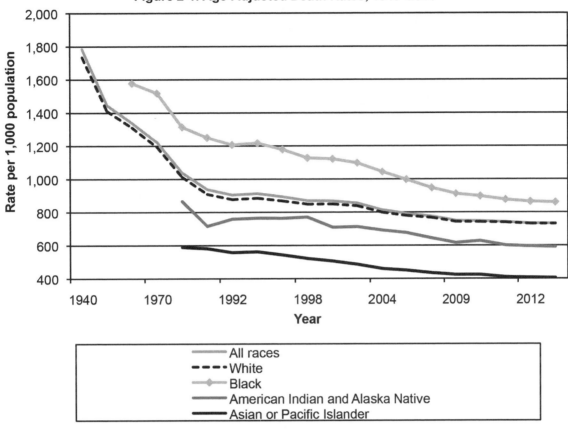

Legend:
- All races
- White
- Black
- American Indian and Alaska Native
- Asian or Pacific Islander

HIGHLIGHTS

- In 2013, 2,596,993 deaths were registered in the United States. The age-adjusted death rate declined to a low of 731.9 per 100,000 standard population. Among all states, Mississippi had the highest age-adjusted death rate at 959.6, while Hawaii had the lowest age-adjusted death rate at 590.8. (Tables 2-1 and 2-27)

- Hispanics had the highest life expectancy of all races and ethnic origins at 81.6 years in 2013. Life expectancy increased for the entire population from 78.2 years in 2008 to 78.8 years in 2013. (Table 2-7)

- The infant mortality rate declined to a record-low in 2013—dropping to 5.96 deaths per 1,000 live births, down from rates of 6.6 in 2008 and 6.4 in 2009. The neonatal mortality rate also declined, falling from 4.3 in 2008 to 4.04 in 2013). The postneonatal mortality rate declined from 2.32 in 2008 to 1.93 in 2013. (Table 2-41)

- The leading cause of infant deaths in 2013 was congenital malformations, deformations, and chromosomal abnormalities, followed by disorders related to length of gestation and fetal malnutrition. (Table 2-42)

Table 2-1. Number of Deaths, Death Rates, and Age-Adjusted Death Rates, by Race and Sex, Selected Years, 1940–2013

(Number, rate per 100,000 population.)

Year	All races[1]			White[2]			Black[2]			American Indian or Alaska Native[2,3]			Asian or Pacific Islander[2,4]		
	Both sexes	Male	Female	Both sexes	Male	Female	Both sexes	Male	Female	Both sexes	Male	Female	Both sexes	Male	Female
Number															
1940	1,417,269	791,003	626,266	1,231,223	690,901	540,322	178,743	95,517	83,226	4,791	2,527	2,264	NA	NA	NA
1950	1,452,454	827,749	624,705	1,276,085	731,366	544,719	169,606	92,004	77,602	4,440	2,497	1,943	NA	NA	NA
1960	1,711,982	975,648	736,334	1,505,335	860,857	644,478	196,010	107,701	88,309	4,528	2,658	1,870	NA	NA	NA
1970	1,921,031	1,078,478	842,553	1,682,096	942,437	739,659	225,647	127,540	98,107	5,675	3,391	2,284	NA	NA	NA
1980	1,989,841	1,075,078	914,763	1,738,607	933,878	804,729	233,135	130,138	102,997	6,923	4,193	2,730	11,071	6,809	4,262
1981	1,977,981	1,063,772	914,209	1,731,233	925,490	805,743	228,560	127,296	101,264	6,608	4,016	2,592	11,475	6,908	4,567
1982	1,974,797	1,056,440	918,357	1,729,085	919,239	809,846	226,513	125,610	100,903	6,679	3,974	2,705	12,430	7,564	4,866
1983	2,019,201	1,071,923	947,278	1,765,582	931,779	833,803	233,124	127,911	105,213	6,839	4,064	2,775	13,554	8,126	5,428
1984	2,039,369	1,076,514	962,855	1,781,897	934,529	847,368	235,884	129,147	106,737	6,949	4,117	2,832	14,483	8,627	5,856
1985	2,086,440	1,097,758	988,682	1,819,054	950,455	868,599	244,207	133,610	110,597	7,154	4,181	2,973	15,887	9,441	6,446
1986	2,105,361	1,104,005	1,001,356	1,831,083	952,554	878,529	250,326	137,214	113,112	7,301	4,365	2,936	16,514	9,795	6,719
1987	2,123,323	1,107,958	1,015,365	1,843,067	953,382	889,685	254,814	139,551	115,263	7,602	4,432	3,170	17,689	10,496	7,193
1988	2,167,999	1,125,540	1,042,459	1,876,906	965,419	911,487	264,019	144,228	119,791	7,917	4,617	3,300	18,963	11,155	7,808
1989	2,150,466	1,114,190	1,036,276	1,853,841	950,852	902,989	267,642	146,393	121,249	8,614	5,066	3,548	20,042	11,688	8,354
1990	2,148,463	1,113,417	1,035,046	1,853,254	950,812	902,442	265,498	145,359	120,139	8,316	4,877	3,439	21,127	12,211	8,916
1991	2,169,518	1,121,665	1,047,853	1,868,904	956,497	912,407	269,525	147,331	122,194	8,621	4,948	3,673	22,173	12,727	9,446
1992	2,175,613	1,122,336	1,053,277	1,873,781	956,957	916,824	269,219	146,630	122,589	8,953	5,181	3,772	23,660	13,568	10,092
1993	2,268,553	1,161,797	1,106,756	1,951,437	988,329	963,108	282,151	153,502	128,649	9,579	5,434	4,145	25,386	14,532	10,854
1994	2,278,994	1,162,747	1,116,247	1,959,875	988,823	971,052	282,379	153,019	129,360	9,637	5,497	4,140	27,103	15,408	11,695
1995	2,312,132	1,172,959	1,139,173	1,987,437	997,277	990,160	286,401	154,175	132,226	9,997	5,574	4,423	28,297	15,933	12,364
1996	2,314,690	1,163,569	1,151,121	1,992,966	991,984	1,000,982	282,089	149,472	132,617	10,127	5,563	4,564	29,508	16,550	12,958
1997	2,314,245	1,154,039	1,160,206	1,996,393	986,884	1,009,509	276,520	144,110	132,410	10,576	5,985	4,591	30,756	17,060	13,696
1998	2,337,256	1,157,260	1,179,996	2,015,984	990,190	1,025,794	278,440	143,417	135,023	10,845	5,994	4,851	31,987	17,659	14,328
1999	2,391,399	1,175,460	1,215,939	2,061,348	1,005,335	1,056,013	285,064	145,703	139,361	11,312	6,092	5,220	33,675	18,330	15,345
2000	2,403,351	1,177,578	1,225,773	2,071,287	1,007,191	1,064,096	285,826	145,184	140,642	11,363	6,185	5,178	34,875	19,018	15,857
2001	2,416,425	1,183,421	1,233,004	2,079,691	1,011,218	1,068,473	287,709	145,908	141,801	11,977	6,466	5,511	37,048	19,829	17,219
2002	2,443,387	1,199,264	1,244,123	2,102,589	1,025,196	1,077,393	290,051	146,835	143,216	12,415	6,750	5,665	38,332	20,483	17,849
2003	2,448,288	1,201,964	1,246,324	2,103,714	1,025,650	1,078,064	291,300	148,022	143,278	13,147	7,106	6,041	40,127	21,186	18,941
2004	2,397,615	1,181,668	1,215,947	2,056,643	1,007,266	1,049,377	287,315	145,970	141,345	13,124	7,134	5,990	40,533	21,298	19,235
2005	2,448,017	1,207,675	1,240,342	2,098,097	1,028,152	1,069,945	292,808	149,108	143,700	13,918	7,607	6,311	43194	22808	20386
2006	2,426,264	1,201,942	1,224,322	2,077,549	1,022,328	1,055,221	289,971	148,602	141,369	14,037	7,630	6,407	44707	23382	21325
2007	2,423,712	1,203,968	1,219,744	2,074,151	1,023,951	1,050,200	289,585	148,309	141,276	14,367	7,885	6,482	45609	23823	21786
2008	2,471,984	1,226,197	1,245,787	2,120,233	1,046,183	1,074,050	289,072	147,143	141,929	14,776	8,163	6,613	47903	24708	23195
2009	2,437,163	1,217,379	1,219,784	2,086,355	1,037,475	1,048,880	286,623	146,239	140,384	14,960	8,105	6,855	49,225	25,560	23,665
2010	2,468,435	1,232,432	1,236,003	2,114,749	1,051,514	1,063,235	286,959	145,802	141,157	15,565	8,516	7,049	51,162	26,600	24,562
2011	2,515,458	1,254,978	1,260,480	2,156,077	1,071,966	1,084,111	290,100	146,884	143,216	15,945	8,638	7,307	53,336	27,490	25,846
2012	2,543,279	1,273,722	1,269,557	2,175,178	1,085,250	1,089,928	295,222	150,586	144,636	16,527	9,067	7,460	56,352	28,819	27,533
2013	2,596,993	1,306,034	1,290,959	2,217,103	1,110,956	1,106,147	302,969	154,767	148,202	17,052	9,331	7,721	59,869	30,890	28,889
Death Rate															
1940	1,076.4	1,197.4	954.6	1,041.5	1,162.2	919.4	NA	NA	NA	NA	NA	NA	NA	NA	NA
1950	963.8	1,106.1	823.5	945.7	1,089.5	803.3	NA	NA	NA	NA	NA	NA	NA	NA	NA
1960	954.7	1,104.5	809.2	947.8	1,098.5	800.9	1,038.6	1,181.7	905.0	NA	NA	NA	NA	NA	NA
1970	945.3	1,090.3	807.8	946.3	1,086.7	812.6	999.3	1,186.6	829.2	NA	NA	NA	NA	NA	NA
1980	878.3	976.9	785.3	892.5	983.3	806.1	875.4	1,034.1	733.3	487.4	597.1	380.1	296.9	375.3	222.5
1981	862.0	954.0	775.0	880.4	965.2	799.8	842.4	992.6	707.7	445.6	547.9	345.6	272.3	336.2	211.5
1982	852.4	938.4	771.2	873.1	951.8	798.2	823.4	966.2	695.5	434.5	522.9	348.1	271.3	338.3	207.4
1983	863.7	943.2	788.4	885.4	957.7	816.4	836.6	971.2	715.9	428.5	515.1	343.9	276.1	339.1	216.1
1984	864.8	938.8	794.7	887.8	954.1	824.6	836.1	968.5	717.4	419.6	502.7	338.4	275.9	336.5	218.1
1985	876.9	948.6	809.1	900.4	963.6	840.1	854.8	989.3	734.2	416.4	492.5	342.5	283.4	344.6	224.9
1986	876.7	944.7	812.3	900.1	958.6	844.3	864.9	1,002.6	741.5	409.5	494.9	325.9	276.2	335.1	219.9
1987	876.4	939.3	816.7	900.1	952.7	849.8	868.9	1,006.2	745.7	410.7	483.8	339.0	278.9	338.3	222.0
1988	886.7	945.1	831.2	910.5	957.9	865.3	888.3	1,026.1	764.6	411.7	485.0	339.9	282.0	339.0	227.7
1989	871.3	926.3	818.9	893.2	936.5	851.8	887.9	1,026.7	763.2	430.5	510.7	351.3	280.9	334.5	229.4
1990	863.8	918.4	812.0	888.0	930.9	846.9	871.0	1,008.0	747.9	402.8	476.4	330.4	283.3	334.3	234.3
1991	857.6	908.8	808.7	883.2	922.7	845.2	861.4	994.8	741.4	405.3	468.9	342.7	278.7	326.9	232.4
1992	848.1	896.1	802.4	875.8	912.2	840.8	841.8	967.6	728.6	406.6	474.1	340.0	282.1	331.1	235.3
1993	872.8	915.0	832.5	902.7	931.8	874.6	864.6	992.2	749.6	419.8	479.6	360.7	288.0	338.1	240.3
1994	866.1	904.2	829.7	897.8	922.6	873.8	849.0	970.2	739.7	408.2	468.8	348.3	294.6	344.0	247.7
1995	868.3	900.8	837.2	901.8	921.0	883.2	846.2	960.2	743.2	409.4	459.4	360.1	294.6	341.4	250.4
1996	859.2	882.8	836.7	896.0	907.1	885.3	819.7	915.3	733.3	399.5	441.5	358.0	294.4	340.2	251.1
1997	848.8	864.6	833.6	889.1	893.3	885.0	789.9	867.1	720.1	402.7	458.2	347.7	294.1	336.8	253.9
1998	847.3	856.4	838.5	889.5	887.3	891.6	782.3	848.2	722.6	397.8	441.9	354.2	293.8	335.4	254.9

Table 2-1. Number of Deaths, Death Rates, and Age-Adjusted Death Rates, by Race and Sex, Selected Years, 1940–2013— continued

(Number, rate per 100,000 population.)

Year	All races[1]			White[2]			Black[2]			American Indian or Alaska Native[2,3]			Asian or Pacific Islander[2,4]		
	Both sexes	Male	Female	Both sexes	Male	Female	Both sexes	Male	Female	Both sexes	Male	Female	Both sexes	Male	Female
1999	857.0	859.2	854.9	901.4	892.1	910.4	788.1	847.4	734.3	399.3	431.8	367.1	296.8	333.2	262.5
2000	854.0	853.0	855.0	900.2	887.8	912.3	781.1	834.1	733.0	380.8	415.6	346.1	296.6	332.9	262.3
2001	848.0	846.0	849.9	895.7	882.5	908.5	772.4	822.7	726.6	386.7	418.5	355.1	298.1	328.9	269.1
2002	849.5	849.2	849.8	899.6	888.5	910.4	768.4	816.8	724.4	387.7	422.4	353.1	295.9	326.5	267.2
2003	843.9	843.9	843.9	894.7	883.6	905.6	762.4	813.6	715.8	396.9	429.9	364.1	298.1	325.6	272.3
2004	818.8	821.6	816.2	869.0	861.6	876.3	741.7	790.7	697.1	382.7	416.5	348.9	290.2	315.9	266.2
2005	828.4	831.7	825.1	880.9	873.5	888.1	745.4	796.1	699.2	391.6	428.4	354.8	298.0	326.6	271.4
2006	813.1	819.6	806.9	866.3	862.3	870.3	727.5	781.4	678.3	380.6	413.7	347.6	297.5	323.4	273.4
2007	804.6	813.1	796.4	859.3	857.8	860.6	715.9	768.1	668.2	375.1	411.1	339.0	293.1	318.7	269.5
2008	812.9	820.3	805.8	872.6	870.6	874.6	704.2	750.6	661.8	370.9	408.7	332.9	297.6	320.0	277.0
2009	794.5	807.2	782.1	853.7	858.2	849.3	688.5	735.3	645.6	361.2	389.9	332.4	296.4	321.2	273.5
2010	799.5	812.0	787.4	861.7	866.1	857.3	682.2	725.4	642.7	365.1	397.5	332.4	301.1	327.0	277.3
2011	807.3	818.7	796.3	872.6	876.4	868.9	679.7	719.4	643.4	366.8	395.1	338.1	321.4	347.4	297.4
2012	810.2	824.5	796.4	876.3	882.8	869.9	683.3	728.0	642.3	375.7	410.2	340.9	311.5	332.8	292.0
2013	821.5	839.1	804.4	889.2	899.1	879.4	693.4	739.3	651.1	382.5	416.5	348.2	321.4	347,4	297.4
Age-Adjusted Death Rate [5]															
1940	1,785.0	1,976.0	1,599.4	1,735.3	1,925.2	1,550.4	NA	NA	NA	NA	NA	NA	NA	NA	NA
1950	1,446.0	1,674.2	1,236.0	1,410.8	1,642.5	1,198.0	NA	NA	NA	NA	NA	NA	NA	NA	NA
1960	1,339.2	1,609.0	1,105.3	1,311.3	1,586.0	1,074.4	1,577.5	1,811.1	1,369.7	NA	NA	NA	NA	NA	NA
1970	1,222.6	1,542.1	971.4	1,193.3	1,513.7	944.0	1,518.1	1,873.9	1,228.7	NA	NA	NA	NA	NA	NA
1980	1,039.1	1,348.1	817.9	1,012.7	1,317.6	796.1	1,314.8	1,697.8	1,033.3	867.0	1,111.5	662.4	589.9	786.5	425.9
1981	1,007.1	1,308.2	792.7	984.0	1,282.2	773.6	1,258.4	1,626.6	986.6	784.6	1,030.2	588.0	544.7	710.3	405.3
1982	985.0	1,279.9	776.6	963.6	1,255.9	758.7	1,221.3	1,580.4	960.1	757.0	940.1	604.4	550.4	738.2	410.3
1983	990.0	1,284.5	783.3	967.3	1,259.4	763.9	1,240.5	1,600.7	980.7	757.3	945.0	605.5	565.1	718.8	428.8
1984	982.5	1,271.4	779.8	959.7	1,245.9	760.7	1,236.7	1,600.8	976.9	761.7	946.0	567.9	574.4	724.7	443.1
1985	988.1	1,278.1	784.5	963.6	1,249.8	764.3	1,261.2	1,634.5	994.4	731.7	926.1	577.2	586.5	755.4	456.7
1986	978.6	1,261.7	778.7	952.8	1,230.5	758.1	1,266.7	1,650.1	994.4	720.8	926.7	549.3	576.4	730.5	445.4
1987	970.0	1,246.1	774.2	943.4	1,213.4	753.3	1,263.1	1,650.3	989.7	719.8	899.3	583.7	577.3	732.4	448.1
1988	975.7	1,250.7	781.0	947.6	1,215.9	759.1	1,284.3	1,677.6	1,006.8	718.6	917.4	563.6	584.2	732.0	451.0
1989	950.5	1,215.0	761.8	920.2	1,176.6	738.8	1,275.5	1,670.1	998.1	761.6	999.8	586.3	581.3	729.6	458.4
1990	938.7	1,202.8	750.9	909.8	1,165.9	728.8	1,250.3	1,644.5	975.1	716.3	916.2	561.8	582.0	716.4	469.3
1991	922.3	1,180.5	738.2	893.2	1,143.1	716.1	1,235.4	1,626.1	963.3	763.9	970.6	608.3	566.2	703.4	453.2
1992	905.6	1,158.3	725.5	877.7	1,122.4	704.1	1,206.7	1,587.8	942.5	759.0	970.4	599.4	558.5	697.3	445.8
1993	926.1	1,177.3	745.9	897.0	1,138.9	724.1	1,241.2	1,632.2	969.5	796.4	1,006.3	641.6	565.8	709.9	450.4
1994	913.5	1,155.5	738.6	885.6	1,118.7	717.5	1,216.9	1,592.8	954.6	764.8	953.3	618.8	562.7	702.5	452.1
1995	909.8	1,143.9	739.4	882.3	1,107.5	718.7	1,213.9	1,585.7	955.9	771.2	932.0	643.9	554.8	693.4	446.7
1996	894.1	1,115.7	733.0	869.0	1,082.9	713.6	1,178.4	1,524.2	940.3	763.6	924.8	641.7	543.2	676.1	439.6
1997	878.1	1,088.1	725.6	855.7	1,059.1	707.8	1,139.8	1,458.8	922.1	774.0	974.8	625.3	531.8	660.2	432.6
1998	870.6	1,069.4	724.7	849.3	1,042.0	707.3	1,127.8	1,430.5	921.6	770.4	943.9	640.5	522.4	646.9	426.7
1999	875.6	1,067.0	734.0	854.6	1,040.0	716.6	1,135.7	1,432.6	933.6	780.9	925.9	668.2	519.7	641.2	427.5
2000	869.0	1,053.8	731.4	849.8	1,029.4	715.3	1,121.4	1,403.5	927.6	709.3	841.5	604.5	506.4	624.2	416.8
2001 [5]	858.8	1,035.4	725.6	840.7	1,012.1	710.4	1,106.2	1,380.5	917.9	714.1	834.4	617.1	495.4	603.7	413.9
2002 [5]	855.9	1,030.6	723.6	839.0	1,009.0	709.3	1,097.3	1,364.8	913.5	713.0	841.3	611.1	486.5	595.3	405.5
2003 [5]	843.5	1,010.3	715.2	827.1	988.8	701.6	1,080.5	1,343.5	898.3	726.3	850.6	628.1	480.5	583.6	404.2
2004 [5]	813.7	973.3	690.5	798.5	953.2	677.7	1,043.8	1,296.8	869.8	691.8	811.4	594.9	460.7	557.4	389.1
2005 [5]	815.0	971.9	692.3	801.1	952.9	680.9	1,035.1	1,281.3	862.7	701.1	824.5	601.8	459.6	560.6	385.2
2006 [5]	791.8	943.5	672.2	779.3	925.8	662.3	997.9	1,239.5	828.4	676.6	780.8	589.0	450.7	544.9	381.2
2007 [5]	775.3	922.9	658.1	764.3	907.1	649.4	972.0	1,204.8	808.1	661.3	780.3	565.2	436.2	525.9	369.2
2008 [5]	774.9	918.8	659.9	767.2	907.1	653.7	947.7	1,168.0	792.0	644.0	757.2	548.7	435.1	518.5	372.4
2009 [5]	749.6	890.9	636.8	742.8	880.5	631.3	912.8	1,123.1	763.3	616.0	709.0	536.4	424.6	509.2	361.1
2010	747.0	887.1	634.9	741.8	878.5	630.8	898.2	1,104.0	752.5	628.3	730.2	541.7	424.3	512.1	359.0
2011	741.3	875.3	632.4	738.8	870.2	630.3	877.1	1,067.1	739.8	600.9	691.7	522.5	410.3	490.7	349.8
2012	732.8	865.1	624.7	730.9	860.0	623.8	864.8	1,058.6	723.9	595.3	690.5	512.3	407.1	484.1	348.8
2013	731.9	863.6	623.5	731.0	859.2	623.6	860.8	1052.8	720.6	591.7	689.2	508.3	405.4	487.8	343.0

NA= Not available.   1 For 1940–1991, data includes deaths among races not shown separately; beginning in 1992, records coded as "other races" and records for which race was unknown, not stated, or not classifiable were assigned to the race of previous record.   2 Multiple-race data were reported by 42 states and the District of Columbia in 2012 and 2013, 38 states and the District of Columbia in 2011, 37 states and the District of Columbia in 2010, 34 states and the District of Columbia in 2008, by 27 states and the District of Columbia in 2007, 25 states and the District of Columbia in 2006, 21 states and the District of Columbia in 2005, 15 states in 2004, and 7 states in 2003. The multiple-race data for these reporting areas were bridged to the single-race categories of the 1977 OMB standards for comparability with other reporting areas.   3 Includes Aleuts and Eskimos.   4 Includes Chinese, Filipinos, Hawaiians, Japanese, and other Asian or Pacific Islander persons.   5 For method of computation, see chapter notes.

Table 2-2. Number of Deaths, Death Rates, and Age-Adjusted Death Rates, by Hispanic Origin, Race for Non-Hispanic Population, and Sex, 1997–2013

(Number, rate per 100,000 population in specified group.)

Year	Hispanic			Non-Hispanic[1]			Non-Hispanic White[2]			Non-Hispanic Black[2]		
	Both sexes	Male	Female	Both sexes	Male	Female	Both sexes	Male	Female	Both sexes	Male	Female
Number												
1997	95,460	54,348	41,112	2,209,450	1,094,541	1,114,909	1,895,461	929,703	965,758	273,381	142,241	131,140
1998	98,406	55,821	42,585	2,230,127	1,096,677	1,133,450	1,912,802	931,844	980,958	275,264	141,627	133,637
1999	103,740	57,991	45,749	2,279,325	1,112,718	1,166,607	1,953,197	944,913	1,008,284	281,979	143,883	138,096
2000	107,254	60,172	47,082	2,287,846	1,112,704	1,175,142	1,959,919	944,781	1,015,138	282,676	143,297	139,379
2001	113,413	63,317	50,096	2,295,244	1,115,683	1,179,561	1,962,810	945,967	1,016,843	284,343	143,971	140,372
2002	117,135	65,703	51,432	2,318,269	1,129,090	1,189,179	1,981,973	957,645	1,024,328	286,573	144,802	141,771
2003	122,026	68,119	53,907	2,319,476	1,129,927	1,189,549	1,979,465	956,194	1,023,271	287,968	146,136	141,832
2004	122,416	68,544	53,872	2,269,583	1,109,848	1,159,735	1,933,382	938,143	995,239	283,859	144,022	139,837
2005	131,161	73,788	57,373	2,312,028	1,131,013	1,181,015	1,967,142	954,402	1,012,740	289,163	147,010	142,153
2006	133,004	74,250	58,754	2,288,424	1,124,813	1,163,611	1,944,617	947,966	996,651	286,581	146,729	139,852
2007	135,519	75,708	59,811	2,284,446	1,125,974	1,158,472	1,939,606	948,662	990,944	286,366	146,474	139,892
2008	139,241	76,861	62,380	2,327,636	1,146,394	1,181,242	1,981,034	969,288	1,011,746	285,522	145,168	140,354
2009	141,576	78,157	63,419	2,289,999	1,135,852	1,154,147	1,944,606	959,014	985,592	282,982	144,197	138,785
2010	144,490	79,622	64,868	2,318,218	1,149,438	1,168,780	1,969,916	971,604	998,312	283,438	143,824	139,614
2011	149,635	81,887	67,748	2,360,643	1,169,971	1,190,672	2,006,319	989,835	1,016,484	286,797	145,052	141,745
2012	156,419	85,238	71,181	2,379,078	1,183,988	1,195,090	2,016,896	998,832	1,018,064	291,179	148,344	142,835
2013	163,241	88,880	74,361	2,426,808	1,212,979	1,213,829	2,052,660	1,021,135	1,031,525	299,227	152,661	146,566
Death Rate												
1997	309	343.2	272.9	913.9	930.4	898.3	967.4	970.6	964.3	813.5	892.9	741.9
1998	303.9	336.0	270.0	916.0	925.3	907.1	972.9	969.2	976.5	805.6	873.7	744.1
1999	305.7	332.6	277.2	929.9	932.2	927.8	990.7	979.6	1001.3	812.1	872.8	757.3
2000	303.8	331.3	274.6	929.6	928.1	931.0	993.2	978.5	1007.3	805.5	859.5	756.7
2001	305.3	331.8	277.4	926.2	923.5	928.7	992.1	976.3	1,007.2	797.9	849.6	751.0
2002	303.3	331.5	273.6	931.0	930.0	932.0	1,000.5	986.7	1,013.8	794.9	844.5	750.0
2003	304.7	332.0	276.0	927.6	926.8	928.3	998.3	984.1	1,011.8	790.6	843.7	742.5
2004	295.0	322.8	265.8	903.1	905.3	901.0	973.4	963.2	983.2	770.3	821.2	724.1
2005	304.9	335.6	272.7	915.7	918.0	913.5	989.1	978.1	999.7	775.8	828.4	728.1
2006	298.2	326.1	269.0	901.8	908.0	895.8	976.2	969.4	982.8	759.8	816.5	708.1
2007	293.4	321.6	264.0	895.7	904.2	887.6	972.3	968.3	976.1	749.9	804.9	699.9
2008	291.3	316.0	265.8	908.2	915.9	900.8	991.6	987.5	995.6	738.7	787.8	694.0
2009	287.0	311.8	261.4	889.5	903.3	876.3	972.3	975.7	969.1	723.7	773.2	678.5
2010	286.2	310.8	260.9	897.6	911.1	884.7	984.3	987.5	981.2	718.7	764.5	676.9
2011	287.5	309.7	264.6	909.5	922.3	897.3	1,001.0	1,004.1	998.1	718.0	760.4	679.2
2012	295.0	316.5	272.7	911.9	928.2	896.4	1,004.9	1,011.2	998.8	720.9	768.5	677.3
2013	301.9	323.7	279.4	926.1	946.2	906.7	1,021.6	1,032.1	1,011.5	733.4	782.5	688.4
Age-Adjusted Death Rate												
1997	669.3	840.5	538.8	885.3	1,096.4	732.6	859.7	1,063.2	712.5	1,154.3	1,476.7	934.2
1998	665.4	833.6	536.9	878.4	1,078.2	732.4	854.1	1,046.7	712.8	1,141.8	1,448.2	932.9
1999	676.4	830.5	555.9	883.9	1,076.4	741.9	859.8	1,045.5	722.3	1,150.1	1,449.4	946.0
2000	665.7	818.1	546.0	877.9	1,063.8	740.0	855.5	1,035.4	721.5	1,137.0	1,422.0	941.2
2001	662.6	808.6	547.0	868.4	1,046.1	734.9	847.1	1,018.8	717.3	1,122.3	1,400.4	931.5
2002	652.2	799.9	535.9	866.4	1,042.1	733.8	846.4	1,016.5	717.1	1,114.1	1,385.1	927.9
2003	645.3	784.0	534.2	854.6	1,022.6	725.8	834.9	996.7	709.8	1,099.0	1,366.8	913.6
2004	616.8	750.1	509.5	825.9	986.7	702.2	807.6	962.5	687.2	1,062.8	1,320.9	885.4
2005	627.6	771.2	513.8	827.3	985.0	704.4	810.1	961.5	690.7	1,055.1	1,306.1	879.4
2006	604.0	732.3	500.2	804.9	958.0	684.6	789.1	935.7	672.4	1,019.3	1,267.0	845.6
2007	586.1	711.4	484.4	789.5	938.7	671.4	775.3	918.4	660.6	994.4	1,233.2	826.4
2008	579.8	695.3	484.7	790.0	935.9	673.7	779.4	920.2	665.4	969.2	1,195.4	809.6
2009	559.7	675.5	466.1	764.7	908.0	650.5	755.1	893.7	643.1	934.4	1,150.5	781.0
2010	558.6	677.7	463.4	762.6	904.6	649.2	755.0	892.5	643.3	920.4	1,131.7	770.8
2011	540.7	647.3	452.8	759.2	895.6	648.4	754.3	887.2	644.6	901.6	1,098.3	759.8
2012	539.1	643.9	452.5	749.8	884.6	639.8	745.8	876.2	637.6	887.1	1,086.4	742.1
2013	535.4	639.8	448.6	750.1	884.4	639.7	747.1	876.8	638.4	885.2	1,083.3	740.6

1 Includes races other than White and Black.   2 Multiple-race data were reported by 42 states and the District of Columbia in 2012 and 2013, 38 states and the District of Columbia in 2011, 37 states and the District of Columbia in 2010, 34 states and the District of Columbia in 2008, by 27 states and the District of Columbia in 2007, 25 states and the District of Columbia in 2006, 21 states and the District of Columbia in 2005, 15 states in 2004, and 7 states in 2003. The multiple-race data for these reporting areas were bridged to the single-race categories of the 1977 OMB standards for comparability with other reporting areas.

Table 2-3. Number of Deaths and Death Rates, by Age, Race, and Sex, 2013

(Number, rate per 100,000 population in specified group.)

Age	All races			White[1]			Black[1]			American Indian or Alaska Native[1,2]			Asian or Pacific Islander[1,3]		
	Both sexes	Male	Female	Both sexes	Male	Female	Both sexes	Male	Female	Both sexes	Male	Female	Both sexes	Male	Female
Number															
All ages	2,596,993	1,306,034	1,290,959	2,217,103	1,110,956	1,106,147	302,969	154,767	148,202	17,052	9,331	7,721	59,869	30,980	28,889
Under 1 year	23,440	13,119	10,321	15,125	8,548	6,577	7,123	3,878	3,245	315	197	118	877	496	381
1 to 4 years	4,068	2,323	1,745	2,774	1,601	1,173	1,006	561	445	104	65	39	184	96	88
5 to 9 years	2,427	1,383	1,044	1,675	967	708	582	321	261	50	26	24	120	69	51
10 to 14 years	2,913	1,694	1,219	2,166	1,252	914	587	354	233	38	21	17	122	67	55
15 to 19 years	9,480	6,759	2,721	6,852	4,767	2,085	2,180	1,685	495	180	128	52	268	179	89
20 to 24 years	19,006	14,105	4,901	13,766	10,113	3,653	4,358	3,356	1,002	368	260	108	514	376	138
25 to 29 years	21,056	15,023	6,033	15,567	11,101	4,466	4,467	3,211	1,256	448	305	143	574	406	168
30 to 34 years	24,407	16,439	7,968	18,210	12,334	5,876	5,064	3,387	1,677	475	310	165	658	408	250
35 to 39 years	27,821	17,544	10,277	20,794	13,215	7,579	5,702	3,523	2,179	518	305	213	807	501	306
40 to 44 years	41,752	25,528	16,224	31,736	19,669	12,067	8,057	4,691	3,366	708	425	283	1,251	743	508
45 to 49 years	66,833	40,531	26,302	51,599	31,717	19,882	12,459	7,142	5,317	1,002	600	402	1,773	1,072	701
50 to 54 years	110,891	67,466	43,425	87,487	54,073	33,414	19,652	11,139	8,513	1,298	775	523	2,454	1,479	975
55 to 59 years	152,981	93,996	58,985	120,916	75,104	45,812	27,213	15,988	11,225	1,536	893	643	3,316	2,011	1,305
60 to 64 years	185,146	112,329	72,817	148,369	90,766	57,603	30,896	18,078	12,818	1,567	922	645	4,314	2,563	1,751
65 to 69 years	214,509	124,324	90,185	179,185	104,448	74,737	28,988	16,278	12,710	1,599	893	706	4,737	2,705	2,032
70 to 74 years	239,920	133,574	106,346	203,937	114,192	89,745	29,142	15,542	13,600	1,569	865	704	5,272	2,975	2,297
75 to 79 years	277,314	146,166	131,148	239,264	127,019	112,245	29,789	14,844	14,945	1,572	783	789	6,689	3,520	3,169
80 to 84 years	347,699	169,174	178,525	308,071	151,438	156,633	30,084	13,108	16,976	1,442	699	743	8,102	3,929	4,173
85 years and over	825,198	304,462	520,736	749,509	278,557	470,952	55,594	17,664	37,930	2,259	856	1,403	17,836	7,385	10,451
Not stated	132	95	37	101	75	26	26	17	9	4	3	1	1	-	1
Rate															
All ages[4]	821.5	839.1	804.4	889.2	899.1	879.4	693.4	739.3	651.1	382.5	416.5	348.2	321.4	347.4	297.4
Under 1 year[5]	594.7	650.5	536.1	512.9	566.4	456.8	1,052.0	1,120.1	980.7	401.3	493.4	305.9	370.0	408.9	329.3
1 to 4 years	25.5	28.6	22.4	23.3	26.2	20.1	37.1	40.6	33.4	33.6	41.5	25.5	18.8	19.3	18.4
5 to 9 years	11.8	13.2	10.4	10.8	12.2	9.3	17.1	18.6	15.6	12.8	13.1	12.4	9.7	11.0	8.3
10 to 14 years	14.1	16.1	12.1	13.8	15.6	11.9	17.4	20.6	14.0	10.1	11.0	*	10.3	11.2	9.3
15 to 19 years	44.8	62.3	26.4	42.6	57.7	26.7	62.0	94.2	28.7	48.0	67.1	28.3	22.7	29.9	15.3
20 to 24 years	83.4	120.8	44.1	80.3	114.6	43.9	113.6	173.7	52.7	93.2	126.8	56.9	36.3	52.5	19.8
25 to 29 years	97.6	137.1	56.8	94.4	131.3	55.6	139.7	205.4	76.9	127.4	165.8	85.3	37.1	53.7	21.2
30 to 34 years	114.8	153.9	75.3	111.7	148.5	73.5	166.2	232.7	105.4	142.3	180.0	102.1	41.6	54.6	29.9
35 to 39 years	141.9	179.3	104.7	138.0	173.2	102.0	207.9	272.2	150.5	174.0	200.3	146.5	53.8	70.8	38.6
40 to 44 years	200.3	246.4	154.7	195.4	240.4	149.8	284.0	351.4	224.1	245.2	290.3	198.7	84.3	106.5	64.5
45 to 49 years	315.1	386.1	245.6	307.1	376.9	237.1	437.3	532.5	352.7	362.2	433.1	291.0	138.3	177.7	103.3
50 to 54 years	491.6	609.4	378.0	480.3	598.7	363.9	680.6	824.0	554.3	478.3	582.8	377.9	207.1	266.9	154.6
55 to 59 years	721.8	914.1	540.5	697.6	883.7	518.6	1,058.6	1,347.6	810.9	668.7	805.2	541.3	312.3	413.7	226.7
60 to 64 years	1,021.7	1,295.0	770.7	986.3	1,245.4	742.8	1,529.1	1,995.1	1,150.1	907.1	1,115.7	715.8	486.9	644.5	358.5
65 to 69 years	1,468.4	1,798.4	1,171.9	1,444.9	1,760.0	1,155.8	2,032.2	2,608.4	1,584.1	1,301.4	1,529.2	1,095.1	719.2	913.5	560.6
70 to 74 years	2,261.7	2,734.7	1,858.0	2,246.5	2,702.7	1,849.4	2,943.6	3,751.2	2,362.4	1,970.6	2,347.9	1,645.7	1,144.6	1,429.4	909.8
75 to 79 years	3,611.9	4,311.2	3,058.8	3,622.8	4,304.0	3,072.5	4,270.6	5,409.0	3,532.3	3,064.0	3,494.4	2,730.2	2,060.6	2,473.7	1,738.2
80 to 84 years	6,027.4	7,137.6	5,253.1	6,094.6	7,194.3	5,309.9	6,479.1	7,949.2	5,669.5	4,603.4	5,515.2	3,983.7	3,713.6	4,484.4	3,196.3
85 years and over	13,660.4	14,911.6	13,021.6	13,965.5	15,220.4	13,316.1	12,428.8	13,657.1	11,929.2	8,368.5	9,034.3	8,008.4	8,934.2	10,142.8	8,240.4

[1] - = Quantity zero.   * = Figure does not meet standards of reliability or precision.   1Race categories are consistent with the 1977 Office of Management and Budget (OMB) standards. In 2013, multiple-race data were reported by 42 states and the District of Columbia. The multiple-race data for these reporting areas were bridged to the single-race categories of the 1977 OMB standards for comparability with other reporting areas.   2Includes Aleuts and Eskimos.   3Includes Chinese, Filipinos, Hawaiians, Japanese, and other Asian or Pacific Islander persons.   4Figures for age not stated are included in "All ages" but not distributed among age groups.   5Death rates for "Under 1 year" (based on population estimates) differ from infant mortality rates (based on live births); for more information, see chapter notes.

Table 2-4. Number of Deaths and Death Rates, by Hispanic Origin, Race for Non-Hispanic Population, Age, and Sex, 2013

(Number, rate per 100,000 population in specified group.)

Age	Hispanic			Non-Hispanic[1]			Non-Hispanic White[2]			Non-Hispanic Black[2]		
	Both sexes	Male	Female	Both sexes	Male	Female	Both sexes	Male	Female	Both sexes	Male	Female
Number												
All ages	163,241	88,880	74,361	2,426,808	1,212,979	1,213,829	2,052,660	1,021,135	1,031,525	299,227	152,661	146,566
Under 1 year	4,751	2,598	2,153	18,439	10,379	8,060	10,563	6,045	4,518	6,781	3,698	3,083
1–4 years	854	483	371	3,200	1,832	1,368	1,977	1,149	828	963	538	425
5–9 years	467	265	202	1,955	1,115	840	1,238	718	520	561	308	253
10–14 years	606	326	280	2,303	1,365	938	1,586	939	647	571	345	226
15–19 years	1,646	1,191	455	7,820	5,558	2,262	5,253	3,611	1,642	2,146	1,660	486
20–24 years	3,011	2,325	686	15,950	11,745	4,205	10,839	7,850	2,989	4,277	3,297	980
25–29 years	2,995	2,266	729	18,003	12,716	5,287	12,634	8,880	3,754	4,394	3,156	1,238
30–34 years	3,346	2,366	980	21,004	14,033	6,971	14,949	10,024	4,925	4,988	3,333	1,655
35–39 years	3,777	2,545	1,232	23,977	14,951	9,026	17,069	10,692	6,377	5,647	3,492	2,155
40–44 years	4,921	3,183	1,738	36,693	22,251	14,442	26,862	16,505	10,357	7,932	4,613	3,319
45–49 years	6,986	4,573	2,413	59,606	35,793	23,813	44,615	27,122	17,493	12,316	7,058	5,258
50–54 years	9,408	6,110	3,298	101,000	61,025	39,975	77,916	47,836	30,080	19,444	11,014	8,430
55–59 years	11,089	7,088	4,001	141,256	86,450	54,806	109,650	67,862	41,788	26,913	15,790	11,123
60–64 years	12,237	7,586	4,651	172,148	104,190	67,958	135,868	82,960	52,908	30,567	17,854	12,713
65–69 years	12,961	7,646	5,315	200,784	116,161	84,623	165,943	96,581	69,362	28,682	16,079	12,603
70–74 years	13,723	7,709	6,014	225,503	125,409	100,094	190,006	106,316	83,690	28,826	15,354	13,472
75–79 years	16,210	8,363	7,847	260,445	137,403	123,042	222,885	118,536	104,349	29,473	14,652	14,821
80–84 years	18,556	8,797	9,759	328,503	160,029	168,474	289,367	142,541	146,826	29,751	12,930	16,821
85 years and over	35,690	13,454	22,236	788,148	290,525	497,623	713,390	264,933	448,457	54,975	17,477	37,498
Not stated	7	6	1	71	49	22	50	35	15	20	13	7
Rate												
All ages[3]	301.9	323.7	279.4	926.1	946.2	906.7	1,021.6	1,032.1	1,011.5	733.4	782.5	688.4
Under 1 year[4]	468.1	501.1	433.7	630.0	692.7	564.2	511.5	571.5	448.5	1,117.3	1,192.3	1,039.0
1–4 years	20.8	23.1	18.4	27.1	30.3	23.7	23.7	26.9	20.4	39.5	43.3	35.4
5–9 years	9.1	10.1	8.1	12.7	14.1	11.1	11.2	12.7	9.7	18.2	19.7	16.7
10–14 years	12.7	13.4	12.0	14.5	16.8	12.1	13.8	16.0	11.6	18.4	21.9	14.8
15–19 years	35.8	50.3	20.4	47.2	65.6	28.0	43.8	58.6	28.2	65.9	100.2	30.3
20–24 years	64.4	94.6	30.9	88.0	127.4	47.3	83.4	118.3	47.0	120.0	183.8	55.4
25–29 years	68.1	96.6	35.5	104.8	147.6	61.7	100.5	139.6	60.5	148.8	218.8	82.0
30–34 years	76.6	103.2	47.3	124.3	167.3	81.9	120.6	160.4	80.1	177.3	248.4	112.5
35–39 years	93.4	122.1	62.9	154.1	194.2	114.8	149.4	186.0	112.4	222.0	291.0	160.3
40–44 years	131.4	166.6	94.7	214.5	263.3	166.9	209.1	256.1	161.9	297.4	367.6	235.0
45–49 years	212.7	273.5	149.6	332.6	405.6	261.8	322.8	393.4	252.5	456.5	556.0	368.1
50–54 years	336.4	437.1	235.8	511.1	630.9	396.2	497.0	616.4	379.9	704.6	852.7	574.3
55–59 years	504.9	662.2	355.4	743.5	938.4	560.0	715.0	901.8	535.0	1,089.7	1,386.3	835.9
60–64 years	754.0	985.3	545.2	1,043.4	1,318.1	790.7	1,002.1	1,260.1	758.5	1,569.2	2,045.3	1,182.6
65–69 years	1,101.2	1,411.4	836.7	1,494.8	1,823.1	1,198.6	1,466.2	1,776.7	1,179.3	2,083.6	2,671.5	1,626.8
70–74 years	1,693.8	2,165.3	1,324.2	2,301.6	2,769.4	1,899.5	2,281.5	2,729.0	1,888.1	3,013.2	3,837.6	2,420.6
75–79 years	2,778.8	3,400.5	2,325.7	3,671.1	4,369.7	3,114.9	3,676.5	4,354.3	3,124.2	4,371.5	5,530.0	3,621.4
80–84 years	4,604.0	5,467.9	4,030.0	6,122.4	7,243.5	5,337.7	6,185.6	7,294.0	5,390.5	6,620.5	8,117.1	5,798.6
85 years and over	9,986.9	10,596.0	9,651.3	13,867.5	15,172.5	13,204.4	14,176.8	15,485.9	13,502.5	12,659.0	13,959.7	12,132.2

- = Quantity zero.   1 Includes races other than White and Black.   2Race categories are consistent with the 1977 Office of Management and Budget (OMB) standards. In 2010, multiple-race data were reported by 42 states and the District of Columbia. The multiple-race data for these reporting areas were bridged to the single-race categories of the 1977 OMB standards for comparability with other reporting areas.   3Figures for age not stated are included in "All ages" but not distributed among age groups.   4Death rates for "Under 1 year" (based on population estimates) differ from infant mortality rates (based on live births); for more information, see chapter notes.

Table 2-5. Number of Deaths and Death Rates, by Age, and Age-Adjusted Death Rates, by Specified Hispanic Origin, Race for Non-Hispanic Population, and Sex, 2010

(Number, rate per 100,000 population in specified group.)

Origin, race, and sex	All ages	Under 1 year[1]	1 to 4 years	5 to 14 years	15 to 24 years	25 to 34 years	35 to 44 years	45 to 54 years	55 to 64 years	65 to 74 years	75 to 84 years	85 years and over	Age not stated	Age-adjusted rate[2]
NUMBER														
All Origins	2,543,279	23,629	4,218	5,200	29,182	44,591	69,162	179,463	329,606	432,346	620,428	805,307	147	X
Male	1,273,722	13,139	2,395	3,036	21,456	30,783	42,929	109,214	200,951	244,935	310,681	294,103	100	X
Female	1,269,557	10,490	1,823	2,164	7,726	13,808	26,233	70,249	128,655	187,411	309,747	511,204	47	X
Hispanic (of any race)	156,419	4,813	899	1,083	4,773	6,216	8,338	15,778	22,620	24,868	33,614	33,410	7	X
Male	85,238	2,662	494	608	3,655	4,578	5,593	10,169	14,258	14,102	16,552	12,560	7	X
Female	71,181	2,151	405	475	1,118	1,638	2,745	5,609	8,362	10,766	17,062	20,850	–	X
Mexican	88,362	3,265	634	747	3,172	3,959	5,274	9,500	13,470	13,768	17,912	16,658	3	X
Male	49,530	1,800	348	416	2,465	2,928	3,589	6,138	8,519	7,827	8,831	6,666	3	X
Female	38,832	1,465	286	331	707	1,031	1,685	3,362	4,951	5,941	9,081	9,992	–	X
Puerto Rican	19,911	501	81	109	468	667	1,002	2,210	3,193	3,594	4,230	3,855	1	X
Male	10,792	290	48	61	351	481	667	1,443	2,034	2,039	2,041	1,336	1	X
Female	9,119	211	33	48	117	186	335	767	1,159	1,555	2,189	2,519	–	X
Cuban	14,620	68	12	22	101	125	230	744	1,216	2,174	4,360	5,568	–	X
Male	7,453	40	4	13	73	86	152	487	827	1,346	2,335	2,090	–	X
Female	7,167	28	8	9	28	39	78	257	389	828	2,025	3,478	–	X
Central and South American	14,876	441	83	100	536	827	941	1,568	2,097	2,364	2,935	2,984	–	X
Male	7,577	239	46	57	409	645	615	1,008	1,209	1,201	1,269	879	–	X
Female	7,299	202	37	43	127	182	326	560	888	1,163	1,666	2,105	–	X
Other and unknown Hispanic	18,650	538	89	105	496	638	891	1,756	2,644	2,968	4,177	4,345	3	X
Male	9,886	293	48	61	357	438	570	1,093	1,669	1,689	2,076	1,589	3	X
Female	8,764	245	41	44	139	200	321	663	975	1,279	2,101	2,756	–	X
Non-Hispanic [3]	2,379,078	18,521	3,305	4,101	24,342	38,235	60,581	162,832	305,530	406,057	585,267	770,206	101	X
Male	1,183,988	10,323	1,892	2,420	17,754	26,107	37,181	98,455	185,700	229,928	293,258	280,906	64	X
Female	1,195,090	8,198	1,413	1,681	6,588	12,128	23,400	64,377	119,830	176,129	292,009	489,300	37	X
White[4]	2,016,896	10,601	2,094	2,667	16,475	27,266	43,940	124,142	240,590	339,392	511,339	698,324	66	X
Male	998,832	5,886	1,202	1,548	11,826	18,606	27,336	76,207	147,634	193,452	258,273	256,821	41	X
Female	1,018,064	4,715	892	1,119	4,649	8,660	16,604	47,935	92,956	145,940	253,066	441,503	25	X
Black[4]	291,179	6,765	989	1,155	6,581	8,948	13,502	32,522	54,983	54,481	57,565	53,657	31	X
Male	148,344	3,792	563	707	5,028	6,155	7,905	18,577	32,243	29,731	26,856	16,766	21	X
Female	142,835	2,973	426	448	1,553	2,793	5,597	13,945	22,740	24,750	30,709	36,891	10	X
Origin Not Stated [5]	7,782	295	14	16	67	140	243	853	1,456	1,421	1,547	1,691	39	X
Male	4,496	154	9	8	47	98	155	590	993	905	871	637	29	X
Female	3,286	141	5	8	20	42	88	263	463	516	676	1,054	10	X
RATE [6]														
All Origins [7]	810.2	599.3	26.3	12.6	66.4	105.4	170.7	405.4	854.2	1,802.5	4,674.5	13,678.6	X	732.8
Male	824.5	651.5	29.2	14.4	95.3	144.3	212.8	500.8	1,080.2	2,186.4	5,500.6	14,974.4	X	865.1
Female	796.4	544.6	23.2	10.8	36.0	65.8	129.0	312.7	643.8	1,466.1	4,062.5	13,030.0	X	624.7
Hispanic	295.0	469.9	21.8	11.1	52.1	71.7	109.0	267.9	622.3	1,330.9	3,552.1	10,157.0	X	539.1
Male	316.5	509.1	23.5	12.3	76.4	100.0	142.7	342.7	816.3	1,679.1	4,250.9	10,799.6	X	643.9
Female	272.7	428.9	20.0	10.0	25.5	40.0	73.6	192.0	442.8	1,046.7	3,063.5	9,805.6	X	452.5
Mexican	259.6	516.7	21.6	11.0	52.2	71.2	107.9	275.6	656.2	1,383.2	3,637.5	10,338.9	X	553.6
Male	283.7	557.0	23.4	12.0	77.9	98.8	141.5	345.5	839.7	1,708.6	4,198.5	10,922.5	X	648.3
Female	234.2	474.5	19.7	9.9	24.3	39.7	71.6	201.3	476.9	1,105.8	3,219.1	9,983.0	X	470.4
Puerto Rican	400.6	574.2	21.8	12.5	52.4	89.5	151.9	374.8	812.1	1,614.8	4,062.6	12,052.9	X	652.2
Male	441.1	663.7	24.8	13.8	77.0	131.2	207.8	499.1	1,122.1	2,036.6	4,938.3	11,710.1	X	777.5
Female	361.3	484.4	18.6	11.1	26.8	49.1	98.9	255.2	546.9	1,269.9	3,486.2	12,243.0	X	548.0
Cuban	746.8	286.3	*	9.8	38.6	50.7	82.2	244.0	591.0	1,402.3	3,868.3	11,597.6	X	562.1
Male	762.9	371.1	*	*	55.1	69.8	102.1	310.3	809.2	1,928.6	5,048.1	11,380.3	X	683.5
Female	730.9	215.8	*	*	21.7	31.7	59.5	173.7	375.6	971.3	3,047.2	11,732.2	X	461.1
Central and South American	188.1	388.5	15.3	8.6	43.3	56.1	71.5	154.9	349.2	817.1	2,339.8	7,475.1	X	358.9
Male	190.2	398.5	17.1	9.6	61.3	81.3	91.1	207.2	459.9	990.1	2,911.6	7,929.6	X	429.2
Female	186.0	377.3	13.6	7.6	22.3	26.7	50.9	106.5	263.0	692.3	2,035.3	7,300.4	X	309.6
Other and unknown Hispanic	456.5	900.6	32.4	15.5	69.3	108.8	166.7	341.8	721.1	1,443.4	3,848.5	10,078.9	X	601.1
Male	496.8	921.7	33.2	17.5	97.5	149.7	227.4	456.1	979.1	1,939.7	4,892.2	10,568.7	X	746.2
Female	418.2	876.7	31.5	13.5	39.7	68.0	113.1	241.8	495.7	1,078.9	3,178.5	9,816.6	X	490.8
Non-Hispanic	911.9	634.6	27.7	13.0	70.0	113.7	184.3	424.3	874.2	1,836.0	4,748.1	13,856.6	X	749.8
Male	928.2	691.0	31.0	15.1	100.1	155.8	228.7	522.6	1,101.7	2,218.7	5,576.5	15,202.7	X	884.6
Female	896.4	575.4	24.2	10.9	38.6	71.9	140.9	329.5	662.2	1,498.5	4,131.7	13,186.3	X	639.8
White	1,004.9	514.8	24.9	11.8	65.5	110.2	179.1	410.9	842.1	1,810.1	4,792.4	14,129.9	X	745.8
Male	1,011.2	558.2	27.9	13.3	92.0	149.0	221.7	508.0	1,058.0	2,175.8	5,599.2	15,504.4	X	876.2
Female	998.8	469.2	21.7	10.1	37.8	70.7	136.0	315.2	635.9	1,480.2	4,178.1	13,437.0	X	637.6
Black	720.9	1,111.6	40.1	18.7	96.8	158.4	259.4	592.0	1,285.3	2,470.1	5,261.4	12,812.2	X	887.1
Male	768.5	1,218.2	45.0	22.5	146.5	226.6	322.4	720.0	1,657.2	3,146.5	6,550.1	14,006.7	X	1,086.4

Table 2-5. Number of Deaths and Death Rates, by Age, and Age-Adjusted Death Rates, by Specified Hispanic Origin, Race for Non-Hispanic Population, and Sex, 2010— continued

(Number, rate per 100,000 population in specified group.)

Origin, race, and sex	All ages	Under 1 year[1]	1 to 4 years	5 to 14 years	15 to 24 years	25 to 34 years	35 to 44 years	45 to 54 years	55 to 64 years	65 to 74 years	75 to 84 years	85 years and over	Age not stated	Age-adjusted rate[2]
Female	677.3	1,000.0	35.2	14.8	46.1	95.2	203.2	478.6	975.0	1,963.1	4,489.1	12,334.1	X	742.1

X = Not applicable.   - = Quantity zero.   * = Figure does not meet standards of reliability or precision.   1Death rates for "Under 1 year" (based on population estimates) differ from infant mortality rates (based on live births); see chapter notes for more information.   2For method of computation, see chapter notes.   3Includes races other than White and Black.   4Race categories are consistent with the 1977 Office of Management and Budget (OMB) standards. In 2012, multiple-race data were reported by 42 states and the District of Columbia. The multiple-race data for these reporting areas were bridged to the single-race categories of the 1977 OMB standards for comparability with other reporting areas.   5Includes deaths for which Hispanic origin was not reported on the death certificate.   6Figures for age not stated are included in "All ages" but not distributed among age groups.   7Figures for origin not stated are included in "All origins" but not distributed among specified origins.

Table 2-6. Abridged Life Table for the Total Population, 2013

(Number.)

Age	Probability of dying be-tween ages x to x+n n q x	Number surviving to age x l x	Number dying between ages x to x+n n d x	Person-years lived between ages x to x+n n L x	Total number of person-years lived above age x T x	Expectancy of life at age x e x
0 to 1 years	0.005958	100,000	596	99,475	7,882,785	78.8
1 to 5 years	0.001021	99,404	102	397,372	7,783,311	78.3
5 to 10 years	0.000590	99,303	59	496,355	7,385,939	74.4
10 to 15 years	0.000705	99,244	70	496,080	6,889,584	69.4
15 to 20 years	0.002227	99,174	221	495,400	6,393,505	64.5
20 to 25 years	0.004158	98,953	411	493,788	5,898,105	59.6
25 to 30 years	0.004869	98,542	480	491,535	5,404,318	54.8
30 to 35 years	0.005727	98,062	562	488,941	4,912,783	50.1
35 to 40 years	0.007072	97,500	690	485,855	4,423,842	45.4
40 to 45 years	0.009949	96,811	963	481,799	3,937,986	40.7
45 to 50 years	0.015604	95,848	1,496	475,781	3,456,188	36.1
50 to 55 years	0.024272	94,352	2,290	466,384	2,980,407	31.6
55 to 60 years	0.035563	92,062	3,274	452,547	2,514,024	27.3
60 to 65 years	0.050060	88,788	4,445	433,361	2,061,477	23.2
65 to 70 years	0.071576	84,343	6,037	407,404	1,628,116	19.3
70 to 75 years	0.109091	78,306	8,543	371,349	1,220,712	15.6
75 to 80 years	0.170567	69,764	11,899	320,641	849,363	12.2
80 to 85 years	0.271135	57,864	15,689	251,503	528,722	9.1
85 to 90 years	0.425836	42,175	17,960	166,078	277,219	6.6
90 to 95 years	0.614587	24,216	14,883	81,352	111,141	4.6
95 to 100 years	0.786379	9,333	7,339	25,247	29,789	3.2
100 years and over	1.000000	1,994	1,994	4,541	4,541	2.3

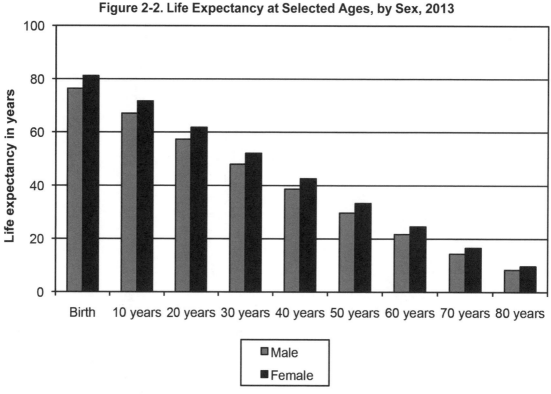

Figure 2-2. Life Expectancy at Selected Ages, by Sex, 2013

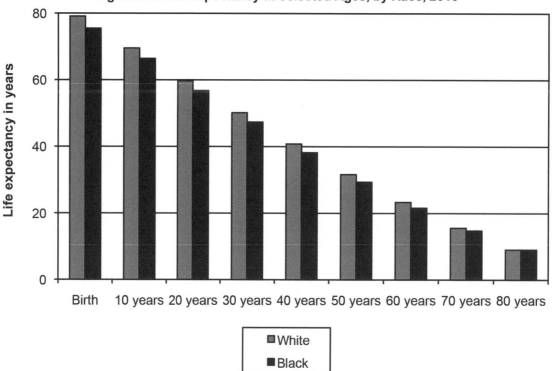

Figure 2-3. Life Expectancy at Selected Ages, by Race, 2013

Table 2-7. Life Expectancy at Birth by Race and Sex, Selected Years, 1940–2013

(Number.)

Year	All races and origins[1]			White[2]			Black[2]			Hispanic[3]			Non-Hispanic White			Non-Hispanic Black		
	Both sexes	Male	Female	Both sexes	Male	Female	Both sexes	Male	Female	Both sexes	Male	Female	Both sexes	Male	Female	Both sexes	Male	Female
1940	62.9	60.8	65.2	64.2	62.1	66.6	NA	NA	NA	NA	NA	NA	NA	NA	NA	NA	NA	NA
1950	68.2	65.6	71.1	69.1	66.5	72.2	NA	NA	NA	NA	NA	NA	NA	NA	NA	NA	NA	NA
1960	69.7	66.6	73.1	70.6	67.4	74.1	NA	NA	NA	NA	NA	NA	NA	NA	NA	NA	NA	NA
1970	70.8	67.1	74.7	71.7	68.0	75.6	64.1	60.0	68.3	NA	NA	NA	NA	NA	NA	NA	NA	NA
1975	72.6	68.8	76.6	73.4	69.5	77.3	66.8	62.4	71.3	NA	NA	NA	NA	NA	NA	NA	NA	NA
1976	72.9	69.1	76.8	73.6	69.9	77.5	67.2	62.9	71.6	NA	NA	NA	NA	NA	NA	NA	NA	NA
1977	73.3	69.5	77.2	74.0	70.2	77.9	67.7	63.4	72.0	NA	NA	NA	NA	NA	NA	NA	NA	NA
1978	73.5	69.6	77.3	74.1	70.4	78.0	68.1	63.7	72.4	NA	NA	NA	NA	NA	NA	NA	NA	NA
1979	73.9	70.0	77.8	74.6	70.8	78.4	68.5	64.0	72.9	NA	NA	NA	NA	NA	NA	NA	NA	NA
1980	73.7	70.0	77.4	74.4	70.7	78.1	68.1	63.8	72.5	NA	NA	NA	NA	NA	NA	NA	NA	NA
1981	74.1	70.4	77.8	74.8	71.1	78.4	68.9	64.5	73.2	NA	NA	NA	NA	NA	NA	NA	NA	NA
1982	74.5	70.8	78.1	75.1	71.5	78.7	69.4	65.1	73.6	NA	NA	NA	NA	NA	NA	NA	NA	NA
1983	74.6	71.0	78.1	75.2	71.6	78.7	69.4	65.2	73.5	NA	NA	NA	NA	NA	NA	NA	NA	NA
1984	74.7	71.1	78.2	75.3	71.8	78.7	69.5	65.3	73.6	NA	NA	NA	NA	NA	NA	NA	NA	NA
1985	74.7	71.1	78.2	75.3	71.8	78.7	69.3	65.0	73.4	NA	NA	NA	NA	NA	NA	NA	NA	NA
1986	74.7	71.2	78.2	75.4	71.9	78.8	69.1	64.8	73.4	NA	NA	NA	NA	NA	NA	NA	NA	NA
1987	74.9	71.4	78.3	75.6	72.1	78.9	69.1	64.7	73.4	NA	NA	NA	NA	NA	NA	NA	NA	NA
1988	74.9	71.4	78.3	75.6	72.2	78.9	68.9	64.4	73.2	NA	NA	NA	NA	NA	NA	NA	NA	NA
1989	75.1	71.7	78.5	75.9	72.5	79.2	68.8	64.3	73.3	NA	NA	NA	NA	NA	NA	NA	NA	NA
1990	75.4	71.8	78.8	76.1	72.7	79.4	69.1	64.5	73.6	NA	NA	NA	NA	NA	NA	NA	NA	NA
1991	75.5	72.0	78.9	76.3	72.9	79.6	69.3	64.6	73.8	NA	NA	NA	NA	NA	NA	NA	NA	NA
1992	75.8	72.3	79.1	76.5	73.2	79.8	69.6	65.0	73.9	NA	NA	NA	NA	NA	NA	NA	NA	NA
1993	75.5	72.2	78.8	76.3	73.1	79.5	69.2	64.6	73.7	NA	NA	NA	NA	NA	NA	NA	NA	NA
1994	75.7	72.4	79.0	76.5	73.3	79.6	69.5	64.9	73.9	NA	NA	NA	NA	NA	NA	NA	NA	NA
1995	75.8	72.5	78.9	76.5	73.4	79.6	69.6	65.2	73.9	NA	NA	NA	NA	NA	NA	NA	NA	NA
1996	76.1	73.1	79.1	76.8	73.9	79.7	70.2	66.1	74.2	NA	NA	NA	NA	NA	NA	NA	NA	NA
1997	76.5	73.6	79.4	77.1	74.3	79.9	71.1	67.2	74.7	NA	NA	NA	NA	NA	NA	NA	NA	NA
1998	76.7	73.8	79.5	77.3	74.5	80.0	71.3	67.6	74.8	NA	NA	NA	NA	NA	NA	NA	NA	NA
1999	76.7	73.9	79.4	77.3	74.6	79.9	71.4	67.8	74.7	NA	NA	NA	NA	NA	NA	NA	NA	NA
2000	76.8	74.1	79.3	77.3	74.7	79.9	71.8	68.2	75.1	NA	NA	NA	NA	NA	NA	NA	NA	NA
2001 [4]	77.0	74.3	79.5	77.5	74.9	80.0	72.0	68.5	75.3	NA	NA	NA	NA	NA	NA	NA	NA	NA
2002 [4]	77.0	74.4	79.6	77.5	74.9	80.1	72.2	68.7	75.4	NA	NA	NA	NA	NA	NA	NA	NA	NA
2003 [4,5]	77.2	74.5	79.7	77.7	75.1	80.2	72.4	68.9	75.7	NA	NA	NA	NA	NA	NA	NA	NA	NA
2004 [4,5]	77.6	75.0	80.1	78.1	75.5	80.5	72.9	69.4	76.1	NA	NA	NA	NA	NA	NA	NA	NA	NA
2005 [4,5]	77.6	75.0	80.1	78.0	75.5	80.5	73.0	69.5	76.2	NA	NA	NA	NA	NA	NA	NA	NA	NA
2006 [4,5]	77.8	75.2	80.3	78.3	75.8	80.7	73.4	69.9	76.7	80.3	77.5	82.9	78.2	75.7	80.6	73.1	69.5	76.4
2007 [4,5]	78.1	75.5	80.6	78.5	76.0	80.9	73.8	70.3	77.0	80.7	77.8	83.2	78.4	75.9	80.8	73.5	69.9	76.7
2008 [4,5]	78.2	75.6	80.6	78.5	76.1	80.9	74.3	70.9	77.3	80.8	78.0	83.3	78.4	76.0	80.7	73.9	70.5	77.0
2009 [4,5]	78.5	76.0	80.9	78.8	76.4	81.2	74.7	71.4	77.7	81.1	78.4	83.5	78.7	76.3	81.1	74.3	70.9	77.4
2010 [4,5]	78.7	76.2	81.0	78.9	76.5	81.3	75.1	71.8	78.0	81.2	78.5	83.8	78.8	76.4	81.1	74.7	71.4	77.7
2011 [4,5]	78.7	76.3	81.1	79.0	76.6	81.3	75.3	72.2	78.2	81.4	78.8	83.7	78.8	76.4	81.1	74.9	71.7	77.8
2012 [4,5]	78.8	76.4	81.2	79.1	76.7	81.4	75.5	72.3	78.4	81.6	79.1	83.9	78.9	76.6	81.2	75.1	71.8	78.1
2013 [4,5]	78.8	76.4	81.2	79.1	76.7	81.4	75.5	72.3	78.4	81.6	79.1	83.8	78.9	76.5	81.2	75.1	71.8	78.1

NA = Not available.   1Includes races other than White and Black.   2Includes Hispanic and non-Hispanic persons.   3Life expectancies for the Hispanic population are based on death rates adjusted for misclassification; please see chapter notes.   4Life table data for 2001–2013 are based on revised life table methodology.   5Race categories are consistent with the 1977 Office of Management and Budget (OMB) standards. Multiple-race data were reported by 42 states and the District of Columbia in 2012 and 2013, by 38 states and the District of Columbia in 2011, by 37 states and the District of Columbia in 2010, by 34 states and the District of Columbia in 2009 and 2008, by 27 states and the District of Columbia in 2007, by 25 states and the District of Columbia in 2006, by 21 states and the District of Columbia in 2005, by 15 states in 2004, and by 7 states in 2003. The multiple-race data for these reporting areas were bridged to the single-race categories of the 1977 OMB standards for comparability with other reporting areas.

Table 2-8. Life Expectancy at Selected Ages by Race, Hispanic Origin, Race for Non-Hispanic Population, and Sex, 2013

(Years.)

Exact age in years	All races and origins[1]			White[2]			Black[2]			Hispanic			Non-Hispanic White[2]			Non-Hispanic Black[2]		
	Both sexes	Male	Female	Both sexes	Male	Female	Both sexes	Male	Female	Both sexes	Male	Female	Both sexes	Male	Female	Both sexes	Male	Female
0 years	78.8	76.4	81.2	79.1	76.7	81.4	75.5	72.3	78.4	81.6	79.1	83.8	78.9	76.5	81.2	75.1	71.8	78.1
1 year	78.3	75.9	80.6	78.5	76.1	80.7	75.4	72.2	78.2	81.0	78.5	83.2	78.3	76.0	80.5	75.0	71.7	77.9
5 years	74.4	72.0	76.7	74.5	72.2	76.8	71.5	68.3	74.3	77.1	74.6	79.3	74.3	72.1	76.6	71.1	67.9	74.0
10 years	69.4	67.1	71.7	69.6	67.3	71.8	66.5	63.4	69.4	72.1	69.6	74.3	69.4	67.1	71.6	66.1	62.9	69.1
15 years	64.5	62.1	66.8	64.6	62.3	66.9	61.6	58.5	64.4	67.2	64.7	69.3	64.4	62.1	66.7	61.2	58.0	64.1
20 years	59.6	57.3	61.8	59.7	57.5	62.0	56.8	53.7	59.5	62.3	59.8	64.4	59.6	57.3	61.7	56.4	53.3	59.2
25 years	54.8	52.6	57.0	55.0	52.8	57.1	52.1	49.2	54.7	57.4	55.1	59.5	54.8	52.6	56.9	51.7	48.7	54.4
30 years	50.1	48.0	52.1	50.2	48.1	52.2	47.4	44.6	49.9	52.6	50.4	54.6	50.1	48.0	52.1	47.1	44.2	49.6
35 years	45.4	43.3	47.3	45.5	43.5	47.4	42.8	40.1	45.1	47.8	45.6	49.7	45.3	43.4	47.3	42.5	39.8	44.9
40 years	40.7	38.7	42.6	40.8	38.8	42.6	38.2	35.7	40.4	43.1	40.9	44.9	40.7	38.7	42.5	37.9	35.3	40.2
45 years	36.1	34.1	37.9	36.2	34.3	37.9	33.7	31.2	35.9	38.4	36.3	40.1	36.1	34.2	37.8	33.5	30.9	35.6
50 years	31.6	29.7	33.3	31.7	29.9	33.4	29.4	27.0	31.5	33.8	31.7	35.4	31.6	29.8	33.3	29.2	26.7	31.2
55 years	27.3	25.6	28.9	27.4	25.7	28.9	25.3	23.0	27.3	29.3	27.4	30.8	27.3	25.7	28.9	25.1	22.8	27.1
60 years	23.2	21.7	24.6	23.3	21.7	24.6	21.6	19.5	23.3	25.0	23.3	26.3	23.2	21.7	24.6	21.4	19.3	23.1
65 years	19.3	17.9	20.5	19.3	18.0	20.5	18.1	16.3	19.5	20.9	19.3	22.0	19.3	17.9	20.4	18.0	16.1	19.4
70 years	15.6	14.4	16.6	15.6	14.4	16.5	14.8	13.2	15.9	17.0	15.7	17.9	15.5	14.4	16.5	14.7	13.1	15.8
75 years	12.2	11.2	12.9	12.1	11.1	12.9	11.8	10.4	12.7	13.4	12.3	14.1	12.1	11.1	12.9	11.7	10.4	12.6
80 years	9.1	8.3	9.7	9.1	8.3	9.7	9.1	8.0	9.7	10.1	9.2	10.6	9.1	8.2	9.6	9.1	8.0	9.7
85 years	6.6	5.9	7.0	6.5	5.9	6.9	6.8	6.0	7.2	7.3	6.6	7.6	6.5	5.9	6.9	6.8	6.0	7.2
90 years	4.6	4.1	4.8	4.5	4.0	4.8	5.1	4.5	5.3	5.1	4.5	5.2	4.5	4.0	4.8	5.1	4.5	5.2
95 years	3.2	2.8	3.3	3.1	2.8	3.2	3.8	3.4	3.8	3.6	3.1	3.5	3.1	2.8	3.2	3.8	3.4	3.8
100 years	2.3	2.0	2.3	2.2	2.0	2.3	2.8	2.6	2.8	2.5	2.2	2.4	2.2	2.0	2.3	2.8	2.6	2.8

1Includes races other than White and Black.   2Race categories are consistent with the 1977 Office of Management and Budget (OMB) standards. Multiple-race data were reported by 42 states and the District of Columbia in 2013; see Technical Notes. The multiple-race data for these reporting areas were bridged to the single-race categories of the 1977 OMB standards for comparability with other reporting areas.

Table 2-9. Death Rates by Age and Age-Adjusted Death Rates for the 15 Leading Causes of Death, 1999–2013

(Rate per 100,000 population in specified group; age-adjusted rates per 100,000 U.S. standard population.)

Cause of death (based on ICD–10) and year	All ages[1]	Under 1 year[2]	1 to 4 years	5 to 14 years	15 to 24 years	25 to 34 years	35 to 44 years	45 to 54 years	55 to 64 years	65 to 74 years	75 to 84 years	85 years and over	Age-adjusted rate[3]
All Causes													
1999	857.0	736.0	34.2	18.6	79.3	102.2	198.0	418.2	1,005.0	2,457.3	5,714.5	15,554.6	875.6
2000	854.0	736.7	32.4	18.0	79.9	101.4	198.9	425.6	992.2	2,399.1	5,666.5	15,524.4	869.0
2001	848.0	687.0	33.4	17.2	80.2	105.6	203.5	426.7	972.5	2,344.2	5,573.7	15,432.6	858.8
2002	849.5	709.5	31.4	17.4	80.9	105.1	204.2	431.0	948.7	2,300.3	5,543.8	15,589.5	855.9
2003	843.9	704.9	31.8	16.9	81.1	105.2	202.6	433.1	937.3	2,235.0	5,451.3	15,401.4	843.5
2004	818.8	695.9	30.3	16.7	79.7	104.1	194.9	426.8	903.2	2,141.0	5,267.4	14,777.6	813.7
2005	828.4	710.2	29.9	16.3	80.7	106.8	194.9	431.9	898.5	2,109.7	5,251.8	14,982.4	815.0
2006	813.1	705.8	29.1	15.2	81.4	109.0	192.0	427.5	881.3	2,031.4	5,096.1	14,426.7	791.8
2007	804.6	702.5	29.4	15.2	78.8	107.2	186.0	420.3	866.7	1,976.0	4,987.1	14,160.9	775.3
2008	812.9	678.9	29.3	13.9	74.2	105.1	181.0	419.6	867.1	1,958.4	4,998.1	14,332.4	774.9
2009	794.5	659.7	27.4	13.8	69.8	104.4	180.0	418.1	856.7	1,888.7	4,820.2	13,660.1	749.6
2010	799.5	623.4	26.5	12.9	67.7	102.9	170.5	407.1	851.9	1,875.1	4,790.2	13,934.3	747.0
2011	807.3	600.1	26.3	13.2	67.7	104.7	172.0	409.8	849.4	1,846.2	4,753.0	13,779.3	741.3
2012	810.2	599.3	26.3	12.6	66.4	105.4	170.7	405.4	854.2	1,802.5	4,674.5	13,678.6	732.8
2013	821.5	594.7	25.5	13.0	64.8	106.1	172.0	406.1	860.0	1,802.1	4,648.1	13,660.4	731.9
Diseases of Heart (I00–I09, I11, I13, I20–I51)													
1999	259.9	13.8	1.2	0.7	2.8	7.6	30.2	95.7	269.9	701.7	1,849.9	6,063.0	266.5
2000	252.6	13.0	1.2	0.7	2.6	7.4	29.2	94.2	261.2	665.6	1,780.3	5,926.1	257.6
2001	245.7	11.9	1.5	0.7	2.5	8.0	29.6	92.4	248.9	632.6	1,723.0	5,784.1	249.5
2002	242.3	12.7	1.1	0.6	2.5	8.0	30.7	93.9	240.5	612.0	1,673.2	5,726.3	244.6
2003	236.1	11.0	1.2	0.6	2.7	8.3	30.8	92.4	232.3	579.8	1,607.7	5,570.7	236.3
2004	222.8	10.5	1.2	0.6	2.5	8.1	29.5	90.2	217.1	535.7	1,504.1	5,233.8	221.6
2005	220.7	8.9	0.9	0.6	2.6	8.3	29.2	89.7	212.8	512.3	1,458.5	5,188.3	216.8
2006	211.7	8.6	1.0	0.6	2.5	8.4	28.5	88.0	205.1	483.0	1,378.0	4,877.6	205.5
2007	204.5	10.2	1.1	0.6	2.5	8.1	27.7	85.2	197.8	454.8	1,308.6	4,668.1	196.1
2008	202.8	9.6	1.2	0.6	2.5	8.1	26.9	85.2	195.3	441.4	1,271.7	4,598.4	192.1
2009	195.4	9.6	0.9	0.5	2.4	7.8	26.7	82.3	190.0	422.8	1,210.8	4,316.9	182.8
2010	193.6	8.3	1.0	0.5	2.4	7.8	25.8	81.6	186.6	409.2	1,172.0	4,285.2	179.1
2011	191.5	7.7	1.0	0.5	2.3	7.9	26.2	80.7	183.2	399.0	1,134.7	4,111.6	173.7
2012	191.0	8.5	1.0	0.4	2.2	7.6	25.9	79.7	184.6	388.3	1,103.7	4,046.1	170.5
2013	193.3	7.8	1.1	0.4	2.1	7.6	25.6	80.3	184.6	390.3	1,095.1	4,013.9	169.8
Malignant Neoplasms (C00–C97)													
1999	197.0	1.8	2.7	2.5	4.5	10.0	37.1	127.6	374.6	827.1	1,331.5	1,805.8	200.8
2000	196.5	2.4	2.7	2.5	4.4	9.8	36.6	127.5	366.7	816.3	1,335.6	1,819.4	199.6
2001	194.3	1.6	2.7	2.4	4.2	10.1	36.8	125.8	359.4	799.7	1,313.7	1,802.9	196.5
2002	193.7	1.9	2.6	2.6	4.2	9.8	36.0	124.1	349.7	787.2	1,308.8	1,812.4	194.3
2003	192.0	1.9	2.5	2.6	4.0	9.5	35.1	122.1	341.6	763.5	1,299.7	1,792.3	190.9
2004	189.2	1.8	2.5	2.5	4.1	9.3	33.6	119.0	330.8	746.8	1,278.6	1,767.4	186.8
2005	189.3	1.9	2.4	2.5	4.0	9.2	33.5	118.6	323.9	733.2	1,272.8	1,778.2	185.1
2006	187.6	1.9	2.4	2.2	3.8	9.3	32.2	116.3	317.7	716.3	1,259.2	1,748.3	181.8
2007	186.9	1.7	2.3	2.4	3.8	8.7	31.0	114.2	311.4	702.9	1,250.1	1,739.4	179.3
2008	186.0	1.7	2.4	2.2	3.8	8.8	30.1	113.4	304.7	688.4	1,230.9	1,724.6	176.4
2009	185.0	1.8	2.2	2.2	3.8	9.0	30.2	112.8	301.7	668.2	1,213.0	1,699.3	173.5
2010	186.2	1.6	2.1	2.2	3.7	8.8	28.8	111.6	300.1	666.1	1,202.2	1,729.5	172.8
2011	185.1	1.8	2.2	2.1	3.7	8.4	28.8	109.3	295.8	647.6	1,179.1	1,676.2	169.0
2012	185.6	1.6	2.4	2.2	3.6	8.7	28.0	108.5	293.2	632.2	1,161.7	1,658.9	166.5
2013	185.0	1.6	2.1	2.2	3.4	8.6	28.1	105.5	288.2	616.9	1,139.4	1,635.4	163.2
Chronic Lower Respiratory Disease (J40-J47)													
1999	44.5	0.9	0.4	0.3	0.5	0.8	2.0	8.5	47.5	177.2	397.8	646.0	45.4
2000	43.4	0.9	0.3	0.3	0.5	0.7	2.1	8.6	44.2	169.4	386.1	648.6	44.2
2001	43.2	1.0	0.3	0.3	0.4	0.7	2.2	8.4	44.5	167.3	379.3	658.3	43.9
2002	43.4	1.0	0.4	0.3	0.5	0.8	2.3	8.7	42.2	162.0	385.8	670.3	43.9
2003	43.6	0.8	0.4	0.3	0.5	0.7	2.2	8.7	43.1	161.7	382.2	670.2	43.7
2004	41.7	0.9	0.3	0.3	0.4	0.6	2.0	8.4	40.1	152.1	366.2	643.2	41.6
2005	44.3	0.8	0.4	0.3	0.3	0.7	2.0	9.4	41.6	158.4	385.0	691.9	43.9
2006	41.8	0.7	0.3	0.3	0.4	0.6	1.9	9.1	38.8	147.0	362.0	641.3	41.0
2007	42.5	1.0	0.4	0.3	0.3	0.7	1.9	9.5	38.6	145.5	367.1	652.0	41.4
2008	46.4	0.8	0.3	0.3	0.4	0.6	1.9	9.9	41.1	155.9	395.4	722.7	44.7
2009	44.8	0.7	0.4	0.3	0.4	0.7	1.8	10.4	40.0	147.5	376.4	684.9	42.7
2010	44.7	0.9	0.3	0.3	0.3	0.7	1.7	9.9	39.0	146.3	369.9	690.7	42.2
2011	45.9	0.8	0.3	0.3	0.4	0.6	1.8	10.4	39.5	144.3	374.9	697.9	42.5
2012	45.7	0.5	0.4	0.3	0.3	0.7	1.8	10.2	39.4	140.0	364.0	687.8	41.5
2013	47.2	0.6	0.4	0.4	0.4	0.7	1.9	10.6	40.5	141.2	367.0	699.3	42.1

Table 2-9. Death Rates by Age and Age-Adjusted Death Rates for the 15 Leading Causes of Death, 1999–2013— continued

(Rate per 100,000 population in specified group; age-adjusted rates per 100,000 U.S. standard population.)

Cause of death (based on ICD–10) and year	All ages[1]	Under 1 year[2]	1 to 4 years	5 to 14 years	15 to 24 years	25 to 34 years	35 to 44 years	45 to 54 years	55 to 64 years	65 to 74 years	75 to 84 years	85 years and over	Age-adjusted rate[3]
Accidents (Unintentional Injuries) (V01–X59, Y85–Y86)													
1999	35.1	22.3	12.4	7.6	35.3	29.6	33.8	31.8	30.6	44.6	100.5	282.4	35.3
2000	34.8	23.1	11.9	7.3	36.0	29.5	34.1	32.6	30.9	41.9	95.1	273.5	34.9
2001	35.6	24.3	11.2	6.9	35.8	30.0	35.4	33.9	30.5	42.6	100.7	282.2	35.7
2002	37.1	23.9	10.6	6.6	37.7	31.9	37.4	36.7	31.3	44.0	101.1	289.6	37.1
2003	37.7	23.8	11.0	6.4	36.9	32.0	38.0	38.8	32.7	43.7	101.6	294.3	37.6
2004	38.3	26.2	10.4	6.5	36.8	33.2	37.6	40.7	32.9	43.5	103.6	295.8	38.1
2005	39.9	27.0	10.5	5.9	37.1	35.7	38.9	43.2	35.4	45.7	106.0	303.5	39.5
2006	40.8	28.4	10.1	5.6	37.9	38.0	40.5	45.5	35.8	43.8	104.7	299.2	40.2
2007	41.1	31.0	9.9	5.4	36.8	37.7	39.6	46.2	36.8	44.4	105.0	313.6	40.4
2008	40.1	31.8	9.1	4.6	32.5	36.3	38.1	45.8	37.4	43.9	105.7	318.3	39.2
2009	38.5	29.5	9.0	4.1	28.6	34.5	36.4	44.5	36.5	42.1	103.5	310.9	37.5
2010	39.1	28.1	8.6	4.0	28.3	35.5	36.0	43.7	38.4	43.3	106.1	328.4	38.0
2011	40.6	29.1	8.5	4.0	28.2	37.1	37.5	46.4	39.8	44.5	107.0	333.8	39.1
2012	40.7	29.6	8.4	3.8	27.1	37.5	37.1	46.1	41.0	44.0	107.8	336.9	39.1
2013	41.3	29.3	8.3	3.7	26.4	37.8	38.0	46.5	43.4	43.5	107.4	340.0	39.4
Cerebrovascular Diseases (I60–I69)													
1999	60.0	2.7	0.3	0.2	0.5	1.4	5.7	15.2	40.6	130.8	469.8	1,614.8	61.6
2000	59.6	3.3	0.3	0.2	0.5	1.5	5.8	16.0	41.0	128.6	461.3	1,589.2	60.9
2001	57.4	2.7	0.4	0.2	0.5	1.5	5.5	15.0	38.3	122.9	443.3	1,532.0	58.4
2002	56.6	3.0	0.3	0.2	0.4	1.4	5.4	15.1	37.1	119.6	430.0	1,520.1	57.2
2003	54.4	2.5	0.3	0.2	0.5	1.5	5.6	15.0	35.5	111.9	409.8	1,446.0	54.6
2004	51.3	3.2	0.3	0.2	0.5	1.4	5.4	14.8	34.0	106.6	385.6	1,331.9	51.2
2005	48.6	3.1	0.4	0.2	0.5	1.4	5.2	15.0	32.7	99.8	358.4	1,239.7	48.0
2006	46.0	3.5	0.3	0.2	0.5	1.3	5.1	14.6	32.9	94.9	333.9	1,131.7	44.8
2007	45.1	3.2	0.3	0.2	0.5	1.3	5.0	14.5	31.7	91.4	320.8	1,110.7	43.5
2008	44.1	3.4	0.4	0.2	0.4	1.3	4.8	13.7	30.6	87.3	313.3	1,071.0	42.1
2009	42.0	3.7	0.3	0.2	0.4	1.3	4.6	13.7	29.7	82.8	294.9	992.2	39.6
2010	41.9	3.3	0.3	0.2	0.4	1.3	4.6	13.1	29.3	81.7	288.3	993.8	39.1
2011	41.4	3.4	0.3	0.2	0.4	1.3	4.2	12.8	29.4	78.2	285.4	943.7	37.9
2012	40.9	2.6	0.3	0.2	0.4	1.3	4.3	12.8	28.7	75.7	272.2	931.2	36.9
2013	40.8	2.7	0.2	0.2	0.3	1.2	4.2	12.4	28.9	74.2	268.9	906.0	36.2
Alzheimer's Disease (G30)													
1999	16.0	*	*	*	*	*	*	0.2	1.9	17.4	129.5	601.3	16.5
2000	17.6	*	*	*	*	*	*	0.2	2.0	18.7	139.6	667.7	18.1
2001	18.9	*	*	*	*	*	*	0.2	2.1	18.6	147.2	725.4	19.3
2002	20.5	*	*	*	*	*	*	0.1	1.9	19.6	157.7	790.9	20.8
2003	21.9	*	*	*	*	*	*	0.2	2.0	20.7	164.1	846.8	22.1
2004	22.5	*	*	*	*	*	*	0.2	1.8	19.5	168.5	875.3	22.6
2005	24.2	*	*	*	*	*	*	0.2	2.1	20.2	177.0	935.5	24.0
2006	24.3	*	*	*	*	*	*	0.2	2.1	19.9	175.0	923.4	23.7
2007	24.8	*	*	*	*	*	*	0.2	2.2	20.2	175.8	928.7	23.8
2008	27.1	*	*	*	*	*	*	0.2	2.2	21.1	192.5	1,002.2	25.8
2009	25.8	*	*	*	*	*	*	0.2	2.0	19.4	179.1	945.3	24.2
2010	27.0	*	*	*	*	*	*	0.3	2.1	19.8	184.5	987.1	25.1
2011	27.3	*	*	*	*	*	*	0.2	2.2	19.2	183.9	967.1	24.7
2012	26.6	*	*	*	*	*	*	0.2	2.2	17.9	175.4	936.1	23.8
2013	26.8	*	*	*	*	*	*	0.2	2.2	18.1	171.6	929.5	23.5
Diabetes Mellitus (E10–E14)[4]													
1999	24.5	*	*	0.1	0.4	1.4	4.3	12.9	38.3	91.8	178.0	317.2	25.0
2000	24.6	*	*	0.1	0.4	1.6	4.3	13.1	37.8	90.7	179.5	319.7	25.0
2001	25.0	*	*	0.1	0.4	1.5	4.3	13.6	38.1	91.0	181.1	328.6	25.4
2002	25.5	*	*	0.1	0.4	1.6	4.8	13.7	37.5	90.9	182.4	337.0	25.6
2003	25.6	*	*	0.1	0.4	1.7	4.6	13.9	38.3	90.0	180.7	335.1	25.5
2004	25.0	*	*	0.1	0.4	1.5	4.6	13.4	36.8	86.2	176.6	328.2	24.7
2005	25.4	*	*	0.1	0.5	1.6	4.7	13.4	36.9	85.7	177.0	338.8	24.9
2006	24.3	*	*	0.1	0.4	1.7	4.8	13.1	35.8	80.6	166.2	310.4	23.6
2007	23.7	*	*	0.1	0.4	1.5	4.6	13.1	34.1	76.7	161.9	302.2	22.8
2008	23.2	*	*	0.1	0.5	1.4	4.4	12.6	33.3	74.7	153.2	298.9	22.0
2009	22.4	*	*	0.1	0.4	1.5	4.5	12.8	32.1	69.6	145.8	282.6	21.0
2010	22.4	*	*	0.1	0.4	1.5	4.4	12.5	32.0	67.6	144.1	285.5	20.8
2011	23.7	*	*	0.1	0.4	1.6	4.5	13.4	33.3	72.0	148.8	289.5	21.6
2012	23.6	*	*	0.1	0.4	1.5	4.6	13.0	32.5	69.7	145.8	285.7	21.2
2013	23.9	*	*	0.1	0.4	1.6	4.8	13.5	33.2	68.5	145.7	279.5	21.2

Table 2-9. Death Rates by Age and Age-Adjusted Death Rates for the 15 Leading Causes of Death, 1999–2013— continued

(Rate per 100,000 population in specified group; age-adjusted rates per 100,000 U.S. standard population.)

Cause of death (based on ICD–10) and year	All ages[1]	Under 1 year[2]	1 to 4 years	5 to 14 years	15 to 24 years	25 to 34 years	35 to 44 years	45 to 54 years	55 to 64 years	65 to 74 years	75 to 84 years	85 years and over	Age-adjusted rate[3]
Influenza and Pneumonia (J09–J18)													
1999	22.8	8.4	0.8	0.2	0.5	0.8	2.4	4.6	11.0	37.2	157.0	751.8	23.5
2000	23.2	7.6	0.7	0.2	0.5	0.9	2.4	4.7	11.9	39.1	160.3	744.1	23.7
2001	21.8	7.5	0.7	0.2	0.5	0.9	2.2	4.6	10.8	36.2	148.3	700.1	22.2
2002	22.8	6.7	0.7	0.2	0.4	0.9	2.2	4.8	11.2	37.2	156.6	732.4	23.2
2003	22.5	8.1	1.0	0.4	0.5	1.0	2.2	5.2	11.2	36.9	150.8	703.0	22.6
2004	20.4	6.8	0.8	0.2	0.4	0.8	2.0	4.6	10.8	34.2	139.1	622.8	20.4
2005	21.3	6.6	0.7	0.3	0.4	0.9	2.1	5.1	11.2	35.1	142.0	644.9	21.0
2006	18.9	6.5	0.8	0.2	0.4	0.9	1.9	4.6	9.9	31.6	127.3	547.0	18.4
2007	17.5	5.4	0.7	0.3	0.4	0.8	1.8	4.3	9.5	28.2	113.5	506.7	16.8
2008	18.5	5.5	0.9	0.2	0.5	0.9	2.1	5.1	10.9	30.5	118.6	512.3	17.6
2009	17.5	6.3	0.9	0.6	1.0	2.0	3.2	6.5	11.7	29.5	107.0	433.8	16.5
2010	16.2	4.9	0.6	0.2	0.4	0.9	1.9	4.3	9.9	27.9	102.4	426.2	15.1
2011	17.3	5.2	0.7	0.3	0.5	1.2	2.1	5.0	11.0	28.9	104.0	439.2	15.7
2012	16.1	4.0	0.6	0.2	0.3	0.8	1.7	4.1	10.2	26.1	98.2	408.4	14.4
2013	18.0	4.5	0.6	0.3	0.4	1.0	2.2	5.1	12.2	29.5	103.7	441.0	15.9
Nephritis, Nephrotic Syndrome and Nephrosis (N00–N07, N17–N19, N25–N27)[4]													
1999	12.7	4.4	*	0.1	0.2	0.6	1.6	4.0	12.0	37.1	97.6	268.9	13.0
2000	13.2	4.3	*	0.1	0.2	0.6	1.6	4.4	12.8	38.0	100.8	277.8	13.5
2001	13.9	3.3	*	*	0.2	0.6	1.7	4.6	13.1	40.0	104.0	293.8	14.1
2002	14.2	4.4	*	0.1	0.2	0.7	1.7	4.7	12.9	39.0	108.9	303.4	14.4
2003	14.6	4.6	*	0.1	0.2	0.7	1.8	4.9	13.6	39.7	109.3	309.3	14.7
2004	14.5	4.3	*	0.1	0.2	0.6	1.8	5.0	13.5	38.1	108.2	306.4	14.5
2005	14.9	4.0	*	0.1	0.2	0.7	1.7	4.8	13.5	38.8	110.2	313.1	14.7
2006	15.2	4.0	*	*	0.2	0.7	1.8	5.2	13.7	38.8	111.0	316.2	14.8
2007	15.4	3.5	0.1	0.1	0.2	0.7	1.8	5.1	13.4	39.4	112.4	317.9	14.9
2008	15.9	3.5	*	*	0.2	0.6	1.8	5.0	14.1	39.9	113.3	325.6	15.1
2009	16.0	2.8	*	*	0.2	0.7	2.0	5.2	13.5	38.7	115.1	321.4	15.1
2010	16.3	2.7	*	0.1	0.2	0.6	1.8	4.9	13.9	39.3	115.7	333.8	15.3
2011	14.6	1.9	*	*	0.2	0.5	1.6	4.4	12.5	34.2	101.4	292.1	13.4
2012	14.5	2.1	*	*	0.2	0.5	1.6	4.7	12.3	33.3	99.9	280.0	13.1
2013	14.9	2.2	*	*	0.1	0.6	1.5	4.6	12.6	33.8	99.0	285.4	13.2
Intentional Self–Harm (Suicide) (*U03, X60–X84, Y87.0)													
1999	10.5	NA	NA	0.6	10.1	12.7	14.3	13.9	12.2	13.4	18.1	19.3	10.5
2000	10.4	NA	NA	0.7	10.2	12.0	14.5	14.4	12.1	12.5	17.6	19.6	10.4
2001[5]	10.7	NA	NA	0.7	9.9	12.8	14.7	15.1	13.2	13.2	17.4	17.7	10.7
2002	11.0	NA	NA	0.6	9.8	12.8	15.3	15.8	13.5	13.4	17.7	18.9	10.9
2003	10.9	NA	NA	0.6	9.6	12.9	15.0	15.9	13.7	12.6	16.4	17.9	10.8
2004	11.1	NA	NA	0.7	10.3	12.9	15.2	16.6	13.7	12.2	16.3	17.6	11.0
2005	11.0	NA	NA	0.7	9.9	12.7	15.1	16.5	13.7	12.4	16.8	18.3	10.9
2006	11.2	NA	NA	0.5	9.8	12.7	15.2	17.2	14.4	12.4	15.8	17.3	11.0
2007	11.5	NA	NA	0.5	9.6	13.3	15.7	17.7	15.3	12.4	16.2	17.0	11.3
2008	11.8	NA	NA	0.5	9.9	13.2	15.9	18.6	16.0	13.6	16.1	16.4	11.6
2009	12.0	NA	NA	0.6	10.0	13.1	16.1	19.2	16.4	13.7	15.8	16.4	11.8
2010	12.4	NA	NA	0.7	10.5	14.0	16.0	19.6	17.5	13.7	15.7	17.6	12.1
2011	12.7	NA	NA	0.7	11.0	14.6	16.2	19.8	17.1	14.1	16.5	16.9	12.3
2012	12.9	NA	NA	0.8	11.1	14.7	16.7	20.0	18.0	14.0	16.8	17.8	12.6
2013	13.0	NA	NA	1.0	11.1	14.8	16.2	19.7	18.1	15.0	17.1	18.6	12.6
Septicemia (A40–A41)													
1999	11.0	7.5	0.6	0.2	0.3	0.7	1.8	4.6	11.4	31.2	79.4	220.7	11.3
2000	11.1	7.2	0.6	0.2	0.3	0.7	1.9	4.9	11.9	31.0	80.4	215.7	11.3
2001	11.3	7.8	0.7	0.2	0.3	0.7	1.8	5.0	12.4	32.6	82.2	210.3	11.5
2002	11.8	7.5	0.5	0.2	0.3	0.8	1.9	5.2	12.6	34.5	86.3	213.4	11.9
2003	11.7	7.0	0.5	0.2	0.4	0.8	2.1	5.3	13.0	32.3	84.8	213.7	11.8
2004	11.4	6.8	0.5	0.2	0.3	0.8	1.9	5.4	12.8	32.1	81.5	199.6	11.3
2005	11.6	7.5	0.5	0.2	0.3	0.8	1.9	5.2	12.8	32.2	81.3	203.4	11.4
2006	11.5	6.7	0.6	0.2	0.3	0.7	2.0	5.2	12.6	31.6	82.1	193.0	11.2
2007	11.6	6.8	0.5	0.2	0.4	0.7	2.1	5.5	12.8	32.2	79.5	190.8	11.2
2008	11.8	7.0	0.6	0.2	0.3	0.9	2.1	5.7	13.3	31.4	82.0	189.8	11.3
2009	11.6	5.5	0.4	0.2	0.3	0.9	2.2	5.4	13.1	31.4	79.2	182.4	11.0
2010	11.3	5.5	0.4	0.2	0.3	0.8	1.9	5.2	12.6	30.1	76.0	179.0	10.6
2011	11.5	4.5	0.4	0.2	0.3	0.8	2.0	5.5	13.0	29.5	74.4	179.7	10.5
2012	11.4	4.5	0.4	0.1	0.3	0.8	1.9	5.3	12.9	29.2	73.9	173.4	10.3
2013	12.1	3.9	0.3	0.1	0.3	0.8	2.0	5.6	13.6	30.5	76.4	179.6	10.7

Table 2-9. Death Rates by Age and Age-Adjusted Death Rates for the 15 Leading Causes of Death, 1999–2013— continued

(Rate per 100,000 population in specified group; age-adjusted rates per 100,000 U.S. standard population.)

Cause of death (based on ICD–10) and year	All ages[1]	Under 1 year[2]	1 to 4 years	5 to 14 years	15 to 24 years	25 to 34 years	35 to 44 years	45 to 54 years	55 to 64 years	65 to 74 years	75 to 84 years	85 years and over	Age-adjusted rate[3]
Chronic Liver Disease and Cirrhosis (K70, K73–K74)													
1999	9.4	*	*	*	0.1	1.0	7.3	17.4	23.7	30.6	31.9	23.2	9.6
2000	9.4	*	*	*	0.1	1.0	7.5	17.7	23.8	29.8	31.0	23.1	9.5
2001	9.5	*	*	*	0.1	1.0	7.4	18.4	22.9	29.8	30.2	22.7	9.5
2002	9.5	*	*	*	0.1	1.0	7.1	18.0	22.8	29.3	31.3	22.5	9.4
2003	9.5	*	*	*	*	0.9	6.8	18.3	22.9	29.2	29.9	21.2	9.3
2004	9.2	*	*	*	*	0.8	6.4	18.0	22.4	27.4	28.7	21.1	9.0
2005	9.3	*	*	*	0.1	0.8	6.2	17.7	23.3	26.8	28.9	21.3	8.9
2006	9.2	*	*	*	0.1	0.8	5.9	17.8	22.6	25.6	28.9	21.1	8.8
2007	9.7	*	*	*	0.1	1.0	6.0	18.7	24.2	26.2	28.2	21.7	9.1
2008	9.9	*	*	*	0.1	1.1	6.1	18.5	25.0	26.3	28.0	21.9	9.2
2009	10.0	*	*	*	0.1	1.1	6.0	18.7	25.9	25.4	27.2	21.1	9.1
2010	10.3	*	*	*	0.1	1.2	5.9	19.2	26.8	26.3	27.7	21.8	9.4
2011	10.8	*	*	*	0.1	1.2	6.0	19.8	28.2	26.3	29.3	22.1	9.7
2012	11.1	*	*	*	0.1	1.4	6.1	20.1	29.1	27.6	29.3	21.4	9.9
2013	11.5	*	*	*	0.1	1.6	6.2	20.1	30.4	28.1	29.9	23.0	10.2
Essential Hypertension and Hypertensive Renal Disease (I10, I12, I15)													
1999	6.1	*	*	*	*	0.2	0.7	2.2	5.5	15.2	43.6	152.1	6.2
2000	6.4	*	*	*	*	0.2	0.8	2.3	5.9	15.1	45.5	162.9	6.5
2001	6.8	*	*	*	0.1	0.3	0.7	2.4	5.8	15.4	47.6	175.6	6.9
2002	7.0	*	*	*	0.1	0.2	0.8	2.3	5.7	15.9	48.1	189.6	7.1
2003	7.6	*	*	*	0.1	0.2	0.8	2.5	6.3	16.8	51.6	199.4	7.6
2004	7.9	*	*	*	0.1	0.3	0.8	2.7	6.3	16.9	52.5	212.2	7.9
2005	8.4	*	*	*	0.1	0.2	0.9	2.7	6.4	17.5	55.5	228.0	8.3
2006	8.0	*	*	*	0.0	0.3	0.9	3.0	6.8	16.5	50.8	206.1	7.7
2007	8.0	*	*	*	0.1	0.2	0.9	2.8	6.4	15.9	49.2	209.1	7.6
2008	8.5	*	*	*	0.1	0.3	1.0	3.0	7.2	16.5	51.9	215.3	8.0
2009	8.4	*	*	*	0.1	0.3	1.0	3.1	7.1	16.3	51.0	208.0	7.8
2010	8.6	*	*	*	0.0	0.3	1.0	3.1	7.3	16.7	51.8	212.0	8.0
2011	8.9	*	*	*	*	0.2	1.0	3.1	7.0	16.6	51.4	222.7	8.1
2012	9.3	*	*	*	*	0.2	0.8	3.0	7.8	16.1	51.7	230.7	8.2
2013	9.7	*	*	*	0.1	0.3	1.0	3.5	8.0	17.3	53.7	231.6	8.5
Parkinson's Disease (G20–G21)													
1999	5.2	*	*	*	*	*	*	0.1	1.0	11.0	58.2	124.4	5.4
2000	5.6	*	*	*	*	*	*	0.1	1.1	11.5	61.9	131.9	5.7
2001	5.8	*	*	*	*	*	*	0.1	1.2	11.7	64.5	137.0	5.9
2002	5.9	*	*	*	*	*	*	0.1	1.2	12.1	63.8	142.2	6.0
2003	6.2	*	*	*	*	*	*	0.2	1.3	12.6	67.6	145.8	6.3
2004	6.1	*	*	*	*	*	*	0.2	1.2	11.9	67.4	145.1	6.2
2005	6.6	*	*	*	*	*	*	0.2	1.4	12.8	71.1	156.0	6.6
2006	6.6	*	*	*	*	*	*	0.2	1.2	12.0	69.5	157.6	6.5
2007	6.7	*	*	*	*	*	*	0.1	1.2	11.7	71.5	157.0	6.5
2008	6.7	*	*	*	*	*	*	0.2	1.2	12.3	71.2	157.4	6.6
2009	6.7	*	*	*	*	*	*	0.2	1.3	11.2	70.8	157.0	6.5
2010	7.1	*	*	*	*	*	*	0.2	1.3	11.8	74.8	165.9	6.8
2011	7.4	*	*	*	*	*	*	0.1	1.3	12.8	76.0	168.1	7.0
2012	7.6	*	*	*	*	*	*	0.1	1.4	12.3	76.2	172.3	7.0
2013	8.0	*	*	*	*	*	*	0.2	1.5	12.7	78.5	178.2	7.3
Pneumonitis due to solids and liquids (J69)													

Table 2-9. Death Rates by Age and Age-Adjusted Death Rates for the 15 Leading Causes of Death, 1999–2013— continued

(Rate per 100,000 population in specified group; age-adjusted rates per 100,000 U.S. standard population.)

| Cause of death (based on ICD–10) and year | All ages[1] | Age | | | | | | | | | | | Age-adjusted rate[3] |
		Under 1 year[2]	1 to 4 years	5 to 14 years	15 to 24 years	25 to 34 years	35 to 44 years	45 to 54 years	55 to 64 years	65 to 74 years	75 to 84 years	85 years and over	
1999	5.5	*	*	*	0.1	0.2	0.4	0.8	2.5	9.5	41.1	175.6	5.6
2000	5.9	*	*	*	0.1	0.2	0.4	1.0	2.5	10.3	44.5	187.6	6.1
2001	6.1	*	*	*	0.1	0.2	0.4	1.0	2.6	10.0	45.7	193.4	6.2
2002	6.1	*	*	*	0.1	0.2	0.4	0.9	2.5	9.8	46.2	195.5	6.2
2003	6.0	*	*	*	0.1	0.2	0.4	1.0	2.8	9.5	44.9	186.0	6.0
2004	5.7	*	*	*	0.1	0.2	0.4	0.9	2.5	9.5	42.8	176.3	5.7
2005	5.8	*	*	*	0.1	0.2	0.4	1.1	2.7	9.2	42.5	178.0	5.8
2006	5.7	*	*	*	0.1	0.2	0.4	1.0	2.7	9.1	40.4	169.6	5.5
2007	5.6	*	*	*	0.1	0.2	0.4	1.0	2.7	8.8	39.6	167.7	5.4
2008	5.5	*	*	*	0.1	0.2	0.4	1.1	2.7	8.2	38.5	157.8	5.2
2009	5.2	*	*	*	0.1	0.2	0.4	1.1	2.8	7.7	35.7	146.7	4.9
2010	5.5	*	*	*	0.1	0.2	0.3	1.1	2.8	8.6	38.2	152.3	5.1
2011	5.8	*	*	*	0.1	0.2	0.4	1.2	2.9	8.8	39.0	158.5	5.3
2012	5.7	*	*	*	0.1	0.2	0.4	1.2	3.1	8.3	36.6	152.9	5.1

NA = Not applicable.   * = Figure does not meet standards of reliability or precision.   1Figures for age not stated included in "All ages" but not distributed among age groups.   2Death rates for "Under 1 year" (based on population estimates) differ from infant mortality rates (based on live births); please see chapter notes for more information.   3For method of computation, please see chapter notes.   4Due to coding rule changes in 2011, fewer deaths are assigned to Nephritis, nephrotic syndrome and nephrosis (N00–N07,N17–N19,N25–N27) and more deaths are assigned to Diabetes mellitus (E10–E14). Trend data for these causes should be interpreted with caution; see chapter notes.   5Figures include September 11, 2001-related deaths for which death certificates were filed as of October 24, 2002; see Technical Notes from ''Deaths: Final Data for 2001,'' National Vital Statistics Reports,Volume 52, Number 3.

Table 2-10A. Number of Deaths from Selected Causes, by Race and Sex, 2013

(Number.)

Cause of death (based on ICD–10, 2004)	All races Both sexes	All races Male	All races Female	White¹ Both sexes	White¹ Male	White¹ Female	Black¹ Both sexes	Black¹ Male	Black¹ Female
All causes	2,596,993	1,306,034	1,290,959	2,217,103	1,110,956	1,106,147	302,969	154,767	148,202
Salmonella infections (A01-A02)	40	28	12	32	20	12	6	6	-
Shigellosis and amebiasis (A03, A06)	6	3	3	2	2	-	2	1	1
Certain other intestinal infections (A04, A07-A09)	10,590	4,148	6,442	9,483	3,639	5,844	879	401	478
Tuberculosis (A16-A19)	555	357	198	346	221	125	88	55	33
Respiratory tuberculosis (A16)	408	267	141	245	159	86	64	42	22
Other tuberculosis (A17-A19)	147	90	57	101	62	39	24	13	11
Whooping cough (A37)	12	5	7	10	4	6	1	-	1
Scarlet fever and erysipelas (A38, A46)	1	1	-	1	1	-	-	-	-
Meningococcal infection (A39)	59	34	25	50	30	20	7	4	3
Septicemia (A40-A41)	38,156	17,994	20,162	30,889	14,602	16,287	6,250	2,882	3,368
Syphilis (A50-A53)	49	28	21	24	13	11	24	14	10
Acute poliomyelitis (A80)	-	-	-	-	-	-	-	-	-
Arthropod-borne viral encephalitis (A83-A84, A85.2)	4	2	2	4	2	2	-	-	-
Measles (B05)	-	-	-	-	-	-	-	-	-
Viral hepatitis (B15-B19)	8,157	5,425	2,732	6,483	4,381	2,102	1,233	797	436
Human immunodeficiency virus (HIV) disease (B20-B24)	6,955	5,096	1,859	3,084	2,518	566	3,742	2,479	1,263
Malaria (B50-B54)	10	9	1	1	1	-	7	6	1
Other and unspecified infectious and parasitic diseases and their sequelae (A00, A05, A20-A36, A42-A44, A48-A49, A54-A79, A81-A82, A85.0-A85.1, A85.8, A86-B04, B06-B09, B25-B49, B55-B99)	6,007	3,105	2,902	4,970	2,575	2,395	834	426	408
Malignant neoplasms (C00-C97)	584,881	307,559	277,322	498,116	263,167	234,949	67,953	34,671	33,282
Malignant neoplasms of lip, oral cavity and pharynx (C00-C14)	8,850	6,227	2,623	7,428	5,217	2,211	1,076	781	295
Malignant neoplasm of esophagus (C15)	14,690	11,732	2,958	13,037	10,526	2,511	1,308	936	372
Malignant neoplasm of stomach (C16)	11,261	6,793	4,468	8,393	5,101	3,292	1,964	1,184	780
Malignant neoplasms of colon, rectum and anus (C18-C21)	52,252	27,354	24,898	43,444	22,726	20,718	6,897	3,620	3,277
Malignant neoplasms of liver and intrahepatic bile ducts (C22)	24,032	16,300	7,732	18,849	12,683	6,166	3,385	2,400	985
Malignant neoplasm of pancreas (C25)	38,996	19,854	19,142	32,947	16,975	15,972	4,737	2,237	2,500
Malignant neoplasm of larynx (C32)	3,729	2,994	735	3,058	2,459	599	599	474	125
Malignant neoplasms of trachea, bronchus and lung(C33-C34)	156,252	85,710	70,542	135,040	73,523	61,517	16,917	9,794	7,123
Malignant melanoma of skin (C43)	9,394	6,239	3,155	9,191	6,129	3,062	141	76	65
Malignant neoplasm of breast (C50)	41,325	464	40,861	33,933	372	33,561	6,167	81	6,086
Malignant neoplasm of cervix uteri (C53)	4,217	X	4,217	3,162	X	3,162	838	X	838
Malignant neoplasms of corpus uteri and uterus, part unspecified (C54-C55)	9,325	X	9,325	7,261	X	7,261	1,764	X	1,764
Malignant neoplasm of ovary (C56)	14,276	X	14,276	12,533	X	12,533	1,254	X	1,254
Malignant neoplasm of prostate (C61)	27,682	27,682	X	22,550	22,550	X	4,528	4,528	X
Malignant neoplasms of kidney and renal pelvis (C64-C65)	13,906	8,967	4,939	12,256	7,918	4,338	1,260	798	462
Malignant neoplasm of bladder (C67)	15,757	11,294	4,463	14,294	10,415	3,879	1,167	684	483
Malignant neoplasms of meninges, brain and other parts of central nervous system (C70-C72)	15,345	8,493	6,852	13,960	7,724	6,236	941	534	407
Malignant neoplasms of lymphoid, hematopoietic and related tissue (C81-C96)	56,936	32,057	24,879	49,521	28,160	21,361	5,744	2,951	2,793
Hodgkin's disease (C81)	1,090	633	457	958	558	400	108	58	50
Non-Hodgkin's lymphoma (C82-C85)	20,114	11,168	8,946	17,979	10,019	7,960	1,460	778	682
Leukemia (C91-C95)	23,428	13,569	9,859	20,785	12,107	8,678	1,962	1,076	886
Multiple myeloma and immunoproliferative neoplasms (C88, C90)	12,225	6,640	5,585	9,730	5,436	4,294	2,205	1,032	1,173
Other and unspecified malignant neoplasms of lymphoid, hematopoietic and related tissue (C96)	79	47	32	69	40	29	9	7	2
All other and unspecified malignant neoplasms (C17, C23-C24, C26-C31, C37-C41, C44-C49, C51-C52, C57-C60, C62-C63, C66, C68-C69, C73-C80, C97)	66,656	35,399	31,257	57,259	30,689	26,570	7,266	3,593	3,673
In situ neoplasms, benign neoplasms and neoplasms of uncertain or unknown behavior (D00-D48)	15,232	8,081	7,151	13,551	7,248	6,303	1,239	615	624
Anemias (D50-D64)	4,894	2,077	2,817	3,803	1,571	2,232	976	446	530
Diabetes mellitus (E10-E14)	75,578	39,841	35,737	58,925	31,745	27,180	13,385	6,378	7,007
Nutritional deficiencies (E40-E64)	3,382	1,350	2,032	2,833	1,103	1,730	446	200	246
Malnutrition (E40-E46)	3,224	1,284	1,940	2,693	1,046	1,647	431	193	238
Other nutritional deficiencies (E50-E64)	158	66	92	140	57	83	15	7	8
Meningitis (G00,G03)	584	326	258	458	257	201	98	49	49
Parkinson's disease (G20-G21)	25,196	15,088	10,108	23,553	14,127	9,426	1,045	623	422
Alzheimer's disease (G30)	84,767	25,836	58,931	77,387	23,648	53,739	5,714	1,664	4,050
Major cardiovascular diseases (I00-I78)	796,494	400,686	395,808	676,822	340,172	336,650	96,545	48,322	48,223
Diseases of heart (I00-I09, I11, I13, I20-I51)	611,105	321,347	289,758	522,645	275,101	247,544	72,010	37,096	34,914
Acute rheumatic fever and chronic rheumatic heart diseases (I00-I09)	3,260	1,141	2,119	2,862	985	1,877	254	100	154
Hypertensive heart disease (I11)	37,144	18,717	18,427	27,809	13,757	14,052	8,325	4,451	3,874
Hypertensive heart and renal disease (I13)	4,028	1,883	2,145	2,867	1,301	1,566	996	519	477
Ischemic heart diseases (I20-I25)	370,213	208,515	161,698	319,783	181,108	138,675	39,784	21,110	18,674
Acute myocardial infarction (I21-I22)	116,793	66,051	50,742	100,928	57,587	43,341	12,592	6,532	6,060
Other acute ischemic heart diseases (I24)	3,936	2,064	1,872	3,283	1,737	1,546	566	287	279
Other forms of chronic ischemic heart disease (I20, I25)	249,484	140,400	109,084	215,572	121,784	93,788	26,626	14,291	12,335
Atherosclerotic cardiovascular disease, so described (I25.0)	59,475	35,906	23,569	48,859	29,458	19,401	8,726	5,275	3,451
All other forms of chronic ischemic heart disease (I20,I25.1-I25.9)	190,009	104,494	85,515	166,713	92,326	74,387	17,900	9,016	8,884
Other heart diseases (I26-I51)	196,460	91,091	105,369	169,324	77,950	91,374	22,651	10,916	11,735
Acute and subacute endocarditis (I33)	1,255	766	489	1,038	629	409	174	113	61
Diseases of pericardium and acute myocarditis (I30-I31, I40)	872	453	419	688	363	325	150	72	78
Heart failure (I50)	65,120	28,513	36,607	57,353	25,005	32,348	6,548	2,946	3,602
All other forms of heart disease (I26-I28, I34-I38, I42-I49, I51)	129,213	61,359	67,854	110,245	51,953	58,292	15,779	7,785	7,994
Essential hypertension and hypertensive renal disease (I10, I12, I15)	30,770	12,963	17,807	24,149	9,940	14,209	5,455	2,496	2,959
Cerebrovascular diseases (I60-I69)	128,978	53,691	75,287	107,909	44,203	63,706	16,269	7,338	8,931
Atherosclerosis (I70)	6,685	2,714	3,971	5,995	2,419	3,576	529	225	304
Other diseases of circulatory system (I71-I78)	18,956	9,971	8,985	16,124	8,509	7,615	2,282	1,167	1,115
Aortic aneurysm and dissection (I71)	9,846	5,753	4,093	8,485	4,980	3,505	1,027	590	437

Table 2-10A. Number of Deaths from Selected Causes, by Race and Sex, 2013— continued

(Number.)

Cause of death (based on ICD–10, 2004)	All races Both sexes	All races Male	All races Female	White[1] Both sexes	White[1] Male	White[1] Female	Black[1] Both sexes	Black[1] Male	Black[1] Female
Other diseases of arteries, arterioles and capillaries (I72-I78)	9,110	4,218	4,892	7,639	3,529	4,110	1,255	577	678
Other disorders of circulatory system (I80-I99)	4,443	2,165	2,278	3,492	1,683	1,809	859	437	422
Influenza and pneumonia (J09-J18)	56,979	26,804	30,175	49,013	22,907	26,106	5,567	2,696	2,871
Influenza (J09-J11)	3,697	1,697	2,000	3,288	1,506	1,782	278	127	151
Pneumonia (J12-J18)	53,282	25,107	28,175	45,725	21,401	24,324	5,289	2,569	2,720
Other acute lower respiratory infections (J20-J22, U04)	285	110	175	252	94	158	30	14	16
Acute bronchitis and bronchiolitis (J20-J21)	226	90	136	199	76	123	24	12	12
Other and unspecified acute lower respiratory infections(J22, U04)	59	20	39	53	18	35	6	2	4
Chronic lower respiratory diseases (J40-J47)	149,205	70,317	78,888	136,682	63,757	72,925	9,918	5,073	4,845
Bronchitis, chronic and unspecified (J40-J42)	664	272	392	580	237	343	66	29	37
Emphysema (J43)	8,284	4,321	3,963	7,589	3,905	3,684	545	317	228
Asthma (J45-J46)	3,630	1,410	2,220	2,415	842	1,573	1,006	470	536
Other chronic lower respiratory diseases (J44, J47)	136,627	64,314	72,313	126,098	58,773	67,325	8,301	4,257	4,044
Pneumoconioses and chemical effects (J60-J66, J68)	806	767	39	764	728	36	32	29	3
Pneumonitis due to solids and liquids (J69)	18,579	10,140	8,439	16,458	8,989	7,469	1,609	857	752
Other diseases of respiratory system (J00-J06, J30-J39, J67, J70-J98)	35,217	17,825	17,392	30,954	15,822	15,132	3,188	1,451	1,737
Peptic ulcer (K25-K28)	2,988	1,535	1,453	2,551	1,286	1,265	295	164	131
Diseases of appendix (K35-K38)	371	216	155	306	176	130	51	34	17
Hernia (K40-K46)	1,932	772	1,160	1,718	687	1,031	173	68	105
Chronic liver disease and cirrhosis (K70, K73-K74)	36,427	23,709	12,718	31,871	20,884	10,987	3,053	1,955	1,098
Alcoholic liver disease (K70)	18,146	12,991	5,155	15,861	11,478	4,383	1,372	930	442
Other chronic liver disease and cirrhosis (K73-K74)	18,281	10,718	7,563	16,010	9,406	6,604	1,681	1,025	656
Cholelithiasis and other disorders of gallbladder (K80-K82)	3,377	1,605	1,772	2,903	1,382	1,521	318	144	174
Nephritis, nephritic syndrome and nephrosis(N00-N07, N17-N19, N25-N27)	47,112	23,493	23,619	37,270	18,800	18,470	8,393	3,976	4,417
Acute and rapidly progressive nephritic and nephritic syndrome (N00-N01,N04)	399	205	194	329	164	165	60	34	26
Chronic glomerulonephritis, nephritis and nephropathy not specified as acute or chronic, and renal sclerosis unspecified (N02-N03, N05-N07, N26)	254	132	122	215	118	97	24	9	15
Renal failure (N17-N19)	46,425	23,136	23,289	36,694	18,500	18,194	8,307	3,931	4,376
Other disorders of kidney (N25, N27)	34	20	14	32	18	14	2	2	-
Infections of kidney (N10-N12,N13.6,N15.1)	641	191	450	534	157	377	73	23	50
Hyperplasia of prostate (N40)	558	558	X	507	507	X	37	37	X
Inflammatory diseases of female pelvic organs (N70-N76)	129	X	129	99	X	99	20	X	20
Pregnancy, childbirth and the puerperium (O00-O99)	1,138	X	1,138	713	X	713	364	X	364
Pregnancy with abortive outcome (O00-O07)	27	X	27	15	X	15	10	X	10
Other complications of pregnancy, childbirth and the puerperium (O10-O99)	1,111	X	1,111	698	X	698	354	X	354
Certain conditions originating in the perinatal period(P00-P96)	12,084	6,723	5,361	7,437	4,162	3,275	4,055	2,215	1,840
Congenital malformations, deformations and chromosomal abnormalities (Q00-Q99)	9,583	5,052	4,531	7,559	3,994	3,565	1,590	815	775
Symptoms, signs and abnormal clinical and laboratory findings, not elsewhere classified (R00-R99)	37,752	16,275	21,477	32,310	13,636	18,674	4,522	2,199	2,323
All other diseases (Residual)	320,065	129,448	190,617	278,876	112,075	166,801	33,391	13,965	19,426
Accidents (unintentional injuries) (V01-X59, Y85-Y86)	130,557	81,916	48,641	112,803	70,161	42,642	13,413	9,017	4,396
Transport accidents (V01-V99, Y85)	37,938	27,102	10,836	31,292	22,410	8,882	5,007	3,647	1,360
Motor vehicle accidents (V02-V04, V09.0, V09.2, V12-V14, V19.0-V19.2, V19.4-V19.6, V20-V79, V80.3-V80.5, V81.0-V81.1, V82.0-V82.1,V83- V86, V87.0-V87.8, V88.0-V88.8, V89.0, V89.2)	35,369	25,048	10,321	29,118	20,662	8,456	4,731	3,431	1,300
Other land transport accidents (V01, V05-V06, V09.1, V09.3-V09.9, V10-V11, V15-V18, V19.3, V19.8-V19.9, V80.0-V80.2, V80.6-V80.9, V81.2- V81.9, V82.2-V82.9, V87.9, V88.9, V89.1, V89.3, V89.9)	1,000	804	196	814	650	164	137	117	20
Water, air and space, and other and unspecified transport accidents and their sequelae (V90-V99, Y85)	1,569	1,250	319	1,360	1,098	262	139	99	40
Nontransport accidents (W00-X59, Y86)	92,619	54,814	37,805	81,511	47,751	33,760	8,406	5,370	3,036
Falls (W00-W19)	30,208	15,205	15,003	27,912	13,880	14,032	1,415	836	579
Accidental discharge of firearms (W32-W34)	505	441	64	399	350	49	93	80	13
Accidental drowning and submersion (W65-W74)	3,391	2,613	778	2,603	1,983	620	532	433	99
Accidental exposure to smoke, fire and flames(X00-X09)	2,760	1,653	1,107	2,136	1,297	839	549	311	238
Accidental poisoning and exposure to noxious substances (X40-X49)	38,851	25,080	13,771	34,035	21,874	12,161	3,823	2,558	1,265
Other and unspecified nontransport accidents and their sequelae (W20-W31, W35-W64, W75-W99, X10-X39, X50-X59, Y86)	16,904	9,822	7,082	14,426	8,367	6,059	1,994	1,152	842
Intentional self-harm (suicide) (*U03, X60-X84, Y87.0)	41,149	32,055	9,094	37,154	28,943	8,211	2,353	1,891	462
Intentional self-harm (suicide) by discharge of firearms (X72-X74)	21,175	18,241	2,934	19,615	16,854	2,761	1,086	975	111
Intentional self-harm (suicide) by other and unspecified means and their sequelae (*U03, X60-X71, X75-X84, Y87.0)	19,974	13,814	6,160	17,539	12,089	5,450	1,267	916	351
Assault (homicide) (*U01-*U02, X85-Y09, Y87.1)	16,121	12,726	3,395	7,523	5,393	2,130	8,059	6,937	1,122
Assault (homicide) by discharge of firearms (*U01.4, X93-X95)	11,208	9,445	1,763	4,484	3,430	1,054	6,442	5,798	644
Assault (homicide) by other and unspecified means and their sequelae (*U01.0-*U01.3, *U01.5-*U01.9, *U02, X85-X92, X96-Y09, Y87.1)	4,913	3,281	1,632	3,039	1,963	1,076	1,617	1,139	478
Legal intervention (Y35, Y89.0)	516	492	24	352	334	18	147	142	5
Events of undetermined intent (Y10-Y34, Y87.2,Y89.9)	4,587	2,708	1,879	3,853	2,224	1,629	586	397	189
Discharge of firearms, undetermined intent (Y22-Y24)	281	221	60	229	181	48	43	34	9
Other and unspecified events of undetermined intent and their sequelae (Y10-Y21, Y25-Y34, Y87.2, Y89.9)	4,306	2,487	1,819	3,624	2,043	1,581	543	363	180
Operations of war and their sequelae (Y36, Y89.1)	15	15	-	14	14	-	1	1	-
Complications of medical and surgical care (Y40-Y84, Y88)	2,768	1,338	1,430	2,308	1,114	1,194	398	191	207
Enterocolitis due to Clostridium difficile (A04.7)[4]	7,665	3,035	4,630	6,933	2,697	4,236	585	264	321
Drug-induced deaths[5,6]	46,471	28,381	18,090	41,053	24,934	16,119	4,376	2,828	1,548
Alcohol-induced deaths[5,7]	29,001	21,361	7,640	25,036	18,509	6,527	2,570	1,897	673
Injury by firearms[5,8]	33,636	28,794	4,842	25,044	21,116	3,928	7,797	7,016	781

Table 2-10B. Number of Deaths from Selected Causes, by Race and Sex, 2013

(Number.)

Cause of death (based on ICD–10, 2004)	American Indian and Alaskan Native[1,2]			Asian or Pacific Islander[1,3]		
	Both sexes	Male	Female	Both sexes	Male	Female
All causes	17,052	9,331	7,721	59,869	30,980	28,889
Salmonella infections (A01-A02)	-	-	-	2	2	-
Shigellosis and amebiasis (A03, A06)	1	-	1	1	-	1
Certain other intestinal infections (A04, A07-A09)	52	22	30	176	86	90
Tuberculosis (A16-A19)	15	8	7	106	73	33
Respiratory tuberculosis (A16)	12	7	5	87	59	28
Other tuberculosis (A17-A19)	3	1	2	19	14	5
Whooping cough (A37)	1	1	-	-	-	-
Scarlet fever and erysipelas (A38, A46)	-	-	-	-	-	-
Meningococcal infection (A39)	1	-	1	1	-	1
Septicemia (A40-A41)	288	139	149	729	371	358
Syphilis (A50-A53)	1	1	-	-	-	-
Acute poliomyelitis (A80)	-	-	-	-	-	-
Arthropod-borne viral encephalitis (A83-A84, A85.2)	-	-	-	-	-	-
Measles (B05)	-	-	-	-	-	-
Viral hepatitis (B15-B19)	133	80	53	308	167	141
Human immunodeficiency virus (HIV) disease (B20-B24)	53	40	13	76	59	17
Malaria (B50-B54)	-	-	-	2	2	-
Other and unspecified infectious and parasitic diseases and their sequelae (A00, A05, A20-A36, A42-A44, A48-A49, A54-A79, A81-A82, A85.0-A85.1, A85.8, A86-B04, B06-B09, B25-B49, B55-B99)	54	29	25	149	75	74
Malignant neoplasms (C00-C97)	3,109	1,650	1,459	15,703	8,071	7,632
Malignant neoplasms of lip, oral cavity and pharynx (C00-C14)	32	23	9	314	206	108
Malignant neoplasm of esophagus (C15)	74	60	14	271	210	61
Malignant neoplasm of stomach (C16)	96	51	45	808	457	351
Malignant neoplasms of colon, rectum and anus (C18-C21)	355	188	167	1,556	820	736
Malignant neoplasms of liver and intrahepatic bile ducts (C22)	256	172	84	1,542	1,045	497
Malignant neoplasm of pancreas (C25)	188	95	93	1,124	547	577
Malignant neoplasm of larynx (C32)	19	12	7	53	49	4
Malignant neoplasms of trachea, bronchus and lung(C33-C34)	754	408	346	3,541	1,985	1,556
Malignant melanoma of skin (C43)	16	9	7	46	25	21
Malignant neoplasm of breast (C50)	166	-	166	1,059	11	1,048
Malignant neoplasm of cervix uteri (C53)	30	X	30	187	X	187
Malignant neoplasms of corpus uteri and uterus, part unspecified (C54-C55)	37	X	37	263	X	263
Malignant neoplasm of ovary (C56)	73	X	73	416	X	416
Malignant neoplasm of prostate (C61)	131	131	X	473	473	X
Malignant neoplasms of kidney and renal pelvis (C64-C65)	118	72	46	272	179	93
Malignant neoplasm of bladder (C67)	48	31	17	248	164	84
Malignant neoplasms of meninges, brain and other parts of central nervous system (C70-C72)	68	35	33	376	200	176
Malignant neoplasms of lymphoid, hematopoietic and related tissue (C81-C96)	259	143	116	1,412	803	609
Hodgkin's disease (C81)	3	2	1	21	15	6
Non-Hodgkin's lymphoma (C82-C85)	88	53	35	587	318	269
Leukemia (C91-C95)	104	55	49	577	331	246
Multiple myeloma and immunoproliferative neoplasms (C88, C90)	64	33	31	226	139	87
Other and unspecified malignant neoplasms of lymphoid, hematopoietic and related tissue (C96)	-	-	-	1	-	1
All other and unspecified malignant neoplasms (C17, C23-C24, C26-C31, C37-C41, C44-C49, C51-C52, C57-C60, C62-C63, C66, C68-C69, C73-C80, C97)	389	220	169	1,742	897	845
In situ neoplasms, benign neoplasms and neoplasms of uncertain or unknown behavior (D00-D48)	62	37	25	380	181	199
Anemias (D50-D64)	23	14	9	92	46	46
Diabetes mellitus (E10-E14)	959	490	469	2,309	1,228	1,081
Nutritional deficiencies (E40-E64)	29	16	13	74	31	43
Malnutrition (E40-E46)	27	14	13	73	31	42
Other nutritional deficiencies (E50-E64)	2	2	-	1	-	1
Meningitis (G00,G03)	5	4	1	23	16	7
Parkinson's disease (G20-G21)	70	39	31	528	299	229
Alzheimer's disease (G30)	238	77	161	1,428	447	981
Major cardiovascular diseases (I00-I78)	4,043	2,247	1,796	19,084	9,945	9,139
Diseases of heart (I00-I09, I11, I13, I20-I51)	3,139	1,843	1,296	13,311	7,307	6,004
Acute rheumatic fever and chronic rheumatic heart diseases (I00-I09)	21	8	13	123	48	75
Hypertensive heart disease (I11)	235	142	93	775	367	408
Hypertensive heart and renal disease (I13)	19	8	11	146	55	91
Ischemic heart diseases (I20-I25)	2,036	1,255	781	8,610	5,042	3,568
Acute myocardial infarction (I21-I22)	618	377	241	2,655	1,555	1,100
Other acute ischemic heart diseases (I24)	21	14	7	66	26	40
Other forms of chronic ischemic heart disease (I20, I25)	1,397	864	533	5,889	3,461	2,428
Atherosclerotic cardiovascular disease, so described (I25.0)	502	317	185	1,388	856	532
All other forms of chronic ischemic heart disease (I20,I25.1-I25.9)	895	547	348	4,501	2,605	1,896
Other heart diseases (I26-I51)	828	430	398	3,657	1,795	1,862
Acute and subacute endocarditis (I33)	18	9	9	25	15	10
Diseases of pericardium and acute myocarditis (I30-I31, I40)	10	7	3	24	11	13

Table 2-10B. Number of Deaths from Selected Causes, by Race and Sex, 2013— continued

(Number.)

Cause of death (based on ICD–10, 2004)	American Indian and Alaskan Native[1,2]			Asian or Pacific Islander[1,3]		
	Both sexes	Male	Female	Both sexes	Male	Female
Heart failure (I50)	241	106	135	978	456	522
All other forms of heart disease (I26-I28, I34-I38, I42-I49, I51)	559	308	251	2,630	1,313	1,317
Essential hypertension and hypertensive renal disease (I10, I12, I15)	183	94	89	983	433	550
Cerebrovascular diseases (I60-I69)	595	253	342	4,205	1,897	2,308
Atherosclerosis (I70)	35	16	19	126	54	72
Other diseases of circulatory system (I71-I78)	91	41	50	459	254	205
Aortic aneurysm and dissection (I71)	39	18	21	295	165	130
Other diseases of arteries, arterioles and capillaries (I72-I78)	52	23	29	164	89	75
Other disorders of circulatory system (I80-I99)	25	15	10	67	30	37
Influenza and pneumonia (J09-J18)	375	190	185	2,024	1,011	1,013
Influenza (J09-J11)	30	9	21	101	55	46
Pneumonia (J12-J18)	345	181	164	1,923	956	967
Other acute lower respiratory infections (J20-J22, U04)	1	-	1	2	2	-
Acute bronchitis and bronchiolitis (J20-J21)	1	-	1	2	2	-
Other and unspecified acute lower respiratory infections(J22, U04)	-	-	-	-	-	-
Chronic lower respiratory diseases (J40-J47)	757	370	387	1,848	1,117	731
Bronchitis, chronic and unspecified (J40-J42)	2	1	1	16	5	11
Emphysema (J43)	41	21	20	109	78	31
Asthma (J45-J46)	34	16	18	175	82	93
Other chronic lower respiratory diseases (J44, J47)	680	332	348	1,548	952	596
Pneumoconioses and chemical effects (J60-J66, J68)	9	9	-	1	1	-
Pneumonitis due to solids and liquids (J69)	76	44	32	436	250	186
Other diseases of respiratory system (J00-J06, J30-J39, J67, J70-J98)	248	124	124	827	428	399
Peptic ulcer (K25-K28)	17	11	6	125	74	51
Diseases of appendix (K35-K38)	5	1	4	9	5	4
Hernia (K40-K46)	12	5	7	29	12	17
Chronic liver disease and cirrhosis (K70, K73-K74)	944	511	433	559	359	200
Alcoholic liver disease (K70)	703	419	284	210	164	46
Other chronic liver disease and cirrhosis (K73-K74)	241	92	149	349	195	154
Cholelithiasis and other disorders of gallbladder (K80-K82)	39	18	21	117	61	56
Nephritis, nephritic syndrome and nephrosis(N00-N07, N17-N19, N25-N27)	302	143	159	1,147	574	573
Acute and rapidly progressive nephritic and nephritic syndrome (N00-N01,N04)	1	-	1	9	7	2
Chronic glomerulonephritis, nephritis and nephropathy not specified as acute or chronic, and renal sclerosis unspecified (N02-N03, N05-N07, N26)	3	1	2	12	4	8
Renal failure (N17-N19)	298	142	156	1,126	563	563
Other disorders of kidney (N25, N27)	-	-	-	-	-	-
Infections of kidney (N10-N12,N13.6,N15.1)	12	3	9	22	8	14
Hyperplasia of prostate (N40)	3	3	X	11	11	X
Inflammatory diseases of female pelvic organs (N70-N76)	3	X	3	7	X	7
Pregnancy, childbirth and the puerperium (O00-O99)	16	X	16	45	X	45
Pregnancy with abortive outcome (O00-O07)	1	X	1	1	X	1
Other complications of pregnancy, childbirth and the puerperium (O10-O99)	15	X	15	44	X	44
Certain conditions originating in the perinatal period(P00-P96)	105	69	36	487	277	210
Congenital malformations, deformations and chromosomal abnormalities (Q00-Q99)	119	77	42	315	166	149
Symptoms, signs and abnormal clinical and laboratory findings, not elsewhere classified (R00-R99)	253	126	127	667	314	353
All other diseases (Residual)	1,915	903	1,012	5,883	2,505	3,378
Accidents (unintentional injuries) (V01-X59, Y85-Y86)	1,833	1,177	656	2,508	1,561	947
Transport accidents (V01-V99, Y85)	715	467	248	924	578	346
Motor vehicle accidents (V02-V04, V09.0, V09.2, V12-V14, V19.0-V19.2, V19.4-V19.6, V20-V79, V80.3-V80.5, V81.0-V81.1, V82.0-V82.1,V83-V86, V87.0-V87.8, V88.0-V88.8, V89.0, V89.2)	664	426	238	856	529	327
Other land transport accidents (V01,V05-V06, V09.1, V09.3-V09.9, V10-V11, V15-V18, V19.3, V19.8-V19.9, V80.0-V80.2, V80.6-V80.9, V81.2-V81.9, V82.2-V82.9, V87.9, V88.9, V89.1, V89.3, V89.9)	20	15	5	29	22	7
Water, air and space, and other and unspecified transport accidents and their sequelae (V90-V99, Y85)	31	26	5	39	27	12
Nontransport accidents (W00-X59, Y86)	1,118	710	408	1,584	983	601
Falls (W00-W19)	189	108	81	692	381	311
Accidental discharge of firearms (W32-W34)	9	8	1	4	3	1
Accidental drowning and submersion (W65-W74)	71	55	16	185	142	43
Accidental exposure to smoke, fire and flames(X00-X09)	42	24	18	33	21	12
Accidental poisoning and exposure to noxious substances (X40-X49)	603	373	230	390	275	115
Other and unspecified nontransport accidents and their sequelae (W20-W31, W35-W64, W75-W99, X10-X39, X50-X59, Y86)	204	142	62	280	161	119
Intentional self-harm (suicide) (*U03, X60-X84, Y87.0)	521	401	120	1,121	820	301
Intentional self-harm (suicide) by discharge of firearms (X72-X74)	202	178	24	272	234	38
Intentional self-harm (suicide) by other and unspecified means and their sequelae (*U03, X60-X71, X75-X84, Y87.0)	319	223	96	849	586	263
Assault (homicide) (*U01-*U02, X85-Y09, Y87.1)	241	187	54	298	209	89
Assault (homicide) by discharge of firearms (*U01.4, X93-X95)	107	88	19	175	129	46

Table 2-10B. Number of Deaths from Selected Causes, by Race and Sex, 2013— continued

(Number.)

Cause of death (based on ICD–10, 2004)	American Indian and Alaskan Native[1,2]			Asian or Pacific Islander[1,3]		
	Both sexes	Male	Female	Both sexes	Male	Female
Assault (homicide) by other and unspecified means and their sequelae (*U01.0-*U01.3, *U01.5-*U01.9, *U02, X85-X92, X96-Y09, Y87.1)	134	99	35	123	80	43
Legal intervention (Y35, Y89.0)	4	4	-	13	12	1
Events of undetermined intent (Y10-Y34, Y87.2,Y89.9)	69	41	28	79	46	33
Discharge of firearms, undetermined intent (Y22-Y24)	4	3	1	5	3	2
Other and unspecified events of undetermined intent and their sequelae (Y10-Y21, Y25-Y34, Y87.2, Y89.9)	65	38	27	74	43	31
Operations of war and their sequelae (Y36, Y89.1)	-	-	-	-	-	-
Complications of medical and surgical care (Y40-Y84, Y88)	11	5	6	51	28	23
Enterocolitis due to Clostridium difficile (A04.7)[4]	37	19	18	110	55	55
Drug-induced deaths[5,6]	559	301	258	483	318	165
Alcohol-induced deaths[5,7]	1,063	694	369	332	261	71
Injury by firearms[5,8]	326	281	45	469	381	88

X = Not applicable.   - = Quantity zero.   1Race categories are consistent with the 1977 Office of Management and Budget (OMB) standards. Multiple-race data were reported by 42 states and the District of Columbia in 2013. The multiple-race data for these reporting areas were bridged to the single-race categories of the 1977 OMB standards for comparability with other reporting areas.   2Includes Aleuts and Eskimos.   3Includes Chinese, Filipinos, Hawaiians, Japanese, and other Asian and Pacific Islander persons.   4Included in certain other intestinal infections (A04, A07–A09). Beginning with data year 2006, Enterocolitis due to Clostridium difficile (A04.7) is shown separately at the bottom of the table and is included in the list of rankable causes.   5Included in selected categories above.   6Includes ICD–10 codes 52.1, D59.0, D59.2, D61.1, D64.2, E06.4, E16.0, E23.1, E24.2, E27.3, E66.1, F11.1-F11.5, F11.7-F11.9, F12.1-F12.5, F12.7-F12.9, F13.1-F13.5, F13.7-F13.9, F14.1-F14.5, F14.7-F14.9, F15.1-F15.5, F15.7-F15.9, F16.1-F16.5, F16.7-F16.9, F17.3-F17.5, F17.7-F17.9, F18.1-F18.5, F18.7- F18.9, F19.1-F19.5, F19.7, F19.9, G21.1, G24.0, G25.1, G25.4, G25.6, G44.4, G62.0, G72.0, I95.2, J70.2-J70.4, K85.3, L10.5, L27.0-L27.1, M10.2, M32.0, M80.4, M81.4, M83.5, M87.1, R50.2, R78.1-R78.5, X40-X44, X60-X64, X85, and Y10-Y14. Trend data for Drug-induced deaths, previously shown in this report, can be found through a link from the online version of this report, available from http://www.cdc.gov/nchs/deaths.htm.   7Includes ICD–10 codes E24.4, F10, G31.2, G62.1, G72.1, I42.6, K29.2, K70, K85.2, K86.0, R78.0, X45, X65, and Y15. Trend data for Alcohol-induced deaths, previously shown in this report, can be found through a link from the online version of this report, available from http://www.cdc.gov/nchs/deaths.htm.   8Includes ICD–10 codes *U01.4, W32-W34, X72-X74, X93-X95, Y22-Y24, and Y35.0. Trend data for Injury by firearms, previously shown in this report, can be found through a link from the online version of this report, available from http://www.cdc.gov/nchs/deaths.htm.

Table 2-11A. Death Rates for Selected Causes, by Race and Sex, 2013

(Rates per 100,000 population in specified group.)

Cause of death (based on ICD-10, 2004)	All races			White[1]			Black[1]		
	Both sexes	Male	Female	Both sexes	Male	Female	Both sexes	Male	Female
All Causes	821.5	839.1	804.4	889.2	899.1	879.4	693.4	739.3	651.1
Salmonella infections (A01-A02)	0.0	0.0	*	0.0	0.0	*	*	*	*
Shigellosis and amebiasis (A03, A06)	*	*	*	*	*	*	*	*	*
Certain other intestinal infections (A04, A07-A09)	3.3	2.7	4.0	3.8	2.9	4.6	2.0	1.9	2.1
Tuberculosis (A16-A19)	0.2	0.2	0.1	0.1	0.2	0.1	0.2	0.3	0.1
Respiratory tuberculosis (A16)	0.1	0.2	0.1	0.1	0.1	0.1	0.1	0.2	0.1
Other tuberculosis (A17-A19)	0.0	0.1	0.0	0.0	0.1	0.0	0.1	*	*
Whooping cough (A37)	*	*	*	*	*	*	*	*	*
Scarlet fever and erysipelas (A38, A46)	*	*	*	*	*	*	*	*	*
Meningococcal infection (A39)	0.0	0.0	0.0	0.0	0.0	0.0	*	*	*
Septicemia (A40-A41)	12.1	11.6	12.6	12.4	11.8	12.9	14.3	13.8	14.8
Syphilis (A50-A53)	0.0	0.0	0.0	0.0	*	*	0.1	*	*
Acute poliomyelitis (A80)	*	*	*	*	*	*	*	*	*
Arthropod-borne viral encephalitis (A83-A84, A85.2)	*	*	*	*	*	*	*	*	*
Measles (B05)	*	*	*	*	*	*	*	*	*
Viral hepatitis (B15-B19)	2.6	3.5	1.7	2.6	3.5	1.7	2.8	3.8	1.9
Human immunodeficiency virus (HIV) disease (B20-B24)	2.2	3.3	1.2	1.2	2.0	0.4	8.6	11.8	5.5
Malaria (B50-B54)	*	*	*	*	*	*	*	*	*
Other and unspecified infectious and parasitic diseases and their sequelae (A00, A05, A20-A36, A42-A44, A48-A49, A54-A79, A81-A82, A85.0-A85.1, A85.8, A86-B04, B06-B09, B25-B49, B55-B99)	1.9	2.0	1.8	2.0	2.1	1.9	1.9	2.0	1.8
Malignant neoplasms (C00-C97)	185.0	197.6	172.8	199.8	213.0	186.8	155.5	165.6	146.2
Malignant neoplasms of lip, oral cavity and pharynx (C00-C14)	2.8	4.0	1.6	3.0	4.2	1.8	2.5	3.7	1.3
Malignant neoplasm of esophagus (C15)	4.6	7.5	1.8	5.2	8.5	2.0	3.0	4.5	1.6
Malignant neoplasm of stomach (C16)	3.6	4.4	2.8	3.4	4.1	2.6	4.5	5.7	3.4
Malignant neoplasms of colon, rectum and anus (C18-C21)	16.5	17.6	15.5	17.4	18.4	16.5	15.8	17.3	14.4
Malignant neoplasms of liver and intrahepatic bile ducts (C22)	7.6	10.5	4.8	7.6	10.3	4.9	7.7	11.5	4.3
Malignant neoplasm of pancreas (C25)	12.3	12.8	11.9	13.2	13.7	12.7	10.8	10.7	11.0
Malignant neoplasm of larynx (C32)	1.2	1.9	0.5	1.2	2.0	0.5	1.4	2.3	0.5
Malignant neoplasm of trachea, bronchus and lung(C33-C34)	49.4	55.1	44.0	54.2	59.5	48.9	38.7	46.8	31.3
Malignant melanoma of skin (C43)	3.0	4.0	2.0	3.7	5.0	2.4	0.3	0.4	0.3
Malignant neoplasm of breast (C50)	13.1	0.3	25.5	13.6	0.3	26.7	14.1	0.4	26.7
Malignant neoplasm of cervix uteri (C53)	1.3	X	2.6	1.3	X	2.5	1.9	X	3.7
Malignant neoplasms of corpus uteri and uterus, part unspecified (C54-C55)	2.9	X	5.8	2.9	X	5.8	4.0	X	7.7
Malignant neoplasm of ovary (C56)	4.5	X	8.9	5.0	X	10.0	2.9	X	5.5
Malignant neoplasm of prostate (C61)	8.8	17.8	X	9.0	18.3	X	10.4	21.6	X
Malignant neoplasms of kidney and renal pelvis (C64-C65)	4.4	5.8	3.1	4.9	6.4	3.4	2.9	3.8	2.0
Malignant neoplasm of bladder (C67)	5.0	7.3	2.8	5.7	8.4	3.1	2.7	3.3	2.1
Malignant neoplasms of meninges, brain and other parts of central nervous system (C70-C72)	4.9	5.5	4.3	5.6	6.3	5.0	2.2	2.6	1.8
Malignant neoplasms of lymphoid, hematopoietic and related tissue (C81-C96)	18.0	20.6	15.5	19.9	22.8	17.0	13.1	14.1	12.3
Hodgkin's disease (C81)	0.3	0.4	0.3	0.4	0.5	0.3	0.2	0.3	0.2
Non-Hodgkin's lymphoma (C82-C85)	6.4	7.2	5.6	7.2	8.1	6.3	3.3	3.7	3.0
Leukemia (C91-C95)	7.4	8.7	6.1	8.3	9.8	6.9	4.5	5.1	3.9
Multiple myeloma and immunoproliferative neoplasms (C88, C90)	3.9	4.3	3.5	3.9	4.4	3.4	5.0	4.9	5.2
Other and unspecified malignant neoplasms of lymphoid, hematopoietic and related tissue (C96)	0.0	0.0	0.0	0.0	0.0	0.0	*	*	*
All other and unspecified malignant neoplasms (C17, C23-C24, C26-C31, C37-C41, C44-C49, C51- C52, C57-C60, C62-C63, C66, C68-C69, C73-C80, C97)	21.1	22.7	19.5	23.0	24.8	21.1	16.6	17.2	16.1
In situ neoplasms, benign neoplasms and neoplasms of uncertain or unknown behavior (D00-D48)	4.8	5.2	4.5	5.4	5.9	5.0	2.8	2.9	2.7
Anemias (D50-D64)	1.5	1.3	1.8	1.5	1.3	1.8	2.2	2.1	2.3
Diabetes mellitus (E10-E14)	23.9	25.6	22.3	23.6	25.7	21.6	30.6	30.5	30.8
Nutritional deficiencies (E40-E64)	1.1	0.9	1.3	1.1	0.9	1.4	1.0	1.0	1.1
Malnutrition (E40-E46)	1.0	0.8	1.2	1.1	0.8	1.3	1.0	0.9	1.0
Other nutritional deficiencies (E50-E64)	0.0	0.0	0.1	0.1	0.0	0.1	*	*	*
Meningitis (G00,G03)	0.2	0.2	0.2	0.2	0.2	0.2	0.2	0.2	0.2
Parkinson's disease (G20-G21)	8.0	9.7	6.3	9.4	11.4	7.5	2.4	3.0	1.9
Alzheimer's disease (G30)	26.8	16.6	36.7	31.0	19.1	42.7	13.1	7.9	17.8
Major cardiovascular diseases (I00-I78)	252.0	257.4	246.6	271.4	275.3	267.6	220.9	230.8	211.9
Diseases of heart (I00-I09, I11, I13, I20-I51)	193.3	206.5	180.6	209.6	222.6	196.8	164.8	177.2	153.4
Acute rheumatic fever and chronic rheumatic heart diseases (I00-I09)	1.0	0.7	1.3	1.1	0.8	1.5	0.6	0.5	0.7
Hypertensive heart disease (I11)	11.7	12.0	11.5	11.2	11.1	11.2	19.1	21.3	17.0
Hypertensive heart and renal disease (I13)	1.3	1.2	1.3	1.1	1.1	1.2	2.3	2.5	2.1
Ischemic heart diseases (I20-I25)	117.1	134.0	100.8	128.2	146.6	110.2	91.0	100.8	82.0
Acute myocardial infarction (I21-I22)	36.9	42.4	31.6	40.5	46.6	34.5	28.8	31.2	26.6
Other acute ischemic heart diseases (I24)	1.2	1.3	1.2	1.3	1.4	1.2	1.3	1.4	1.2
Other forms of chronic ischemic heart disease (I20, I25)	78.9	90.2	68.0	86.5	98.6	74.6	60.9	68.3	54.2
Atherosclerotic cardiovascular disease, so described (I25.0)	18.8	23.1	14.7	19.6	23.8	15.4	20.0	25.2	15.2
All other forms of chronic ischemic heart disease (I20,I25.1-I25.9)	60.1	67.1	53.3	66.9	74.7	59.1	41.0	43.1	39.0
Other heart diseases (I26-I51)	62.1	58.5	65.7	67.9	63.1	72.6	51.8	52.1	51.6
Acute and subacute endocarditis (I33)	0.4	0.5	0.3	0.4	0.5	0.3	0.4	0.5	0.3
Diseases of pericardium and acute myocarditis (I30-I31, I40)	0.3	0.3	0.3	0.3	0.3	0.3	0.3	0.3	0.3
Heart failure (I50)	20.6	18.3	22.8	23.0	20.2	25.7	15.0	14.1	15.8
All other forms of heart disease (I26-I28, I34-I38, I42-I49, I51)	40.9	39.4	42.3	44.2	42.0	46.3	36.1	37.2	35.1
Essential hypertension and hypertensive renal disease (I10, I12, I15)	9.7	8.3	11.1	9.7	8.0	11.3	12.5	11.9	13.0
Cerebrovascular diseases (I60-I69)	40.8	34.5	46.9	43.3	35.8	50.6	37.2	35.1	39.2
Atherosclerosis (I70)	2.1	1.7	2.5	2.4	2.0	2.8	1.2	1.1	1.3

Table 2-11A. Death Rates for Selected Causes, by Race and Sex, 2013— continued

(Rates per 100,000 population in specified group.)

Cause of death (based on ICD-10, 2004)	All races			White[1]			Black[1]		
	Both sexes	Male	Female	Both sexes	Male	Female	Both sexes	Male	Female
Other diseases of circulatory system (I71-I78)	6.0	6.4	5.6	6.5	6.9	6.1	5.2	5.6	4.9
Aortic aneurysm and dissection (I71)	3.1	3.7	2.6	3.4	4.0	2.8	2.4	2.8	1.9
Other diseases of arteries, arterioles and capillaries (I72-I78)	2.9	2.7	3.0	3.1	2.9	3.3	2.9	2.8	3.0
Other disorders of circulatory system (I80-I99)	1.4	1.4	1.4	1.4	1.4	1.4	2.0	2.1	1.9
Influenza and pneumonia (J09-J18)	18.0	17.2	18.8	19.7	18.5	20.8	12.7	12.9	12.6
Influenza (J09-J11)	1.2	1.1	1.2	1.3	1.2	1.4	0.6	0.6	0.7
Pneumonia (J12-J18)	16.9	16.1	17.6	18.3	17.3	19.3	12.1	12.3	11.9
Other acute lower respiratory infections (J20-J22, U04)	0.1	0.1	0.1	0.1	0.1	0.1	0.1	*	*
Acute bronchitis and bronchiolitis (J20-J21)	0.1	0.1	0.1	0.1	0.1	0.1	0.1	*	*
Other and unspecified acute lower respiratory infections(J22, U04)	0.0	0.0	0.0	0.0	*	0.0	*	*	*
Chronic lower respiratory diseases (J40-J47)	47.2	45.2	49.2	54.8	51.6	58.0	22.7	24.2	21.3
Bronchitis, chronic and unspecified (J40-J42)	0.2	0.2	0.2	0.2	0.2	0.3	0.2	0.1	0.2
Emphysema (J43)	2.6	2.8	2.5	3.0	3.2	2.9	1.2	1.5	1.0
Asthma (J45-J46)	1.1	0.9	1.4	1.0	0.7	1.3	2.3	2.2	2.4
Other chronic lower respiratory diseases (J44, J47)	43.2	41.3	45.1	50.6	47.6	53.5	19.0	20.3	17.8
Pneumoconioses and chemical effects (J60-J66, J68)	0.3	0.5	0.0	0.3	0.6	0.0	0.1	0.1	*
Pneumonitis due to solids and liquids (J69)	5.9	6.5	5.3	6.6	7.3	5.9	3.7	4.1	3.3
Other diseases of respiratory system (J00-J06, J30-J39, J67, J70-J98)	11.1	11.5	10.8	12.4	12.8	12.0	7.3	6.9	7.6
Peptic ulcer (K25-K28)	0.9	1.0	0.9	1.0	1.0	1.0	0.7	0.8	0.6
Diseases of appendix (K35-K38)	0.1	0.1	0.1	0.1	0.1	0.1	0.1	0.2	*
Hernia (K40-K46)	0.6	0.5	0.7	0.7	0.6	0.8	0.4	0.3	0.5
Chronic liver disease and cirrhosis (K70, K73-K74)	11.5	15.2	7.9	12.8	16.9	8.7	7.0	9.3	4.8
Alcoholic liver disease (K70)	5.7	8.3	3.2	6.4	9.3	3.5	3.1	4.4	1.9
Other chronic liver disease and cirrhosis (K73-K74)	5.8	6.9	4.7	6.4	7.6	5.3	3.8	4.9	2.9
Cholelithiasis and other disorders of gallbladder (K80-K82)	1.1	1.0	1.1	1.2	1.1	1.2	0.7	0.7	0.8
Nephritis, nephrotic syndrome and nephrosis(N00-N07, N17-N19, N25-N27)	14.9	15.1	14.7	14.9	15.2	14.7	19.2	19.0	19.4
Acute and rapidly progressive nephritic and nephrotic syndrome (N00-N01,N04)	0.1	0.1	0.1	0.1	0.1	0.1	0.1	0.2	0.1
Chronic glomerulonephritis, nephritis and nephropathy not specified as acute or chronic, and renal sclerosis unspecified (N02-N03, N05-N07, N26)	0.1	0.1	0.1	0.1	0.1	0.1	0.1	*	*
Renal failure (N17-N19)	14.7	14.9	14.5	14.7	15.0	14.5	19.0	18.8	19.2
Other disorders of kidney (N25, N27)	0.0	0.0	*	0.0	*	*	*	*	*
Infections of kidney (N10-N12,N13.6,N15.1)	0.2	0.1	0.3	0.2	0.1	0.3	0.2	0.1	0.2
Hyperplasia of prostate (N40)	0.2	0.4	X	0.2	0.4	X	0.1	0.2	X
Inflammatory diseases of female pelvic organs (N70-N76)	0.0	X	0.1	0.0	X	0.1	0.0	X	0.1
Pregnancy, childbirth and the puerperium (O00-O99)	0.4	X	0.7	0.3	X	0.6	0.8	X	1.6
Pregnancy with abortive outcome (O00-O07)	0.0	X	0.0	*	X	*	*	X	*
Other complications of pregnancy, childbirth and the puerperium (O10-O99)	0.4	X	0.7	0.3	X	0.6	0.8	X	1.6
Certain conditions originating in the perinatal period(P00-P96)	3.8	4.3	3.3	3.0	3.4	2.6	9.3	10.6	8.1
Congenital malformations, deformations and chromosomal abnormalities (Q00-Q99)	3.0	3.2	2.8	3.0	3.2	2.8	3.6	3.9	3.4
Symptoms, signs and abnormal clinical and laboratory findings, not elsewhere classified (R00-R99)	11.9	10.5	13.4	13.0	11.0	14.8	10.3	10.5	10.2
All other diseases (Residual)	101.2	83.2	118.8	111.8	90.7	132.6	76.4	66.7	85.3
Accidents (unintentional injuries) (V01-X59, Y85-Y86)	41.3	52.6	30.3	45.2	56.8	33.9	30.7	43.1	19.3
Transport accidents (V01-V99, Y85)	12.0	17.4	6.8	12.5	18.1	7.1	11.5	17.4	6.0
Motor vehicle accidents (V02-V04, V09.0, V09.2, V12-V14, V19.0-V19.2, V19.4-V19.6, V20-V79, V80.3-V80.5, V81.0-V81.1, V82.0-V82.1,V83-V86, V87.0-V87.8, V88.0-V88.8, V89.0, V89.2)	11.2	16.1	6.4	11.7	16.7	6.7	10.8	16.4	5.7
Other land transport accidents (V01,V05-V06, V09.1, V09.3-V09.9, V10-V11, V15-V18, V19.3, V19.8-V19.9, V80.0-V80.2, V80.6-V80.9, V81.2-V81.9, V82.2-V82.9, V87.9, V88.9, V89.1, V89.3, V89.9)	0.3	0.5	0.1	0.3	0.5	0.1	0.3	0.6	0.1
Water, air and space, and other and unspecified transport accidents and their sequelae (V90-V99, Y85)	0.5	0.8	0.2	0.5	0.9	0.2	0.3	0.5	0.2
Nontransport accidents (W00-X59, Y86)	29.3	35.2	23.6	32.7	38.6	26.8	19.2	25.7	13.3
Falls (W00-W19)	9.6	9.8	9.3	11.2	11.2	11.2	3.2	4.0	2.5
Accidental discharge of firearms (W32-W34)	0.2	0.3	0.0	0.2	0.3	0.0	0.2	0.4	*
Accidental drowning and submersion (W65-W74)	1.1	1.7	0.5	1.0	1.6	0.5	1.2	2.1	0.4
Accidental exposure to smoke, fire and flames(X00-X09)	0.9	1.1	0.7	0.9	1.0	0.7	1.3	1.5	1.0
Accidental poisoning and exposure to noxious substances (X40-X49)	12.3	16.1	8.6	13.6	17.7	9.7	8.7	12.2	5.6
Other and unspecified nontransport accidents and their sequelae (W20-W31, W35-W64, W75-W99, X10-X39, X50-X59, Y86)	5.3	6.3	4.4	5.8	6.8	4.8	4.6	5.5	3.7
Intentional self-harm (suicide) (*U03, X60-X84, Y87.0)	13.0	20.6	5.7	14.9	23.4	6.5	5.4	9.0	2.0
Intentional self-harm (suicide) by discharge of firearms (X72-X74)	6.7	11.7	1.8	7.9	13.6	2.2	2.5	4.7	0.5
Intentional self-harm (suicide) by other and unspecified means and their sequelae (*U03, X60-X71, X75-X84, Y87.0)	6.3	8.9	3.8	7.0	9.8	4.3	2.9	4.4	1.5
Assault (homicide) (*U01-*U02, X85-Y09, Y87.1)	5.1	8.2	2.1	3.0	4.4	1.7	18.4	33.1	4.9
Assault (homicide) by discharge of firearms (*U01.4, X93-X95)	3.5	6.1	1.1	1.8	2.8	0.8	14.7	27.7	2.8
Assault (homicide) by other and unspecified means and their sequelae (*U01.0-*U01.3, *U01.5-*U01.9, *U02, X85-X92, X96-Y09, Y87.1)	1.6	2.1	1.0	1.2	1.6	0.9	3.7	5.4	2.1
Legal intervention (Y35, Y89.0)	0.2	0.3	0.0	0.1	0.3	*	0.3	0.7	*
Events of undetermined intent (Y10-Y34, Y87.2,Y89.9)	1.5	1.7	1.2	1.5	1.8	1.3	1.3	1.9	0.8
Discharge of firearms, undetermined intent (Y22-Y24)	0.1	0.1	0.0	0.1	0.1	0.0	0.1	0.2	*
Other and unspecified events of undetermined intent and their sequelae (Y10-Y21, Y25-Y34, Y87.2, Y89.9)	1.4	1.6	1.1	1.5	1.7	1.3	1.2	1.7	0.8
Operations of war and their sequelae (Y36, Y89.1)	*	*	*	*	*	*	*	*	*
Complications of medical and surgical care (Y40-Y84, Y88)	0.9	0.9	0.9	0.9	0.9	0.9	0.9	0.9	0.9
Enterocolitis due to Clostridium difficile (A04.7)[4]	2.4	1.9	2.9	2.8	2.2	3.4	1.3	1.3	1.4
Drug-induced deaths[5,6]	14.7	18.2	11.3	16.5	20.2	12.8	10.0	13.5	6.8
Alcohol-induced deaths[5,7]	9.2	13.7	4.8	10.0	15.0	5.2	5.9	9.1	3.0
Injury by firearms[5,8]	10.6	18.5	3.0	10.0	17.1	3.1	17.8	33.5	3.4

Table 2-11B. Death Rates for Selected Causes, by Race and Sex, 2013

(Rates per 100,000 population in specified group.)

Cause of death (based on ICD-10, 2004)	American Indian or Alaska Native[1,2]			Asian or Pacific Islander[1,3]		
	Both sexes	Male	Female	Both sexes	Male	Female
All Causes	382.5	416.5	348.2	321.4	347.4	297.4
Salmonella infections (A01-A02)	*	*	*	*	*	*
Shigellosis and amebiasis (A03, A06)	*	*	*	*	*	*
Certain other intestinal infections (A04, A07-A09)	1.2	1.0	1.4	0.9	1.0	0.9
Tuberculosis (A16-A19)	*	*	*	0.6	0.8	0.3
Respiratory tuberculosis (A16)	*	*	*	0.5	0.7	0.3
Other tuberculosis (A17-A19)	*	*	*	*	*	*
Whooping cough (A37)	*	*	*	*	*	*
Scarlet fever and erysipelas (A38, A46)	*	*	*	*	*	*
Meningococcal infection (A39)	*	*	*	*	*	*
Septicemia (A40-A41)	6.5	6.2	6.7	3.9	4.2	3.7
Syphilis (A50-A53)	*	*	*	*	*	*
Acute poliomyelitis (A80)	*	*	*	*	*	*
Arthropod-borne viral encephalitis (A83-A84, A85.2)	*	*	*	*	*	*
Measles (B05)	*	*	*	*	*	*
Viral hepatitis (B15-B19)	3.0	3.6	2.4	1.7	1.9	1.5
Human immunodeficiency virus (HIV) disease (B20-B24)	1.2	1.8	*	0.4	0.7	*
Malaria (B50-B54)	*	*		*	*	
Other and unspecified infectious and parasitic diseases and their sequelae (A00, A05, A20-A36, A42-A44, A48-A49, A54-A79, A81-A82, A85.0-A85.1, A85.8, A86-B04, B06-B09, B25-B49, B55-B99)	1.2	1.3	1.1	0.8	0.8	0.8
Malignant neoplasms (C00-C97)	69.7	73.6	65.8	84.3	90.5	78.6
Malignant neoplasms of lip, oral cavity and pharynx (C00-C14)	0.7	1.0	*	1.7	2.3	1.1
Malignant neoplasm of esophagus (C15)	1.7	2.7	*	1.5	2.4	0.6
Malignant neoplasm of stomach (C16)	2.2	2.3	2.0	4.3	5.1	3.6
Malignant neoplasms of colon, rectum and anus (C18-C21)	8.0	8.4	7.5	8.4	9.2	7.6
Malignant neoplasms of liver and intrahepatic bile ducts (C22)	5.7	7.7	3.8	8.3	11.7	5.1
Malignant neoplasm of pancreas (C25)	4.2	4.2	4.2	6.0	6.1	5.9
Malignant neoplasm of larynx (C32)	*	*	*	0.3	0.5	*
Malignant neoplasms of trachea, bronchus and lung(C33-C34)	16.9	18.2	15.6	19.0	22.3	16.0
Malignant melanoma of skin (C43)	*	*	*	0.2	0.3	0.2
Malignant neoplasm of breast (C50)	3.7	*	7.5	5.7	*	10.8
Malignant neoplasm of cervix uteri (C53)	0.7	X	1.4	1.0	X	1.9
Malignant neoplasms of corpus uteri and uterus, part unspecified (C54-C55)	0.8	X	1.7	1.4	X	2.7
Malignant neoplasm of ovary (C56)	1.6	X	3.3	2.2	X	4.3
Malignant neoplasm of prostate (C61)	2.9	5.8	X	2.5	5.3	X
Malignant neoplasms of kidney and renal pelvis (C64-C65)	2.6	3.2	2.1	1.5	2.0	1.0
Malignant neoplasm of bladder (C67)	1.1	1.4	*	1.3	1.8	0.9
Malignant neoplasms of meninges, brain and other parts of central nervous system (C70-C72)	1.5	1.6	1.5	2.0	2.2	1.8
Malignant neoplasms of lymphoid, hematopoietic and related tissue (C81-C96)	5.8	6.4	5.2	7.6	9.0	6.3
Hodgkin's disease (C81)	*	*	*	0.1	*	*
Non-Hodgkin's lymphoma (C82-C85)	2.0	2.4	1.6	3.2	3.6	2.8
Leukemia (C91-C95)	2.3	2.5	2.2	3.1	3.7	2.5
Multiple myeloma and immunoproliferative neoplasms (C88, C90)	1.4	1.5	1.4	1.2	1.6	0.9
Other and unspecified malignant neoplasms of lymphoid, hematopoietic and related tissue (C96)	*	*	*	*	*	*
All other and unspecified malignant neoplasms (C17, C23-C24, C26-C31, C37-C41, C44-C49, C51-C52, C57-C60, C62-C63, C66, C68-C69, C73-C80, C97)	8.7	9.8	7.6	9.4	10.1	8.7
In situ neoplasms, benign neoplasms and neoplasms of uncertain or unknown behavior (D00-D48)	1.4	1.7	1.1	2.0	2.0	2.0
Anemias (D50-D64)	0.5	*	*	0.5	0.5	0.5
Diabetes mellitus (E10-E14)	21.5	21.9	21.2	12.4	13.8	11.1
Nutritional deficiencies (E40-E64)	0.7	*	*	0.4	0.3	0.4
Malnutrition (E40-E46)	0.6	*	*	0.4	0.3	0.4
Other nutritional deficiencies (E50-E64)	*	*	*	*	*	*
Meningitis (G00,G03)	*	*	*	0.1	*	*
Parkinson's disease (G20-G21)	1.6	1.7	1.4	2.8	3.4	2.4
Alzheimer's disease (G30)	5.3	3.4	7.3	7.7	5.0	10.1
Major cardiovascular diseases (I00-I78)	90.7	100.3	81.0	102.4	111.5	94.1
Diseases of heart (I00-I09, I11, I13, I20-I51)	70.4	82.3	58.4	71.4	81.9	61.8
Acute rheumatic fever and chronic rheumatic heart diseases (I00-I09)	0.5	*	*	0.7	0.5	0.8
Hypertensive heart disease (I11)	5.3	6.3	4.2	4.2	4.1	4.2
Hypertensive heart and renal disease (I13)	*	*	*	0.8	0.6	0.9
Ischemic heart diseases (I20-I25)	45.7	56.0	35.2	46.2	56.5	36.7
Acute myocardial infarction (I21-I22)	13.9	16.8	10.9	14.3	17.4	11.3
Other acute ischemic heart diseases (I24)	0.5	*	*	0.4	0.3	0.4
Other forms of chronic ischemic heart disease (I20, I25)	31.3	38.6	24.0	31.6	38.8	25.0
Atherosclerotic cardiovascular disease, so described (I25.0)	11.3	14.1	8.3	7.5	9.6	5.5
All other forms of chronic ischemic heart disease (I20,I25.1-I25.9)	20.1	24.4	15.7	24.2	29.2	19.5
Other heart diseases (I26-I51)	18.6	19.2	17.9	19.6	20.1	19.2
Acute and subacute endocarditis (I33)	*	*	*	0.1	*	*
Diseases of pericardium and acute myocarditis (I30-I31, I40)	*	*	*	0.1	*	*

Table 2-11B. Death Rates for Selected Causes, by Race and Sex, 2013— continued

(Rates per 100,000 population in specified group.)

Cause of death (based on ICD-10, 2004)	American Indian or Alaska Native[1,2]			Asian or Pacific Islander[1,3]		
	Both sexes	Male	Female	Both sexes	Male	Female
Heart failure (I50)	5.4	4.7	6.1	5.2	5.1	5.4
All other forms of heart disease (I26-I28, I34-I38, I42-I49, I51)	12.5	13.7	11.3	14.1	14.7	13.6
Essential hypertension and hypertensive renal disease (I10, I12, I15)	4.1	4.2	4.0	5.3	4.9	5.7
Cerebrovascular diseases (I60-I69)	13.3	11.3	15.4	22.6	21.3	23.8
Atherosclerosis (I70)	0.8	*	*	0.7	0.6	0.7
Other diseases of circulatory system (I71-I78)	2.0	1.8	2.3	2.5	2.8	2.1
Aortic aneurysm and dissection (I71)	0.9	*	0.9	1.6	1.9	1.3
Other diseases of arteries, arterioles and capillaries (I72-I78)	1.2	1.0	1.3	0.9	1.0	0.8
Other disorders of circulatory system (I80-I99)	0.6	*	*	0.4	0.3	0.4
Influenza and pneumonia (J09-J18)	8.4	8.5	8.3	10.9	11.3	10.4
Influenza (J09-J11)	0.7	*	0.9	0.5	0.6	0.5
Pneumonia (J12-J18)	7.7	8.1	7.4	10.3	10.7	10.0
Other acute lower respiratory infections (J20-J22, U04)	*	*	*	*	*	*
Acute bronchitis and bronchiolitis (J20-J21)	*	*	*	*	*	*
Other and unspecified acute lower respiratory infections(J22, U04)	*	*	*	*	*	*
Chronic lower respiratory diseases (J40-J47)	17.0	16.5	17.5	9.9	12.5	7.5
Bronchitis, chronic and unspecified (J40-J42)	*	*	*	*	*	*
Emphysema (J43)	0.9	0.9	0.9	0.6	0.9	0.3
Asthma (J45-J46)	0.8	*	*	0.9	0.9	1.0
Other chronic lower respiratory diseases (J44, J47)	15.3	14.8	15.7	8.3	10.7	6.1
Pneumoconioses and chemical effects (J60-J66, J68)	*	*	*	*	*	*
Pneumonitis due to solids and liquids (J69)	1.7	2.0	1.4	2.3	2.8	1.9
Other diseases of respiratory system (J00-J06, J30-J39, J67, J70-J98)	5.6	5.5	5.6	4.4	4.8	4.1
Peptic ulcer (K25-K28)	*	*	*	0.7	0.8	0.5
Diseases of appendix (K35-K38)	*	*	*	*	*	*
Hernia (K40-K46)	*	*	*	0.2	*	*
Chronic liver disease and cirrhosis (K70, K73-K74)	21.2	22.8	19.5	3.0	4.0	2.1
Alcoholic liver disease (K70)	15.8	18.7	12.8	1.1	1.8	0.5
Other chronic liver disease and cirrhosis (K73-K74)	5.4	4.1	6.7	1.9	2.2	1.6
Cholelithiasis and other disorders of gallbladder (K80-K82)	0.9	*	0.9	0.6	0.7	0.6
Nephritis, nephrotic syndrome and nephrosis(N00-N07, N17-N19, N25-N27)	6.8	6.4	7.2	6.2	6.4	5.9
Acute and rapidly progressive nephritic and nephrotic syndrome (N00-N01,N04)	*	*	*	*	*	*
Chronic glomerulonephritis, nephritis and nephropathy not specified as acute or chronic, and renal sclerosis unspecified (N02-N03, N05-N07, N26)	*	*	*	*	*	*
Renal failure (N17-N19)	6.7	6.3	7.0	6.0	6.3	5.8
Other disorders of kidney (N25, N27)	*	*	*	*	*	*
Infections of kidney (N10-N12,N13.6,N15.1)	*	*	*	0.1	*	*
Hyperplasia of prostate (N40)	*	*	X	*	*	X
Inflammatory diseases of female pelvic organs (N70-N76)	*	X	*	*	X	*
Pregnancy, childbirth and the puerperium (O00-O99)	*	X	*	0.2	X	0.5
Pregnancy with abortive outcome (O00-O07)	*	X	*	*	X	*
Other complications of pregnancy, childbirth and the puerperium (O10-O99)	*	X	*	0.2	X	0.5
Certain conditions originating in the perinatal period(P00-P96)	2.4	3.1	1.6	2.6	3.1	2.2
Congenital malformations, deformations and chromosomal abnormalities (Q00-Q99)	2.7	3.4	1.9	1.7	1.9	1.5
Symptoms, signs and abnormal clinical and laboratory findings, not elsewhere classified (R00-R99)	5.7	5.6	5.7	3.6	3.5	3.6
All other diseases (Residual)	43.0	40.3	45.6	31.6	28.1	34.8
Accidents (unintentional injuries) (V01-X59, Y85-Y86)	41.1	52.5	29.6	13.5	17.5	9.7
Transport accidents (V01-V99, Y85)	16.0	20.8	11.2	5.0	6.5	3.6
Motor vehicle accidents (V02-V04, V09.0, V09.2, V12-V14, V19.0-V19.2, V19.4-V19.6, V20-V79, V80.3-V80.5, V81.0-V81.1, V82.0-V82.1,V83-V86, V87.0-V87.8, V88.0-V88.8, V89.0, V89.2)	14.9	19.0	10.7	4.6	5.9	3.4
Other land transport accidents (V01,V05-V06, V09.1, V09.3-V09.9, V10-V11, V15-V18, V19.3, V19.8-V19.9, V80.0-V80.2, V80.6-V80.9, V81.2-V82.9, V87.9, V88.9, V89.1, V89.3, V89.9)	0.4	*	*	0.2	0.2	*
Water, air and space, and other and unspecified transport accidents and their sequelae (V90-V99, Y85)	0.7	1.2	*	0.2	0.3	*
Nontransport accidents (W00-X59, Y86)	25.1	31.7	18.4	8.5	11.0	6.2
Falls (W00-W19)	4.2	4.8	3.7	3.7	4.3	3.2
Accidental discharge of firearms (W32-W34)	*	*	*	*	*	*
Accidental drowning and submersion (W65-W74)	1.6	2.5	*	1.0	1.6	0.4
Accidental exposure to smoke, fire and flames(X00-X09)	0.9	1.1	*	0.2	0.2	*
Accidental poisoning and exposure to noxious substances (X40-X49)	13.5	16.6	10.4	2.1	3.1	1.2
Other and unspecified nontransport accidents and their sequelae (W20-W31, W35-W64, W75-W99, X10-X39, X50-X59, Y86)	4.6	6.3	2.8	1.5	1.8	1.2
Intentional self-harm (suicide) (*U03, X60-X84, Y87.0)	11.7	17.9	5.4	6.0	9.2	3.1
Intentional self-harm (suicide) by discharge of firearms (X72-X74)	4.5	7.9	1.1	1.5	2.6	0.4
Intentional self-harm (suicide) by other and unspecified means and their sequelae (*U03, X60-X71, X75-X84, Y87.0)	7.2	10.0	4.3	4.6	6.6	2.7
Assault (homicide) (*U01-*U02, X85-Y09, Y87.1)	5.4	8.3	2.4	1.6	2.3	0.9
Assault (homicide) by discharge of firearms (*U01.4, X93-X95)	2.4	3.9	*	0.9	1.4	0.5

Table 2-11B. Death Rates for Selected Causes, by Race and Sex, 2013— continued

(Rates per 100,000 population in specified group.)

Cause of death (based on ICD-10, 2004)	American Indian or Alaska Native[1,2]			Asian or Pacific Islander[1,3]		
	Both sexes	Male	Female	Both sexes	Male	Female
Assault (homicide) by other and unspecified means and their sequelae (*U01.0-*U01.3, *U01.5-*U01.9, *U02, X85-X92, X96-Y09, Y87.1)	3.0	4.4	1.6	0.7	0.9	0.4
Legal intervention (Y35, Y89.0)	*	*	*	*	*	*
Events of undetermined intent (Y10-Y34, Y87.2,Y89.9)	1.5	1.8	1.3	0.4	0.5	0.3
Discharge of firearms, undetermined intent (Y22-Y24)	*	*	*	*	*	*
Other and unspecified events of undetermined intent and their sequelae (Y10-Y21, Y25-Y34, Y87.2, Y89.9)	1.5	1.7	1.2	0.4	0.5	0.3
Operations of war and their sequelae (Y36, Y89.1)	*	*	*	*	*	*
Complications of medical and surgical care (Y40-Y84, Y88)	*	*	*	0.3	0.3	0.2
Enterocolitis due to Clostridium difficile (A04.7)[4]	0.8	*	*	0.6	0.6	0.6
Drug-induced deaths[5,6]	12.5	13.4	11.6	2.6	3.6	1.7
Alcohol-induced deaths[5,7]	23.8	31.0	16.6	1.8	2.9	0.7
Injury by firearms[5,8]	7.3	12.5	2.0	2.5	4.3	0.9

X = Not applicable.   0.0 = Quantity more than zero but less than 0.05.   * = Figure does not meet standards of reliability or precision.   1Race categories are consistent with the 1977 Office of Management and Budget (OMB) standards. Multiple-race data were reported by 42 states and the District of Columbia in 2013. The multiple-race data for these reporting areas were bridged to the single-race categories of the 1977 OMB standards for comparability with other reporting areas.   2Includes Aleuts and Eskimos.   3Includes Chinese, Filipino, Hawaiian, Japanese, and Other Asian and Pacific Islander.   4Included in certain other intestinal infections (A04, A07–A09). Beginning with data year 2006, Enterocolitis due to Clostridium difficile (A04.7) is shown separately at the bottom of the table and is included in the list of rankable causes.   5Included in selected categories above.   6Includes ICD–10 codes D52.1, D59.0, D59.2, D61.1, D64.2, E06.4, E16.0, E23.1, E24.2, E27.3, E66.1, F11.1-F11.5, F11.7-F11.9, F12.1-F12.5, F12.7-F12.9, F13.1-F13.5, F13.7-F13.9, F14.1-F14.5, F14.7-F14.9, F15.1-F15.5, F15.7-F15.9, F16.1-F16.5, F16.7-F16.9, F17.3-F17.5, F17.7-17.9, F18.1-F18.5, F18.7-F18.9, F19.1-F19.5, F19.7-F19.9, G21.1, G24.0, G25.1, G25.4, G25.6, G44.4, G62.0, G72.0, I95.2, J70.2-J70.4, K85.3, L10.5, L27.0-L27.1, M10.2, M32.0, M80.4, M81.4, M83.5, M87.1, R50.2, R78.1-R78.5, X40-X44, X60-X64, X85, and Y10-Y14. Trend data for Drug-induced deaths, previously shown in this report, can be found through a link from the online version of this report, available from http://www.cdc.gov/nchs/deaths.htm.   7Includes ICD–10 codes E24.4, F10, G31.2, G62.1, G72.1, I42.6, K29.2, K70, K85.2, K86.0, R78.0, X45, X65, and Y15. Trend data for Alcohol-induced deaths, previously shown in this report, can be found through a link from the online version of this report, available from http://www.cdc.gov/nchs/deaths.htm.   8Includes ICD–10 codes *U01.4, W32-W34, X72-X74, X93-X95, Y22-Y24, and Y35.0. Trend data for Injury by firearms, previously shown in this report, can be found through a link from the online version of this report, available from http://www.cdc.gov/nchs/deaths.htm.

Table 2-12A. Number of Deaths from Selected Causes, by Hispanic Origin and, Race for Non-Hispanic Population, and Sex, 2013

(Number.)

Cause of death (based on ICD–10, 2004)	All origins			Hispanic			Non–Hispanic[1]		
	Both sexes	Male	Female	Both sexes	Male	Female	Both sexes	Male	Female
All causes	2,596,993	1,306,034	1,290,959	163,241	88,880	74,361	2,426,808	1,212,979	1,213,829
Salmonella infections (A01-A02)	40	28	12	6	5	1	34	23	11
Shigellosis and amebiasis (A03, A06)	6	3	3	2	1	1	4	2	2
Certain other intestinal infections (A04, A07-A09)	10,590	4,148	6,442	642	270	372	9,912	3,864	6,048
Tuberculosis (A16-A19)	555	357	198	97	61	36	454	294	160
Respiratory tuberculosis (A16)	408	267	141	77	47	30	328	218	110
Other tuberculosis (A17-A19)	147	90	57	20	14	6	126	76	50
Whooping cough (A37)	12	5	7	3	2	1	9	3	6
Scarlet fever and erysipelas (A38, A46)	1	1	-	-	-	-	1	1	-
Meningococcal infection (A39)	59	34	25	9	8	1	50	26	24
Septicemia (A40-A41)	38,156	17,994	20,162	2,435	1,226	1,209	35,618	16,715	18,903
Syphilis (A50-A53)	49	28	21	6	2	4	43	26	17
Acute poliomyelitis (A80)	-	-	-	-	-	-	-	-	-
Arthropod-borne viral encephalitis (A83-A84, A85.2)	4	2	2	-	-	-	4	2	2
Measles (B05)	-	-	-	-	-	-	-	-	-
Viral hepatitis (B15-B19)	8,157	5,425	2,732	1,237	839	398	6,875	4,557	2,318
Human immunodeficiency virus (HIV) disease (B20-B24)	6,955	5,096	1,859	927	742	185	5,949	4,293	1,656
Malaria (B50-B54)	10	9	1	-	-	-	10	9	1
Other and unspecified infectious and parasitic diseases and their sequelae (A00, A05, A20-A36, A42-A44, A48- A49, A54-A79, A81-A82, A85.0-A85.1, A85.8, A86-B04, B06-B09, B25-B49, B55-B99)	6,007	3,105	2,902	518	276	242	5,471	2,821	2,650
Malignant neoplasms (C00-C97)	584,881	307,559	277,322	35,147	18,371	16,776	548,524	288,471	260,053
Malignant neoplasms of lip, oral cavity and pharynx (C00-C14)	8,850	6,227	2,623	455	332	123	8,364	5,869	2,495
Malignant neoplasm of esophagus (C15)	14,690	11,732	2,958	593	475	118	14,061	11,227	2,834
Malignant neoplasm of stomach (C16)	11,261	6,793	4,468	1,633	941	692	9,605	5,835	3,770
Malignant neoplasms of colon, rectum and anus (C18-C21)	52,252	27,354	24,898	3,577	2,032	1,545	48,559	25,256	23,303
Malignant neoplasms of liver and intrahepatic bile ducts (C22)	24,032	16,300	7,732	2,994	1,996	998	20,974	14,253	6,721
Malignant neoplasm of pancreas (C25)	38,996	19,854	19,142	2,473	1,207	1,266	36,458	18,608	17,850
Malignant neoplasm of larynx (C32)	3,729	2,994	735	219	196	23	3,498	2,787	711
Malignant neoplasm of trachea, bronchus and lung(C33-C34)	156,252	85,710	70,542	5,359	3,229	2,130	150,572	82,284	68,288
Malignant melanoma of skin (C43)	9,394	6,239	3,155	236	135	101	9,151	6,099	3,052
Malignant neoplasm of breast (C50)	41,325	464	40,861	2,695	24	2,671	38,541	436	38,105
Malignant neoplasm of cervix uteri (C53)	4,217	X	4,217	521	X	521	3,682	X	3,682
Malignant neoplasms of corpus uteri and uterus, part unspecified (C54-C55)	9,325	X	9,325	679	X	679	8,629	X	8,629
Malignant neoplasm of ovary (C56)	14,276	X	14,276	942	X	942	13,312	X	13,312
Malignant neoplasm of prostate (C61)	27,682	27,682	X	1,634	1,634	X	25,983	25,983	X
Malignant neoplasms of kidney and renal pelvis (C64-C65)	13,906	8,967	4,939	1,053	665	388	12,820	8,276	4,544
Malignant neoplasm of bladder (C67)	15,757	11,294	4,463	630	451	179	15,098	10,821	4,277
Malignant neoplasms of meninges, brain and other parts of central nervous system (C70-C72)	15,345	8,493	6,852	1,046	548	498	14,281	7,935	6,346
Malignant neoplasms of lymphoid, hematopoietic and related tissue (C81-C96)	56,936	32,057	24,879	4,054	2,251	1,803	52,780	29,754	23,026
Hodgkin's disease (C81)	1,090	633	457	134	80	54	954	551	403
Non-Hodgkin's lymphoma (C82-C85)	20,114	11,168	8,946	1,459	817	642	18,618	10,331	8,287
Leukemia (C91-C95)	23,428	13,569	9,859	1,667	923	744	21,722	12,627	9,095
Multiple myeloma and immunoproliferative neoplasms (C88, C90)	12,225	6,640	5,585	787	428	359	11,414	6,201	5,213
Other and unspecified malignant neoplasms of lymphoid, hemato-poietic and related tissue (C96)	79	47	32	7	3	4	72	44	28
All other and unspecified malignant neoplasms (C17, C23-C24, C26-C31, C37-C41, C44-C49, C51- C52, C57-C60, C62-C63, C66, C68-C69, C73-C80, C97)	66,656	35,399	31,257	4,354	2,255	2,099	62,156	33,048	29,108
In situ neoplasms, benign neoplasms and neoplasms of uncertain or unknown behavior (D00-D48)	15,232	8,081	7,151	831	435	396	14,379	7,630	6,749
Anemias (D50-D64)	4,894	2,077	2,817	269	122	147	4,615	1,952	2,663
Diabetes mellitus (E10-E14)	75,578	39,841	35,737	7,632	3,934	3,698	67,729	35,779	31,950
Nutritional deficiencies (E40-E64)	3,382	1,350	2,032	173	75	98	3,199	1,268	1,931
Malnutrition (E40-E46)	3,224	1,284	1,940	169	73	96	3,045	1,204	1,841
Other nutritional deficiencies (E50-E64)	158	66	92	4	2	2	154	64	90
Meningitis (G00,G03)	584	326	258	70	45	25	512	279	233
Parkinson's disease (G20-G21)	25,196	15,088	10,108	1,302	752	550	23,856	14,314	9,542
Alzheimer's disease (G30)	84,767	25,836	58,931	4,127	1,298	2,829	80,528	24,502	56,026
Major cardiovascular diseases (I00-I78)	796,494	400,686	395,808	44,599	23,774	20,825	749,619	375,522	374,097
Diseases of heart (I00-I09, I11, I13, I20-I51)	611,105	321,347	289,758	33,243	18,377	14,866	575,985	301,784	274,201
Acute rheumatic fever and chronic rheumatic heart diseases (I00-I09)	3,260	1,141	2,119	162	52	110	3,091	1,086	2,005
Hypertensive heart disease (I11)	37,144	18,717	18,427	2,512	1,410	1,102	34,400	17,160	17,240
Hypertensive heart and renal disease (I13)	4,028	1,883	2,145	304	164	140	3,709	1,709	2,000
Ischemic heart diseases (I20-I25)	370,213	208,515	161,698	21,788	12,518	9,270	347,126	195,143	151,983
Acute myocardial infarction (I21-I22)	116,793	66,051	50,742	6,957	4,099	2,858	109,560	61,776	47,784
Other acute ischemic heart diseases (I24)	3,936	2,064	1,872	137	67	70	3,789	1,991	1,798
Other forms of chronic ischemic heart disease (I20, I25)	249,484	140,400	109,084	14,694	8,352	6,342	233,777	131,376	102,401
Atherosclerotic cardiovascular disease, so described (I25.0)	59,475	35,906	23,569	3,812	2,517	1,295	55,192	33,042	22,150
All other forms of chronic ischemic heart disease (I20,I25.1-I25.9)	190,009	104,494	85,515	10,882	5,835	5,047	178,585	98,334	80,251
Other heart diseases (I26-I51)	196,460	91,091	105,369	8,477	4,233	4,244	187,659	86,686	100,973
Acute and subacute endocarditis (I33)	1,255	766	489	94	60	34	1,155	702	453
Diseases of pericardium and acute myocarditis (I30-I31, I40)	872	453	419	81	44	37	785	406	379
Heart failure (I50)	65,120	28,513	36,607	2,544	1,144	1,400	62,489	27,328	35,161
All other forms of heart disease (I26-I28, I34-I38, I42-I49, I51)	129,213	61,359	67,854	5,758	2,985	2,773	123,230	58,250	64,980
Essential hypertension and hypertensive renal disease (I10, I12, I15)	30,770	12,963	17,807	2,092	972	1,120	28,598	11,944	16,654
Cerebrovascular diseases (I60-I69)	128,978	53,691	75,287	8,127	3,841	4,286	120,586	49,723	70,863
Atherosclerosis (I70)	6,685	2,714	3,971	265	107	158	6,407	2,601	3,806

Table 2-12A. Number of Deaths from Selected Causes, by Hispanic Origin and, Race for Non-Hispanic Population, and Sex, 2013—continued

(Number.)

Cause of death (based on ICD-10, 2004)	All origins			Hispanic			Non-Hispanic[1]		
	Both sexes	Male	Female	Both sexes	Male	Female	Both sexes	Male	Female
Other diseases of circulatory system (I71-I78)	18,956	9,971	8,985	872	477	395	18,043	9,470	8,573
Aortic aneurysm and dissection (I71)	9,846	5,753	4,093	407	260	147	9,419	5,480	3,939
Other diseases of arteries, arterioles and capillaries (I72-I78)	9,110	4,218	4,892	465	217	248	8,624	3,990	4,634
Other disorders of circulatory system (I80-I99)	4,443	2,165	2,278	269	118	151	4,151	2,032	2,119
Influenza and pneumonia (J09-J18)	56,979	26,804	30,175	3,592	1,816	1,776	53,188	24,885	28,303
Influenza (J09-J11)	3,697	1,697	2,000	247	129	118	3,444	1,564	1,880
Pneumonia (J12-J18)	53,282	25,107	28,175	3,345	1,687	1,658	49,744	23,321	26,423
Other acute lower respiratory infections (J20-J22, U04)	285	110	175	27	12	15	258	98	160
Acute bronchitis and bronchiolitis (J20-J21)	226	90	136	24	12	12	202	78	124
Other and unspecified acute lower respiratory infections(J22, U04)	59	20	39	3	-	3	56	20	36
Chronic lower respiratory diseases (J40-J47)	149,205	70,317	78,888	4,827	2,536	2,291	144,041	67,590	76,451
Bronchitis, chronic and unspecified (J40-J42)	664	272	392	39	20	19	623	252	371
Emphysema (J43)	8,284	4,321	3,963	261	160	101	8,000	4,149	3,851
Asthma (J45-J46)	3,630	1,410	2,220	327	144	183	3,295	1,263	2,032
Other chronic lower respiratory diseases (J44, J47)	136,627	64,314	72,313	4,200	2,212	1,988	132,123	61,926	70,197
Pneumoconioses and chemical effects (J60-J66, J68)	806	767	39	22	21	1	782	744	38
Pneumonitis due to solids and liquids (J69)	18,579	10,140	8,439	824	454	370	17,726	9,670	8,056
Other diseases of respiratory system (J00-J06, J30-J39, J67, J70-J98)	35,217	17,825	17,392	2,417	1,197	1,220	32,732	16,593	16,139
Peptic ulcer (K25-K28)	2,988	1,535	1,453	174	100	74	2,802	1,427	1,375
Diseases of appendix (K35-K38)	371	216	155	30	18	12	341	198	143
Hernia (K40-K46)	1,932	772	1,160	142	53	89	1,781	714	1,067
Chronic liver disease and cirrhosis (K70, K73-K74)	36,427	23,709	12,718	5,141	3,552	1,589	31,132	20,035	11,097
Alcoholic liver disease (K70)	18,146	12,991	5,155	2,712	2,191	521	15,332	10,717	4,615
Other chronic liver disease and cirrhosis (K73-K74)	18,281	10,718	7,563	2,429	1,361	1,068	15,800	9,318	6,482
Cholelithiasis and other disorders of gallbladder (K80-K82)	3,377	1,605	1,772	267	135	132	3,099	1,467	1,632
Nephritis, nephrotic syndrome and nephrosis(N00-N07, N17-N19, N25-N27)	47,112	23,493	23,619	3,083	1,583	1,500	43,925	21,855	22,070
Acute and rapidly progressive nephritic and nephrotic syndrome (N00-N01,N04)	399	205	194	17	6	11	381	198	183
Chronic glomerulonephritis, nephritis and nephropathy not specified as acute or chronic, and renal sclerosis unspecified (N02-N03, N05-N07, N26)	254	132	122	32	12	20	221	119	102
Renal failure (N17-N19)	46,425	23,136	23,289	3,032	1,563	1,469	43,291	21,520	21,771
Other disorders of kidney (N25, N27)	34	20	14	2	2	-	32	18	14
Infections of kidney (N10-N12,N13.6,N15.1)	641	191	450	50	13	37	591	178	413
Hyperplasia of prostate (N40)	558	558	X	36	36	X	521	521	X
Inflammatory diseases of female pelvic organs (N70-N76)	129	X	129	6	X	6	123	X	123
Pregnancy, childbirth and the puerperium (O00-O99)	1,138	X	1,138	165	X	165	971	X	971
Pregnancy with abortive outcome (O00-O07)	27	X	27	6	X	6	20	X	20
Other complications of pregnancy, childbirth and the puerperium (O10-O99)	1,111	X	1,111	159	X	159	951	X	951
Certain conditions originating in the perinatal period(P00-P96)	12,084	6,723	5,361	2,428	1,320	1,108	9,471	5,294	4,177
Congenital malformations, deformations and chromosomal abnormalities (Q00-Q99)	9,583	5,052	4,531	1,726	913	813	7,822	4,122	3,700
Symptoms, signs and abnormal clinical and laboratory findings, not elsewhere classified (R00-R99)	37,752	16,275	21,477	2,197	1,195	1,002	35,379	14,980	20,399
All other diseases (Residual)	320,065	129,448	190,617	17,702	7,977	9,725	301,669	121,090	180,579
Accidents (unintentional injuries) (V01-X59, Y85-Y86)	130,557	81,916	48,641	12,015	8,760	3,255	118,080	72,836	45,244
Transport accidents (V01-V99, Y85)	37,938	27,102	10,836	5,191	3,872	1,319	32,646	23,151	9,495
Motor vehicle accidents (V02-V04, V09.0, V09.2, V12-V14, V19.0-V19.2, V19.4-V19.8, V20-V79, V80.3-V80.5, V81.0-V81.1, V82.0-V82.1,V83- V86, V87.0-V87.8, V88.0-V88.8, V89.0, V89.2)	35,369	25,048	10,321	4,931	3,653	1,278	30,352	21,329	9,023
Other land transport accidents (V01,V05-V06, V09.1, V09.3-V09.9, V10-V11, V15-V18, V19.3, V19.8-V19.9, V80.0-V80.2, V80.6-V80.9, V81.2- V81.9, V82.2-V82.9, V87.9, V88.9, V89.1, V89.3, V89.9)	1,000	804	196	139	123	16	849	671	178
Water, air and space, and other and unspecified transport accidents and their sequelae (V90-V99, Y85)	1,569	1,250	319	121	96	25	1,445	1,151	294
Nontransport accidents (W00-X59, Y86)	92,619	54,814	37,805	6,824	4,888	1,936	85,434	49,685	35,749
Falls (W00-W19)	30,208	15,205	15,003	1,584	991	593	28,543	14,172	14,371
Accidental discharge of firearms (W32-W34)	505	441	64	49	46	3	456	395	61
Accidental drowning and submersion (W65-W74)	3,391	2,613	778	436	365	71	2,941	2,239	702
Accidental exposure to smoke, fire and flames(X00-X09)	2,760	1,653	1,107	181	105	76	2,570	1,541	1,029
Accidental poisoning and exposure to noxious substances (X40-X49)	38,851	25,080	13,771	3,337	2,498	839	35,310	22,433	12,877
Other and unspecified nontransport accidents and their sequelae (W20-W31, W35-W64, W75-W99, X10-X39, X50-X59, Y86)	16,904	9,822	7,082	1,237	883	354	15,614	8,905	6,709
Intentional self-harm (suicide) (*U03, X60-X84, Y87.0)	41,149	32,055	9,094	2,865	2,279	586	38,117	29,640	8,477
Intentional self-harm (suicide) by discharge of firearms (X72-X74)	21,175	18,241	2,934	1,034	910	124	20,087	17,282	2,805
Intentional self-harm (suicide) by other and unspecified means and their sequelae (*U03, X60-X71, X75-X84, Y87.0)	19,974	13,814	6,160	1,831	1,369	462	18,030	12,358	5,672
Assault (homicide) (*U01-*U02, X85-Y09, Y87.1)	16,121	12,726	3,395	2,571	2,132	439	13,484	10,539	2,945
Assault (homicide) by discharge of firearms (*U01.4, X93-X95)	11,208	9,445	1,763	1,750	1,530	220	9,426	7,885	1,541
Assault (homicide) by other and unspecified means and their sequelae (*U01.0-*U01.3, *U01.5-*U01.9, *U02, X85-X92, X96-Y09, Y87.1)	4,913	3,281	1,632	821	602	219	4,058	2,654	1,404
Legal intervention (Y35, Y89.0)	516	492	24	90	86	4	425	405	20
Events of undetermined intent (Y10-Y34, Y87.2,Y89.9)	4,587	2,708	1,879	347	247	100	4,217	2,450	1,767
Discharge of firearms, undetermined intent (Y22-Y24)	281	221	60	32	27	5	246	192	54
Other and unspecified events of undetermined intent and their sequelae (Y10-Y21, Y25-Y34, Y87.2, Y89.9)	4,306	2,487	1,819	315	220	95	3,971	2,258	1,713
Operations of war and their sequelae (Y36, Y89.1)	15	15	-	1	1	-	14	14	-
Complications of medical and surgical care (Y40-Y84, Y88)	2,768	1,338	1,430	195	88	107	2,571	1,249	1,322
Enterocolitis due to Clostridium difficile (A04.7)[4]	7,665	3,035	4,630	431	181	250	7,210	2,847	4,363
Drug-induced deaths[5,6]	46,471	28,381	18,090	3,616	2,546	1,070	42,606	25,665	16,941

Table 2-12A. Number of Deaths from Selected Causes, by Hispanic Origin and, Race for Non-Hispanic Population, and Sex, 2013— continued

(Number.)

Cause of death (based on ICD–10, 2004)	All origins			Hispanic			Non–Hispanic[1]		
	Both sexes	Male	Female	Both sexes	Male	Female	Both sexes	Male	Female
Alcohol-induced deaths[5,7]	29,001	21,361	7,640	3,698	3,034	664	25,113	18,173	6,940
Injury by firearms[5,8]	33,636	28,794	4,842	2,951	2,595	356	30,595	26,117	4,478

Table 2-12B. Number of Deaths from Selected Causes, by Hispanic Origin and, Race for Non-Hispanic Population, and Sex, 2013

(Number.)

Cause of death (based on ICD–10, 2004)	Non–Hispanic White[2]			Non–Hispanic Black[2]			Origin not stated[3]		
	Both sexes	Male	Female	Both sexes	Male	Female	Both sexes	Male	Female
All causes	2,052,660	1,021,135	1,031,525	299,227	152,661	146,566	6,944	4,175	2,769
Salmonella infections (A01-A02)	26	15	11	6	6	-	-	-	-
Shigellosis and amebiasis (A03, A06)	1	1	-	2	1	1	-	-	-
Certain other intestinal infections (A04, A07-A09)	8,826	3,365	5,461	866	394	472	36	14	22
Tuberculosis (A16-A19)	249	160	89	87	54	33	4	2	2
Respiratory tuberculosis (A16)	169	112	57	63	41	22	3	2	1
Other tuberculosis (A17-A19)	80	48	32	24	13	11	1	-	1
Whooping cough (A37)	7	2	5	1	-	1	-	-	-
Scarlet fever and erysipelas (A38, A46)	1	1	-	-	-	-	-	-	-
Meningococcal infection (A39)	42	23	19	6	3	3	-	-	-
Septicemia (A40-A41)	28,431	13,364	15,067	6,193	2,854	3,339	103	53	50
Syphilis (A50-A53)	18	11	7	24	14	10	-	-	-
Acute poliomyelitis (A80)	-	-	-	-	-	-	-	-	-
Arthropod-borne viral encephalitis (A83-A84, A85.2)	4	2	2	-	-	-	-	-	-
Measles (B05)	-	-	-	-	-	-	-	-	-
Viral hepatitis (B15-B19)	5,250	3,543	1,707	1,212	785	427	45	29	16
Human immunodeficiency virus (HIV) disease (B20-B24)	2,161	1,774	387	3,673	2,429	1,244	79	61	18
Malaria (B50-B54)	1	1	-	7	6	1	-	-	-
Other and unspecified infectious and parasitic diseases and their sequelae (A00, A05, A20-A36, A42-A44, A48- A49, A54-A79, A81-A82, A85.0-A85.1, A85.8, A86-B04, B06-B09, B25-B49, B55-B99)	4,452	2,298	2,154	824	423	401	18	8	10
Malignant neoplasms (C00-C97)	462,850	244,646	218,204	67,272	34,319	32,953	1,210	717	493
Malignant neoplasms of lip, oral cavity and pharynx (C00-C14)	6,960	4,872	2,088	1,061	769	292	31	26	5
Malignant neoplasm of esophagus (C15)	12,429	10,040	2,389	1,298	928	370	36	30	6
Malignant neoplasm of stomach (C16)	6,770	4,163	2,607	1,943	1,172	771	23	17	6
Malignant neoplasms of colon, rectum and anus (C18-C21)	39,851	20,682	19,169	6,832	3,582	3,250	116	66	50
Malignant neoplasms of liver and intrahepatic bile ducts (C22)	15,885	10,701	5,184	3,345	2,376	969	64	51	13
Malignant neoplasm of pancreas (C25)	30,477	15,761	14,716	4,692	2,214	2,478	65	39	26
Malignant neoplasm of larynx (C32)	2,839	2,263	576	592	468	124	12	11	1
Malignant neoplasms of trachea, bronchus and lung(C33-C34)	129,562	70,230	59,332	16,779	9,699	7,080	321	197	124
Malignant melanoma of skin (C43)	8,950	5,990	2,960	140	76	64	7	5	2
Malignant neoplasm of breast (C50)	31,241	344	30,897	6,104	81	6,023	89	4	85
Malignant neoplasm of cervix uteri (C53)	2,642	X	2,642	827	X	827	14	X	14
Malignant neoplasms of corpus uteri and uterus, part unspecified (C54-C55)	6,592	X	6,592	1,747	X	1,747	17	X	17
Malignant neoplasm of ovary (C56)	11,599	X	11,599	1,239	X	1,239	22	X	22
Malignant neoplasm of prostate (C61)	20,914	20,914	X	4,477	4,477	X	65	65	X
Malignant neoplasm of kidney and renal pelvis (C64-C65)	11,193	7,242	3,951	1,250	792	458	33	26	7
Malignant neoplasm of bladder (C67)	13,653	9,953	3,700	1,155	677	478	29	22	7
Malignant neoplasms of meninges, brain and other parts of central nervous system (C70-C72)	12,918	7,174	5,744	930	531	399	18	10	8
Malignant neoplasms of lymphoid, hematopoietic and related tissue (C81-C96)	45,482	25,910	19,572	5,674	2,921	2,753	102	52	50
Hodgkin's disease (C81)	825	478	347	106	57	49	2	2	-
Non-Hodgkin's lymphoma (C82-C85)	16,520	9,198	7,322	1,437	770	667	37	20	17
Leukemia (C91-C95)	19,128	11,188	7,940	1,937	1,064	873	39	19	20
Multiple myeloma and immunoproliferative neoplasms (C88, C90)	8,947	5,009	3,938	2,185	1,023	1,162	24	11	13
Other and unspecified malignant neoplasms of lymphoid, hemato-poietic and related tissue (C96)	62	37	25	9	7	2	-	-	-
All other and unspecified malignant neoplasms (C17, C23-C24, C26-C31, C37-C41, C44-C49, C51- C52, C57-C60, C62-C63, C66, C68-C69, C73-C80, C97)	52,893	28,407	24,486	7,187	3,556	3,631	146	96	50
In situ neoplasms, benign neoplasms and neoplasms of uncertain or unknown behavior (D00-D48)	12,725	6,812	5,913	1,219	604	615	22	16	6
Anemias (D50-D64)	3,532	1,450	2,082	970	443	527	10	3	7
Diabetes mellitus (E10-E14)	51,297	27,807	23,490	13,239	6,298	6,941	217	128	89
Nutritional deficiencies (E40-E64)	2,656	1,023	1,633	442	199	243	10	7	3
Malnutrition (E40-E46)	2,520	968	1,552	427	192	235	10	7	3
Other nutritional deficiencies (E50-E64)	136	55	81	15	7	8	-	-	-
Meningitis (G00,G03)	391	214	177	95	47	48	2	2	-
Parkinson's disease (G20-G21)	22,241	13,370	8,871	1,030	615	415	38	22	16
Alzheimer's disease (G30)	73,234	22,345	50,889	5,664	1,646	4,018	112	36	76
Major cardiovascular diseases (I00-I78)	631,595	315,936	315,659	95,395	47,672	47,723	2,276	1,390	886
Diseases of heart (I00-I09, I11, I13, I20-I51)	488,817	256,294	232,523	71,102	36,562	34,540	1,877	1,186	691
Acute rheumatic fever and chronic rheumatic heart diseases (I00-I09)	2,697	932	1,765	251	98	153	7	3	4
Hypertensive heart disease (I11)	25,228	12,296	12,932	8,190	4,368	3,822	232	147	85
Hypertensive heart and renal disease (I13)	2,567	1,141	1,426	984	509	475	15	10	5
Ischemic heart diseases (I20-I25)	297,501	168,228	129,273	39,199	20,758	18,441	1,299	854	445
Acute myocardial infarction (I21-I22)	93,895	53,434	40,461	12,460	6,456	6,004	276	176	100
Other acute ischemic heart diseases (I24)	3,141	1,665	1,476	563	286	277	10	6	4
Other forms of chronic ischemic heart disease (I20, I25)	200,465	113,129	87,336	26,176	14,016	12,160	1,013	672	341
Atherosclerotic cardiovascular disease, so described (I25.0)	44,804	26,750	18,054	8,543	5,153	3,390	471	347	124
All other forms of chronic ischemic heart disease (I20,I25.1-I25.9)	155,661	86,379	69,282	17,633	8,863	8,770	542	325	217
Other heart diseases (I26-I51)	160,824	73,697	87,127	22,478	10,829	11,649	324	172	152
Acute and subacute endocarditis (I33)	942	568	374	170	110	60	6	4	2
Diseases of pericardium and acute myocarditis (I30-I31, I40)	609	318	291	147	71	76	6	3	3
Heart failure (I50)	54,787	23,847	30,940	6,518	2,933	3,585	87	41	46
All other forms of heart disease (I26-I28, I34-I38, I42-I49, I51)	104,486	48,964	55,522	15,643	7,715	7,928	225	124	101
Essential hypertension and hypertensive renal disease (I10, I12, I15)	22,043	8,955	13,088	5,400	2,467	2,933	80	47	33
Cerebrovascular diseases (I60-I69)	99,759	40,350	59,409	16,111	7,266	8,845	265	127	138
Atherosclerosis (I70)	5,727	2,309	3,418	523	224	299	13	6	7

Table 2-12B. Number of Deaths from Selected Causes, by Hispanic Origin and, Race for Non-Hispanic Population, and Sex, 2013—continued

(Number.)

Cause of death (based on ICD–10, 2004)	Non–Hispanic White[2]			Non–Hispanic Black[2]			Origin not stated[3]		
	Both sexes	Male	Female	Both sexes	Male	Female	Both sexes	Male	Female
Other diseases of circulatory system (I71-I78)	15,249	8,028	7,221	2,259	1,153	1,106	41	24	17
Aortic aneurysm and dissection (I71)	8,079	4,718	3,361	1,015	582	433	20	13	7
Other diseases of arteries, arterioles and capillaries (I72-I78)	7,170	3,310	3,860	1,244	571	673	21	11	10
Other disorders of circulatory system (I80-I99)	3,225	1,563	1,662	841	426	415	23	15	8
Influenza and pneumonia (J09-J18)	45,350	21,059	24,291	5,494	2,657	2,837	199	103	96
Influenza (J09-J11)	3,046	1,378	1,668	273	125	148	6	4	2
Pneumonia (J12-J18)	42,304	19,681	22,623	5,221	2,532	2,689	193	99	94
Other acute lower respiratory infections (J20-J22, U04)	226	83	143	29	13	16	-	-	-
Acute bronchitis and bronchiolitis (J20-J21)	176	65	111	23	11	12	-	-	-
Other and unspecified acute lower respiratory infections(J22, U04)	50	18	32	6	2	4	-	-	-
Chronic lower respiratory diseases (J40-J47)	131,667	61,106	70,561	9,816	5,019	4,797	337	191	146
Bronchitis, chronic and unspecified (J40-J42)	539	217	322	66	29	37	2	-	2
Emphysema (J43)	7,315	3,738	3,577	539	314	225	23	12	11
Asthma (J45-J46)	2,100	703	1,397	991	464	527	8	3	5
Other chronic lower respiratory diseases (J44, J47)	121,713	56,448	65,265	8,220	4,212	4,008	304	176	128
Pneumoconioses and chemical effects (J60-J66, J68)	740	705	35	32	29	3	2	2	-
Pneumonitis due to solids and liquids (J69)	15,630	8,534	7,096	1,601	852	749	29	16	13
Other diseases of respiratory system (J00-J06, J30-J39, J67, J70-J98)	28,533	14,623	13,910	3,151	1,433	1,718	68	35	33
Peptic ulcer (K25-K28)	2,369	1,180	1,189	293	163	130	12	8	4
Diseases of appendix (K35-K38)	279	160	119	50	33	17	-	-	-
Hernia (K40-K46)	1,573	634	939	168	64	104	9	5	4
Chronic liver disease and cirrhosis (K70, K73-K74)	26,692	17,290	9,402	2,998	1,915	1,083	154	122	32
Alcoholic liver disease (K70)	13,119	9,254	3,865	1,340	906	434	102	83	19
Other chronic liver disease and cirrhosis (K73-K74)	13,573	8,036	5,537	1,658	1,009	649	52	39	13
Cholelithiasis and other disorders of gallbladder (K80-K82)	2,636	1,251	1,385	313	139	174	11	3	8
Nephritis, nephrotic syndrome and nephrosis(N00-N07, N17-N19, N25-N27)	34,173	17,213	16,960	8,340	3,944	4,396	104	55	49
Acute and rapidly progressive nephritic and nephrotic syndrome (N00-N01,N04)	311	157	154	60	34	26	1	1	-
Chronic glomerulonephritis, nephritis and nephropathy not specified as acute or chronic, and renal sclerosis unspecified (N02-N03, N05-N07, N26)	182	105	77	24	9	15	1	1	-
Renal failure (N17-N19)	33,650	16,935	16,715	8,254	3,899	4,355	102	53	49
Other disorders of kidney (N25, N27)	30	16	14	2	2	-	-	-	-
Infections of kidney (N10-N12,N13.6,N15.1)	486	144	342	72	23	49	-	-	-
Hyperplasia of prostate (N40)	471	471	X	37	37	X	1	1	X
Inflammatory diseases of female pelvic organs (N70-N76)	93	X	93	20	X	20	-	X	-
Pregnancy, childbirth and the puerperium (O00-O99)	551	X	551	362	X	362	2	X	2
Pregnancy with abortive outcome (O00-O07)	8	X	8	10	X	10	1	X	1
Other complications of pregnancy, childbirth and the puerperium (O10-O99)	543	X	543	352	X	352	1	X	1
Certain conditions originating in the perinatal period(P00-P96)	5,077	2,872	2,205	3,854	2,102	1,752	185	109	76
Congenital malformations, deformations and chromosomal abnormalities (Q00-Q99)	5,887	3,109	2,778	1,526	787	739	35	17	18
Symptoms, signs and abnormal clinical and laboratory findings, not elsewhere classified (R00-R99)	30,056	12,405	17,651	4,440	2,153	2,287	176	100	76
All other diseases (Residual)	261,010	103,978	157,032	33,038	13,795	19,243	694	381	313
Accidents (unintentional injuries) (V01-X59, Y85-Y86)	100,773	61,391	39,382	13,169	8,845	4,324	462	320	142
Transport accidents (V01-V99, Y85)	26,158	18,564	7,594	4,932	3,594	1,338	101	79	22
Motor vehicle accidents (V02-V04, V09.0, V09.2, V12-V14, V19.0-V19.2, V19.4-V19.6, V20-V79, V80.3-V80.5, V81.0-V81.1, V82.0-V82.1, V83- V86, V87.0-V87.8, V88.0-V88.8, V89.0, V89.2)	24,249	17,043	7,206	4,658	3,379	1,279	86	66	20
Other land transport accidents (V01, V05-V06, V09.1, V09.3-V09.9, V10-V11, V15-V18, V19.3, V19.8-V19.9, V80.0-V80.2, V80.6-V80.9, V81.2- V81.9, V82.2-V82.9, V87.9, V88.9, V89.1, V89.3, V89.9)	671	521	150	135	116	19	12	10	2
Water, air and space, and other and unspecified transport accidents and their sequelae (V90-V99, Y85)	1,238	1,000	238	139	99	40	3	3	-
Nontransport accidents (W00-X59, Y86)	74,615	42,827	31,788	8,237	5,251	2,986	361	241	120
Falls (W00-W19)	26,283	12,865	13,418	1,395	826	569	81	42	39
Accidental discharge of firearms (W32-W34)	356	309	47	91	79	12	-	-	-
Accidental drowning and submersion (W65-W74)	2,183	1,632	551	514	419	95	14	9	5
Accidental exposure to smoke, fire and flames(X00-X09)	1,950	1,189	761	546	308	238	9	7	2
Accidental poisoning and exposure to noxious substances (X40-X49)	30,651	19,343	11,308	3,735	2,492	1,243	204	149	55
Other and unspecified nontransport accidents and their sequelae (W20-W31, W35-W64, W75-W99, X10-X39, X50-X59, Y86)	13,192	7,489	5,703	1,956	1,127	829	53	34	19
Intentional self-harm (suicide) (*U03, X60-X84, Y87.0)	34,253	26,621	7,632	2,293	1,850	443	167	136	31
Intentional self-harm (suicide) by discharge of firearms (X72-X74)	18,561	15,921	2,640	1,072	965	107	54	49	5
Intentional self-harm (suicide) by other and unspecified means and their sequelae (*U03, X60-X71, X75-X84, Y87.0)	15,692	10,700	4,992	1,221	885	336	113	87	26
Assault (homicide) (*U01-*U02, X85-Y09, Y87.1)	5,024	3,311	1,713	7,950	6,851	1,099	66	55	11
Assault (homicide) by discharge of firearms (*U01.4, X93-X95)	2,799	1,950	849	6,364	5,732	632	32	30	2
Assault (homicide) by other and unspecified means and their sequelae (*U01.0-*U01.3, *U01.5-*U01.9, *U02, X85-X92, X96-Y09, Y87.1)	2,225	1,361	864	1,586	1,119	467	34	25	9
Legal intervention (Y35, Y89.0)	268	254	14	142	137	5	1	1	-
Events of undetermined intent (Y10-Y34, Y87.2,Y89.9)	3,497	1,975	1,522	576	391	185	23	11	12
Discharge of firearms, undetermined intent (Y22-Y24)	196	153	43	42	34	8	3	2	1
Other and unspecified events of undetermined intent and their sequelae (Y10-Y21, Y25-Y34, Y87.2, Y89.9)	3,301	1,822	1,479	534	357	177	20	9	11
Operations of war and their sequelae (Y36, Y89.1)	13	13	-	1	1	-	-	-	-
Complications of medical and surgical care (Y40-Y84, Y88)	2,118	1,027	1,091	394	190	204	2	1	1
Enterocolitis due to Clostridium difficile (A04.7)[4]	6,490	2,515	3,975	578	259	319	24	7	17
Drug-induced deaths[5,6]	37,359	22,332	15,027	4,282	2,766	1,516	249	170	79

Table 2-12B. Number of Deaths from Selected Causes, by Hispanic Origin and, Race for Non-Hispanic Population, and Sex, 2013—continued

(Number.)

Cause of death (based on ICD–10, 2004)	Non–Hispanic White[2]			Non–Hispanic Black[2]			Origin not stated[3]		
	Both sexes	Male	Female	Both sexes	Male	Female	Both sexes	Male	Female
Alcohol-induced deaths[5,7]	21,260	15,401	5,859	2,519	1,862	657	190	154	36
Injury by firearms[5,8]	22,149	18,558	3,591	7,697	6,934	763	90	82	8

X = Not applicable.   – = Quantity zero.   1Includes races other than White and Black.   2Race categories are consistent with the 1977 Office of Management and Budget (OMB) standards. Multiple-race data were reported by 42 states and the District of Columbia in 2013. The multiple-race data for these reporting areas were bridged to the single-race categories of the 1977 OMB standards for comparability with other reporting areas.   3Includes deaths for which Hispanic origin was not reported on the death certificate.   4Included in certain other intestinal infections (A04, A07–A09). Beginning with data year 2006, Enterocolitis due to Clostridium difficile (A04.7) is shown separately at the bottom of the table and is included in the list of rankable causes.   5Included in selected categories above.   6Includes ICD–10 codes D52.1, D59.0, D59.2, D61.1, D64.2, E06.4, E16.0, E23.1, E24.2, E27.3, E66.1, F11.1–F11.5, F11.7–F11.9, F12.1–F12.5, F12.7–F12.9, F13.1–F13.5, F13.7–F13.9, F14.1–F14.5, F14.7–F14.9, F15.1–F15.5, F15.7–F15.9, F16.1–F16.5, F16.7–F16.9, F17.3–F17.5, F17.7–F17.9, F18.1–F18.5, F18.7–F18.9, F19.1–F19.5, F19.7–F19.9, G21.1, G24.0, G25.1, G25.4, G25.6, G44.4, G62.0, G72.0, I95.2, J70.2–J70.4, K85.3, L10.5, L27.0–L27.1, M10.2, M32.0, M80.4, M81.4, M83.5, M87.1, R50.2, R78.1–R78.5, X40–X44, X60–X64, X85, and Y10–Y14. Trend data for drug-induced deaths, previously shown in this report, can be found at http://www.cdc.gov/nchs/deaths.htm.   7Includes ICD–10 codes E24.4, F10, G31.2, G62.1, G72.1, I42.6, K29.2, K70, K85.2, K86.0, R78.0, X45, X65, and Y15. Trend data for alcohol-induced deaths, previously shown in this report, can be found at http://www.cdc.gov/nchs/deaths.htm.   8Includes ICD–10 codes *U01.4, W32–W34, X72–X74, X93–X95, Y22–Y24, and Y35.0. Trend data for Injury by firearms, previously shown in this report, can be found at http://www.cdc.gov/nchs/deaths.htm.

Table 2-13A. Death Rates from Selected Causes, by Hispanic Origin, Race for Non-Hispanic Population, and Sex, 2010

(Rates per 100,000 population in specified group.)

Cause of death (based on ICD-10, 2004)	All origins[1]			Hispanic[2]			Non-Hispanic		
	Both sexes	Male	Female	Both sexes	Male	Female	Both sexes	Male	Female
All Causes	821.5	839.1	804.4	301.9	323.7	279.4	926.1	946.2	906.7
Salmonella infections (A01-A02)	0.0	0.0	*	*	*	*	0.0	0.0	*
Shigellosis and amebiasis (A03, A06)	*	*	*	*	*	*	*	*	*
Certain other intestinal infections (A04, A07-A09)	3.3	2.7	4.0	1.2	1.0	1.4	3.8	3.0	4.5
Tuberculosis (A16-A19)	0.2	0.2	0.1	0.2	0.2	0.1	0.2	0.2	0.1
Respiratory tuberculosis (A16)	0.1	0.2	0.1	0.1	0.2	0.1	0.1	0.2	0.1
Other tuberculosis (A17-A19)	0.0	0.1	0.0	0.0	*	*	0.0	0.1	0.0
Whooping cough (A37)	*	*	*	*	*	*	*	*	*
Scarlet fever and erysipelas (A38, A46)	*	*	*	*	*	*	*	*	*
Meningococcal infection (A39)	0.0	0.0	0.0	*	*	*	0.0	0.0	0.0
Septicemia (A40-A41)	12.1	11.6	12.6	4.5	4.5	4.5	13.6	13.0	14.1
Syphilis (A50-A53)	0.0	0.0	0.0	*	*	*	0.0	0.0	*
Acute poliomyelitis (A80)	*	*	*	*	*	*	*	*	*
Arthropod-borne viral encephalitis (A83-A84, A85.2)	*	*	*	*	*	*	*	*	*
Measles (B05)	*	*	*	*	*	*	*	*	*
Viral hepatitis (B15-B19)	2.6	3.5	1.7	2.3	3.1	1.5	2.6	3.6	1.7
Human immunodeficiency virus (HIV) disease (B20-B24)	2.2	3.3	1.2	1.7	2.7	0.7	2.3	3.3	1.2
Malaria (B50-B54)	*	*	*	*	*	*	*	*	*
Other and unspecified infectious and parasitic diseases and their sequelae (A00, A05, A20-A36, A42-A44, A48- A49, A54-A79, A81-A82, A85.0-A85.1, A85.8, A86-B04, B06-B09, B25-B49, B55-B99)	1.9	2.0	1.8	1.0	1.0	0.9	2.1	2.2	2.0
Malignant neoplasms (C00-C97)	185.0	197.6	172.8	65.0	66.9	63.0	209.3	225.0	194.3
Malignant neoplasms of lip, oral cavity and pharynx (C00-C14)	2.8	4.0	1.6	0.8	1.2	0.5	3.2	4.6	1.9
Malignant neoplasm of esophagus (C15)	4.6	7.5	1.8	1.1	1.7	0.4	5.4	8.8	2.1
Malignant neoplasm of stomach (C16)	3.6	4.4	2.8	3.0	3.4	2.6	3.7	4.6	2.8
Malignant neoplasms of colon, rectum and anus (C18-C21)	16.5	17.6	15.5	6.6	7.4	5.8	18.5	19.7	17.4
Malignant neoplasms of liver and intrahepatic bile ducts (C22)	7.6	10.5	4.8	5.5	7.3	3.8	8.0	11.1	5.0
Malignant neoplasm of pancreas (C25)	12.3	12.8	11.9	4.6	4.4	4.8	13.9	14.5	13.3
Malignant neoplasm of larynx (C32)	1.2	1.9	0.5	0.4	0.7	0.1	1.3	2.2	0.5
Malignant neoplasms of trachea, bronchus and lung(C33-C34)	49.4	55.1	44.0	9.9	11.8	8.0	57.5	64.2	51.0
Malignant melanoma of skin (C43)	3.0	4.0	2.0	0.4	0.5	0.4	3.5	4.8	2.3
Malignant neoplasm of breast (C50)	13.1	0.3	25.5	5.0	0.1	10.0	14.7	0.3	28.5
Malignant neoplasm of cervix uteri (C53)	1.3	X	2.6	1.0	X	2.0	1.4	X	2.8
Malignant neoplasms of corpus uteri and uterus, part unspecified (C54-C55)	2.9	X	5.8	1.3	X	2.6	3.3	X	6.4
Malignant neoplasm of ovary (C56)	4.5	X	8.9	1.7	X	3.5	5.1	X	9.9
Malignant neoplasm of prostate (C61)	8.8	17.8	X	3.0	6.0	X	9.9	20.3	X
Malignant neoplasms of kidney and renal pelvis (C64-C65)	4.4	5.8	3.1	1.9	2.4	1.5	4.9	6.5	3.4
Malignant neoplasm of bladder (C67)	5.0	7.3	2.8	1.2	1.6	0.7	5.8	8.4	3.2
Malignant neoplasms of meninges, brain and other parts of central nervous system (C70-C72)	4.9	5.5	4.3	1.9	2.0	1.9	5.4	6.2	4.7
Malignant neoplasms of lymphoid, hematopoietic and related tissue (C81-C96)	18.0	20.6	15.5	7.5	8.2	6.8	20.1	23.2	17.2
Hodgkin's disease (C81)	0.3	0.4	0.3	0.2	0.3	0.2	0.4	0.4	0.3
Non-Hodgkin's lymphoma (C82-C85)	6.4	7.2	5.6	2.7	3.0	2.4	7.1	8.1	6.2
Leukemia (C91-C95)	7.4	8.7	6.1	3.1	3.4	2.8	8.3	9.9	6.8
Multiple myeloma and immunoproliferative neoplasms (C88, C90)	3.9	4.3	3.5	1.5	1.6	1.3	4.4	4.8	3.9
Other and unspecified malignant neoplasms of lymphoid, hemato-poietic and related tissue (C96)	0.0	0.0	0.0	*	*	*	0.0	0.0	0.0
All other and unspecified malignant neoplasms (C17, C23-C24, C26-C31, C37-C41, C44-C49, C51- C52, C57-C60, C62-C63, C66, C68-C69, C73-C80, C97)	21.1	22.7	19.5	8.1	8.2	7.9	23.7	25.8	21.7
In situ neoplasms, benign neoplasms and neoplasms of uncertain or unknown behavior (D00-D48)	4.8	5.2	4.5	1.5	1.6	1.5	5.5	6.0	5.0
Anemias (D50-D64)	1.5	1.3	1.8	0.5	0.4	0.6	1.8	1.5	2.0
Diabetes mellitus (E10-E14)	23.9	25.6	22.3	14.1	14.3	13.9	25.8	27.9	23.9
Nutritional deficiencies (E40-E64)	1.1	0.9	1.3	0.3	0.3	0.4	1.2	1.0	1.4
Malnutrition (E40-E46)	1.0	0.8	1.2	0.3	0.3	0.4	1.2	0.9	1.4
Other nutritional deficiencies (E50-E64)	0.0	0.0	0.1	*	*	*	0.1	0.0	0.1
Meningitis (G00,G03)	0.2	0.2	0.2	0.1	0.2	0.1	0.2	0.2	0.2
Parkinson's disease (G20-G21)	8.0	9.7	6.3	2.4	2.7	2.1	9.1	11.2	7.1
Alzheimer's disease (G30)	26.8	16.6	36.7	7.6	4.7	10.6	30.7	19.1	41.9
Major cardiovascular diseases (I00-I78)	252.0	257.4	246.6	82.5	86.6	78.3	286.1	292.9	279.5
Diseases of heart (I00-I09, I11, I13, I20-I51)	193.3	206.5	180.6	61.5	66.9	55.9	219.8	235.4	204.8
Acute rheumatic fever and chronic rheumatic heart diseases (I00-I09)	1.0	0.7	1.3	0.3	0.2	0.4	1.2	0.8	1.5
Hypertensive heart disease (I11)	11.7	12.0	11.5	4.6	5.1	4.1	13.1	13.4	12.9
Hypertensive heart and renal disease (I13)	1.3	1.2	1.3	0.6	0.6	0.5	1.4	1.3	1.5
Ischemic heart diseases (I20-I25)	117.1	134.0	100.8	40.3	45.6	34.8	132.5	152.2	113.5
Acute myocardial infarction (I21-I22)	36.9	42.4	31.6	12.9	14.9	10.7	41.8	48.2	35.7
Other acute ischemic heart diseases (I24)	1.2	1.3	1.2	0.3	0.2	0.3	1.4	1.6	1.3
Other forms of chronic ischemic heart disease (I20, I25)	78.9	90.2	68.0	27.2	30.4	23.8	89.2	102.5	76.5
Atherosclerotic cardiovascular disease, so described (I25.0)	18.8	23.1	14.7	7.0	9.2	4.9	21.1	25.8	16.5
All other forms of chronic ischemic heart disease (I20,I25.1-I25.9)	60.1	67.1	53.3	20.1	21.2	19.0	68.1	76.7	59.9
Other heart diseases (I26-I51)	62.1	58.5	65.7	15.7	15.4	15.9	71.6	67.6	75.4
Acute and subacute endocarditis (I33)	0.4	0.5	0.3	0.2	0.2	0.1	0.4	0.5	0.3
Diseases of pericardium and acute myocarditis (I30-I31, I40)	0.3	0.3	0.3	0.1	0.2	0.1	0.3	0.3	0.3
Heart failure (I50)	20.6	18.3	22.8	4.7	4.2	5.3	23.8	21.3	26.3
All other forms of heart disease (I26-I28, I34-I38, I42-I49, I51)	40.9	39.4	42.3	10.6	10.9	10.4	47.0	45.4	48.5
Essential hypertension and hypertensive renal disease (I10, I12, I15)	9.7	8.3	11.1	3.9	3.5	4.2	10.9	9.3	12.4
Cerebrovascular diseases (I60-I69)	40.8	34.5	46.9	15.0	14.0	16.1	46.0	38.8	52.9

Table 2-13A. Death Rates from Selected Causes, by Hispanic Origin, Race for Non-Hispanic Population, and Sex, 2010 — continued

(Rates per 100,000 population in specified group.)

Cause of death (based on ICD-10, 2004)	All origins[1]			Hispanic[2]			Non-Hispanic		
	Both sexes	Male	Female	Both sexes	Male	Female	Both sexes	Male	Female
Atherosclerosis (I70)	2.1	1.7	2.5	0.5	0.4	0.6	2.4	2.0	2.8
Other diseases of circulatory system (I71-I78)	6.0	6.4	5.6	1.6	1.7	1.5	6.9	7.4	6.4
Aortic aneurysm and dissection (I71)	3.1	3.7	2.6	0.8	0.9	0.6	3.6	4.3	2.9
Other diseases of arteries, arterioles and capillaries (I72-I78)	2.9	2.7	3.0	0.9	0.8	0.9	3.3	3.1	3.5
Other disorders of circulatory system (I80-I99)	1.4	1.4	1.4	0.5	0.4	0.6	1.6	1.6	1.6
Influenza and pneumonia (J09-J18)[1]	18.0	17.2	18.8	6.6	6.6	6.7	20.3	19.4	21.1
Influenza (J09-J11)[1]	1.2	1.1	1.2	0.5	0.5	0.4	1.3	1.2	1.4
Pneumonia (J12-J18)	16.9	16.1	17.6	6.2	6.1	6.2	19.0	18.2	19.7
Other acute lower respiratory infections (J20-J22, U04)[2]	0.1	0.1	0.1	0.0	*	*	0.1	0.1	0.1
Acute bronchitis and bronchiolitis (J20-J21)	0.1	0.1	0.1	0.0	*	*	0.1	0.1	0.1
Other and unspecified acute lower respiratory infections(J22, U04)[2,3]	0.0	0.0	0.0	*	*	*	0.0	0.0	0.0
Chronic lower respiratory diseases (J40-J47)	47.2	45.2	49.2	8.9	9.2	8.6	55.0	52.7	57.1
Bronchitis, chronic and unspecified (J40-J42)	0.2	0.2	0.2	0.1	0.1	*	0.2	0.2	0.3
Emphysema (J43)	2.6	2.8	2.5	0.5	0.6	0.4	3.1	3.2	2.9
Asthma (J45-J46)	1.1	0.9	1.4	0.6	0.5	0.7	1.3	1.0	1.5
Other chronic lower respiratory diseases (J44, J47)	43.2	41.3	45.1	7.8	8.1	7.5	50.4	48.3	52.4
Pneumoconioses and chemical effects (J60-J66, J68)	0.3	0.5	0.0	0.0	0.1	*	0.3	0.6	0.0
Pneumonitis due to solids and liquids (J69)	5.9	6.5	5.3	1.5	1.7	1.4	6.8	7.5	6.0
Other diseases of respiratory system (J00-J06, J30-J39, J67, J70-J98)	11.1	11.5	10.8	4.5	4.4	4.6	12.5	12.9	12.1
Peptic ulcer (K25-K28)	0.9	1.0	0.9	0.3	0.4	0.3	1.1	1.1	1.0
Diseases of appendix (K35-K38)	0.1	0.1	0.1	0.1	*	*	0.1	0.2	0.1
Hernia (K40-K46)	0.6	0.5	0.7	0.3	0.2	0.3	0.7	0.6	0.8
Chronic liver disease and cirrhosis (K70, K73-K74)	11.5	15.2	7.9	9.5	12.9	6.0	11.9	15.6	8.3
Alcoholic liver disease (K70)	5.7	8.3	3.2	5.0	8.0	2.0	5.9	8.4	3.4
Other chronic liver disease and cirrhosis (K73-K74)	5.8	6.9	4.7	4.5	5.0	4.0	6.0	7.3	4.8
Cholelithiasis and other disorders of gallbladder (K80-K82)	1.1	1.0	1.1	0.5	0.5	0.5	1.2	1.1	1.2
Nephritis, nephrotic syndrome and nephrosis(N00-N07, N17-N19, N25-N27)	14.9	15.1	14.7	5.7	5.8	5.6	16.8	17.0	16.5
Acute and rapidly progressive nephritic and nephrotic syndrome (N00-N01,N04)	0.1	0.1	0.1	*	*	*	0.1	0.2	0.1
Chronic glomerulonephritis, nephritis and nephropathy not specified as acute or chronic, and renal sclerosis unspecified (N02-N03, N05-N07, N26)	0.1	0.1	0.1	0.1	*	0.1	0.1	0.1	0.1
Renal failure (N17-N19)	14.7	14.9	14.5	5.6	5.7	5.5	16.5	16.8	16.3
Other disorders of kidney (N25, N27)	0.0	0.0	*	*	*	*	0.0	*	*
Infections of kidney (N10-N12,N13.6,N15.1)	0.2	0.1	0.3	0.1	*	0.1	0.2	0.1	0.3
Hyperplasia of prostate (N40)	0.2	0.4	X	0.1	0.1	X	0.2	0.4	X
Inflammatory diseases of female pelvic organs (N70-N76)	0.0	X	0.1	*	X	*	0.0	X	0.1
Pregnancy, childbirth and the puerperium (O00-O99)	0.4	X	0.7	0.3	X	0.6	0.4	X	0.7
Pregnancy with abortive outcome (O00-O07)	0.0	X	0.0	*	X	*	0.0	X	0.0
Other complications of pregnancy, childbirth and the puerperium (O10-O99)	0.4	X	0.7	0.3	X	0.6	0.4	X	0.7
Certain conditions originating in the perinatal period(P00-P96)	3.8	4.3	3.3	4.5	4.8	4.2	3.6	4.1	3.1
Congenital malformations, deformations and chromosomal abnormalities (Q00-Q99)	3.0	3.2	2.8	3.2	3.3	3.1	3.0	3.2	2.8
Symptoms, signs and abnormal clinical and laboratory findings, not elsewhere classified (R00-R99)	11.9	10.5	13.4	4.1	4.4	3.8	13.5	11.7	15.2
All other diseases (Residual)	101.2	83.2	118.8	32.7	29.0	36.5	115.1	94.5	134.9
Accidents (unintentional injuries) (V01-X59, Y85-Y86)	41.3	52.6	30.3	22.2	31.9	12.2	45.1	56.8	33.8
Transport accidents (V01-V99, Y85)	12.0	17.4	6.8	9.6	14.1	5.0	12.5	18.1	7.1
Motor vehicle accidents (V02-V04, V09.0, V09.2, V12-V14, V19.0-V19.2, V19.4-V19.6, V20-V79, V80.3-V80.5, V81.0-V81.1, V82.0-V82.1, V83-V86, V87.0-V87.8, V88.0-V88.8, V89.0, V89.2)	11.2	16.1	6.4	9.1	13.3	4.8	11.6	16.6	6.7
Other land transport accidents (V01,V05-V06, V09.1, V09.3-V09.9, V10-V11,V15-V18, V19.3, V19.8-V19.9, V80.0-V80.2, V80.6-V80.9, V81.2-V81.9, V82.2-V82.9, V87.9, V88.9, V89.1, V89.3, V89.9)	0.3	0.5	0.1	0.3	0.4	*	0.3	0.5	0.1
Water, air and space, and other and unspecified transport accidents and their sequelae (V90-V99, Y85)	0.5	0.8	0.2	0.2	0.3	0.1	0.6	0.9	0.2
Nontransport accidents (W00-X59, Y86)	29.3	35.2	23.6	12.6	17.8	7.3	32.6	38.8	26.7
Falls (W00-W19)	9.6	9.8	9.3	2.9	3.6	2.2	10.9	11.1	10.7
Accidental discharge of firearms (W32-W34)	0.2	0.3	0.0	0.1	0.2	*	0.2	0.3	0.0
Accidental drowning and submersion (W65-W74)	1.1	1.7	0.5	0.8	1.3	0.3	1.1	1.7	0.5
Accidental exposure to smoke, fire and flames(X00-X09)	0.9	1.1	0.7	0.3	0.4	0.3	1.0	1.2	0.8
Accidental poisoning and exposure to noxious substances (X40-X49)	12.3	16.1	8.6	6.2	9.1	3.2	13.5	17.5	9.6
Other and unspecified nontransport accidents and their sequelae (W20-W31, W35-W64, W75-W99, X10-X39, X50-X59, Y86)	5.3	6.3	4.4	2.3	3.2	1.3	6.0	6.9	5.0
Intentional self-harm (suicide) (*U03, X60-X84, Y87.0)	13.0	20.6	5.7	5.3	8.3	2.2	14.5	23.1	6.3
Intentional self-harm (suicide) by discharge of firearms (X72-X74)	6.7	11.7	1.8	1.9	3.3	0.5	7.7	13.5	2.1
Intentional self-harm (suicide) by other and unspecified means and their sequelae (*U03, X60-X71, X75-X84, Y87.0)	6.3	8.9	3.8	3.4	5.0	1.7	6.9	9.6	4.2
Assault (homicide) (*U01-*U02, X85-Y09, Y87.1)	5.1	8.2	2.1	4.8	7.8	1.6	5.1	8.2	2.2
Assault (homicide) by discharge of firearms (*U01.4, X93-X95)	3.5	6.1	1.1	3.2	5.6	0.8	3.6	6.2	1.2
Assault (homicide) by other and unspecified means and their sequelae (*U01.0-*U01.3, *U01.5-*U01.9, *U02, X85-X92, X96-Y09, Y87.1)	1.6	2.1	1.0	1.5	2.2	0.8	1.5	2.1	1.0
Legal intervention (Y35, Y89.0)	0.2	0.3	0.0	0.2	0.3	*	0.2	0.3	0.0
Events of undetermined intent (Y10-Y34, Y87.2,Y89.9)	1.5	1.7	1.2	0.6	0.9	0.4	1.6	1.9	1.3
Discharge of firearms, undetermined intent (Y22-Y24)	0.1	0.1	0.0	0.1	0.1	*	0.1	0.1	0.0
Other and unspecified events of undetermined intent and their sequelae (Y10-Y21, Y25-Y34, Y87.2, Y89.9)	1.4	1.6	1.1	0.6	0.8	0.4	1.5	1.8	1.3
Operations of war and their sequelae (Y36, Y89.1)	*	*	*	*	*	*	*	*	*
Complications of medical and surgical care (Y40-Y84, Y88)	0.9	0.9	0.9	0.4	0.3	0.4	1.0	1.0	1.0
Enterocolitis due to Clostridium difficile (A04.7)[3]	2.4	1.9	2.9	0.8	0.7	0.9	2.8	2.2	3.3

Table 2-13A. Death Rates from Selected Causes, by Hispanic Origin, Race for Non-Hispanic Population, and Sex, 2010 — continued

(Rates per 100,000 population in specified group.)

Cause of death (based on ICD-10, 2004)	All origins[1]			Hispanic[2]			Non-Hispanic		
	Both sexes	Male	Female	Both sexes	Male	Female	Both sexes	Male	Female
Drug-induced deaths[4,5]	14.7	18.2	11.3	6.7	9.3	4.0	16.3	20.0	12.7
Alcohol-induced deaths[4,6]	9.2	13.7	4.8	6.8	11.0	2.5	9.6	14.2	5.2
Injury by firearms[4,7]	10.6	18.5	3.0	5.5	9.4	1.3	11.7	20.4	3.3

Table 2-13B. Death Rates from Selected Causes, by Hispanic Origin, Race for Non-Hispanic Population, and Sex, 2010

(Rates per 100,000 population in specified group.)

Cause of death (based on ICD-10, 2004)	Non-Hispanic White			Non-Hispanic Black		
	Both sexes	Male	Female	Both sexes	Male	Female
All Causes	1,021.6	1,032.1	1,011.5	733.4	782.5	688.4
Salmonella infections (A01-A02)	0.0	*	*	*	*	*
Shigellosis and amebiasis (A03, A06)	*	*	*	*	*	*
Certain other intestinal infections (A04, A07-A09)	4.4	3.4	5.4	2.1	2.0	2.2
Tuberculosis (A16-A19)	0.1	0.2	0.1	0.2	0.3	0.2
Respiratory tuberculosis (A16)	0.1	0.1	0.1	0.2	0.2	0.1
Other tuberculosis (A17-A19)	0.0	0.0	0.0	0.1	*	*
Whooping cough (A37)	*	*	*	*	*	*
Scarlet fever and erysipelas (A38, A46)	*	*	*	*	*	*
Meningococcal infection (A39)	0.0	0.0	*	*	*	*
Septicemia (A40-A41)	14.2	13.5	14.8	15.2	14.6	15.7
Syphilis (A50-A53)	*	*	*	0.1	*	*
Acute poliomyelitis (A80)	*	*	*	*	*	*
Arthropod-borne viral encephalitis (A83-A84, A85.2)	*	*	*	*	*	*
Measles (B05)	*	*	*	*	*	*
Viral hepatitis (B15-B19)	2.6	3.6	1.7	3.0	4.0	2.0
Human immunodeficiency virus (HIV) disease (B20-B24)	1.1	1.8	0.4	9.0	12.4	5.8
Malaria (B50-B54)	*	*	*	*	*	*
Other and unspecified infectious and parasitic diseases and their sequelae (A00, A05, A20-A36, A42-A44, A48-A49, A54-A79, A81-A82, A85.0-A85.1, A85.8, A86-B04, B06-B09, B25-B49, B55-B99)	2.2	2.3	2.1	2.0	2.2	1.9
Malignant neoplasms (C00-C97)	230.4	247.3	214.0	164.9	175.9	154.8
Malignant neoplasms of lip, oral cavity and pharynx (C00-C14)	3.5	4.9	2.0	2.6	3.9	1.4
Malignant neoplasm of esophagus (C15)	6.2	10.1	2.3	3.2	4.8	1.7
Malignant neoplasm of stomach (C16)	3.4	4.2	2.6	4.8	6.0	3.6
Malignant neoplasms of colon, rectum and anus (C18-C21)	19.8	20.9	18.8	16.7	18.4	15.3
Malignant neoplasms of liver and intrahepatic bile ducts (C22)	7.9	10.8	5.1	8.2	12.2	4.6
Malignant neoplasm of pancreas (C25)	15.2	15.9	14.4	11.5	11.3	11.6
Malignant neoplasm of larynx (C32)	1.4	2.3	0.6	1.5	2.4	0.6
Malignant neoplasms of trachea, bronchus and lung(C33-C34)	64.5	71.0	58.2	41.1	49.7	33.3
Malignant melanoma of skin (C43)	4.5	6.1	2.9	0.3	0.4	0.3
Malignant neoplasm of breast (C50)	15.5	0.3	30.3	15.0	0.4	28.3
Malignant neoplasm of cervix uteri (C53)	1.3	X	2.6	2.0	X	3.9
Malignant neoplasms of corpus uteri and uterus, part unspecified (C54-C55)	3.3	X	6.5	4.3	X	8.2
Malignant neoplasm of ovary (C56)	5.8	X	11.4	3.0	X	5.8
Malignant neoplasm of prostate (C61)	10.4	21.1	X	11.0	22.9	X
Malignant neoplasms of kidney and renal pelvis (C64-C65)	5.6	7.3	3.9	3.1	4.1	2.2
Malignant neoplasm of bladder (C67)	6.8	10.1	3.6	2.8	3.5	2.2
Malignant neoplasms of meninges, brain and other parts of central nervous system (C70-C72)	6.4	7.3	5.6	2.3	2.7	1.9
Malignant neoplasms of lymphoid, hematopoietic and related tissue (C81-C96)	22.6	26.2	19.2	13.9	15.0	12.9
Hodgkin's disease (C81)	0.4	0.5	0.3	0.3	0.3	0.2
Non-Hodgkin's lymphoma (C82-C85)	8.2	9.3	7.2	3.5	3.9	3.1
Leukemia (C91-C95)	9.5	11.3	7.8	4.7	5.5	4.1
Multiple myeloma and immunoproliferative neoplasms (C88, C90)	4.5	5.1	3.9	5.4	5.2	5.5
Other and unspecified malignant neoplasms of lymphoid, hematopoietic and related tissue (C96)	0.0	0.0	0.0	*	*	*
All other and unspecified malignant neoplasms (C17, C23-C24, C26-C31, C37-C41, C44-C49, C51-C52, C57-C60, C62-C63, C66, C68-C69; C73-C80; C97)	26.3	28.7	24.0	17.6	18.2	17.1
In situ neoplasms, benign neoplasms and neoplasms of uncertain or unknown behavior (D00-D48)	6.3	6.9	5.8	3.0	3.1	2.9
Anemias (D50-D64)	1.8	1.5	2.0	2.4	2.3	2.5
Diabetes mellitus (E10-E14)	25.5	28.1	23.0	32.4	32.3	32.6
Nutritional deficiencies (E40-E64)	1.3	1.0	1.6	1.1	1.0	1.1
Malnutrition (E40-E46)	1.3	1.0	1.5	1.0	1.0	1.1
Other nutritional deficiencies (E50-E64)	0.1	0.1	0.1	*	*	*
Meningitis (G00,G03)	0.2	0.2	0.2	0.2	0.2	0.2
Parkinson's disease (G20-G21)	11.1	13.5	8.7	2.5	3.2	1.9
Alzheimer's disease (G30)	36.4	22.6	49.9	13.9	8.4	18.9
Major cardiovascular diseases (I00-I78)	314.4	319.3	309.5	233.8	244.3	224.1
Diseases of heart (I00-I09, I11, I13, I20-I51)	243.3	259.0	228.0	174.3	187.4	162.2
Acute rheumatic fever and chronic rheumatic heart diseases (I00-I09)	1.3	0.9	1.7	0.6	0.5	0.7
Hypertensive heart disease (I11)	12.6	12.4	12.7	20.1	22.4	18.0
Hypertensive heart and renal disease (I13)	1.3	1.2	1.4	2.4	2.6	2.2
Ischemic heart diseases (I20-I25)	148.1	170.0	126.8	96.1	106.4	86.6
Acute myocardial infarction (I21-I22)	46.7	54.0	39.7	30.5	33.1	28.2
Other acute ischemic heart diseases (I24)	1.6	1.7	1.4	1.4	1.5	1.3
Other forms of chronic ischemic heart disease (I20, I25)	99.8	114.3	85.6	64.2	71.8	57.1
Atherosclerotic cardiovascular disease, so described (I25.0)	22.3	27.0	17.7	20.9	26.4	15.9
All other forms of chronic ischemic heart disease (I20,I25.1-I25.9)	77.5	87.3	67.9	43.2	45.4	41.2
Other heart diseases (I26-I51)	80.0	74.5	85.4	55.1	55.5	54.7
Acute and subacute endocarditis (I33)	0.5	0.6	0.4	0.4	0.6	0.3
Diseases of pericardium and acute myocarditis (I30-I31, I40)	0.3	0.3	0.3	0.4	0.4	0.4

Table 2-13B. Death Rates from Selected Causes, by Hispanic Origin, Race for Non-Hispanic Population, and Sex, 2010 — continued

(Rates per 100,000 population in specified group.)

Cause of death (based on ICD-10, 2004)	Non-Hispanic White			Non-Hispanic Black		
	Both sexes	Male	Female	Both sexes	Male	Female
Heart failure (I50)	27.3	24.1	30.3	16.0	15.0	16.8
All other forms of heart disease (I26-I28, I34-I38, I42-I49, I51)	52.0	49.5	54.4	38.3	39.5	37.2
Essential hypertension and hypertensive renal disease (I10, I12, I15)	11.0	9.1	12.8	13.2	12.6	13.8
Cerebrovascular diseases (I60-I69)	49.7	40.8	58.3	39.5	37.2	41.5
Atherosclerosis (I70)	2.9	2.3	3.4	1.3	1.1	1.4
Other diseases of circulatory system (I71-I78)	7.6	8.1	7.1	5.5	5.9	5.2
Aortic aneurysm and dissection (I71)	4.0	4.8	3.3	2.5	3.0	2.0
Other diseases of arteries, arterioles and capillaries (I72-I78)	3.6	3.3	3.8	3.0	2.9	3.2
Other disorders of circulatory system (I80-I99)	1.6	1.6	1.6	2.1	2.2	1.9
Influenza and pneumonia (J09-J18)[1]	22.6	21.3	23.8	13.5	13.6	13.3
Influenza (J09-J11)[1]	1.5	1.4	1.6	0.7	0.6	0.7
Pneumonia (J12-J18)	21.1	19.9	22.2	12.8	13.0	12.6
Other acute lower respiratory infections (J20-J22, U04)[2]	0.1	0.1	0.1	0.1	*	*
Acute bronchitis and bronchiolitis (J20-J21)	0.1	0.1	0.1	0.1	*	*
Other and unspecified acute lower respiratory infections (J22, U04)[2,3]	0.0	*	0.0	*	*	*
Chronic lower respiratory diseases (J40-J47)	65.5	61.8	69.2	24.1	25.7	22.5
Bronchitis, chronic and unspecified (J40-J42)	0.3	0.2	0.3	0.2	0.1	0.2
Emphysema (J43)	3.6	3.8	3.5	1.3	1.6	1.1
Asthma (J45-J46)	1.0	0.7	1.4	2.4	2.4	2.5
Other chronic lower respiratory diseases (J44, J47)	60.6	57.1	64.0	20.1	21.6	18.8
Pneumoconioses and chemical effects (J60-J66, J68)	0.4	0.7	0.0	0.1	0.1	*
Pneumonitis due to solids and liquids (J69)	7.8	8.6	7.0	3.9	4.4	3.5
Other diseases of respiratory system (J00-J06, J30-J39, J67, J70-J98)	14.2	14.8	13.6	7.7	7.3	8.1
Peptic ulcer (K25-K28)	1.2	1.2	1.2	0.7	0.8	0.6
Diseases of appendix (K35-K38)	0.1	0.2	0.1	0.1	0.2	*
Hernia (K40-K46)	0.8	0.6	0.9	0.4	0.3	0.5
Chronic liver disease and cirrhosis (K70, K73-K74)	13.3	17.5	9.2	7.3	9.8	5.1
Alcoholic liver disease (K70)	6.5	9.4	3.8	3.3	4.6	2.0
Other chronic liver disease and cirrhosis (K73-K74)	6.8	8.1	5.4	4.1	5.2	3.0
Cholelithiasis and other disorders of gallbladder (K80-K82)	1.3	1.3	1.4	0.8	0.7	0.8
Nephritis, nephrotic syndrome and nephrosis(N00-N07, N17-N19, N25-N27)	17.0	17.4	16.6	20.4	20.2	20.6
Acute and rapidly progressive nephritic and nephrotic syndrome (N00-N01,N04)	0.2	0.2	0.2	0.1	0.2	0.1
Chronic glomerulonephritis, nephritis and nephropathy not specified as acute or chronic, and renal sclerosis unspecified (N02-N03, N05-N07, N26)	0.1	0.1	0.1	0.1	*	*
Renal failure (N17-N19)	16.7	17.1	16.4	20.2	20.0	20.5
Other disorders of kidney (N25, N27)	0.0	*	*	*	*	*
Infections of kidney (N10-N12,N13.6,N15.1)	0.2	0.1	0.3	0.2	0.1	0.2
Hyperplasia of prostate (N40)	0.2	0.5	X	0.1	0.2	X
Inflammatory diseases of female pelvic organs (N70-N76)	0.0	X	0.1	0.0	X	0.1
Pregnancy, childbirth and the puerperium (O00-O99)	0.3	X	0.5	0.9	X	1.7
Pregnancy with abortive outcome (O00-O07)	*	X	*	*	X	*
Other complications of pregnancy, childbirth and the puerperium (O10-O99)	0.3	X	0.5	0.9	X	1.7
Certain conditions originating in the perinatal period(P00-P96)	2.5	2.9	2.2	9.4	10.8	8.2
Congenital malformations, deformations and chromosomal abnormalities (Q00-Q99)	2.9	3.1	2.7	3.7	4.0	3.5
Symptoms, signs and abnormal clinical and laboratory findings, not elsewhere classified (R00-R99)	15.0	12.5	17.3	10.9	11.0	10.7
All other diseases (Residual)	129.9	105.1	154.0	81.0	70.7	90.4
Accidents (unintentional injuries) (V01-X59, Y85-Y86)	50.2	62.1	38.6	32.3	45.3	20.3
Transport accidents (V01-V99, Y85)	13.0	18.8	7.4	12.1	18.4	6.3
Motor vehicle accidents (V02-V04, V09.0, V09.2, V12-V14, V19.0-V19.2, V19.4-V19.6, V20-V79, V80.3-V80.5, V81.0-V81.1, V82.0-V82.1,V83-V86, V87.0-V87.8, V88.0-V88.8, V89.0, V89.2)	12.1	17.2	7.1	11.4	17.3	6.0
Other land transport accidents (V01, V05-V06, V09.1, V09.3-V09.9, V10-V11, V15-V18, V19.3, V19.8-V19.9, V80.0-V80.2, V80.6-V80.9, V81.2-V81.9, V82.2-V82.9, V87.9, V88.9, V89.1, V89.3, V89.9)	0.3	0.5	0.1	0.3	0.6	*
Water, air and space, and other and unspecified transport accidents and their sequelae (V90-V99, Y85)	0.6	1.0	0.2	0.3	0.5	0.2
Nontransport accidents (W00-X59, Y86)	37.1	43.3	31.2	20.2	26.9	14.0
Falls (W00-W19)	13.1	13.0	13.2	3.4	4.2	2.7
Accidental discharge of firearms (W32-W34)	0.2	0.3	0.0	0.2	0.4	*
Accidental drowning and submersion (W65-W74)	1.1	1.6	0.5	1.3	2.1	0.4
Accidental exposure to smoke, fire and flames(X00-X09)	1.0	1.2	0.7	1.3	1.6	1.1
Accidental poisoning and exposure to noxious substances (X40-X49)	15.3	19.6	11.1	9.2	12.8	5.8
Other and unspecified nontransport accidents and their sequelae (W20-W31, W35-W64, W75-W99, X10-X39, X50-X59, Y86)	6.6	7.6	5.6	4.8	5.8	3.9
Intentional self-harm (suicide) (*U03, X60-X84, Y87.0)	17.0	26.9	7.5	5.6	9.5	2.1
Intentional self-harm (suicide) by discharge of firearms (X72-X74)	9.2	16.1	2.6	2.6	4.9	0.5
Intentional self-harm (suicide) by other and unspecified means and their sequelae (*U03, X60-X71, X75-X84, Y87.0)	7.8	10.8	4.9	3.0	4.5	1.6
Assault (homicide) (*U01-*U02, X85-Y09, Y87.1)	2.5	3.3	1.7	19.5	35.1	5.2
Assault (homicide) by discharge of firearms (*U01.4, X93-X95)	1.4	2.0	0.8	15.6	29.4	3.0

Table 2-13B. Death Rates from Selected Causes, by Hispanic Origin, Race for Non-Hispanic Population, and Sex, 2010 — continued

(Rates per 100,000 population in specified group.)

Cause of death (based on ICD-10, 2004)	Non-Hispanic White			Non-Hispanic Black		
	Both sexes	Male	Female	Both sexes	Male	Female
Assault (homicide) by other and unspecified means and their sequelae (*U01.0-*U01.3, *U01.5-*U01.9, *U02, X85-X92, X96-Y09, Y87.1)	1.1	1.4	0.8	3.9	5.7	2.2
Legal intervention (Y35, Y89.0)	0.1	0.3	*	0.3	0.7	*
Events of undetermined intent (Y10-Y34, Y87.2,Y89.9)	1.7	2.0	1.5	1.4	2.0	0.9
Discharge of firearms, undetermined intent (Y22-Y24)	0.1	0.2	0.0	0.1	0.2	*
Other and unspecified events of undetermined intent and their sequelae (Y10-Y21, Y25-Y34, Y87.2, Y89.9)	1.6	1.8	1.5	1.3	1.8	0.8
Operations of war and their sequelae (Y36, Y89.1)	*	*	*	*	*	*
Complications of medical and surgical care (Y40-Y84, Y88)	1.1	1.0	1.1	1.0	1.0	1.0
Enterocolitis due to Clostridium difficile (A04.7)[3]	3.2	2.5	3.9	1.4	1.3	1.5
Drug-induced deaths[4,5]	18.6	22.6	14.7	10.5	14.2	7.1
Alcohol-induced deaths[4,6]	10.6	15.6	5.7	6.2	9.5	3.1
Injury by firearms[4,7]	11.0	18.8	3.5	18.9	35.5	3.6

X = Not applicable.   - = Quantity zero.   * = Figure does not meet standards of reliability or precision.   1 Figures for origin not stated are included in "All origins" but not distributed among specified origins.   2 Includes races other than White and Black.   3 Included in certain other intestinal infections (A04, A07–A09). Beginning with data year 2006, Enterocolitis due to Clostridium difficile (A04.7) is shown separately at the bottom of the table and is included in the list of rankable causes.   4 Included in selected categories above.   5 Includes ICD–10 codes D52.1, D59.0, D59.2, D61.1, D64.2, E06.4, E16.0, E23.1, E24.2, E27.3, E66.1, F11.1-F11.5, F11.7-F11.9, F12.1-F12.5, F12.7-F12.9, F13.1-F13.5, F13.7-F13.9, F14.1-F14.5, F14.7-F14.9, F15.1-F15.5, F15.7-F15.9, F16.1-F16.5, F16.7-16.9, F17.3-F17.5, F17.7-F17.9, F18.1-F18.5, F18.7-F18.9, F19.1-F19.5, F19.7-F19.9, G21.1, G24.0, G25.1, G25.4, G25.6, G44.4, G62.0, G72.0, I95.2, J70.2-J70.4, K85.3, L10.5, L27.0-L27.1, M10.2, M32.0, M80.4, M81.4, M83.5, M87.1, R50.2, R78.1-R78.5, X40-X44, X60-X64, X85, and Y10-Y14. Trend data for Drug-induced deaths, previously shown in this report, can be found through a link from the online version of this report, available from http://www.cdc.gov/nchs/deaths.htm.   6 Includes ICD–10 codes E24.4, F10, G31.2, G62.1, G72.1, I42.6, K29.2, K70, K85.2, K86.0, R78.0, X45, X65, and Y15. Trend data for Alcohol-induced deaths, previously shown in this report, can be found through a link from the online version of this report, available from http://www.cdc.gov/nchs/deaths.htm.   7 Includes ICD–10 codes *U01.4, W32-W34, X72-X74, X93-X95, Y22-Y24, and Y35.0. Trend data for Injury by firearms, previously shown in this report, can be found through a link from the online version of this report, available from http://www.cdc.gov/nchs/deaths.htm.

Figure 2-4. Age-Adjusted Death Rates for Selected Causes, 2013

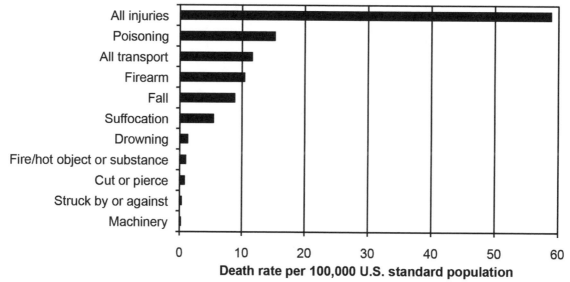

Death rate per 100,000 U.S. standard population

Figure 2.5. Age-Adjusted Death Rates for Injury Deaths, by Mechanism, 2013

Death rate per 100,000 U.S. standard population

Table 2-14A. Age-Adjusted Death Rates from Selected Causes, by Race and Sex, 2013

(Age-adjusted rates per 100,000 U.S. standard population.)

Cause of death (based on ICD-10, 2004)	All races			White[1]			Black[1]		
	Both sexes	Male	Female	Both sexes	Male	Female	Both sexes	Male	Female
All Causes	731.9	863.6	623.5	731.0	859.2	623.6	860.8	1,052.8	720.6
Salmonella infections (A01-A02)	0.0	0.0	*	0.0	0.0	*	*	*	*
Shigellosis and amebiasis (A03, A06)	*	*	*	*	*	*	*	*	*
Certain other intestinal infections (A04, A07-A09)	3.0	2.9	3.1	3.1	2.9	3.2	2.6	2.9	2.4
Tuberculosis (A16-A19)	0.1	0.2	0.1	0.1	0.2	0.1	0.3	0.4	0.2
Respiratory tuberculosis (A16)	0.1	0.2	0.1	0.1	0.1	0.0	0.2	0.3	0.1
Other tuberculosis (A17-A19)	0.0	0.0	0.0	0.0	0.0	0.0	0.1	*	*
Whooping cough (A37)	*	*	*	*	*	*	*	*	*
Scarlet fever and erysipelas (A38, A46)	*	*	*	*	*	*	*	*	*
Meningococcal infection (A39)	0.0	0.0	0.0	0.0	0.0	0.0	*	*	*
Septicemia (A40-A41)	10.7	11.9	9.9	10.1	11.2	9.3	18.3	21.0	16.5
Syphilis (A50-A53)	0.0	0.0	0.0	0.0	*	*	0.1	*	*
Acute poliomyelitis (A80)	*	*	*	*	*	*	*	*	*
Arthropod-borne viral encephalitis (A83-A84, A85.2)	*	*	*	*	*	*	*	*	*
Measles (B05)	*	*	*	*	*	*	*	*	*
Viral hepatitis (B15-B19)	2.1	3.0	1.4	2.1	2.9	1.3	2.9	4.1	1.9
Human immunodeficiency virus (HIV) disease (B20-B24)	2.1	3.1	1.1	1.2	1.9	0.4	8.9	12.7	5.7
Malaria (B50-B54)	*	*	*	*	*	*	*	*	*
Other and unspecified infectious and parasitic diseases and their sequelae (A00, A05, A20-A36, A42-A44, A48-A49, A54-A79, A81-A82, A85.0-A85.1, A85.8, A86-B04, B06-B09, B25-B49, B55-B99)	1.7	2.0	1.5	1.7	2.0	1.4	2.3	2.7	1.9
Malignant neoplasms (C00-C97)	163.2	196.0	139.5	163.7	195.5	140.2	189.2	238.7	158.5
Malignant neoplasms of lip, oral cavity and pharynx (C00-C14)	2.4	3.7	1.3	2.4	3.7	1.3	2.8	4.8	1.4
Malignant neoplasm of esophagus (C15)	4.0	7.2	1.5	4.2	7.5	1.5	3.5	5.9	1.8
Malignant neoplasm of stomach (C16)	3.2	4.3	2.3	2.8	3.8	2.0	5.6	8.2	3.8
Malignant neoplasms of colon, rectum and anus (C18-C21)	14.6	17.4	12.3	14.3	16.9	12.1	19.4	24.7	15.8
Malignant neoplasms of liver and intrahepatic bile ducts (C22)	6.5	9.6	3.9	6.1	8.8	3.6	8.4	13.5	4.5
Malignant neoplasm of pancreas (C25)	10.8	12.4	9.5	10.7	12.4	9.3	13.4	14.8	12.2
Malignant neoplasm of larynx (C32)	1.0	1.8	0.4	1.0	1.8	0.4	1.6	3.1	0.6
Malignant neoplasms of trachea, bronchus and lung(C33-C34)	43.4	53.7	35.5	44.1	53.7	36.7	46.8	65.7	34.1
Malignant melanoma of skin (C43)	2.7	4.0	1.6	3.1	4.6	1.9	0.4	0.5	0.3
Malignant neoplasm of breast (C50)	11.5	0.3	20.8	11.2	0.3	20.4	16.6	0.5	28.3
Malignant neoplasm of cervix uteri (C53)	1.2	X	2.3	1.1	X	2.2	2.2	X	3.9
Malignant neoplasms of corpus uteri and uterus, part unspecified (C54-C55)	2.6	X	4.7	2.3	X	4.3	4.9	X	8.3
Malignant neoplasm of ovary (C56)	4.0	X	7.2	4.1	X	7.5	3.5	X	6.0
Malignant neoplasm of prostate (C61)	7.8	19.2	X	7.3	17.9	X	14.1	38.7	X
Malignant neoplasms of kidney and renal pelvis (C64-C65)	3.9	5.6	2.5	4.0	5.8	2.5	3.5	5.3	2.3
Malignant neoplasm of bladder (C67)	4.4	7.7	2.1	4.6	8.1	2.2	3.5	5.3	2.4
Malignant neoplasms of meninges, brain and other parts of central nervous system (C70-C72)	4.3	5.2	3.6	4.7	5.6	4.0	2.4	3.2	1.9
Malignant neoplasms of lymphoid, hematopoietic and related tissue (C81-C96)	16.2	21.1	12.5	16.5	21.6	12.6	16.5	20.7	13.7
Hodgkin's disease (C81)	0.3	0.4	0.3	0.3	0.4	0.3	0.3	0.3	0.2
Non-Hodgkin's lymphoma (C82-C85)	5.7	7.3	4.5	6.0	7.6	4.6	4.1	5.2	3.3
Leukemia (C91-C95)	6.7	9.0	5.0	7.0	9.4	5.2	5.6	7.6	4.3
Multiple myeloma and immunoproliferative neoplasms (C88, C90)	3.4	4.3	2.8	3.2	4.1	2.5	6.5	7.5	5.8
Other and unspecified malignant neoplasms of lymphoid, hematopoietic and related tissue (C96)	0.0	0.0	0.0	0.0	0.0	0.0	*	*	*
All other and unspecified malignant neoplasms (C17, C23-C24, C26-C31, C37-C41, C44-C49, C51- C52, C57-C60, C62-C63, C66, C68-C69, C73-C80, C97)	18.7	22.7	15.6	18.9	23.0	15.7	20.1	23.9	17.5
In situ neoplasms, benign neoplasms and neoplasms of uncertain or unknown behavior (D00-D48)	4.3	5.5	3.5	4.5	5.7	3.6	3.7	4.6	3.1
Anemias (D50-D64)	1.4	1.4	1.4	1.2	1.3	1.2	2.6	2.8	2.5
Diabetes mellitus (E10-E14)	21.2	25.6	17.6	19.4	23.9	15.7	38.4	44.0	34.3
Nutritional deficiencies (E40-E64)	0.9	0.9	0.9	0.9	0.9	0.9	1.4	1.5	1.2
Malnutrition (E40-E46)	0.9	0.9	0.9	0.9	0.8	0.9	1.3	1.5	1.2
Other nutritional deficiencies (E50-E64)	0.0	0.0	0.0	0.0	0.0	0.0	*	*	*
Meningitis (G00,G03)	0.2	0.2	0.1	0.2	0.2	0.1	0.2	0.2	0.2
Parkinson's disease (G20-G21)	7.3	11.0	4.8	7.8	11.7	5.1	3.6	5.9	2.2
Alzheimer's disease (G30)	23.5	19.3	25.9	24.4	19.9	27.1	20.1	17.3	21.2
Major cardiovascular diseases (I00-I78)	221.7	268.4	183.6	218.0	264.4	179.7	284.1	345.3	238.6
Diseases of heart (I00-I09, I11, I13, I20-I51)	169.8	214.5	134.3	168.2	213.1	132.0	210.4	262.8	172.1
Acute rheumatic fever and chronic rheumatic heart diseases (I00-I09)	0.9	0.8	1.0	0.9	0.8	1.0	0.7	0.6	0.7
Hypertensive heart disease (I11)	10.3	11.9	8.7	9.0	10.3	7.6	22.9	28.5	18.5
Hypertensive heart and renal disease (I13)	1.1	1.3	1.0	0.9	1.0	0.8	2.9	3.6	2.4
Ischemic heart diseases (I20-I25)	102.6	138.2	74.9	102.9	139.2	74.2	117.5	152.0	92.7
Acute myocardial infarction (I21-I22)	32.4	42.9	24.0	32.7	43.4	23.8	36.9	46.2	30.1
Other acute ischemic heart diseases (I24)	1.1	1.3	0.9	1.0	1.3	0.8	1.6	2.0	1.4
Other forms of chronic ischemic heart disease (I20, I25)	69.1	94.0	50.1	69.2	94.4	49.5	78.9	103.8	61.3
Atherosclerotic cardiovascular disease, so described (I25.0)	16.3	22.4	11.1	15.7	21.6	10.6	24.2	34.5	16.6
All other forms of chronic ischemic heart disease (I20,I25.1-I25.9)	52.8	71.6	39.0	53.4	72.8	38.9	54.7	69.3	44.6
Other heart diseases (I26-I51)	54.8	62.4	48.7	54.5	61.9	48.4	66.4	78.0	57.8
Acute and subacute endocarditis (I33)	0.4	0.5	0.3	0.3	0.5	0.2	0.4	0.7	0.3
Diseases of pericardium and acute myocarditis (I30-I31, I40)	0.2	0.3	0.2	0.2	0.3	0.2	0.4	0.4	0.4
Heart failure (I50)	18.0	20.2	16.3	18.1	20.3	16.4	20.4	23.5	18.2
All other forms of heart disease (I26-I28, I34-I38, I42-I49, I51)	36.2	41.4	31.8	35.8	40.8	31.5	45.3	53.5	39.0

Table 2-14A. Age-Adjusted Death Rates from Selected Causes, by Race and Sex, 2013— continued

(Age-adjusted rates per 100,000 U.S. standard population.)

Cause of death (based on ICD-10, 2004)	All races			White[1]			Black[1]		
	Both sexes	Male	Female	Both sexes	Male	Female	Both sexes	Male	Female
Essential hypertension and hypertensive renal disease (I10, I12, I15)	8.5	8.7	8.1	7.7	7.7	7.4	16.4	18.3	14.7
Cerebrovascular diseases (I60-I69)	36.2	36.7	35.2	34.9	35.0	34.2	49.0	54.1	44.7
Atherosclerosis (I70)	1.8	1.9	1.7	1.9	1.9	1.8	1.7	1.9	1.5
Other diseases of circulatory system (I71-I78)	5.3	6.6	4.3	5.2	6.6	4.2	6.7	8.2	5.5
Aortic aneurysm and dissection (I71)	2.8	3.8	2.0	2.8	3.8	2.0	2.9	3.8	2.2
Other diseases of arteries, arterioles and capillaries (I72-I78)	2.5	2.8	2.3	2.5	2.7	2.2	3.8	4.4	3.4
Other disorders of circulatory system (I80-I99)	1.3	1.4	1.2	1.2	1.3	1.1	2.3	2.6	2.0
Influenza and pneumonia (J09-J18)[1]	15.9	18.6	14.0	15.8	18.3	14.0	16.7	20.8	14.2
Influenza (J09-J11)[1]	1.1	1.2	1.0	1.1	1.2	1.0	0.8	0.8	0.7
Pneumonia (J12-J18)	14.8	17.5	13.0	14.7	17.1	13.0	16.0	20.0	13.5
Other acute lower respiratory infections (J20-J22, U04)[2]	0.1	0.1	0.1	0.1	0.1	0.1	0.1	*	*
Acute bronchitis and bronchiolitis (J20-J21)	0.1	0.1	0.1	0.1	0.1	0.1	0.1	*	*
Other and unspecified acute lower respiratory infections(J22, U04)[2,3]	0.0	0.0	0.0	0.0	*	0.0	*	*	*
Chronic lower respiratory diseases (J40-J47)	42.1	47.5	38.5	44.8	49.5	41.6	29.5	39.1	23.8
Bronchitis, chronic and unspecified (J40-J42)	0.2	0.2	0.2	0.2	0.2	0.2	0.2	0.2	0.2
Emphysema (J43)	2.3	2.9	2.0	2.5	3.0	2.1	1.6	2.4	1.1
Asthma (J45-J46)	1.1	0.9	1.2	0.8	0.7	1.0	2.5	2.5	2.4
Other chronic lower respiratory diseases (J44, J47)	38.5	43.5	35.2	41.2	45.6	38.3	25.2	34.0	20.0
Pneumoconioses and chemical effects (J60-J66, J68)	0.2	0.5	0.0	0.2	0.6	0.0	0.1	0.2	*
Pneumonitis due to solids and liquids (J69)	5.2	7.2	3.9	5.3	7.3	4.0	5.0	7.2	3.8
Other diseases of respiratory system (J00-J06, J30-J39, J67, J70-J98)	10.0	12.0	8.5	10.2	12.3	8.6	9.1	10.3	8.4
Peptic ulcer (K25-K28)	0.8	1.0	0.7	0.8	1.0	0.7	0.8	1.1	0.6
Diseases of appendix (K35-K38)	0.1	0.1	0.1	0.1	0.1	0.1	0.1	0.2	*
Hernia (K40-K46)	0.5	0.5	0.5	0.6	0.5	0.6	0.5	0.5	0.5
Chronic liver disease and cirrhosis (K70, K73-K74)	10.2	13.8	6.8	10.7	14.7	7.1	7.3	10.4	4.8
Alcoholic liver disease (K70)	5.1	7.5	2.9	5.5	8.1	3.0	3.2	4.7	1.9
Other chronic liver disease and cirrhosis (K73-K74)	5.0	6.3	3.9	5.3	6.6	4.1	4.1	5.6	3.0
Cholelithiasis and other disorders of gallbladder (K80-K82)	1.0	1.1	0.8	0.9	1.1	0.8	1.0	1.1	0.9
Nephritis, nephrotic syndrome and nephrosis(N00-N07, N17-N19, N25-N27)	13.2	16.1	11.3	12.1	14.9	10.2	25.0	29.8	22.0
Acute and rapidly progressive nephritic and nephrotic syndrome (N00-N01,N04)	0.1	0.1	0.1	0.1	0.1	0.1	0.2	0.3	0.1
Chronic glomerulonephritis, nephritis and nephropathy not specified as acute or chronic, and renal sclerosis unspecified (N02-N03, N05-N07, N26)	0.1	0.1	0.0	0.1	0.1	0.0	0.1	*	*
Renal failure (N17-N19)	13.0	15.8	11.1	11.9	14.7	10.0	24.8	29.4	21.8
Other disorders of kidney (N25, N27)	0.0	0.0	*	0.0	*	*	*	*	*
Infections of kidney (N10-N12,N13.6,N15.1)	0.2	0.1	0.2	0.2	0.1	0.2	0.2	0.2	0.2
Hyperplasia of prostate (N40)	0.1	0.4	X	0.2	0.4	X	0.1	0.3	X
Inflammatory diseases of female pelvic organs (N70-N76)	0.0	X	0.1	0.0	X	0.0	0.0	X	0.1
Pregnancy, childbirth and the puerperium (O00-O99)	0.4	X	0.8	0.3	X	0.6	0.8	X	1.6
Pregnancy with abortive outcome (O00-O07)	0.0	X	0.0	*	X	*	*	X	*
Other complications of pregnancy, childbirth and the puerperium (O10-O99)	0.4	X	0.7	0.3	X	0.6	0.8	X	1.6
Certain conditions originating in the perinatal period(P00-P96)	4.2	4.6	3.8	3.5	3.8	3.1	8.3	8.8	7.7
Congenital malformations, deformations and chromosomal abnormalities (Q00-Q99)	3.1	3.3	2.9	3.2	3.4	3.0	3.5	3.6	3.3
Symptoms, signs and abnormal clinical and laboratory findings, not elsewhere classified (R00-R99)	10.7	11.1	10.1	10.7	11.0	10.2	12.4	13.9	11.1
All other diseases (Residual)	89.4	88.1	88.5	90.2	88.4	89.5	100.8	105.7	96.2
Accidents (unintentional injuries) (V01-X59, Y85-Y86)	39.4	53.1	26.6	41.9	55.9	28.5	32.6	47.8	19.9
Transport accidents (V01-V99, Y85)	11.7	17.2	6.5	12.2	17.7	6.7	11.6	18.1	5.9
Motor vehicle accidents (V02-V04, V09.0, V09.2, V12-V14, V19.0-V19.2, V19.4-V19.6, V20-V79, V80.3-V80.5, V81.0-V81.1, V82.0-V82.1,V83- V86, V87.0-V87.8, V88.0-V88.8, V89.0, V89.2)	10.9	15.9	6.2	11.3	16.3	6.4	10.9	17.0	5.7
Other land transport accidents (V01,V05-V06, V09.1, V09.3-V09.9, V10-V11,V15-V18, V19.3,V19.8-V19.9,V80.0-V80.2, V80.6-V80.9, V81.2- V81.9, V82.2-V82.9, V87.9, V88.9, V89.1, V89.3, V89.9)	0.3	0.5	0.1	0.3	0.5	0.1	0.3	0.6	0.1
Water, air and space, and other and unspecified transport accidents and their sequelae (V90-V99, Y85)	0.5	0.8	0.2	0.5	0.8	0.2	0.3	0.5	0.2
Nontransport accidents (W00-X59, Y86)	27.7	36.0	20.1	29.7	38.2	21.8	21.0	29.8	14.0
Falls (W00-W19)	8.5	10.6	6.9	9.1	11.1	7.4	4.2	6.1	2.9
Accidental discharge of firearms (W32-W34)	0.2	0.3	0.0	0.2	0.3	0.0	0.2	0.4	*
Accidental drowning and submersion (W65-W74)	1.1	1.6	0.5	1.0	1.6	0.5	1.2	2.0	0.4
Accidental exposure to smoke, fire and flames(X00-X09)	0.8	1.0	0.6	0.8	1.0	0.6	1.4	1.7	1.1
Accidental poisoning and exposure to noxious substances (X40-X49)	12.2	16.0	8.5	13.7	17.6	9.7	8.9	12.8	5.6
Other and unspecified nontransport accidents and their sequelae (W20-W31, W35-W64, W75-W99, X10-X39, X50-X59, Y86)	4.9	6.5	3.5	5.0	6.6	3.5	5.2	6.8	3.9
Intentional self-harm (suicide) (*U03, X60-X84, Y87.0)	12.6	20.3	5.5	14.2	22.6	6.3	5.4	9.3	2.0
Intentional self-harm (suicide) by discharge of firearms (X72-X74)	6.4	11.5	1.8	7.4	13.0	2.1	2.6	4.9	0.5
Intentional self-harm (suicide) by other and unspecified means and their sequelae (*U03, X60-X71, X75-X84, Y87.0)	6.2	8.8	3.7	6.9	9.6	4.2	2.9	4.4	1.5
Assault (homicide) (*U01-*U02, X85-Y09, Y87.1)	5.2	8.2	2.1	3.1	4.4	1.7	17.8	31.6	4.9
Assault (homicide) by discharge of firearms (*U01.4, X93-X95)	3.6	6.1	1.1	1.8	2.8	0.8	14.1	26.0	2.8
Assault (homicide) by other and unspecified means and their sequelae (*U01.0-*U01.3, *U01.5-*U01.9, *U02, X85-X92, X96-Y09, Y87.1)	1.5	2.1	1.0	1.2	1.6	0.9	3.7	5.6	2.1
Legal intervention (Y35, Y89.0)	0.2	0.3	0.0	0.1	0.3	*	0.3	0.7	*
Events of undetermined intent (Y10-Y34, Y87.2,Y89.9)	1.4	1.7	1.1	1.5	1.8	1.3	1.3	1.9	0.9
Discharge of firearms, undetermined intent (Y22-Y24)	0.1	0.1	0.0	0.1	0.1	0.0	0.1	0.2	*
Other and unspecified events of undetermined intent and their sequelae (Y10-Y21, Y25-Y34, Y87.2, Y89.9)	1.3	1.6	1.1	1.4	1.6	1.2	1.3	1.8	0.8

Table 2-14A. Age-Adjusted Death Rates from Selected Causes, by Race and Sex, 2013— continued

(Age-adjusted rates per 100,000 U.S. standard population.)

Cause of death (based on ICD-10, 2004)	All races			White[1]			Black[1]		
	Both sexes	Male	Female	Both sexes	Male	Female	Both sexes	Male	Female
Operations of war and their sequelae (Y36, Y89.1)	*	*	*	*	*	*	*	*	*
Complications of medical and surgical care (Y40-Y84, Y88)	0.8	0.9	0.7	0.8	0.9	0.7	1.1	1.2	1.0
Enterocolitis due to Clostridium difficile (A04.7)[4]	2.1	2.1	2.2	2.2	2.2	2.3	1.8	2.1	1.6
Drug-induced deaths[5,6]	14.6	18.0	11.1	16.4	20.0	12.7	10.2	14.0	6.8
Alcohol-induced deaths[5,7]	8.2	12.5	4.3	8.7	13.1	4.5	6.0	9.9	2.9
Injury by firearms[5,8]	10.4	18.3	3.0	9.6	16.5	3.0	17.2	32.1	3.4

Table 2-14B. Age-Adjusted Death Rates from Selected Causes, by Race and Sex, 2013

(Age-adjusted rates per 100,000 U.S. standard population.)

Cause of death (based on ICD-10, 2004)	American Indian or Alaska Native[1,2]			Asian or Pacific Islander[1,3]		
	Both sexes	Male	Female	Both sexes	Male	Female
All Causes	591.7	689.2	508.3	405.4	487.8	343.0
Salmonella infections (A01-A02)	*	*	*	*	*	*
Shigellosis and amebiasis (A03, A06)	*	*	*	*	*	*
Certain other intestinal infections (A04, A07-A09)	1.9	1.7	2.0	1.3	1.5	1.2
Tuberculosis (A16-A19)	*	*	*	0.7	1.2	0.4
Respiratory tuberculosis (A16)	*	*	*	0.6	1.0	0.3
Other tuberculosis (A17-A19)	*	*	*	*	*	*
Whooping cough (A37)	*	*	*	*	*	*
Scarlet fever and erysipelas (A38, A46)	*	*	*	*	*	*
Meningococcal infection (A39)	*	*	*	*	*	*
Septicemia (A40-A41)	10.2	10.6	9.8	5.0	5.9	4.3
Syphilis (A50-A53)	*	*	*	*	*	*
Acute poliomyelitis (A80)	*	*	*	*	*	*
Arthropod-borne viral encephalitis (A83-A84, A85.2)	*	*	*	*	*	*
Measles (B05)	*	*	*	*	*	*
Viral hepatitis (B15-B19)	3.3	4.1	2.6	1.9	2.2	1.6
Human immunodeficiency virus (HIV) disease (B20-B24)	1.3	2.1	*	0.4	0.7	*
Malaria (B50-B54)	*	*	*	*	*	*
Other and unspecified infectious and parasitic diseases and their sequelae (A00, A05, A20-A36, A42-A44, A48-A49, A54-A79, A81-A82, A85.0-A85.1, A85.8, A86-B04, B06-B09, B25-B49, B55-B99)	1.7	2.0	1.5	1.0	1.1	0.9
Malignant neoplasms (C00-C97)	110.2	132.3	94.3	100.5	120.9	86.0
Malignant neoplasms of lip, oral cavity and pharynx (C00-C14)	1.1	1.7	*	1.9	2.7	1.2
Malignant neoplasm of esophagus (C15)	2.5	4.5	*	1.7	3.0	0.7
Malignant neoplasm of stomach (C16)	3.4	4.1	3.0	5.2	6.9	3.9
Malignant neoplasms of colon, rectum and anus (C18-C21)	12.6	15.0	10.9	9.8	11.8	8.2
Malignant neoplasms of liver and intrahepatic bile ducts (C22)	8.0	10.8	5.5	9.5	14.2	5.8
Malignant neoplasm of pancreas (C25)	6.8	7.3	6.2	7.5	8.3	6.9
Malignant neoplasm of larynx (C32)	*	*	*	0.4	0.8	*
Malignant neoplasms of trachea, bronchus and lung(C33-C34)	27.7	34.4	22.9	23.3	30.6	18.0
Malignant melanoma of skin (C43)	*	*	*	0.3	0.4	0.2
Malignant neoplasm of breast (C50)	5.5	*	10.1	6.3	*	11.1
Malignant neoplasm of cervix uteri (C53)	0.9	X	1.7	1.1	X	1.9
Malignant neoplasms of corpus uteri and uterus, part unspecified (C54-C55)	1.2	X	2.3	1.6	X	2.9
Malignant neoplasm of ovary (C56)	2.4	X	4.5	2.5	X	4.5
Malignant neoplasm of prostate (C61)	5.7	14.0	X	3.5	8.6	X
Malignant neoplasms of kidney and renal pelvis (C64-C65)	4.3	5.7	3.2	1.7	2.6	1.0
Malignant neoplasm of bladder (C67)	1.7	2.5	*	1.8	2.8	1.0
Malignant neoplasms of meninges, brain and other parts of central nervous system (C70-C72)	2.0	2.1	1.9	2.2	2.6	1.9
Malignant neoplasms of lymphoid, hematopoietic and related tissue (C81-C96)	9.5	11.7	7.9	9.2	12.2	7.0
Hodgkin's disease (C81)	*	*	*	0.1	*	*
Non-Hodgkin's lymphoma (C82-C85)	3.4	4.2	2.6	3.9	5.0	3.2
Leukemia (C91-C95)	3.6	4.3	3.1	3.7	4.9	2.7
Multiple myeloma and immunoproliferative neoplasms (C88, C90)	2.4	2.9	2.1	1.5	2.1	1.0
Other and unspecified malignant neoplasms of lymphoid, hematopoietic and related tissue (C96)	*	*	*	*	*	*
All other and unspecified malignant neoplasms (C17, C23-C24, C26-C31, C37-C41, C44-C49, C51-C52, C57-C60, C62-C63, C66, C68-C69, C73-C80, C97)	13.7	16.9	11.0	11.2	13.1	9.6
In situ neoplasms, benign neoplasms and neoplasms of uncertain or unknown behavior (D00-D48)	2.3	3.3	1.6	2.6	3.0	2.3
Anemias (D50-D64)	0.9	*	*	0.6	0.8	0.6
Diabetes mellitus (E10-E14)	34.1	37.9	30.9	15.8	19.4	13.1
Nutritional deficiencies (E40-E64)	1.3	*	*	0.6	0.6	0.5
Malnutrition (E40-E46)	1.2	*	*	0.5	0.6	0.5
Other nutritional deficiencies (E50-E64)	*	*	*	*	*	*
Meningitis (G00,G03)	*	*	*	0.1	*	*
Parkinson's disease (G20-G21)	3.5	4.9	2.5	4.0	5.6	2.9
Alzheimer's disease (G30)	12.7	10.0	14.3	11.1	9.0	12.4
Major cardiovascular diseases (I00-I78)	157.5	187.4	131.3	133.5	162.2	111.4
Diseases of heart (I00-I09, I11, I13, I20-I51)	120.6	152.3	93.9	92.8	118.4	73.3
Acute rheumatic fever and chronic rheumatic heart diseases (I00-I09)	0.8	*	*	0.8	0.7	0.8
Hypertensive heart disease (I11)	8.3	10.0	6.5	5.3	5.6	4.9
Hypertensive heart and renal disease (I13)	*	*	*	1.1	1.0	1.1
Ischemic heart diseases (I20-I25)	78.2	104.8	56.5	59.9	81.5	43.8
Acute myocardial infarction (I21-I22)	23.0	30.2	17.1	18.3	24.8	13.4
Other acute ischemic heart diseases (I24)	0.8	*	*	0.5	0.4	0.5
Other forms of chronic ischemic heart disease (I20, I25)	54.4	73.4	38.9	41.2	56.3	29.9
Atherosclerotic cardiovascular disease, so described (I25.0)	17.4	22.5	12.7	9.1	12.3	6.4
All other forms of chronic ischemic heart disease (I20,I25.1-I25.9)	37.0	50.9	26.2	32.1	44.0	23.5
Other heart diseases (I26-I51)	32.6	36.1	29.1	25.7	29.6	22.7
Acute and subacute endocarditis (I33)	*	*	*	0.1	*	*
Diseases of pericardium and acute myocarditis (I30-I31, I40)	*	*	*	0.1	*	*

Table 2-14B. Age-Adjusted Death Rates from Selected Causes, by Race and Sex, 2013— continued

(Age-adjusted rates per 100,000 U.S. standard population.)

Cause of death (based on ICD-10, 2004)	American Indian or Alaska Native[1,2]			Asian or Pacific Islander[1,3]		
	Both sexes	Male	Female	Both sexes	Male	Female
Heart failure (I50)	11.1	10.9	10.9	7.2	8.1	6.5
All other forms of heart disease (I26-I28, I34-I38, I42-I49, I51)	20.7	24.4	17.4	18.2	21.1	15.9
Essential hypertension and hypertensive renal disease (I10, I12, I15)	7.5	8.0	7.0	7.2	7.7	6.8
Cerebrovascular diseases (I60-I69)	24.6	22.7	25.5	29.4	31.2	27.9
Atherosclerosis (I70)	1.4	*	*	1.0	1.0	0.9
Other diseases of circulatory system (I71-I78)	3.4	3.4	3.5	3.1	4.0	2.4
Aortic aneurysm and dissection (I71)	1.5	*	1.5	2.0	2.5	1.5
Other diseases of arteries, arterioles and capillaries (I72-I78)	2.0	2.1	1.9	1.2	1.5	0.9
Other disorders of circulatory system (I80-I99)	0.9	*	*	0.4	0.4	0.5
Influenza and pneumonia (J09-J18)	15.0	17.6	13.3	15.0	18.6	12.5
Influenza (J09-J11)	1.0	*	1.2	0.7	0.09	0.6
Pneumonia (J12-J18)	14.0	16.9	12.1	14.3	17.8	12.0
Other acute lower respiratory infections (J20-J22, U04)	*	*	*	*	*	*
Acute bronchitis and bronchiolitis (J20-J21)	*	*	*	*	*	*
Other and unspecified acute lower respiratory infections(J22, U04)	*	*	*	*	*	*
Chronic lower respiratory diseases (J40-J47)	30.8	36.3	27.4	13.6	20.4	9.1
Bronchitis, chronic and unspecified (J40-J42)	*	*	*	*	*	*
Emphysema (J43)	1.6	2.0	1.4	0.8	1.4	0.4
Asthma (J45-J46)	1.1	*	*	1.1	1.2	1.1
Other chronic lower respiratory diseases (J44, J47)	28.0	33.2	24.9	11.5	17.7	7.4
Pneumoconioses and chemical effects (J60-J66, J68)	*	*	*	*	*	*
Pneumonitis due to solids and liquids (J69)	3.4	4.6	2.5	3.3	4.7	2.3
Other diseases of respiratory system (J00-J06, J30-J39, J67, J70-J98)	9.5	10.9	8.6	5.8	7.2	4.9
Peptic ulcer (K25-K28)	*	*	*	0.9	1.2	0.6
Diseases of appendix (K35-K38)	*	*	*	*	*	*
Hernia (K40-K46)	*	*	*	0.2	*	*
Chronic liver disease and cirrhosis (K70, K73-K74)	24.8	27.2	22.5	3.3	4.6	2.2
Alcoholic liver disease (K70)	17.8	21.7	14.1	1.1	1.9	0.4
Other chronic liver disease and cirrhosis (K73-K74)	7.0	5.5	8.4	2.2	2.7	1.8
Cholelithiasis and other disorders of gallbladder (K80-K82)	1.6	*	1.5	0.8	1.1	0.7
Nephritis, nephrotic syndrome and nephrosis(N00-N07, N17-N19, N25-N27)	11.4	12.8	10.7	8.1	9.8	6.9
Acute and rapidly progressive nephritic and nephrotic syndrome (N00-N01,N04)	*	*	*	*	*	*
Chronic glomerulonephritis, nephritis and nephropathy not specified as acute or chronic, and renal sclerosis unspecified (N02-N03, N05-N07, N26)	*	*	*	*	*	*
Renal failure (N17-N19)	11.3	12.7	10.5	7.9	9.6	6.8
Other disorders of kidney (N25, N27)	*	*	*	*	*	*
Infections of kidney (N10-N12,N13.6,N15.1)	*	*	*	0.2	*	*
Hyperplasia of prostate (N40)	*	*	X	*	*	X
Inflammatory diseases of female pelvic organs (N70-N76)	*	X	*	*	X	*
Pregnancy, childbirth and the puerperium (O00-O99)	*	X	*	0.2	X	0.4
Pregnancy with abortive outcome (O00-O07)	*	X	*	*	X	*
Other complications of pregnancy, childbirth and the puerperium (O10-O99)	*	X	*	0.2	X	0.4
Certain conditions originating in the perinatal period(P00-P96)	1.8	2.4	1.3	2.8	3.2	2.5
Congenital malformations, deformations and chromosomal abnormalities (Q00-Q99)	2.4	3.2	1.7	1.8	1.9	1.7
Symptoms, signs and abnormal clinical and laboratory findings, not elsewhere classified (R00-R99)	7.4	7.5	7.1	4.6	4.7	4.3
All other diseases (Residual)	72.0	71.5	71.0	41.8	42.0	41.1
Accidents (unintentional injuries) (V01-X59, Y85-Y86)	47.1	60.8	34.1	15.2	20.8	10.6
Transport accidents (V01-V99, Y85)	16.6	22.0	11.4	5.2	7.0	3.6
Motor vehicle accidents (V02-V04, V09.0, V09.2, V12-V14, V19.0-V19.2, V19.4-V19.6, V20-V79, V80.3-V80.5, V81.0-V81.1, V82.0-V82.1,V83-V86, V87.0-V87.8, V88.0-V88.8, V89.0, V89.2)	15.4	20.0	11.0	4.8	6.4	3.4
Other land transport accidents (V01,V05-V06, V09.1, V09.3-V09.9, V10-V11,V15-V18, V19.3, V19.8-V19.9, V80.0-V80.2, V80.6-V80.9, V81.2-V81.9, V82.2-V82.9, V87.9, V88.9, V89.1, V89.3, V89.9)	0.4	*	*	0.2	0.3	*
Water, air and space, and other and unspecified transport accidents and their sequelae (V90-V99, Y85)	0.7	1.3	*	0.2	0.3	*
Nontransport accidents (W00-X59, Y86)	30.5	38.8	22.7	10.0	13.8	7.0
Falls (W00-W19)	7.3	9.0	5.9	4.9	6.4	3.9
Accidental discharge of firearms (W32-W34)	*	*	*	*	*	*
Accidental drowning and submersion (W65-W74)	1.6	2.5	*	1.0	1.6	0.5
Accidental exposure to smoke, fire and flames(X00-X09)	1.3	1.5	*	0.2	0.3	*
Accidental poisoning and exposure to noxious substances (X40-X49)	14.2	17.3	11.0	2.0	3.0	1.1
Other and unspecified nontransport accidents and their sequelae (W20-W31, W35-W64, W75-W99, X10-X39, X50-X59, Y86)	6.0	8.2	3.9	1.9	2.5	1.4
Intentional self-harm (suicide) (*U03, X60-X84, Y87.0)	11.7	18.1	5.3	5.9	9.1	3.0
Intentional self-harm (suicide) by discharge of firearms (X72-X74)	4.7	8.6	1.1	1.4	2.5	0.4
Intentional self-harm (suicide) by other and unspecified means and their sequelae (*U03, X60-X71, X75-X84, Y87.0)	6.9	9.6	4.3	4.5	6.5	2.6
Assault (homicide) (*U01-*U02, X85-Y09, Y87.1)	5.3	8.2	2.4	1.5	2.3	0.9
Assault (homicide) by discharge of firearms (*U01.4, X93-X95)	2.4	3.9	*	0.9	1.4	0.4

Table 2-14B. Age-Adjusted Death Rates from Selected Causes, by Race and Sex, 2013— continued

(Age-adjusted rates per 100,000 U.S. standard population.)

Cause of death (based on ICD-10, 2004)	American Indian or Alaska Native[1,2]			Asian or Pacific Islander[1,3]		
	Both sexes	Male	Female	Both sexes	Male	Female
Assault (homicide) by other and unspecified means and their sequelae (*U01.0-*U01.3, *U01.5-*U01.9, *U02, X85-X92, X96-Y09, Y87.1)	2.9	4.4	1.5	0.7	0.9	0.4
Legal intervention (Y35, Y89.0)	*	*	*	*	*	*
Events of undetermined intent (Y10-Y34, Y87.2,Y89.9)	1.5	1.8	1.3	0.4	0.5	0.3
Discharge of firearms, undetermined intent (Y22-Y24)	*	*	*	*	*	*
Other and unspecified events of undetermined intent and their sequelae (Y10-Y21, Y25-Y34, Y87.2, Y89.9)	1.5	1.7	1.3	0.4	0.5	0.3
Operations of war and their sequelae (Y36, Y89.1)	*	*	*	*	*	*
Complications of medical and surgical care (Y40-Y84, Y88)	*	*	*	0.3	0.4	0.3
Enterocolitis due to Clostridium difficile (A04.7)[4]	1.5	*	*	0.8	1.0	0.7
Drug-induced deaths[5,6]	13.2	13.8	12.5	2.5	3.5	1.6
Alcohol-induced deaths[5,7]	26.8	35.6	18.3	1.8	3.0	0.7
Injury by firearms[5,8]	7.4	12.9	2.0	2.4	4.1	0.9

X = Not applicable.   0.0 = Quantity more than zero but less than 0.05.   * = Figure does not meet standards of reliability or precision.   1Race categories are consistent with the 1977 Office of Management and Budget (OMB) standards. Multiple-race data were reported by 42 states and the District of Columbia in 2013. The multiple-race data for these reporting areas were bridged to the single-race categories of the 1977 OMB standards for comparability with other reporting areas.   2Includes Aleuts and Eskimos.   3Includes Chinese, Filipinos, Hawaiians, Japanese, and other Asian and Pacific Islander persons.   4Included in certain other intestinal infections (A04, A07–A09). Beginning with data year 2006, Enterocolitis due to Clostridium difficile (A04.7) is shown separately at the bottom of the table and is included in the list of rankable causes.   5Included in selected categories above.   6Includes ICD–10 codes D52.1, D59.0, D59.2, D61.1, D64.2, E06.4, E16.0, E23.1, E24.2, E27.3, E66.1, F11.1-F11.5, F11.7-F11.9, F12.1-F12.5, F12.7-F12.9, F13.1-F13.5, F13.7-F13.9, F14.1-F14.5, F14.7-F14.9, F15.1-F15.5, F15.7-F15.9, F16.1-F16.5, F16.7-16.9, F17.3-F17.5, F17.7-F17.9, F18.1-F18.5, F18.7-F18.9, F19.1-F19.5, F19.7-F19.9, G21.1, G24.0, G25.1, G25.4, G25.6, G44.4, G62.0, G72.0, I95.2, J70.2-J70.4, K85.3, L10.5, L27.0-L27.1, M10.2, M32.0, M80.4, M81.4, M83.5, M87.1, R50.2, R78.1-R78.5, X40-X44, X60-X64, X85, and Y10-Y14. Trend data for Drug-induced deaths, previously shown in this report, can be found through a link from the online version of this report, available from http://www.cdc.gov/nchs/deaths.htm.   7Includes ICD–10 codes E24.4, F10, G31.2, G62.1, G72.1, I42.6, K29.2, K70, K85.2, K86.0, R78.0, X45, X65, and Y15. Trend data for Alcohol-induced deaths, previously shown in this report, can be found through a link from the online version of this report, available from http://www.cdc.gov/nchs/deaths.htm.   8Includes ICD–10 codes *U01.4, W32-W34, X72-X74, X93-X95, Y22-Y24, and Y35.0. Trend data for Injury by firearms, previously shown in this report, can be found through a link from the online version of this report, available from http://www.cdc.gov/nchs/deaths.htm.

Table 2-15A. Age-Adjusted Death Rates from Selected Causes, by Hispanic Origin, Race for Non-Hispanic Population, and Sex, 2013

(Age-adjusted rates per 100,000 U.S. standard population.)

Cause of death (based on ICD-10, 2004)	All origins[1]			Hispanic (of any race)			Non-Hispanic[2]		
	Both sexes	Male	Female	Both sexes	Male	Female	Both sexes	Male	Female
All Causes	731.9	863.6	623.5	535.4	639.8	448.6	750.1	884.4	639.7
Salmonella infections (A01-A02)	0.0	0.0	*	*	*	*	0.0	0.0	*
Shigellosis and amebiasis (A03, A06)	*	*	*	*	*	*	*	*	*
Certain other intestinal infections (A04, A07-A09)	3.0	2.9	3.1	2.4	2.3	2.4	3.1	2.9	3.1
Tuberculosis (A16-A19)	0.1	0.2	0.1	0.3	0.4	0.2	0.1	0.2	0.1
Respiratory tuberculosis (A16)	0.1	0.2	0.1	0.2	0.3	0.2	0.1	0.1	0.0
Other tuberculosis (A17-A19)	0.0	0.0	0.0	0.0	*	*	0.0	0.0	0.0
Whooping cough (A37)	*	*	*	*	*	*	*	*	*
Scarlet fever and erysipelas (A38, A46)	*	*	*	*	*	*	*	*	*
Meningococcal infection (A39)	0.0	0.0	0.0	*	*	*	0.0	0.0	0.0
Septicemia (A40-A41)	10.7	11.9	9.9	8.4	9.8	7.4	10.9	12.1	10.1
Syphilis (A50-A53)	0.0	0.0	0.0	*	*	*	0.0	0.0	*
Acute poliomyelitis (A80)	*	*	*	*	*	*	*	*	*
Arthropod-borne viral encephalitis (A83-A84, A85.2)	*	*	*	*	*	*	*	*	*
Measles (B05)	*	*	*	*	*	*	*	*	*
Viral hepatitis (B15-B19)	2.1	3.0	1.4	3.2	4.4	2.1	2.0	2.8	1.3
Human immunodeficiency virus (HIV) disease (B20-B24)	2.1	3.1	1.1	2.1	3.4	0.9	2.1	3.1	1.2
Malaria (B50-B54)	*	*	*	*	*	*	*	*	*
Other and unspecified infectious and parasitic diseases and their sequelae (A00, A05, A20-A36, A42-A44, A48- A49, A54-A79, A81-A82, A85.0-A85.1, A85.8, A86-B04, B06-B09, B25-B49, B55-B99)	1.7	2.0	1.5	1.6	1.8	1.3	1.7	2.0	1.5
Malignant neoplasms (C00-C97)	163.2	196.0	139.5	114.5	138.8	97.3	167.5	200.8	143.4
Malignant neoplasms of lip, oral cavity and pharynx (C00-C14)	2.4	3.7	1.3	1.4	2.3	0.7	2.5	3.9	1.4
Malignant neoplasm of esophagus (C15)	4.0	7.2	1.5	1.9	3.5	0.7	4.2	7.5	1.5
Malignant neoplasm of stomach (C16)	3.2	4.3	2.3	5.1	6.7	3.9	2.9	4.1	2.1
Malignant neoplasms of colon, rectum and anus (C18-C21)	14.6	17.4	12.3	11.7	15.0	9.1	14.9	17.6	12.7
Malignant neoplasms of liver and intrahepatic bile ducts (C22)	6.5	9.6	3.9	9.4	13.3	6.0	6.2	9.2	3.7
Malignant neoplasm of pancreas (C25)	10.8	12.4	9.5	8.4	9.0	7.8	11.0	12.7	9.6
Malignant neoplasm of larynx (C32)	1.0	1.8	0.4	0.7	1.5	0.1	1.0	1.8	0.4
Malignant neoplasms of trachea, bronchus and lung(C33-C34)	43.4	53.7	35.5	18.7	26.2	13.2	45.6	56.2	37.5
Malignant melanoma of skin (C43)	2.7	4.0	1.6	0.7	0.9	0.6	2.9	4.3	1.7
Malignant neoplasm of breast (C50)	11.5	0.3	20.8	8.1	0.2	14.6	11.9	0.3	21.4
Malignant neoplasm of cervix uteri (C53)	1.2	X	2.3	1.4	X	2.5	1.2	X	2.3
Malignant neoplasms of corpus uteri and uterus, part unspecified (C54-C55)	2.6	X	4.7	2.1	X	3.8	2.6	X	4.7
Malignant neoplasm of ovary (C56)	4.0	X	7.2	3.0	X	5.4	4.1	X	7.4
Malignant neoplasm of prostate (C61)	7.8	19.2	X	6.4	15.7	X	7.9	19.4	X
Malignant neoplasms of kidney and renal pelvis (C64-C65)	3.9	5.6	2.5	3.4	4.7	2.3	3.9	5.7	2.5
Malignant neoplasm of bladder (C67)	4.4	7.7	2.1	2.4	4.1	1.2	4.6	7.9	2.2
Malignant neoplasms of meninges, brain and other parts of central nervous system (C70-C72)	4.3	5.2	3.6	2.9	3.2	2.6	4.5	5.5	3.7
Malignant neoplasms of lymphoid, hematopoietic and related tissue (C81-C96)	16.2	21.1	12.5	13.0	16.6	10.5	16.4	21.4	12.6
Hodgkin's disease (C81)	0.3	0.4	0.3	0.4	0.5	0.3	0.3	0.4	0.2
Non-Hodgkin's lymphoma (C82-C85)	5.7	7.3	4.5	4.9	6.3	3.9	5.7	7.4	4.5
Leukemia (C91-C95)	6.7	9.0	5.0	5.0	6.3	4.1	6.8	9.2	5.0
Multiple myeloma and immunoproliferative neoplasms (C88, C90)	3.4	4.3	2.8	2.7	3.4	2.2	3.5	4.4	2.8
Other and unspecified malignant neoplasms of lymphoid, hemato-poietic and related tissue (C96)	0.0	0.0	0.0	*	*	*	0.0	0.0	0.0
All other and unspecified malignant neoplasms (C17, C23-C24, C26-C31, C37-C41, C44-C49, C51- C52, C57-C60, C62-C63, C66, C68-C69, C73-C80, C97)	18.7	22.7	15.6	13.9	15.9	12.3	19.1	23.2	15.9
In situ neoplasms, benign neoplasms and neoplasms of uncertain or unknown behavior (D00-D48)	4.3	5.5	3.5	2.9	3.5	2.4	4.4	5.7	3.6
Anemias (D50-D64)	1.4	1.4	1.4	0.9	0.9	0.9	1.4	1.5	1.4
Diabetes mellitus (E10-E14)	21.2	25.6	17.6	26.3	30.4	23.0	20.8	25.2	17.2
Nutritional deficiencies (E40-E64)	0.9	0.9	0.9	0.7	0.7	0.6	1.0	0.9	1.0
Malnutrition (E40-E46)	0.9	0.9	0.9	0.6	0.7	0.6	0.9	0.9	0.9
Other nutritional deficiencies (E50-E64)	0.0	0.0	0.0	*	*	*	0.0	0.0	0.0
Meningitis (G00,G03)	0.2	0.2	0.1	0.1	0.2	0.1	0.2	0.2	0.1
Parkinson's disease (G20-G21)	7.3	11.0	4.8	5.5	7.9	3.8	7.4	11.2	4.9
Alzheimer's disease (G30)	23.5	19.3	25.9	17.7	14.4	19.6	23.9	19.6	26.4
Major cardiovascular diseases (I00-I78)	221.7	268.4	183.6	162.9	196.6	135.5	226.4	274.3	187.4
Diseases of heart (I00-I09, I11, I13, I20-I51)	169.8	214.5	134.3	121.2	151.5	97.0	173.9	219.8	137.3
Acute rheumatic fever and chronic rheumatic heart diseases (I00-I09)	0.9	0.8	1.0	0.5	0.4	0.6	0.9	0.8	1.0
Hypertensive heart disease (I11)	10.3	11.9	8.7	8.5	10.0	7.0	10.5	12.1	8.8
Hypertensive heart and renal disease (I13)	1.1	1.3	1.0	1.1	1.4	0.9	1.1	1.3	1.0
Ischemic heart diseases (I20-I25)	102.6	138.2	74.9	80.3	104.7	61.3	104.5	141.0	76.0
Acute myocardial infarction (I21-I22)	32.4	42.9	24.0	25.1	33.4	18.6	33.1	43.8	24.5
Other acute ischemic heart diseases (I24)	1.1	1.3	0.9	0.5	0.5	0.5	1.1	1.4	0.9
Other forms of chronic ischemic heart disease (I20, I25)	69.1	94.0	50.1	54.8	70.8	42.2	70.2	95.8	50.6
Atherosclerotic cardiovascular disease, so described (I25.0)	16.3	22.4	11.1	12.6	17.8	8.3	16.6	22.8	11.3
All other forms of chronic ischemic heart disease (I20,I25.1-I25.9)	52.8	71.6	39.0	42.1	53.0	33.9	53.6	73.0	39.3
Other heart diseases (I26-I51)	54.8	62.4	48.7	30.7	34.9	27.2	56.8	64.7	50.4
Acute and subacute endocarditis (I33)	0.4	0.5	0.3	0.3	0.4	0.2	0.4	0.5	0.3
Diseases of pericardium and acute myocarditis (I30-I31, I40)	0.2	0.3	0.2	0.2	0.2	0.2	0.3	0.3	0.2
Heart failure (I50)	18.0	20.2	16.3	10.1	11.1	9.5	18.6	20.9	16.8
All other forms of heart disease (I26-I28, I34-I38, I42-I49, I51)	36.2	41.4	31.8	20.1	23.2	17.4	37.6	43.0	33.1
Essential hypertension and hypertensive renal disease (I10, I12, I15)	8.5	8.7	8.1	8.0	8.6	7.4	8.6	8.7	8.2
Cerebrovascular diseases (I60-I69)	36.2	36.7	35.2	29.6	31.8	27.6	36.6	36.9	35.7

Table 2-15A. Age-Adjusted Death Rates from Selected Causes, by Hispanic Origin, Race for Non-Hispanic Population, and Sex, 2013 — continued

(Age-adjusted rates per 100,000 U.S. standard population.)

Cause of death (based on ICD-10, 2004)	All origins[1]			Hispanic (of any race)			Non-Hispanic[2]		
	Both sexes	Male	Female	Both sexes	Male	Female	Both sexes	Male	Female
Atherosclerosis (I70)	1.8	1.9	1.7	1.1	1.0	1.1	1.9	2.0	1.8
Other diseases of circulatory system (I71-I78)	5.3	6.6	4.3	3.1	3.8	2.5	5.5	6.9	4.4
Aortic aneurysm and dissection (I71)	2.8	3.8	2.0	1.4	1.9	0.9	2.9	4.0	2.1
Other diseases of arteries, arterioles and capillaries (I72-I78)	2.5	2.8	2.3	1.7	1.9	1.6	2.6	2.9	2.3
Other disorders of circulatory system (I80-I99)	1.3	1.4	1.2	0.8	0.7	0.8	1.3	1.4	1.2
Influenza and pneumonia (J09-J18)	15.9	18.6	14.0	13.2	15.6	11.3	16.1	18.8	14.2
Influenza (J09-J11)	1.1	1.2	1.0	0.7	0.8	0.6	1.1	1.2	1.0
Pneumonia (J12-J18)	14.8	17.5	13.0	12.4	14.7	10.7	15.0	17.6	13.2
Other acute lower respiratory infections (J20-J22, U04)	0.1	0.1	0.1	0.1	*	*	0.1	0.1	0.1
Acute bronchitis and bronchiolitis (J20-J21)	0.1	0.1	0.1	0.1	*	*	0.1	0.1	0.1
Other and unspecified acute lower respiratory infections(J22, U04)	0.0	0.0	0.0	*	*	*	0.0	0.0	0.0
Chronic lower respiratory diseases (J40-J47)	42.1	47.5	38.5	18.7	24.0	15.1	44.1	49.3	40.5
Bronchitis, chronic and unspecified (J40-J42)	0.2	0.2	0.2	0.1	0.2	*	0.2	0.2	0.2
Emphysema (J43)	2.3	2.9	2.0	1.0	1.5	0.7	2.4	3.0	2.1
Asthma (J45-J46)	1.1	0.9	1.2	0.9	0.7	1.0	1.1	1.0	1.2
Other chronic lower respiratory diseases (J44, J47)	38.5	43.5	35.2	16.6	21.6	13.3	40.3	45.2	37.1
Pneumoconioses and chemical effects (J60-J66, J68)	0.2	0.5	0.0	0.1	0.2	*	0.2	0.6	0.0
Pneumonitis due to solids and liquids (J69)	5.2	7.2	3.9	3.2	4.3	2.5	5.3	7.4	4.0
Other diseases of respiratory system (J00-J06, J30-J39, J67, J70-J98)	10.0	12.0	8.5	8.6	9.8	7.7	10.1	12.2	8.6
Peptic ulcer (K25-K28)	0.8	1.0	0.7	0.6	0.7	0.5	0.8	1.0	0.7
Diseases of appendix (K35-K38)	0.1	0.1	0.1	0.1	*	*	0.1	0.1	0.1
Hernia (K40-K46)	0.5	0.5	0.5	0.5	0.4	0.6	0.5	0.5	0.5
Chronic liver disease and cirrhosis (K70, K73-K74)	10.2	13.8	6.8	14.0	19.7	8.8	9.7	13.1	6.7
Alcoholic liver disease (K70)	5.1	7.5	2.9	6.7	11.5	2.5	4.9	7.0	2.9
Other chronic liver disease and cirrhosis (K73-K74)	5.0	6.3	3.9	7.3	8.2	6.3	4.8	6.1	3.7
Cholelithiasis and other disorders of gallbladder (K80-K82)	1.0	1.1	0.8	1.0	1.1	0.9	0.9	1.1	0.8
Nephritis, nephrotic syndrome and nephrosis(N00-N07, N17-N19, N25-N27)	13.2	16.1	11.3	11.1	13.4	9.4	13.3	16.3	11.4
Acute and rapidly progressive nephritic and nephrotic syndrome (N00-N01,N04)	0.1	0.1	0.1	*	*	*	0.1	0.1	0.1
Chronic glomerulonephritis, nephritis and nephropathy not specified as acute or chronic, and renal sclerosis unspecified (N02-N03, N05-N07, N26)	0.1	0.1	0.0	0.1	*	0.1	0.1	0.1	0.0
Renal failure (N17-N19)	13.0	15.8	11.1	10.9	13.3	9.2	13.2	16.0	11.2
Other disorders of kidney (N25, N27)	0.0	0.0	*	*	*	*	0.0	*	*
Infections of kidney (N10-N12,N13.6,N15.1)	0.2	0.1	0.2	0.2	*	0.2	0.2	0.1	0.2
Hyperplasia of prostate (N40)	0.1	0.4	X	0.1	0.4	X	0.1	0.4	X
Inflammatory diseases of female pelvic organs (N70-N76)	0.0	X	0.1	*	X	*	0.0	X	0.1
Pregnancy, childbirth and the puerperium (O00-O99)	0.4	X	0.8	0.3	X	0.6	0.4	X	0.8
Pregnancy with abortive outcome (O00-O07)	0.0	X	0.0	*	X	*	0.0	X	0.0
Other complications of pregnancy, childbirth and the puerperium (O10-O99)	0.4	X	0.7	0.3	X	0.6	0.4	X	0.8
Certain conditions originating in the perinatal period(P00-P96)	4.2	4.6	3.8	3.3	3.5	3.1	4.5	4.9	4.0
Congenital malformations, deformations and chromosomal abnormalities (Q00-Q99)	3.1	3.3	2.9	2.7	2.8	2.5	3.2	3.4	3.0
Symptoms, signs and abnormal clinical and laboratory findings, not elsewhere classified (R00-R99)	10.7	11.1	10.1	6.4	7.2	5.5	11.2	11.5	10.6
All other diseases (Residual)	89.4	88.1	88.5	62.4	62.6	61.0	91.6	90.2	90.8
Accidents (unintentional injuries) (V01-X59, Y85-Y86)	39.4	53.1	26.6	26.9	39.2	15.2	41.3	55.4	28.3
Transport accidents (V01-V99, Y85)	11.7	17.2	6.5	10.2	15.1	5.3	12.0	17.5	6.7
Motor vehicle accidents (V02-V04, V09.0, V09.2, V12-V14, V19.0-V19.2, V19.4-V19.8, V20-V79, V80.3-V80.5, V81.0-V81.1, V82.0-V82.1, V83- V86, V87.0-V87.8, V88.0-V88.8, V89.0, V89.2)	10.9	15.9	6.2	9.7	14.2	5.2	11.2	16.2	6.4
Other land transport accidents (V01,V05-V06, V09.1, V09.3-V09.9, V10-V11, V15-V18, V19.3, V19.9, V80.0-V80.2, V80.6-V80.9, V81.2- V81.9, V82.2-V82.9, V87.9, V88.9, V89.1, V89.3, V89.9)	0.3	0.5	0.1	0.3	0.5	*	0.3	0.5	0.1
Water, air and space, and other and unspecified transport accidents and their sequelae (V90-V99, Y85)	0.5	0.8	0.2	0.3	0.4	0.1	0.5	0.8	0.2
Nontransport accidents (W00-X59, Y86)	27.7	36.0	20.1	16.7	24.0	9.8	29.3	37.9	21.6
Falls (W00-W19)	8.5	10.6	6.9	5.5	7.6	3.9	8.7	10.7	7.1
Accidental discharge of firearms (W32-W34)	0.2	0.3	0.0	0.1	0.2	*	0.2	0.3	0.1
Accidental drowning and submersion (W65-W74)	1.1	1.6	0.5	0.8	1.3	0.3	1.1	1.7	0.5
Accidental exposure to smoke, fire and flames(X00-X09)	0.8	1.0	0.6	0.5	0.5	0.4	0.9	1.1	0.7
Accidental poisoning and exposure to noxious substances (X40-X49)	12.2	16.0	8.5	6.7	9.8	3.5	13.3	17.3	9.5
Other and unspecified nontransport accidents and their sequelae (W20-W31, W35-W64, W75-W99, X10-X39, X50-X59, Y86)	4.9	6.5	3.5	3.1	4.7	1.8	5.1	6.7	3.7
Intentional self-harm (suicide) (*U03, X60-X84, Y87.0)	12.6	20.3	5.5	5.7	9.3	2.3	13.8	22.2	6.0
Intentional self-harm (suicide) by discharge of firearms (X72-X74)	6.4	11.5	1.8	2.1	3.8	0.5	7.1	12.8	2.0
Intentional self-harm (suicide) by other and unspecified means and their sequelae (*U03, X60-X71, X75-X84, Y87.0)	6.2	8.8	3.7	3.6	5.5	1.8	6.7	9.4	4.1
Assault (homicide) (*U01-*U02, X85-Y09, Y87.1)	5.2	8.2	2.1	4.5	7.3	1.6	5.3	8.4	2.2
Assault (homicide) by discharge of firearms (*U01.4, X93-X95)	3.6	6.1	1.1	3.0	5.1	0.8	3.8	6.4	1.2
Assault (homicide) by other and unspecified means and their sequelae (*U01.0-*U01.3, *U01.5-*U01.9, *U02, X85-X92, X96-Y09, Y87.1)	1.5	2.1	1.0	1.5	2.2	0.8	1.5	2.1	1.1
Legal intervention (Y35, Y89.0)	0.2	0.3	0.0	0.2	0.3	*	0.2	0.3	0.0
Events of undetermined intent (Y10-Y34, Y87.2,Y89.9)	1.4	1.7	1.1	0.7	1.0	0.4	1.6	1.9	1.3
Discharge of firearms, undetermined intent (Y22-Y24)	0.1	0.1	0.0	0.1	0.1	*	0.1	0.1	0.0
Other and unspecified events of undetermined intent and their sequelae (Y10-Y21, Y25-Y34, Y87.2, Y89.9)	1.3	1.6	1.1	0.7	0.9	0.4	1.5	1.7	1.2
Operations of war and their sequelae (Y36, Y89.1)	*	*	*	*	*	*	*	*	*
Complications of medical and surgical care (Y40-Y84, Y88)	0.8	0.9	0.7	0.6	0.6	0.6	0.8	0.9	0.8
Enterocolitis due to Clostridium difficile (A04.7)[4]	2.1	2.1	2.2	1.7	1.7	1.7	2.2	2.2	2.2

Table 2-15A. Age-Adjusted Death Rates from Selected Causes, by Hispanic Origin, Race for Non-Hispanic Population, and Sex, 2013 — continued

(Age-adjusted rates per 100,000 U.S. standard population.)

Cause of death (based on ICD-10, 2004)	All origins[1]			Hispanic (of any race)			Non-Hispanic[2]		
	Both sexes	Male	Female	Both sexes	Male	Female	Both sexes	Male	Female
Drug-induced deaths[5,6]	14.6	18.0	11.1	7.3	10.0	4.4	16.0	19.7	12.3
Alcohol-induced deaths[5,7]	8.2	12.5	4.3	9.0	15.3	3.1	8.1	12.1	4.5
Injury by firearms[5,8]	10.4	18.3	3.0	5.4	9.4	1.3	11.3	19.9	3.2

Table 2-15B. Age-Adjusted Death Rates from Selected Causes, by Hispanic Origin, Race for Non-Hispanic Population, and Sex, 2013

(Age-adjusted rates per 100,000 U.S. standard population.)

Cause of death (based on ICD-10, 2004)	Non-Hispanic White[2]			Non-Hispanic Black[2]		
	Both sexes	Male	Female	Both sexes	Male	Female
All Causes	747.1	876.8	638.4	885.2	1,083.3	740.6
Salmonella infections (A01-A02)	0.0	*	*	*	*	*
Shigellosis and amebiasis (A03, A06)	*	*	*	*	*	*
Certain other intestinal infections (A04, A07-A09)	3.1	3.0	3.3	2.7	3.0	2.4
Tuberculosis (A16-A19)	0.1	0.1	0.0	0.3	0.4	0.2
Respiratory tuberculosis (A16)	0.1	0.1	0.0	0.2	0.3	0.1
Other tuberculosis (A17-A19)	0.0	0.0	0.0	0.1	*	*
Whooping cough (A37)	*	*	*	*	*	*
Scarlet fever and erysipelas (A38, A46)	*	*	*	*	*	*
Meningococcal infection (A39)	0.0	0.0	*	*	*	*
Septicemia (A40-A41)	10.2	11.3	9.5	18.8	21.7	17.0
Syphilis (A50-A53)	*	*	*	0.1	*	*
Acute poliomyelitis (A80)	*	*	*	*	*	*
Arthropod-borne viral encephalitis (A83-A84, A85.2)	*	*	*	*	*	*
Measles (B05)	*	*	*	*	*	*
Viral hepatitis (B15-B19)	1.9	2.6	1.2	2.9	4.2	1.9
Human immunodeficiency virus (HIV) disease (B20-B24)	0.9	1.6	0.3	9.2	13.1	5.9
Malaria (B50-B54)	*	*	*	*	*	*
Other and unspecified infectious and parasitic diseases and their sequelae (A00, A05, A20-A36, A42-A44, A48-A49, A54-A79, A81-A82, A85.0-A85.1, A85.8, A86-B04, B06-B09, B25-B49, B55-B99)	1.7	1.9	1.4	2.3	2.8	2.0
Malignant neoplasms (C00-C97)	167.7	200.0	143.9	194.4	245.4	163.0
Malignant neoplasms of lip, oral cavity and pharynx (C00-C14)	2.5	3.8	1.3	2.9	4.9	1.4
Malignant neoplasm of esophagus (C15)	4.5	7.9	1.5	3.6	6.0	1.8
Malignant neoplasm of stomach (C16)	2.5	3.4	1.7	5.8	8.4	3.9
Malignant neoplasms of colon, rectum and anus (C18-C21)	14.5	17.0	12.4	19.9	25.4	16.2
Malignant neoplasms of liver and intrahepatic bile ducts (C22)	5.7	8.3	3.4	8.6	13.9	4.6
Malignant neoplasm of pancreas (C25)	10.9	12.7	9.4	13.8	15.2	12.5
Malignant neoplasm of larynx (C32)	1.0	1.8	0.4	1.7	3.2	0.6
Malignant neoplasms of trachea, bronchus and lung(C33-C34)	46.6	56.3	39.0	48.2	67.5	35.1
Malignant melanoma of skin (C43)	3.4	5.0	2.1	0.4	0.5	0.3
Malignant neoplasm of breast (C50)	11.5	0.3	20.9	17.1	0.6	29.2
Malignant neoplasm of cervix uteri (C53)	1.1	X	2.1	2.2	X	4.0
Malignant neoplasms of corpus uteri and uterus, part unspecified (C54-C55)	2.4	X	4.3	5.0	X	8.5
Malignant neoplasm of ovary (C56)	4.2	X	7.7	3.6	X	6.1
Malignant neoplasm of prostate (C61)	7.4	18.0	X	14.5	39.6	X
Malignant neoplasms of kidney and renal pelvis (C64-C65)	4.0	5.8	2.6	3.6	5.4	2.3
Malignant neoplasm of bladder (C67)	4.9	8.4	2.3	3.6	5.5	2.4
Malignant neoplasms of meninges, brain and other parts of central nervous system (C70-C72)	5.0	6.0	4.1	2.5	3.3	1.9
Malignant neoplasms of lymphoid, hematopoietic and related tissue (C81-C96)	16.6	21.8	12.7	16.9	21.3	14.0
Hodgkin's disease (C81)	0.3	0.4	0.2	0.3	0.4	0.2
Non-Hodgkin's lymphoma (C82-C85)	6.0	7.7	4.6	4.2	5.4	3.4
Leukemia (C91-C95)	7.1	9.5	5.2	5.8	7.8	4.4
Multiple myeloma and immunoproliferative neoplasms (C88, C90)	3.2	4.1	2.5	6.7	7.7	6.0
Other and unspecified malignant neoplasms of lymphoid, hematopoietic and related tissue (C96)	0.0	0.0	0.0	*	*	*
All other and unspecified malignant neoplasms (C17, C23-C24, C26-C31, C37-C41, C44-C49, C51- C52, C57-C60, C62-C63, C66, C68-C69, C73-C80, C97)	19.3	23.5	15.9	20.6	24.6	18.0
In situ neoplasms, benign neoplasms and neoplasms of uncertain or unknown behavior (D00-D48)	4.6	5.9	3.7	3.7	4.7	3.2
Anemias (D50-D64)	1.3	1.3	1.2	2.7	3.0	2.6
Diabetes mellitus (E10-E14)	18.6	23.1	14.9	39.5	45.1	35.2
Nutritional deficiencies (E40-E64)	0.9	0.9	1.0	1.4	1.6	1.2
Malnutrition (E40-E46)	0.9	0.8	0.9	1.4	1.5	1.2
Other nutritional deficiencies (E50-E64)	0.0	0.0	0.0	*	*	*
Meningitis (G00,G03)	0.2	0.2	0.1	0.2	0.2	0.2
Parkinson's disease (G20-G21)	8.0	12.0	5.2	3.6	6.0	2.3
Alzheimer's disease (G30)	24.8	20.2	27.5	20.5	17.7	21.6
Major cardiovascular diseases (I00-I78)	221.9	269.3	182.7	291.2	354.0	244.6
Diseases of heart (I00-I09, I11, I13, I20-I51)	171.8	217.9	134.6	215.5	269.1	176.4
Acute rheumatic fever and chronic rheumatic heart diseases (I00-I09)	1.0	0.8	1.1	0.7	0.7	0.8
Hypertensive heart disease (I11)	9.0	10.3	7.6	23.5	29.2	19.0
Hypertensive heart and renal disease (I13)	0.9	1.0	0.8	3.0	3.7	2.4
Ischemic heart diseases (I20-I25)	104.6	141.8	75.0	119.9	155.1	94.7
Acute myocardial infarction (I21-I22)	33.3	44.4	24.2	37.8	47.4	30.8
Other acute ischemic heart diseases (I24)	1.1	1.4	0.9	1.7	2.0	1.4
Other forms of chronic ischemic heart disease (I20, I25)	70.1	96.1	49.9	80.4	105.7	62.4
Atherosclerotic cardiovascular disease, so described (I25.0)	15.9	21.8	10.8	24.6	35.0	16.9
All other forms of chronic ischemic heart disease (I20,I25.1-I25.9)	54.2	74.2	39.1	55.8	70.7	45.5
Other heart diseases (I26-I51)	56.4	64.1	50.1	68.5	80.5	59.5
Acute and subacute endocarditis (I33)	0.4	0.5	0.3	0.5	0.7	0.3
Diseases of pericardium and acute myocarditis (I30-I31, I40)	0.2	0.3	0.2	0.4	0.4	0.4

Table 2-15B. Age-Adjusted Death Rates from Selected Causes, by Hispanic Origin, Race for Non-Hispanic Population, and Sex, 2013 — continued

(Age-adjusted rates per 100,000 U.S. standard population.)

Cause of death (based on ICD-10, 2004)	Non-Hispanic White[2]			Non-Hispanic Black[2]		
	Both sexes	Male	Female	Both sexes	Male	Female
Heart failure (I50)	18.7	21.0	16.9	21.0	24.2	18.7
All other forms of heart disease (I26-I28, I34-I38, I42-I49, I51)	37.2	42.3	32.7	46.6	55.2	40.2
Essential hypertension and hypertensive renal disease (I10, I12, I15)	7.6	7.6	7.4	16.8	18.8	15.1
Cerebrovascular diseases (I60-I69)	35.0	34.9	34.5	50.3	55.6	45.9
Atherosclerosis (I70)	1.9	2.0	1.9	1.7	1.9	1.5
Other diseases of circulatory system (I71-I78)	5.5	6.8	4.3	6.9	8.5	5.7
Aortic aneurysm and dissection (I71)	2.9	4.0	2.1	3.0	3.9	2.2
Other diseases of arteries, arterioles and capillaries (I72-I78)	2.5	2.8	2.3	3.9	4.5	3.5
Other disorders of circulatory system (I80-I99)	1.2	1.3	1.1	2.4	2.7	2.1
Influenza and pneumonia (J09-J18)	15.9	18.5	14.1	17.1	21.3	14.5
Influenza (J09-J11)	1.1	1.2	1.0	0.8	0.8	0.8
Pneumonia (J12-J18)	14.8	17.2	13.1	16.4	20.5	13.8
Other acute lower respiratory infections (J20-J22, U04)[2]	0.1	0.1	0.1	0.1	*	*
Acute bronchitis and bronchiolitis (J20-J21)	0.1	0.1	0.1	0.1	*	*
Other and unspecified acute lower respiratory infections (J22, U04)[2,3]	0.0	*	0.0	*	*	*
Chronic lower respiratory diseases (J40-J47)	47.0	51.5	44.1	30.2	40.1	24.4
Bronchitis, chronic and unspecified (J40-J42)	0.2	0.2	0.2	0.2	0.2	0.2
Emphysema (J43)	2.6	3.1	2.3	1.7	2.4	1.2
Asthma (J45-J46)	0.8	0.7	1.0	2.6	2.6	2.5
Other chronic lower respiratory diseases (J44, J47)	43.4	47.6	40.6	25.8	34.9	20.5
Pneumoconioses and chemical effects (J60-J66, J68)	0.3	0.6	0.0	0.1	0.2	*
Pneumonitis due to solids and liquids (J69)	5.4	7.5	4.1	5.2	7.4	3.9
Other diseases of respiratory system (J00-J06, J30-J39, J67, J70-J98)	10.3	12.5	8.7	9.3	10.6	8.6
Peptic ulcer (K25-K28)	0.9	1.0	0.7	0.8	1.1	0.6
Diseases of appendix (K35-K38)	0.1	0.1	0.1	0.1	0.2	*
Hernia (K40-K46)	0.6	0.6	0.6	0.5	0.5	0.5
Chronic liver disease and cirrhosis (K70, K73-K74)	10.3	13.8	7.0	7.5	10.6	5.0
Alcoholic liver disease (K70)	5.2	7.5	3.1	3.2	4.8	2.0
Other chronic liver disease and cirrhosis (K73-K74)	5.0	6.3	3.8	4.2	5.7	3.0
Cholelithiasis and other disorders of gallbladder (K80-K82)	0.9	1.1	0.8	1.0	1.2	0.9
Nephritis, nephrotic syndrome and nephrosis (N00-N07, N17-N19, N25-N27)	12.1	14.9	10.1	25.8	30.7	22.7
Acute and rapidly progressive nephritic and nephrotic syndrome (N00-N01,N04)	0.1	0.1	0.1	0.2	0.3	0.1
Chronic glomerulonephritis, nephritis and nephropathy not specified as acute or chronic, and renal sclerosis unspecified (N02-N03, N05-N07, N26)	0.1	0.1	0.0	0.1	*	*
Renal failure (N17-N19)	11.9	14.7	10.0	25.5	30.3	22.5
Other disorders of kidney (N25, N27)	0.0	*	*	*	*	*
Infections of kidney (N10-N12,N13.6,N15.1)	0.2	0.1	0.2	0.2	0.2	0.2
Hyperplasia of prostate (N40)	0.2	0.4	X	0.1	0.4	X
Inflammatory diseases of female pelvic organs (N70-N76)	0.0	X	0.0	0.1	X	0.1
Pregnancy, childbirth and the puerperium (O00-O99)	0.3	X	0.6	0.9	X	1.7
Pregnancy with abortive outcome (O00-O07)	*	X	*	*	X	*
Other complications of pregnancy, childbirth and the puerperium (O10-O99)	0.3	X	0.6	0.9	X	1.7
Certain conditions originating in the perinatal period (P00-P96)	3.4	3.7	3.0	8.8	9.4	8.2
Congenital malformations, deformations and chromosomal abnormalities (Q00-Q99)	3.2	3.4	3.0	3.6	3.8	3.5
Symptoms, signs and abnormal clinical and laboratory findings, not elsewhere classified (R00-R99)	11.2	11.3	10.7	12.9	14.3	11.5
All other diseases (Residual)	92.3	90.4	91.7	103.6	108.7	98.8
Accidents (unintentional injuries) (V01-X59, Y85-Y86)	44.2	58.6	30.7	33.9	49.7	20.7
Transport accidents (V01-V99, Y85)	12.4	17.9	7.0	12.1	19.0	6.2
Motor vehicle accidents (V02-V04, V09.0, V09.2, V12-V14, V19.0-V19.2, V19.4-V19.6, V20-V79, V80.3-V80.5, V81.0-V81.1, V82.0-V82.1,V83- V86, V87.0-V87.8, V88.0-V88.8, V89.0, V89.2)	11.5	16.5	6.6	11.5	17.8	6.0
Other land transport accidents (V01,V05-V06, V09.1, V09.3-V09.9, V10-V11, V15-V18, V19.3, V19.8-V19.9, V80.0-V80.2, V80.6-V80.9, V81.2-V81.9, V82.2-V82.9, V87.9, V88.9, V89.1, V89.3, V89.9)	0.3	0.5	0.1	0.3	0.6	*
Water, air and space, and other and unspecified transport accidents and their sequelae (V90-V99, Y85)	0.6	0.9	0.2	0.3	0.5	0.2
Nontransport accidents (W00-X59, Y86)	31.9	40.7	23.7	21.7	30.8	14.5
Falls (W00-W19)	9.3	11.3	7.7	4.3	6.2	2.9
Accidental discharge of firearms (W32-W34)	0.2	0.3	0.0	0.2	0.4	*
Accidental drowning and submersion (W65-W74)	1.1	1.6	0.5	1.2	2.0	0.4
Accidental exposure to smoke, fire and flames (X00-X09)	0.8	1.1	0.6	1.5	1.8	1.2
Accidental poisoning and exposure to noxious substances (X40-X49)	15.3	19.6	11.1	9.2	13.2	5.8
Other and unspecified nontransport accidents and their sequelae (W20-W31, W35-W64, W75-W99, X10-X39, X50-X59, Y86)	5.2	6.8	3.7	5.4	7.1	4.1
Intentional self-harm (suicide) (*U03, X60-X84, Y87.0)	15.9	25.3	7.1	5.6	9.7	2.0
Intentional self-harm (suicide) by discharge of firearms (X72-X74)	8.4	14.8	2.4	2.7	5.2	0.5
Intentional self-harm (suicide) by other and unspecified means and their sequelae (*U03, X60-X71, X75-X84, Y87.0)	7.5	10.5	4.7	3.0	4.6	1.5
Assault (homicide) (*U01-*U02, X85-Y09, Y87.1)	2.5	3.4	1.7	18.8	33.5	5.1
Assault (homicide) by discharge of firearms (*U01.4, X93-X95)	1.4	2.0	0.8	15.0	27.7	2.9

Table 2-15B. Age-Adjusted Death Rates from Selected Causes, by Hispanic Origin, Race for Non-Hispanic Population, and Sex, 2013 — continued

(Age-adjusted rates per 100,000 U.S. standard population.)

Cause of death (based on ICD-10, 2004)	Non-Hispanic White[2]			Non-Hispanic Black[2]		
	Both sexes	Male	Female	Both sexes	Male	Female
Assault (homicide) by other and unspecified means and their sequelae (*U01.0-*U01.3, *U01.5-*U01.9, *U02, X85-X92, X96-Y09, Y87.1)	1.1	1.3	0.8	3.9	5.8	2.2
Legal intervention (Y35, Y89.0)	0.1	0.2	*	0.3	0.7	*
Events of undetermined intent (Y10-Y34, Y87.2,Y89.9)	1.7	2.0	1.5	1.4	2.0	0.9
Discharge of firearms, undetermined intent (Y22-Y24)	0.1	0.2	0.0	0.1	0.2	*
Other and unspecified events of undetermined intent and their sequelae (Y10-Y21, Y25-Y34, Y87.2, Y89.9)	1.6	1.8	1.4	1.3	1.9	0.8
Operations of war and their sequelae (Y36, Y89.1)	*	*	*	*	*	*
Complications of medical and surgical care (Y40-Y84, Y88)	0.8	0.9	0.7	1.1	1.2	1.0
Enterocolitis due to Clostridium difficile (A04.7)[4]	2.3	2.2	2.4	1.8	2.1	1.7
Drug-induced deaths[5,6]	18.5	22.5	14.5	10.5	14.5	7.1
Alcohol-induced deaths[5,7]	8.6	12.6	4.8	6.2	10.2	3.0
Injury by firearms[5,8]	10.2	17.5	3.3	18.2	34.0	3.6

X = Not applicable.   - = Quantity zero.   * = Figure does not meet standards of reliability or precision.   1Figures for origin not stated are included in ''All origins'' but not distributed among specified origins. 2Includes races other than White and Black.   3Race categories are consistent with the 1977 Office of Management and Budget (OMB) standards. Multiple-race data were reported by 42 states and the District of Columbia in 2013. The multiple-race data for these reporting areas were bridged to the single-race categories of the 1977 OMB standards for comparability with other reporting areas.   4Included in certain other intestinal infections (A04, A07–A09). Beginning with data year 2006, Enterocolitis due to Clostridium difficile (A04.7) is shown separately at the bottom of the table and is included in the list of rankable causes.   5Included in selected categories above.   6Includes ICD–10 codes D52.1, D59.0, D59.2, D61.1, D64.2, E06.4, E16.0, E23.1, E24.2, E27.3, E66.1, F11.1-F11.5, F11.7-F11.9, F12.1-F12.5, F12.7-F12.9, F13.1-F13.5, F13.7-F13.9, F14.1-F14.5, F14.7-F14.9, F15.1-F15.5, F15.7-F15.9, F16.1-F16.5, F16.7-16.9, F17.3-F17.5, F17.7-F17.9, F18.1-F18.5, F18.7-F18.9, F19.1-F19.5, F19.7-F19.9, G21.1, G24.0, G25.1, G25.4, G25.6, G44.4, G62.0, G72.0, I95.2, J70.2-J70.4, K85.3, L10.5, L27.0-L27.1, M10.2, M32.0, M80.4, M81.4, M83.5, M87.1, R50.2, R78.1-R78.5, X40-X44, X60-X64, X85, and Y10-Y14. Trend data for Drug-induced deaths, previously shown in this report, can be found through a link from the online version of this report, available from http://www.cdc.gov/nchs/deaths.htm.   7Includes ICD–10 codes E24.4, F10, G31.2, G62.1, G72.1, I42.6, K29.2, K70, K85.2, K86.0, R78.0, X45, X65, and Y15. Trend data for Alcohol-induced deaths, previously shown in this report, can be found through a link from the online version of this report, available from http://www.cdc.gov/nchs/deaths.htm.   8Includes ICD–10 codes *U01.4, W32-W34, X72-X74, X93-X95, Y22-Y24, and Y35.0. Trend data for Injury by firearms, previously shown in this report, can be found through a link from the online version of this report, available from http://www.cdc.gov/nchs/deaths.htm.

Table 2-16. Age-Adjusted Death Rates, by Race, Hispanic Origin, Average Annual 1979–1981, 1989–1991, and 2011–2013

(Age-adjusted death rate per 100,000 population. [1])

State	All persons			White	Black	American Indian, or Alaska Native[2]	Asian or Pacific Islander[c]	Hispanic, or Latino[c]	White, not Hispanic or Latino[2]
	1979–1981	1989–1991	2011–2013	2011–2013	2011–2013	2011–2013	2011–2013	2011–2013	2011–2013
United States [3]	1,022.8	942.2	735.3	733.5	867.4	595.8	407.5	538.3	749.0
Alabama	1,091.2	1,037.9	928.4	910.6	1,016.5	325.7	296.6	346.7	919.0
Alaska	1,087.4	944.6	734.0	682.6	664.9	1,129.2	486.6	385.6	690.6
Arizona	951.5	873.5	681.8	676.8	783.7	828.6	394.8	604.6	686.4
Arkansas	1,017.0	996.3	895.6	883.4	1,026.9	288.7	507.3	354.7	893.3
California	975.5	911.0	633.8	663.4	825.8	371.7	408.8	527.9	696.3
Colorado	941.1	856.1	666.0	670.7	765.2	449.7	404.8	657.1	665.6
Connecticut	961.5	857.5	651.7	654.1	691.6	210.1	334.0	511.2	655.4
Delaware	1,069.7	1,001.9	745.0	740.6	813.3	*	338.2	415.5	746.7
District of Columbia	1,243.1	1,255.3	755.1	468.1	967.9	*	365.3	378.9	462.8
Florida	960.8	870.9	670.0	663.7	758.7	277.6	316.3	520.1	696.8
Georgia	1,094.3	1,037.4	810.0	797.9	879.2	185.9	392.5	298.0	816.6
Hawaii	801.2	752.2	587.4	632.6	492.6	*	572.9	769.7	631.2
Idaho	936.7	856.6	733.9	736.5	554.1	711.1	500.1	491.5	745.1
Illinois	1,063.7	973.8	729.9	713.6	923.9	178.2	385.2	465.1	728.9
Indiana	1,048.3	962.0	828.3	821.9	963.1	180.6	379.2	466.3	829.9
Iowa	919.9	848.2	721.5	719.0	922.2	623.7	506.8	398.6	722.4
Kansas	940.1	867.2	761.9	754.9	926.0	1,079.3	465.3	550.4	761.5
Kentucky	1,088.9	1,024.5	908.7	911.7	935.2	229.6	420.1	302.4	918.1
Louisiana	1,132.6	1,074.6	894.3	854.3	1,013.4	451.8	414.3	362.8	869.9
Maine	1,002.9	918.7	745.7	748.6	467.0	731.1	355.6	269.9	744.9
Maryland	1,063.3	985.2	711.7	695.6	810.2	217.5	351.2	330.1	708.7
Massachusetts	982.6	884.8	665.8	680.4	612.3	272.4	342.5	453.1	682.1
Michigan	1,050.2	966.0	780.2	758.2	966.6	829.6	348.1	608.5	758.9
Minnesota	892.9	825.2	653.1	647.1	718.1	1,009.4	485.3	391.1	649.3
Mississippi	1,108.7	1,071.4	952.9	914.0	1,045.3	769.5	504.4	296.1	921.1
Missouri	1,033.7	952.4	807.5	796.9	942.2	387.5	446.1	400.7	802.5
Montana	1,013.6	890.2	751.5	729.3	*	1,209.1	*	484.4	727.0
Nebraska	930.6	867.9	717.7	710.3	937.1	886.4	405.9	439.9	716.2
Nevada	1,077.4	1,017.4	777.8	805.0	836.3	551.1	439.9	470.9	859.2
New Hampshire	982.3	891.7	692.0	699.1	376.6	*	315.5	285.6	702.1
New Jersey	1,047.5	956.0	681.5	685.0	813.5	181.2	334.0	469.4	702.2
New Mexico	967.1	891.9	741.6	740.9	706.6	781.0	344.5	720.8	727.4
New York	1,051.8	973.7	655.5	672.7	674.4	179.7	359.2	510.4	669.4
North Carolina	1,050.4	986.0	784.8	765.6	888.6	777.7	347.8	276.1	778.5
North Dakota	922.4	818.4	702.9	681.1	370.2	1,319.9	*	454.8	679.6
Ohio	1,070.6	967.4	816.9	807.0	940.6	235.4	369.6	466.8	809.6
Oklahoma	1,025.6	961.4	904.3	893.8	1,020.0	978.3	468.7	533.4	905.5
Oregon	953.9	893.0	716.0	723.5	809.6	658.1	435.7	437.9	733.0
Pennsylvania	1,076.4	963.4	765.4	754.8	926.4	285.5	393.5	547.3	750.5
Rhode Island	990.8	889.6	701.1	714.9	486.0	477.3	414.2	413.6	720.0
South Carolina	1,104.6	1,030.0	837.5	807.3	948.7	437.4	399.6	357.4	815.1
South Dakota	941.9	846.4	703.7	666.9	320.4	1,280.2	498.7	284.1	669.9
Tennessee	1,045.5	1,011.8	880.3	871.1	976.8	247.2	414.3	298.4	879.1
Texas	1,014.9	947.6	752.1	750.9	901.2	148.1	399.6	633.3	786.9
Utah	924.9	823.2	703.4	706.3	660.9	723.3	534.4	528.1	715.0
Vermont	990.2	908.6	707.2	710.7	*	*	*	359.9	712.9
Virginia	1,054.0	963.1	732.0	721.5	864.3	315.0	377.1	354.8	731.1
Washington	947.7	869.4	683.6	695.5	738.4	856.3	431.3	448.8	703.8
West Virginia	1,100.3	1,031.5	938.6	940.3	1,026.8	*	279.4	232.4	944.7
Wisconsin	956.4	879.1	716.2	702.7	973.3	990.5	491.9	445.0	706.6
Wyoming	1,016.1	897.4	744.5	742.7	356.7	1,155.3	*	588.4	749.3
American Samoa[4]	NA	NA	1,080.6	NA	NA	NA	NA	NA	NA
Guam[4]	NA	NA	767.3	NA	NA	NA	NA	NA	NA
Northern Marianas[4]	NA	NA	746.1	NA	NA	NA	NA	NA	NA
Puerto Rico[4]	NA	NA	692.0	NA	NA	NA	NA	NA	NA
Virgin Islands[4]	NA	NA	†644.0	NA	NA	NA	NA	NA	NA

NOTE: The race groups, white, black, American Indian or Alaska Native, and Asian or Pacific Islander, include persons of Hispanic and non-Hispanic origin. Prior to 2001, age-adjusted rates were calculated using standard million proportions based on rounded population numbers. Starting with 2001 data, unrounded population numbers are used to calculate age-adjusted rates. People of Hispanic origin may be of any race.   NA = Not available.   † = Rate shown is for 2010-2012 because death data were not available for the Virgin Islands for 2013.   1 Age-adjusted average annual death rates are calculated using the year 2000 standard population. Prior to 2001, age-adjusted rates were calculated using standard million proportions based on rounded population numbers. Starting with 2001 data, unrounded population numbers are used to calculate age-adjusted rates. Age-adjusted rates for Puerto Rico, Virgin Islands, Guam, American Samoa, and Northern Marianas were computed by applying the age-specific death rates to the U.S. standard population combining the age groups for age 75 and over. For the territories, age groups were not available for those age 75 and over by age. Prior to 2011-2013, denominators for rates are resident population estimates for the middle year of each 3-year period, multiplied by 3. Starting with 2011-2013, denominators for rates are the 3-year average population.   2 Death rates for Hispanic, American Indian or Alaska Native, and Asian or Pacific Islander persons should be interpreted with caution because of inconsistencies in reporting Hispanic origin or race on the death certificate (death rate numerators) compared with population figures (death rate denominators). The net effect of misclassification is an underestimation of deaths and death rates for races other than White and Black.   3 Excludes data for American Samoa, Guam, Northern Marianas, Puerto Rico, and Virgin Islands.   4 Comparable population data were not available for all time periods and for all racial and ethnicity groups. Therefore, only selected rates are presented for the territories.

Table 2-17. Age-Adjusted Death Rates for Selected Causes of Death, by Sex, Race, and Hispanic Origin, Selected Years, 1950–2013

(Age-adjusted rate per 100,000 population.)

Sex, race, Hispanic origin, and cause of death[1]	1950[2,3]	1960[2,3]	1970[3]	1980[3]	1990[3]	2000[4]	2010[4]	2012[4]	2013[4]
All Persons[5]									
All causes	1,446.0	1,339.2	1,222.6	1,039.1	938.7	869.0	747.0	732.8	731.9
Diseases of heart	588.8	559.0	492.7	412.1	321.8	257.6	179.1	170.5	169.8
Ischemic heart disease	NA	NA	NA	345.2	249.6	186.8	113.6	105.4	102.6
Cerebrovascular diseases	180.7	177.9	147.7	96.2	65.3	60.9	39.1	36.9	36.2
Malignant neoplasms	193.9	193.9	198.6	207.9	216.0	199.6	172.8	166.5	163.2
Trachea, bronchus, and lung	15.0	24.1	37.1	49.9	59.3	56.1	47.6	44.9	43.4
Colon, rectum, and anus	NA	30.3	28.9	27.4	24.5	20.8	15.8	14.9	14.6
Chronic lower respiratory diseases	NA	NA	NA	28.3	37.2	44.2	42.2	41.5	42.1
Influenza and pneumonia	48.1	53.7	41.7	31.4	36.8	23.7	15.1	14.4	15.9
Chronic liver disease and cirrhosis	11.3	13.3	17.8	15.1	11.1	9.5	9.4	9.9	10.2
Diabetes mellitus[6]	23.1	22.5	24.3	18.1	20.7	25.0	20.8	21.2	21.2
Alzheimer's disease	NA	NA	NA	V	V	18.1	25.1	23.8	23.5
Human immunodeficiency virus (HIV) disease	X	X	X	X	10.2	5.2	2.6	2.2	2.1
Unintentional injuries	78.0	62.3	60.1	46.4	36.3	34.9	38.0	39.1	39.4
Motor vehicle-related injuries	24.6	23.1	27.6	22.3	18.5	15.4	11.3	11.4	10.9
Poisoning	2.5	1.7	2.8	1.9	2.3	4.5	10.6	11.5	12.2
Nephritis, nephrotic syndrome, and nephrosis[6]	NA	NA	NA	9.1	9.3	13.5	15.3	13.1	13.2
Suicide[7]	13.2	12.5	13.1	12.2	12.5	10.4	12.1	12.6	12.6
Homicide[7]	5.1	5.0	8.8	10.4	9.4	5.9	5.3	5.4	5.2
Male									
All causes	1,674.2	1,609.0	1,542.1	1,348.1	1,202.8	1,053.8	887.1	865.1	863.6
Diseases of heart	699.0	687.6	634.0	538.9	412.4	320.0	225.1	214.7	214.5
Ischemic heart disease	NA	NA	NA	459.7	328.2	241.4	151.3	141.1	138.2
Cerebrovascular diseases	186.4	186.1	157.4	102.2	68.5	62.4	39.3	37.1	36.7
Malignant neoplasms	208.1	225.1	247.6	271.2	280.4	248.9	209.9	200.3	196.0
Trachea, bronchus, and lung	24.6	43.6	67.5	85.2	91.1	76.7	60.3	56.1	53.7
Colon, rectum, and anus	NA	31.8	32.3	32.8	30.4	25.1	19.0	17.7	17.4
Prostate	28.6	28.7	28.8	32.8	38.4	30.4	21.9	19.5	19.2
Chronic lower respiratory diseases	NA	NA	NA	49.9	55.4	55.8	48.7	47.2	47.5
Influenza and pneumonia	55.0	65.8	54.0	42.1	47.8	28.9	18.2	17.3	18.6
Chronic liver disease and cirrhosis	15.0	18.5	24.8	21.3	15.9	13.4	12.9	13.4	13.8
Diabetes mellitus[6]	18.8	19.9	23.0	18.1	21.7	27.8	24.9	25.5	25.6
Alzheimer's disease	NA	NA	NA	V	V	15.2	21.0	19.8	19.3
Human immunodeficiency virus (HIV) disease	X	X	X	X	18.5	7.9	3.8	3.2	3.1
Unintentional injuries	101.8	85.5	87.4	69.0	52.9	49.3	51.5	52.6	53.1
Motor vehicle-related injuries	38.5	35.4	41.5	33.6	26.5	21.7	16.2	16.5	15.9
Poisoning	3.3	2.3	3.9	2.7	3.5	6.6	13.8	15.0	16.0
Nephritis, nephrotic syndrome, and nephrosis[6]	NA	NA	NA	12.2	12.1	16.9	18.7	16.0	16.1
Suicide[7]	21.2	20.0	19.8	19.9	21.5	17.7	19.8	20.4	20.3
Homicide[7]	7.9	7.5	14.3	16.6	14.8	9.0	8.4	8.5	8.2
Female									
All causes	1,236.0	1,105.3	971.4	817.9	750.9	731.4	634.9	624.7	623.5
Diseases of heart	486.6	447.0	381.6	320.8	257.0	210.9	143.3	135.5	134.3
Ischemic heart disease	NA	NA	NA	263.1	193.9	146.5	84.9	77.8	74.9
Cerebrovascular diseases	175.8	170.7	140.0	91.7	62.6	59.1	38.3	36.1	35.2
Malignant neoplasms	182.3	168.7	163.2	166.7	175.7	167.6	146.7	142.1	139.5
Trachea, bronchus, and lung	5.8	7.5	13.1	24.4	37.1	41.3	38.1	36.4	35.5
Colon, rectum, and anus	NA	29.1	26.5	23.8	20.6	17.7	13.3	12.6	12.3
Breast	31.9	31.7	32.1	31.9	33.3	26.8	22.1	21.3	20.8
Chronic lower respiratory diseases	NA	NA	NA	14.9	26.6	37.4	38.0	37.8	38.5
Influenza and pneumonia	41.9	43.8	32.7	25.1	30.5	20.7	13.1	12.5	14.0
Chronic liver disease and cirrhosis	7.8	8.7	11.9	9.9	7.1	6.2	6.2	6.7	6.8
Diabetes mellitus[6]	27.0	24.7	25.1	18.0	19.9	23.0	17.6	17.7	17.6
Alzheimer's disease	NA	NA	NA	V	V	19.3	27.3	26.1	25.9
Human immunodeficiency virus (HIV) disease	X	X	X	X	2.2	2.5	1.4	1.2	1.1
Unintentional injuries	54.0	40.0	35.1	26.1	21.5	22.0	25.6	26.4	26.6
Motor vehicle-related injuries	11.5	11.7	14.9	11.8	11.0	9.5	6.5	6.5	6.2
Poisoning	1.7	1.1	1.8	1.3	1.2	2.5	7.5	8.1	8.5
Nephritis, nephrotic syndrome, and nephrosis[6]	NA	NA	NA	7.3	7.7	11.5	13.0	11.1	11.3
Suicide[7]	5.6	5.6	7.4	5.7	4.8	4.0	5.0	5.4	5.5
Homicide[7]	2.4	2.6	3.7	4.4	4.0	2.8	2.3	2.2	2.1
White[8]									
All causes	1,410.8	1,311.3	1,193.3	1,012.7	909.8	849.8	741.8	730.9	731.0
Diseases of heart	586.0	559.0	492.2	409.4	317.0	253.4	176.9	168.9	168.2
Ischemic heart disease	NA	NA	NA	347.6	249.7	185.6	113.5	105.6	102.9
Cerebrovascular diseases	175.5	172.7	143.5	93.2	62.8	58.8	37.7	35.6	34.9
Malignant neoplasms	194.6	193.1	196.7	204.2	211.6	197.2	172.4	166.6	163.7
Trachea, bronchus, and lung	15.2	24.0	36.7	49.2	58.6	56.2	48.3	45.6	44.1

Table 2-17. Age-Adjusted Death Rates for Selected Causes of Death, by Sex, Race, and Hispanic Origin, Selected Years, 1950–2013—continued

(Age-adjusted rate per 100,000 population.)

Sex, race, Hispanic origin, and cause of death[1]	1950[2,3]	1960[2,3]	1970[3]	1980[3]	1990[3]	2000[4]	2010[4]	2012[4]	2013[4]
Colon, rectum, and anus	NA	30.9	29.2	27.4	24.1	20.3	15.3	14.5	14.3
Chronic lower respiratory diseases	NA	NA	NA	29.3	38.3	46.0	44.6	44.1	44.8
Influenza and pneumonia	44.8	50.4	39.8	30.9	36.4	23.5	14.9	14.3	15.8
Chronic liver disease and cirrhosis	11.5	13.2	16.6	13.9	10.5	9.6	9.9	10.5	10.7
Diabetes mellitus[6]	22.9	21.7	22.9	16.7	18.8	22.8	19.0	19.4	19.4
Alzheimer's disease	NA	NA	NA	V	V	18.8	26.0	24.7	24.4
Human immunodeficiency virus (HIV) disease	X	X	X	X	8.3	2.8	1.4	1.2	1.2
Unintentional injuries	77.0	60.4	57.8	45.3	35.5	35.1	40.3	41.5	41.9
Motor vehicle-related injuries	24.4	22.9	27.1	22.6	18.5	15.6	11.7	11.8	11.3
Poisoning	2.4	1.6	2.4	1.8	2.1	4.5	11.9	12.9	13.7
Nephritis, nephrotic syndrome, and nephrosis[6]	NA	NA	NA	8.0	8.3	12.1	14.0	12.0	12.1
Suicide[7]	13.9	13.1	13.8	13.0	13.4	11.3	13.6	14.1	14.2
Homicide[7]	2.6	2.7	4.7	6.7	5.5	3.6	3.3	3.2	3.1
Black or African American [8]									
All causes	1,722.1	1,577.5	1,518.1	1,314.8	1,250.3	1,121.4	898.2	864.8	860.8
Diseases of heart	588.7	548.3	512.0	455.3	391.5	324.8	224.9	211.7	210.4
Ischemic heart disease	NA	NA	NA	334.5	267.0	218.3	131.2	121.3	117.5
Cerebrovascular diseases	233.6	235.2	197.1	129.1	91.6	81.9	53.0	49.3	49.0
Malignant neoplasms	176.4	199.1	225.3	256.4	279.5	248.5	203.8	193.8	189.2
Trachea, bronchus, and lung	11.1	23.7	41.3	59.7	72.4	64.0	51.4	48.3	46.8
Colon, rectum, and anus	NA	22.8	26.1	28.3	30.6	28.2	21.8	20.0	19.4
Chronic lower respiratory diseases	NA	NA	NA	19.2	28.1	31.6	29.0	29.0	29.5
Influenza and pneumonia	76.7	81.1	57.2	34.4	39.4	25.6	16.8	15.7	16.7
Chronic liver disease and cirrhosis	9.0	13.6	28.1	25.0	16.5	9.4	6.7	6.9	7.3
Diabetes mellitus[6]	23.5	30.9	38.8	32.7	40.5	49.5	38.7	38.7	38.4
Alzheimer's disease	NA	NA	NA	V	V	13.0	20.6	19.9	20.1
Human immunodeficiency virus (HIV) disease	X	X	X	X	26.7	23.3	11.6	9.5	8.9
Unintentional injuries	79.9	74.0	78.3	57.6	43.8	37.7	31.3	31.4	32.6
Motor vehicle-related injuries	26.0	24.2	31.1	20.2	18.8	15.7	10.9	11.3	10.9
Poisoning	2.8	2.9	5.8	3.1	4.1	6.0	7.3	8.1	8.9
Nephritis, nephrotic syndrome, and nephrosis[6]	NA	NA	NA	20.9	19.8	28.7	29.3	25.2	25.0
Suicide[7]	4.5	5.0	6.2	6.5	7.1	5.5	5.2	5.6	5.4
Homicide[7]	28.3	26.0	44.0	39.0	36.3	20.5	17.7	18.4	17.8
American Indian or Alaska Native [8]									
All causes	NA	NA	NA	867.0	716.3	709.3	628.3	595.3	591.7
Diseases of heart	NA	NA	NA	240.6	200.6	178.2	128.6	119.6	120.6
Ischemic heart disease	NA	NA	NA	173.6	139.1	129.1	84.9	79.2	78.2
Cerebrovascular diseases	NA	NA	NA	57.8	40.7	45.0	28.1	25.2	24.6
Malignant neoplasms	NA	NA	NA	113.7	121.8	127.8	122.4	111.4	110.2
Trachea, bronchus, and lung	NA	NA	NA	20.7	30.9	32.3	33.1	30.1	27.7
Colon, rectum, and anus	NA	NA	NA	9.5	12.0	13.4	11.7	11.1	12.6
Chronic lower respiratory diseases	NA	NA	NA	14.2	25.4	32.8	33.8	29.8	30.8
Influenza and pneumonia	NA	NA	NA	44.4	36.1	22.3	15.9	13.1	15.0
Chronic liver disease and cirrhosis	NA	NA	NA	45.3	24.1	24.3	22.8	25.3	24.8
Diabetes mellitus[6]	NA	NA	NA	29.6	34.1	41.5	36.4	36.9	34.1
Alzheimer's disease	NA	NA	NA	V	V	9.1	17.2	12.3	12.7
Human immunodeficiency virus (HIV) disease	X	X	X	X	1.8	2.2	1.6	1.0	1.3
Unintentional injuries	NA	NA	NA	99.0	62.6	51.3	46.9	49.5	47.1
Motor vehicle-related injuries	NA	NA	NA	54.5	32.5	27.3	15.7	16.3	15.4
Poisoning	NA	NA	NA	2.3	3.2	4.7	13.0	15.1	14.2
Nephritis, nephrotic syndrome, and nephrosis[6]	NA	NA	NA	12.2	11.6	15.0	16.4	12.6	11.4
Suicide[7]	NA	NA	NA	11.9	11.7	9.8	10.8	10.8	11.7
Homicide[7]	NA	NA	NA	15.5	10.4	6.8	5.7	5.8	5.3
Asian or Pacific Islander [8]									
All causes	NA	NA	NA	589.9	582.0	506.4	424.3	407.1	405.4
Diseases of heart	NA	NA	NA	202.1	181.7	146.0	100.9	92.2	92.8
Ischemic heart disease	NA	NA	NA	168.2	139.6	109.6	68.7	60.5	59.9
Cerebrovascular diseases	NA	NA	NA	66.1	56.9	52.9	33.2	30.8	29.4
Malignant neoplasms	NA	NA	NA	126.1	134.2	121.9	108.9	104.2	100.5
Trachea, bronchus, and lung	NA	NA	NA	28.4	30.2	28.1	24.8	24.0	23.3
Colon, rectum, and anus	NA	NA	NA	16.4	14.4	12.7	11.4	10.8	9.8
Chronic lower respiratory diseases	NA	NA	NA	12.9	19.4	18.6	13.9	12.8	13.6
Influenza and pneumonia	NA	NA	NA	24.0	31.4	19.7	14.4	14.0	15.0
Chronic liver disease and cirrhosis	NA	NA	NA	6.1	5.2	3.5	3.2	3.3	3.3
Diabetes mellitus[6]	NA	NA	NA	12.6	14.6	16.4	15.5	15.7	15.8
Alzheimer's disease	NA	NA	NA	V	V	5.5	10.9	11.7	11.1
Human immunodeficiency virus (HIV) disease	X	X	X	X	2.2	0.6	0.4	0.4	0.4
Unintentional injuries	NA	NA	NA	27.0	23.9	17.9	15.0	15.1	15.2

Table 2-17. Age-Adjusted Death Rates for Selected Causes of Death, by Sex, Race, and Hispanic Origin, Selected Years, 1950–2013—continued

(Age-adjusted rate per 100,000 population.)

Sex, race, Hispanic origin, and cause of death[1]	1950[2,3]	1960[2,3]	1970[3]	1980[3]	1990[3]	2000[4]	2010[4]	2012[4]	2013[4]
Motor vehicle-related injuries	NA	NA	NA	13.9	14.0	8.6	5.1	4.6	4.8
Poisoning	NA	NA	NA	0.5	0.7	0.7	1.4	1.8	2.0
Nephritis, nephrotic syndrome, and nephrosis[6]	NA	NA	NA	7.2	7.1	8.4	9.6	8.0	8.1
Suicide[7]	NA	NA	NA	7.8	6.7	5.5	6.2	6.3	5.9
Homicide[7]	NA	NA	NA	5.9	5.0	3.0	1.8	1.9	1.5
Hispanic or Latino [8,9]									
All causes	NA	NA	NA	NA	692.0	665.7	558.6	539.1	535.4
Diseases of heart	NA	NA	NA	NA	217.1	196.0	132.8	122.0	121.2
Ischemic heart disease	NA	NA	NA	NA	173.3	153.2	92.3	81.1	80.3
Cerebrovascular diseases	NA	NA	NA	NA	45.2	46.4	32.1	30.0	29.6
Malignant neoplasms	NA	NA	NA	NA	136.8	134.9	119.7	116.9	114.5
Trachea, bronchus, and lung	NA	NA	NA	NA	26.5	24.8	20.4	19.2	18.7
Colon, rectum, and anus	NA	NA	NA	NA	14.7	14.1	12.3	11.7	11.7
Chronic lower respiratory diseases	NA	NA	NA	NA	19.3	21.1	19.6	18.5	18.7
Influenza and pneumonia	NA	NA	NA	NA	29.7	20.6	13.7	12.0	13.2
Chronic liver disease and cirrhosis	NA	NA	NA	NA	18.3	16.5	13.7	14.1	14.0
Diabetes mellitus[6]	NA	NA	NA	NA	28.2	36.9	27.1	26.9	26.3
Alzheimer's disease	NA	NA	NA	NA	V	10.4	18.5	17.4	17.7
Human immunodeficiency virus (HIV) disease	X	X	X	X	16.3	6.7	2.8	2.2	2.1
Unintentional injuries	NA	NA	NA	NA	34.6	30.1	25.8	26.5	26.9
Motor vehicle-related injuries	NA	NA	NA	NA	19.5	14.7	9.6	9.6	9.7
Poisoning	NA	NA	NA	NA	3.2	4.1	5.6	6.2	6.7
Nephritis, nephrotic syndrome, and nephrosis[6]	NA	NA	NA	NA	8.4	11.8	14.1	11.3	11.1
Suicide[7]	NA	NA	NA	NA	7.8	5.9	5.9	5.8	5.7
Homicide[7]	NA	NA	NA	NA	16.2	7.5	5.3	4.9	4.5
White, not Hispanic or Latino [9]									
All causes	NA	NA	NA	NA	914.5	855.5	755.0	745.8	747.1
Diseases of heart	NA	NA	NA	NA	319.7	255.5	179.9	172.3	171.8
Ischemic heart disease	NA	NA	NA	NA	251.9	186.6	115.0	107.4	104.6
Cerebrovascular diseases	NA	NA	NA	NA	63.5	59.0	37.8	35.8	35.0
Malignant neoplasms	NA	NA	NA	NA	215.4	200.6	176.5	170.6	167.7
Trachea, bronchus, and lung	NA	NA	NA	NA	60.3	58.2	50.8	48.0	46.6
Colon, rectum, and anus	NA	NA	NA	NA	24.6	20.5	15.5	14.7	14.5
Chronic lower respiratory diseases	NA	NA	NA	NA	39.2	47.2	46.6	46.3	47.0
Influenza and pneumonia	NA	NA	NA	NA	36.5	23.5	14.9	14.4	15.9
Chronic liver disease and cirrhosis	NA	NA	NA	NA	9.9	9.0	9.4	10.0	10.3
Diabetes mellitus[6]	NA	NA	NA	NA	18.3	21.8	18.2	18.5	18.6
Alzheimer's disease	NA	NA	NA	NA	V	19.1	26.4	25.1	24.8
Human immunodeficiency virus (HIV) disease	X	X	X	X	7.4	2.2	1.1	1.0	0.9
Unintentional injuries	NA	NA	NA	NA	35.0	35.3	42.4	43.9	44.2
Motor vehicle-related injuries	NA	NA	NA	NA	18.2	15.6	11.9	12.1	11.5
Poisoning	NA	NA	NA	NA	2.0	4.6	13.3	14.4	15.3
Nephritis, nephrotic syndrome, and nephrosis[6]	NA	NA	NA	NA	8.1	12.0	13.8	11.9	12.1
Suicide[7]	NA	NA	NA	NA	13.8	12.0	15.0	15.7	15.9
Homicide[7]	NA	NA	NA	NA	4.0	2.8	2.5	2.6	2.5

NA = Not available.   V = Data for Alzheimer's disease are only presented for data years 1999 and beyond due to large differences in death rates caused by changes in the coding of the causes of death between ICD-9 and ICD-10.   X = Not applicable.   1 Underlying cause of death code numbers are based on the applicable revision of the International Classification of Diseases (ICD) for data years shown.   2 Includes deaths of persons who were not residents of the 50 states and the District of Columbia.   3 Underlying cause of death was coded according to the 6th Revision of the ICD in 1950, 7th Revision in 1960, 8th Revision in 1970, and 9th Revision in 1980-1998.   4 Starting with 1999 data, cause of death is coded according to ICD-10.   5 Age-adjusted rates are calculated using the year 2000 standard population. Prior to 2001, age-adjusted rates were calculated using standard million proportions based on rounded population numbers. Starting with 2001 data, unrounded population numbers are used to calculate age-adjusted rates.   6 Starting with 2011 data, the rules for selecting Renal failure as the underlying cause of death were changed, affecting the number of deaths in the Nephritis, nephrotic syndrome and nephrosis and Diabetes categories. These changes directly affect deaths with mention of Renal failure and other associated conditions, such as Diabetes mellitus with renal complications. The result is a decrease in the number of deaths for Nephritis, nephrotic syndrome and nephrosis and an increase in the number of deaths for Diabetes mellitus. Therefore, trend data for these two causes of death should be interpreted with caution.   7 Figures for 2001 include September 11-related deaths, for which death certificates were filed as of October 24, 2002.   8 The race groups White, Black, Asian or Pacific Islander, and American Indian or Alaska Native, include persons of Hispanic and non-Hispanic origin. Persons of Hispanic origin may be of any race. Death rates for the American Indian or Alaska Native, Asian or Pacific Islander, and Hispanic populations are known to be underestimated.   9 Prior to 1997, data from states that did not report Hispanic origin on the death certificate were excluded.

Table 2-18. Number of Deaths, Death Rates, and Age-Adjusted Death Rates for Injury Deaths, by Mechanism and Intent of Death, 2013

(Number; rates per 100,000 population; age-adjusted rates per 100,000 U.S. standard population.)

Mechanism and intent of death (based on the ICD, Tenth Revision)	Number	Rate	Age-adjusted rate[1]
All Injury (*U01'-*U03, V01'-Y36, Y85'-Y87, Y89)	192,945	61.0	58.8
Unintentional (V01'-X59, Y85'-Y86)	130,557	41.3	39.4
Suicide (*U03,X60'-X84, Y87.0)	41,149	13.0	12.6
Homicide (*U01'-*U02, X85'-Y09, Y87.1)	16,121	5.1	5.2
Undetermined (Y10'-Y34, Y87.2, Y89.9)	4,587	1.5	1.4
Legal intervention/war (Y35'-Y36, Y89[.0,.1])	531	0.2	0.2
Cut/Pierce (W25'-W29, W45, X78, X99, Y28, Y35.4)	2,576	0.8	0.8
Unintentional (W25'-W29, W45)	134	0.0	0.0
Suicide (X78)	783	0.2	0.2
Homicide (X99)	1,639	0.5	0.5
Undetermined (Y28)	20	0.0	0.0
Legal intervention/war (Y35.4)	-	*	*
Drowning (W65'-W74, X71, X92, Y21)	4,056	1.3	1.3
Unintentional (W65'-W74)	3,391	1.1	1.1
Suicide (X71)	397	0.1	0.1
Homicide (X92)	30	0.0	0.0
Undetermined (Y21)	238	0.1	0.1
Fall (W00'-W19, X80, Y01, Y30)	31,240	9.9	8.8
Unintentional (W00'-W19)	30,208	9.6	8.5
Suicide (X80)	976	0.3	0.3
Homicide (Y01)	11	*	*
Undetermined (Y30)	45	0.0	0.0
Fire/Hot Object or Substance (*U01.3, X00'-X19, X76'-X77, X97'-X98, Y26'-Y27, Y36.3)[2]	3,220	1.0	1.0
Unintentional (X00'-X19)	2,818	0.9	0.8
Suicide (X76'-X77)	173	0.1	0.1
Homicide (*U01.3, X97'-X98)	97	0.0	0.0
Undetermined (Y26'-Y27)	132	0.0	0.1
Legal intervention/war (Y36.3)	-	*	*
Fire/flame (X00'-X09, X76, X97, Y26)	3,160	1.0	0.9
Unintentional (X00'-X09)	2,760	0.9	0.8
Suicide (X76)	173	0.1	0.1
Homicide (X97)	95	0.0	0.0
Undetermined (Y26)	132	0.0	0.1
Hot object/substance (X10'-X19, X77, X98,Y27)	60	0.0	0.0
Unintentional (X10'-X19)	58	0.0	0.0
Suicide (X77)	-	*	*
Homicide (X98)	2	*	*
Undetermined (Y27)	-	*	*
Firearm (*U01.4, W32'-W34, X72'-X74, X93'-X95, Y22'-Y24, Y35.0)	33,636	10.6	10.4
Unintentional (W32'-W34)	505	0.2	0.2
Suicide (X72'-X74)	21,175	6.7	6.4
Homicide (*U01.4, X93'-X95)	11,208	3.5	3.6
Undetermined (Y22'-Y24)	281	0.1	0.1
Legal intervention/war (Y35.0)	467	0.1	0.2
Machinery (W24,W30'-W31)[3]	588	0.2	0.2
All Transport (*U01.1, V01'-V99, X82, Y03, Y32, Y36.1)	37,427	11.8	11.6
Unintentional (V01'-V99)	37,184	11.8	11.5
Suicide (X82)	191	0.1	0.1
Homicide (*U01.1,Y03)	38	0.0	0.0
Undetermined (Y32)	14	*	*
Legal intervention/war (Y36.1)	-	*	*
Motor vehicle traffic (V02'-V04[.1,.9], V09.2, V12'-V14[.3'-.9], V19[.4'-.6], V20'-V28[.3'-.9], V29'-V79[.4'-.9], V80[.3'- .5],V81.1, V82.1,V83'-V86[.0'-.3], V87[.0'-.8],V89.2)[3]	33,804	10.7	10.5
Occupant (V30'-V79[.4'-.9], V83'-V86[.0'-.3])[3]	8,629	2.7	2.7
Motorcyclist (V20'-V28[.3'-.9], V29[.4'-.9])[3]	4,169	1.3	1.3
Pedal cyclist (V12'-V14[.3'-.9], V19[.4'-.6])[3]	623	0.2	0.2
Pedestrian (V02'-V04[.1,.9], V09.2)[3]	4,989	1.6	1.5
Other (V80[.3'-.5], V81.1, V82.1)[3]	6	*	*
Unspecified (V87[.0'-.8], V89.2)[3]	15,388	4.9	4.8
Pedal cyclist, other (V10'-V11, V12'-V14[.0'-.2], V15'-V18, V19[.0'-.3,.8,.9])[3]	302	0.1	0.1
Pedestrian, other (V01, V02'-V04[.0], V05, V06, V09[.0,.1,.3,.9])[3]	985	0.3	0.3
Other land transport (V20'-V28[.0'-.2], V29'-V79[.0'-.3],V80'-V82[.0,.2'-.9], V81'-V82[.0,.2'-.9], V83'-V86[.4'-.9],V87.9,V88[.0'-.9], V89[.0,.1,.3,.8],X82, Y03, Y32)[3]	1,521	0.5	0.5
Unintentional (V20'-V28[.0'-.2], V29'-V79[.0'-.3], V80(.0'-.2,.6'-.9), V81'-V82[.0,.2'-.9], V83'-V86[.4'-.9], V87.9, V88[.0'-.9], V89[.0,.1,.3,.9])	1,278	0.4	0.4
Suicide (X82)	191	0.1	0.1
Homicide (Y03)	38	0.0	0.0
Undetermined (Y32)	14	*	*
Other transport (*U01.1, V90'-V99, Y36.1)	815	0.3	0.3
Unintentional (V90'-V99)	815	0.3	0.3
Homicide (*U01.1)	-	*	*
Legal intervention/war (Y36.1)	-	*	*

Table 2-18. Number of Deaths, Death Rates, and Age-Adjusted Death Rates for Injury Deaths, by Mechanism and Intent of Death, 2013— continued

(Number; rates per 100,000 population; age-adjusted rates per 100,000 U.S. standard population.)

Mechanism and intent of death (based on the ICD, Tenth Revision)	Number	Rate	Age-adjusted rate[1]
Natural/Environmental (W42'-W43, W53'-W64, W92'-W99, X20'-X39, X51'-X57) [2]	1,535	0.5	0.5
Overexertion (X50) [2]	13	*	*
Poisoning (*U01[.6'-.7], X40'-X49, X60'-X69, X85'-X90, Y10'-Y19, Y35.2)	48,545	15.4	15.2
Unintentional (X40'-X49)	38,851	12.3	12.2
Suicide (X60'-X69)	6,637	2.1	2.0
Homicide (*U01[.6'-.7], X85'-X90)	97	0.0	0.0
Undetermined (Y10'-Y19)	2,960	0.9	0.9
Legal intervention/war (Y35.2)	-	*	*
Struck by or Against (W20'-W22, W50'-W52, X79, Y00, Y04, Y29, Y35.3)	936	0.3	0.3
Unintentional (W20'-W22, W50'-W52)	823	0.3	0.2
Suicide (X79)	-	*	*
Homicide (Y00,Y04)	111	0.0	0.0
Undetermined (Y29)	2	*	*
Legal intervention/war (Y35.3)	-	*	*
Suffocation (W75'-W84, X70, X91,Y20)	17,316	5.5	5.4
Unintentional (W75'-W84)	6,601	2.1	2.0
Suicide (X70)	10,062	3.2	3.2
Homicide (X91)	533	0.2	0.2
Undetermined (Y20)	120	0.0	0.0
Other Specified, Classifiable (*U01[.0,.2,.5], *U03.0, W23, W35'-W41, W44,W49, W85'-W91, X75, X81, X96, Y02, Y05'- Y07, Y25, Y31, Y35[.1,.5], Y36[.0,.2,.4'-.8], Y85)	2,100	0.7	0.6
Unintentional (W23, W35'-W41, W44, W49, W85'-W91, Y85)	1,325	0.4	0.4
Suicide (*U03.0, X75, X81)	525	0.2	0.2
Homicide (*U01[.0,.2,.5], X96, Y02, Y05'-Y07)	197	0.1	0.0
Undetermined (Y25, Y31)	15	*	*
Legal intervention/war (Y35[.1,.5], Y36[.0,.2,.4'-.8])	38	0.0	0.0
Other Specified, Not Elsewhere Classified (*U01.8, *U02, X58, X83, Y08, Y33, Y35.6, Y86'-Y87, Y89[.0'-.1])	1,981	0.6	0.6
Unintentional (X58, Y86)	1,174	0.4	0.3
Suicide (X83, Y87.0)	163	0.1	0.1
Homicide (*U01.8, *U02, Y08, Y87.1)	440	0.1	0.1
Undetermined (Y33, Y87.2)	180	0.1	0.1
Legal intervention/war (Y35.6, Y89[.0,.1])	24	0.0	0.0
Unspecified (*U01.9, *U03.9, X59, X84, Y09, Y34, Y35.7, Y36.9, Y89.9)	7,776	2.5	2.2
Unintentional (X59)	5,407	1.7	1.5
Suicide (*U03.9, X84)	67	0.0	0.0
Homicide (*U01.9, Y09)	1,720	0.5	0.5
Undetermined (Y34, Y89.9)	580	0.2	0.2
Legal intervention/war (Y35.7, Y36.9)	2	*	*

- = Quantity zero.   * = Figure does not meet standard of reliability or precision.   0.0 = Quantity more than zero but less than 0.05.   1 For method of computation, see chapter notes.   2 Codes *U01.3 and Y36.3 cannot be divided separately into the subcategories shown below; therefore, subcategories may not add to the total.   3 Intent of death is unintentional.

Table 2-19. Leading Causes of Death and Numbers of Death, by Sex, Race, and Hispanic Origin, 1980 and 2013

(Number.)

Sex, race, Hispanic origin, and rank order	1980 Cause	Cause of death	Sex, race, Hispanic origin, and rank order	2013[1] Cause	Cause of death
All Persons			**All Persons**		
Rank	All causes	1,989,841	Rank	All causes	2,596,993
1	Diseases of heart	761,085	1	Diseases of heart	611,105
2	Malignant neoplasms	416,509	2	Malignant neoplasms	584,881
3	Cerebrovascular diseases	170,225	3	Chronic lower respiratory diseases	149,205
4	Unintentional injuries	105,718	4	Unintentional injuries	130,557
5	Chronic obstructive pulmonary diseases	56,050	5	Cerebrovascular diseases	128,978
6	Pneumonia and influenza	54,619	6	Alzheimer's disease	84,767
7	Diabetes mellitus	34,851	7	Diabetes mellitus[1]	75,578
8	Chronic liver disease and cirrhosis	30,583	8	Influenza and pneumonia	56,979
9	Atherosclerosis	29,449	9	Nephritis, nephrotic syndrome and nephrosis[1]	47,112
10	Suicide	26,869	10	Suicide	41,149
Male			**Male**		
Rank	All causes	1,075,078	Rank	All causes	1,306,034
1	Diseases of heart	405,661	1	Diseases of heart	321,347
2	Malignant neoplasms	225,948	2	Malignant neoplasms	307,559
3	Unintentional injuries	74,180	3	Unintentional injuries	81,916
4	Cerebrovascular diseases	69,973	4	Chronic lower respiratory diseases	70,317
5	Chronic obstructive pulmonary diseases	38,625	5	Cerebrovascular diseases	53,691
6	Pneumonia and influenza	27,574	6	Diabetes mellitus[1]	39,841
7	Suicide	20,505	7	Suicide	32,055
8	Chronic liver disease and cirrhosis	19,768	8	Influenza and pneumonia	26,804
9	Homicide	18,779	9	Alzheimer's disease	25,836
10	Diabetes mellitus	14,325	10	Chronic liver disease and cirrhosis	23,709
Female			**Female**		
Rank	All causes	914,763	Rank	All causes	1,290,959
1	Diseases of heart	355,424	1	Diseases of heart	289,758
2	Malignant neoplasms	190,561	2	Malignant neoplasms	277,322
3	Cerebrovascular diseases	100,252	3	Chronic lower respiratory diseases	78,888
4	Unintentional injuries	31,538	4	Cerebrovascular diseases	75,287
5	Pneumonia and influenza	27,045	5	Alzheimer's disease	58,931
6	Diabetes mellitus	20,526	6	Unintentional injuries	48,641
7	Atherosclerosis	17,848	7	Diabetes mellitus[1]	35,737
8	Chronic obstructive pulmonary diseases	17,425	8	Influenza and pneumonia	30,175
9	Chronic liver disease and cirrhosis	10,815	9	Nephritis, nephrotic syndrome and nephrosis[1]	23,619
10	Certain conditions originating in the perinatal period	9,815	10	Septicemia	20,162
White			**White**		
Rank	All causes	1,738,607	Rank	All causes	2,217,103
1	Diseases of heart	683,347	1	Diseases of heart	522,645
2	Malignant neoplasms	368,162	2	Malignant neoplasms	498,116
3	Cerebrovascular diseases	148,734	3	Chronic lower respiratory diseases	136,682
4	Unintentional injuries	90,122	4	Unintentional injuries	112,803
5	Chronic obstructive pulmonary diseases	52,375	5	Cerebrovascular diseases	107,909
6	Pneumonia and influenza	48,369	6	Alzheimer's disease	77,387
7	Diabetes mellitus	28,868	7	Diabetes mellitus[1]	58,925
8	Atherosclerosis	27,069	8	Influenza and pneumonia	49,013
9	Chronic liver disease and cirrhosis	25,240	9	Nephritis, nephrotic syndrome and nephrosis[1]	37,270
10	Suicide	24,829	10	Suicide	37,154
Black			**Black**		
Rank	All causes	233,135	Rank	All causes	302,969
1			1		
2	Diseases of heart	72,956	2	Diseases of heart	72,010
3	Malignant neoplasms	45,037	3	Malignant neoplasms	67,953
4	Cerebrovascular diseases	20,135	4	Cerebrovascular diseases	16,269
5	Unintentional injuries	13,480	5	Unintentional injuries	13,413
6	Homicide	10,172	6	Diabetes mellitus[1]	13,385
7	Certain conditions originating in the perinatal period	6,961	7	Chronic lower respiratory diseases	9,918
8	Pneumonia and influenza	5,648	8	Nephritis, nephrotic syndrome and nephrosis[1]	8,393
9	Diabetes mellitus	5,544	9	Homicide	8,059
10	Chronic liver disease and cirrhosis	4,790	10	Septicemia	6,250
	Nephritis, nephrotic syndrome, and nephrosis	3,416		Alzheimer's disease	5,714

Table 2-19. Leading Causes of Death and Numbers of Death, by Sex, Race, and Hispanic Origin, 1980 and 2013 — continued

(Number.)

Sex, race, Hispanic origin, and rank order	1980	Cause of death	Sex, race, Hispanic origin, and rank order	2013[1]	Cause of death
American Indian or Alaska Native			**American Indian or Alaska Native**		
Rank	All causes	6,923	Rank	All causes	17,052
1	Diseases of heart	1,494	1	Diseases of heart	3,139
2	Unintentional injuries	1,290	2	Malignant neoplasms	3,109
3	Malignant neoplasms	770	3	Unintentional injuries	1,833
4	Chronic liver disease and cirrhosis	410	4	Diabetes mellitus[1]	959
5	Cerebrovascular diseases	322	5	Chronic liver disease and cirrhosis	944
6	Pneumonia and influenza	257	6	Chronic lower respiratory diseases	757
7	Homicide	217	7	Cerebrovascular diseases	595
8	Diabetes mellitus	210	8	Suicide	521
9	Certain conditions originating in the perinatal period	199	9	Influenza and pneumonia	375
10	Suicide	181	10	Nephritis, nephrotic syndrome and nephrosis[1]	302
Asian or Pacific Islander			**Asian or Pacific Islander**		
Rank	All causes	11,071	Rank	All causes	59,869
1	Diseases of heart	3,265	1	Malignant neoplasms	15,703
2	Malignant neoplasms	2,522	2	Diseases of heart	13,311
3	Cerebrovascular diseases	1,028	3	Cerebrovascular diseases	4,205
4	Unintentional injuries	810	4	Unintentional injuries	2,508
5	Pneumonia and influenza	342	5	Diabetes mellitus[1]	2,309
6	Suicide	249	6	Influenza and pneumonia	2,024
7	Certain conditions originating in the perinatal period	246	7	Chronic lower respiratory diseases	1,848
8	Diabetes mellitus	227	8	Alzheimer's disease	1,428
9	Homicide	211	9	Nephritis, nephrotic syndrome and nephrosis[1]	1,147
10	Chronic obstructive pulmonary diseases	207	10	Suicide	1,121
Hispanic or Latino			**Hispanic or Latino**		
Rank	NA	NA	Rank	All causes	163,241
1	NA	NA	1	Malignant neoplasms	35,147
2	NA	NA	2	Diseases of heart	33,243
3	NA	NA	3	Unintentional injuries	12,015
4	NA	NA	4	Cerebrovascular diseases	8,127
5	NA	NA	5	Diabetes mellitus[1]	7,632
6	NA	NA	6	Chronic liver disease and cirrhosis	5,141
7	NA	NA	7	Chronic lower respiratory diseases	4,827
8	NA	NA	8	Alzheimer's disease	4,127
9	NA	NA	9	Influenza and pneumonia	3,592
10	NA	NA	10	Nephritis, nephrotic syndrome and nephrosis[1]	3,083
White Male			**White Male**		
Rank	All causes	933,878	Rank	All causes	1,110,956
1	Diseases of heart	364,679	1	Diseases of heart	275,101
2	Malignant neoplasms	198,188	2	Malignant neoplasms	263,167
3	Unintentional injuries	62,963	3	Unintentional injuries	70,161
4	Cerebrovascular diseases	60,095	4	Chronic lower respiratory diseases	63,757
5	Chronic obstructive pulmonary diseases	35,977	5	Cerebrovascular diseases	44,203
6	Pneumonia and influenza	23,810	6	Diabetes mellitus[1]	31,745
7	Suicide	18,901	7	Suicide	28,943
8	Chronic liver disease and cirrhosis	16,407	8	Alzheimer's disease	23,648
9	Diabetes mellitus	12,125	9	Influenza and pneumonia	22,907
10	Atherosclerosis	10,543	10	Chronic liver disease and cirrhosis	20,884
Black or African American Male			**Black or African American male**		
Rank	All causes	130,138	Rank	All causes	154,767
1	Diseases of heart	37,877	1	Diseases of heart	37,096
2	Malignant neoplasms	25,861	2	Malignant neoplasms	34,671
3	Unintentional injuries	9,701	3	Unintentional injuries	9,017
4	Cerebrovascular diseases	9,194	4	Cerebrovascular diseases	7,338
5	Homicide	8,274	5	Homicide	6,937
6	Certain conditions originating in the perinatal period	3,869	6	Diabetes mellitus[1]	6,378
7	Pneumonia and influenza	3,386	7	Chronic lower respiratory diseases	5,073
8	Chronic liver disease and cirrhosis	3,020	8	Nephritis, nephrotic syndrome and nephrosis[1]	3,976
9	Chronic obstructive pulmonary diseases	2,429	9	Septicemia	2,882
10	Diabetes mellitus	2,010	10	Influenza and pneumonia	2,696

Table 2-19. Leading Causes of Death and Numbers of Death, by Sex, Race, and Hispanic Origin, 1980 and 2013 — continued

(Number.)

Sex, race, Hispanic origin, and rank order	1980	Cause of death	Sex, race, Hispanic origin, and rank order	2013[1]	Cause of death
American Indian or Alaska Native Male			**American Indian or Alaska Native Male**		
Rank	All causes	4,193	Rank	All causes	9,331
1	Unintentional injuries	946	1	Diseases of heart	1,843
2	Diseases of heart	917	2	Malignant neoplasms	1,650
3	Malignant neoplasms	408	3	Unintentional injuries	1,177
4	Chronic liver disease and cirrhosis	239	4	Chronic liver disease and cirrhosis	511
5	Cerebrovascular diseases	163	5	Diabetes mellitus[1]	490
6	Homicide	162	6	Suicide	401
71	Pneumonia and influenza	148	71	Chronic lower respiratory diseases	370
8	Suicide	147	8	Cerebrovascular diseases	253
9	Certain conditions originating in the perinatal period	107	9	Influenza and pneumonia	190
10	Diabetes mellitus	86	10	Homicide	187
Asian or Pacific Islander Male			**Asian or Pacific Islander Male**		
Rank	All causes	6,809	Rank	All causes	30,980
1	Diseases of heart	2,174	1	Malignant neoplasms	8,071
2	Malignant neoplasms	1,485	2	Diseases of heart	7,307
3	Unintentional injuries	556	3	Cerebrovascular diseases	1,897
4	Cerebrovascular diseases	521	4	Unintentional injuries	1,561
5	Pneumonia and influenza	227	5	Diabetes mellitus[1]	1,228
6	Suicide	159	6	Chronic lower respiratory diseases	1,117
7	Chronic obstructive pulmonary diseases	158	7	Influenza and pneumonia	1,011
8	Homicide	151	8	Suicide	820
9	Certain conditions originating in the perinatal period	128	9	Nephritis, nephrotic syndrome and nephrosis[1]	574
10	Diabetes mellitus	103	10	Alzheimer's disease	447
Hispanic or Latino Male			**Hispanic or Latino Male**		
Rank	NA	NA	Rank	All causes	30,980
1	NA	NA	1	Malignant neoplasms	8,071
2	NA	NA	2	Diseases of heart	7,307
3	NA	NA	3	Cerebrovascular diseases	1,897
4	NA	NA	4	Unintentional injuries	1,561
5	NA	NA	5	Diabetes mellitus[1]	1,228
6	NA	NA	6	Chronic lower respiratory diseases	1,117
7	NA	NA	7	Influenza and pneumonia	1,011
8	NA	NA	8	Suicide	820
9	NA	NA	9	Nephritis, nephrotic syndrome and nephrosis[1]	574
10	NA	NA	10	Alzheimer's disease	447
White Female			**White Female**		
Rank	All causes	804,729	Rank	All causes	1,106,147
1	Diseases of heart	318,668	1	Diseases of heart	247,544
2	Malignant neoplasms	169,974	2	Malignant neoplasms	234,949
3	Cerebrovascular diseases	88,639	3	Chronic lower respiratory diseases	72,925
4	Unintentional injuries	27,159	4	Cerebrovascular diseases	63,706
5	Pneumonia and influenza	24,559	5	Alzheimer's disease	53,739
6	Diabetes mellitus	16,743	6	Unintentional injuries	42,642
7	Atherosclerosis	16,526	7	Diabetes mellitus[1]	27,180
8	Chronic obstructive pulmonary diseases	16,398	8	Influenza and pneumonia	26,106
9	Chronic liver disease and cirrhosis	8,833	9	Nephritis, nephrotic syndrome and nephrosis[1]	18,470
10	Certain conditions originating in the perinatal period	6,512	10	Septicemia	16,287
Black or African American Female			**Black or African American Female**		
Rank	All causes	102,997	Rank	All causes	148,202
1	Diseases of heart	35,079	1	Diseases of heart	34,914
2	Malignant neoplasms	19,176	2	Malignant neoplasms	33,282
3	Cerebrovascular diseases	10,941	3	Cerebrovascular diseases	8,931
4	Unintentional injuries	3,779	4	Diabetes mellitus[1]	7,007
5	Diabetes mellitus	3,534	5	Chronic lower respiratory diseases	4,845
6	Certain conditions originating in the perinatal period	3,092	6	Nephritis, nephrotic syndrome and nephrosis[1]	4,417
7	Pneumonia and influenza	2,262	7	Unintentional injuries	4,396
8	Homicide	1,898	8	Alzheimer's disease	4,050
9	Chronic liver disease and cirrhosis	1,770	9	Septicemia	3,368
10	Nephritis, nephrotic syndrome, and nephrosis	1,722	10	Essential hypertension and hypertensive renal disease	2,959

Table 2-19. Leading Causes of Death and Numbers of Death, by Sex, Race, and Hispanic Origin, 1980 and 2013 — continued

(Number.)

Sex, race, Hispanic origin, and rank order	1980	Cause of death	Sex, race, Hispanic origin, and rank order	2013[1]	Cause of death
American Indian or Alaska Native Female			**American Indian or Alaska Native Female**		
Rank	All causes	2,730	Rank	All causes	7,721
1	Diseases of heart	577	1	Malignant neoplasms	1,459
2	Malignant neoplasms	362	2	Diseases of heart	1,296
3	Unintentional injuries	344	3	Unintentional injuries	656
4	Chronic liver disease and cirrhosis	171	4	Diabetes mellitus[1]	469
5	Cerebrovascular diseases	159	5	Chronic liver disease and cirrhosis	433
6	Diabetes mellitus	124	6	Chronic lower respiratory diseases	387
7	Pneumonia and influenza	109	7	Cerebrovascular diseases	342
8	Certain conditions originating in the perinatal period	92	8	Influenza and pneumonia	185
9	Nephritis, nephrotic syndrome, and nephrosis	56	9	Alzheimer's disease	161
10	Homicide	55	10	Nephritis, nephrotic syndrome and nephrosis[1]	159
Asian or Pacific Islander Female			**Asian or Pacific Islander Female**		
Rank	All causes	4,262	Rank	All causes	28,889
1	Diseases of heart	1,091	1	Malignant neoplasms	7,632
2	Malignant neoplasms	1,037	2	Diseases of heart	6,004
3	Cerebrovascular diseases	507	3	Cerebrovascular diseases	2,308
4	Unintentional injuries	254	4	Diabetes mellitus[1]	1,081
5	Diabetes mellitus	124	5	Influenza and pneumonia	1,013
6	Certain conditions originating in the perinatal period	118	6	Alzheimer's disease	981
7	Pneumonia and influenza	115	7	Unintentional injuries	947
8	Congenital anomalies	104	8	Chronic lower respiratory diseases	731
9	Suicide	90	9	Nephritis, nephrotic syndrome and nephrosis[1]	573
10	Homicide	60	10	Essential hypertension and hypertensive renal disease	550
Hispanic or Latina Female			**Hispanic or Latina Female**		
Rank	NA	NA	Rank	All causes	74,361
1	NA	NA	1	Malignant neoplasms	16,776
2	NA	NA	2	Diseases of heart	14,866
3	NA	NA	3	Cerebrovascular diseases	4,286
4	NA	NA	4	Diabetes mellitus[1]	3,698
5	NA	NA	5	Unintentional injuries	3,255
6	NA	NA	6	Alzheimer's disease	2,829
7	NA	NA	7	Chronic lower respiratory diseases	2,291
8	NA	NA	8	Influenza and pneumonia	1,776
9	NA	NA	9	Chronic liver disease and cirrhosis	1,589
10	NA	NA	10	Nephritis, nephrotic syndrome and nephrosis[1]	1,500

NA = Not available. Complete coverage of all states for the Hispanic origin variable began in 1997.   1 Starting with 2011 data, the rules for selecting renal failure as the underlying cause of death were changed, affecting the number of deaths in the nephritis, nephrotic syndrome and nephrosis and diabetes categories. These changes directly affect deaths with mention of renal failure and other associated conditions, such as diabetes mellitus with renal complications. The result is a decrease in the number of deaths for nephritis, nephrotic syndrome and nephrosis and an increase in the number of deaths for diabetes mellitus. Therefore, trend data for these two causes of death should be interpreted with caution.

Table 2-20. Leading Causes of Death and Numbers of Deaths, by Age, 1980 and 2013

(Number.)

Age and rank order	1980 Cause of death	Deaths	Age and rank order	2013[1] Cause of death	Deaths
Under 1 Year			**Under 1 Year**		
Rank	All causes	45,526	Rank	All causes	23,440
1	Congenital anomalies	9,220	1	Congenital malformations, deformations and chromosomal abnormalities	4,758
2	Sudden infant death syndrome	5,510	2	Disorders related to short gestation and low birthweight, not elsewhere classified	4,202
3	Respiratory distress syndrome	4,989	3	Newborn affected by maternal complications of pregnancy	1,595
4	Disorders relating to short gestation and unspecified low birthweight	3,648	4	Sudden infant death syndrome	1,563
5	Newborn affected by maternal complications of pregnancy	1,572	5	Unintentional injuries	1,156
6	Intrauterine hypoxia and birth asphyxia	1,497	6	Newborn affected by complications of placenta, cord and membranes	953
7	Unintentional injuries	1,166	7	Bacterial sepsis of newborn	578
8	Birth trauma	1,058	8	Respiratory distress of newborn	522
9	Pneumonia and influenza	1,012	9	Diseases of circulatory system	458
10	Newborn affected by complications of placenta, cord, and membranes	985	10	Neonatal hemorrhage	389
1 to 4 Years			**1 to 4 Years**		
Rank	All causes	8,187	Rank	All causes	4,068
1	Unintentional injuries	3,313	1	Unintentional injuries	1,316
2	Congenital anomalies	1,026	2	Congenital malformations, deformations and chromosomal abnormalities	476
3	Malignant neoplasms	573	3	Homicide	337
4	Diseases of heart	338	4	Malignant neoplasms	328
5	Homicide	319	5	Diseases of heart	169
6	Pneumonia and influenza	267	6	Influenza and pneumonia	102
7	Meningitis	223	7	Chronic lower respiratory diseases	64
8	Meningococcal infection	110	8	Septicemia	53
9	Certain conditions originating in the perinatal period	84	9	In situ neoplasms, benign neoplasms and neoplasms of uncertain or unknown behavior	47
10	Septicemia	71	10	Certain conditions originating in the perinatal period	45
5 to 14 Years			**5 to 14 Years**		
Rank	All causes	10,689	Rank	All causes	5,340
1	Unintentional injuries	5,224	1	Unintentional injuries	1,521
2	Malignant neoplasms	1,497	2	Malignant neoplasms	895
3	Congenital anomalies	561	3	Suicide	395
4	Homicide	415	4	Congenital malformations, deformations and chromosomal abnormalities	340
5	Diseases of heart	330	5	Homicide	277
6	Pneumonia and influenza	194	6	Diseases of heart	173
7	Suicide	142	7	Chronic lower respiratory diseases	155
8	Benign neoplasms	104	8	Influenza and pneumonia	128
9	Cerebrovascular diseases	95	9	Cerebrovascular diseases	89
10	Chronic obstructive pulmonary diseases	85	10	In situ neoplasms, benign neoplasms and neoplasms of uncertain or unknown behavior	65
15 to 24 Years			**15 to 24 Years**		
Rank	All causes	49,027	Rank	All causes	28,486
1	Unintentional injuries	26,206	1	Unintentional injuries	11,619
2	Homicide	6,537	2	Suicide	4,878
3	Suicide	5,239	3	Homicide	4,329
4	Malignant neoplasms	2,683	4	Malignant neoplasms	1,496
5	Diseases of heart	1,223	5	Diseases of heart	941
6	Congenital anomalies	600	6	Congenital malformations, deformations and chromosomal abnormalities	362
7	Cerebrovascular diseases	418	7	Influenza and pneumonia	197
8	Pneumonia and influenza	348	8	Diabetes mellitus[1]	193
9	Chronic obstructive pulmonary diseases	141	9	Pregnancy, childbirth, and the puerperium	178
10	Anemias	133	10	Chronic lower respiratory diseases	155
25 to 44 Years			**25 to 44 Years**		
Rank	All causes	108,658	Rank	All causes	115,036
1			1		
2	Unintentional injuries	26,722	2	Unintentional injuries	31,563
3	Malignant neoplasms	17,551	3	Malignant neoplasms	15,022
4	Diseases of heart	14,513	4	Diseases of heart	13,599
5	Homicide	10,983	5	Suicide	12,899
6	Suicide	9,855	6	Homicide	6,817
7	Chronic liver disease and cirrhosis	4,782	7	Chronic liver disease and cirrhosis	3,167
8	Cerebrovascular diseases	3,154	8	Diabetes mellitus[1]	2,636
9	Diabetes mellitus	1,472	9	Cerebrovascular diseases	2,195
10	Pneumonia and influenza	1,467	10	Human immunodeficiency virus (HIV) disease	1,877
101	Congenital anomalies	817	101	Influenza and pneumonia	1,330

Table 2-20. Leading Causes of Death and Numbers of Deaths, by Age, 1980 and 2013— continued

(Number.)

Age and rank order	1980		Age and rank order	2013[1]	
	Cause of death	Deaths		Cause of death	Deaths
45 to 64 Years			**45 to 64 Years**		
Rank	All causes	425,338	Rank	All causes	515,851
1	Diseases of heart	148,322	1	Malignant neoplasms	159,509
2	Malignant neoplasms	135,675	2	Diseases of heart	107,735
3	Cerebrovascular diseases	19,909	3	Unintentional injuries	37,414
4	Unintentional injuries	18,140	4	Chronic liver disease and cirrhosis	20,736
5	Chronic liver disease and cirrhosis	16,089	5	Chronic lower respiratory diseases	20,561
6	Chronic obstructive pulmonary diseases	11,514	6	Diabetes mellitus[1]	18,960
7	Diabetes mellitus	7,977	7	Cerebrovascular diseases	16,789
8	Suicide	7,079	8	Suicide	15,756
9	Pneumonia and influenza	5,804	9	Septicemia	7,790
10	Homicide	4,019	10	Influenza and pneumonia	7,012
65 Years and Over			**65 Years and Over**		
Rank	All causes	1,341,848	Rank	All causes	1,904,640
1	Diseases of heart	595,406	1	Diseases of heart	488,156
2	Malignant neoplasms	258,389	2	Malignant neoplasms	407,558
3	Cerebrovascular diseases	146,417	3	Chronic lower respiratory diseases	127,194
4	Pneumonia and influenza	45,512	4	Cerebrovascular diseases	109,602
5	Chronic obstructive pulmonary diseases	43,587	5	Alzheimer's disease	83,786
6	Atherosclerosis	28,081	6	Diabetes mellitus[1]	53,751
7	Diabetes mellitus	25,216	7	Influenza and pneumonia	48,031
8	Unintentional injuries	24,844	8	Unintentional injuries	45,942
9	Nephritis, nephrotic syndrome, and nephrosis	12,968	9	Nephritis, nephrotic syndrome and nephrosis[1]	39,080
10	Chronic liver disease and cirrhosis	9,519	10	Septicemia	28,815

1 Starting with 2011 data, the rules for selecting renal failure as the underlying cause of death were changed, affecting the number of deaths in the nephritis, nephrotic syndrome and nephrosis and diabetes categories. These changes directly affect deaths with mention of renal failure and other associated conditions, such as diabetes mellitus with renal complications. The result is a decrease in the number of deaths for nephritis, nephrotic syndrome and nephrosis and an increase in the number of deaths for diabetes mellitus. Therefore, trend data for these two causes of death should be interpreted with caution.

Table 2-21. Deaths from Selected Occupational Diseases Among Persons 15 Years of Age and Over, Selected Years, 1980–2013

(Number of deaths.)

Cause of death	1980[1]	1990[1]	2000[2]	2010[2]	2011[2]	2012[2]	2013[2]
Multiple Cause of Death (Number of Death Certificates with Cause of Death Code(s) Mentioned)							
Angiosarcoma of liver[3]	NA	NA	16	29	22	29	22
Malignant mesothelioma[4]	699	874	2,531	2,744	2,832	2,874	2,686
Pneumoconiosis[5]	4,151	3,644	2,859	2,028	1,890	1,850	1,859
Coal workers' pneumoconiosis	2,576	1,990	949	486	409	399	361
Asbestosis	339	948	1,486	1,308	1,243	1,208	1,229
Silicosis	448	308	151	101	88	103	111
Other (including unspecified)	814	413	290	146	166	153	170
Underlying Cause of Death							
Angiosarcoma of liver[3]	NA	NA	15	28	20	27	19
Malignant mesothelioma[4]	531	725	2,384	2,573	2,651	2,686	2,497
Pneumoconiosis	1,581	1,335	1,142	820	752	755	781
Coal workers' pneumoconiosis	982	734	389	213	160	158	151
Asbestosis	101	302	558	486	460	466	475
Silicosis	207	150	71	52	56	58	70
Other (including unspecified)	291	149	124	69	76	73	85

NA = Not available.   Note: Multiple cause of death includes underlying and nonunderlying causes of death. Cause-of-death titles for selected occupational diseases and corresponding code numbers according to the International Classification of Diseases, 9th and 10th Revisions.   1 For the period 1980-1998, underlying cause of death was coded according to the 9th Revision of the International Classification of Diseases (ICD).   2 Starting with 1999 data, ICD-10 was introduced for coding cause of death. Discontinuities exist between 1998 and 1999 due to ICD-10 coding and classification changes.   3 Prior to 1999, there was no discrete code for this condition.   4 Prior to 1999, the combined ICD-9 categories of malignant neoplasm of peritoneum and malignant neoplasm of pleura served as a crude surrogate for malignant mesothelioma category under ICD-10.   5 For multiple cause of death, counts for pneumoconiosis subgroups may sum to slightly more than total pneumoconiosis due to the reporting of more than one type of pneumoconiosis on some death certificates. Multiple cause of death includes underlying and nonunderlying causes of death.

Figure 2-6. Number of Fatal Occupational Injuries by Selected Industry, 2012

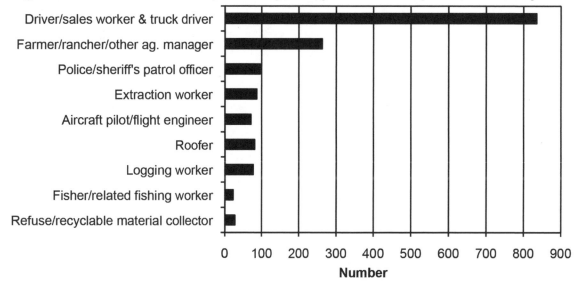

Figure 2-7. Number of Fatal Occupational Injuries by Selected Occupation, Preliminary 2014

Table 2-22. Occupational Fatal Injuries, by Industry, Sex, Age, Race, and Hispanic Origin, Selected Years 2005–2012

(Number.)

Characteristic	2005	2006	2007	2008	2009	2010	2011	2012
Rate								
Total workforce	5,734	5,840	5,657	5,214	4,551	4,690	4,693	4,628
Sex								
Male	5,328	5,396	5,228	4,827	4,216	4,322	4,308	4,277
Female	406	444	429	387	335	368	385	351
Age								
Under 16 years	23	11	18	11	13	16	10	19
16-17 years	31	21	20	23	14	18	13	10
18-19 years	111	106	97	66	57	56	61	59
20-24 years	403	390	424	353	275	245	292	287
25-34 years	1,017	1,041	991	850	704	785	714	736
35-44 years	1,243	1,288	1,168	1,113	908	868	875	829
45-54 years	1,389	1,417	1,425	1,292	1,173	1,169	1,222	1,161
55-64 years	933	963	934	920	853	948	936	936
65 years and over	578	599	574	580	551	582	569	588
Unspecified	6	4	6	6	3	3	1	3
Race and Hispanic origin								
Hispanic or Latino (may be of any race)	923	990	937	804	713	707	749	748
Not Hispanic or Latino	4,811	4,850	4,720	4,410	3,838	3,983	3,944	3,880
White	3,977	4,019	3,867	3,663	3,204	3,363	3,323	3,177
Black or African American	584	565	609	533	421	412	440	486
American Indian or Alaska Native	50	46	29	32	33	32	30	37
Asian	154	148	166	145	141	143	121	147
Native Hawaiian or Other Pacific Islander	9	11	6	7	7	6	3	7
Multiple races	*	11	10	6	7	8	15	5
Other races or not reported	35	50	33	24	25	19	12	21
Industry [1]								
Private sector	5,214	5,320	5,112	4,670	4,090	4,206	4,188	4,175
Agriculture, forestry, fishing, and hunting	715	655	585	672	575	621	566	509
Mining[2]	159	192	183	176	99	172	155	181
Utilities	30	53	34	37	16	26	39	23
Construction	1,192	1,239	1,204	975	834	774	738	806
Manufacturing	393	456	400	411	319	329	327	327
Wholesale trade	209	222	207	180	190	191	190	204
Retail trade	400	359	348	301	307	311	268	273
Transportation and warehousing	885	860	890	796	633	661	749	741
Information	65	66	79	47	33	43	56	42
Finance and insurance	42	44	46	24	33	24	36	21
Real estate and rental and leasing	57	82	73	82	75	89	62	64
Professional and technical services	83	78	77	69	85	76	74	57
Management, administrative, and waste services[3]	NA	NA	NA	NA	NA	NA	359	352
Educational services	46	49	34	28	27	30	37	34
Health care and social assistance	104	129	115	113	123	141	117	107
Arts, entertainment, and recreation	77	80	96	92	80	84	93	80
Accommodation and food services	136	185	164	146	151	154	138	152
Other services (except public administration)	210	183	175	178	173	192	183	199
Government[4]	520	520	545	544	461	484	505	453

NA = Not available.   * = Estimates are unreliable or data do not meet publication criteria.   Note: Fatal work injuries are based on revised data and may differ from originally published data from the Census of Fatal Occupational Injuries (CFOI).   1 Industry data from 2003 to 2008 are based on the North American Industry Classification System (NAICS), 2002. Industry data from 2009 to the present are based on NAICS 2007. NAICS replaces the Standard Industrial Classification (SIC) system. Because of substantial differences between these systems, industry data classified by these two systems are not comparable. 2 Includes fatal injuries at all establishments categorized as Mining (Sector 21) in the NAICS, including establishments not governed by the Mine Safety and Health Administration (MSHA) rules and reporting, such as those in Oil and Gas Extraction.   3 Starting with 2011 data, CFOI combined the categories "Management of companies and enterprises" and "Administrative and support and waste management and remediation services" into one category entitled "Management, administrative, and waste services."   4 Includes fatal work injuries to workers employed by governmental organizations, regardless of industry.

Table 2-23. Number of Fatal Work Injuries, by Most Frequent Type, 1992–Preliminary 2014

(Number.)

Year	Total	Roadway incidents	Homicides	Falls, slips, trips	Struck by object
1992	6,217	1,158	1,044	600	557
1993	6,331	1,242	1,074	618	565
1994	6,632	1,343	1,080	665	591
1995	6,275	1,346	1,036	651	547
1996	6,202	1,346	927	691	582
1997	6,238	1,393	860	716	579
1998	6,055	1,442	714	706	520
1999	6,054	1,496	651	721	585
2000	5,920	1,365	677	734	571
2001	5,915	1,409	643	810	553
2002	5,534	1,373	609	719	505
2003	5,575	1,353	632	696	531
2004	5,764	1,398	559	822	602
2005	5,734	1,437	567	770	607
2006	5,840	1,356	540	827	589
2007	5,657	1,414	628	847	504
2008	5,214	1,215	526	700	520
2009	4,551	985	542	645	420
2010	4,690	1,044	518	646	404
2011	4,693	1,103	468	681	NA
2012	4,383	1,044	463	668	NA
2013	4,585	1,099	404	724	721
2014[1]	4,679	1,076	421	795	515

NA = Not available.   1 Preliminary.

Table 2-24. Number of Fatal Occupational Injuries, by Selected Industry Sector and Occupation, and Percentage of Fatal Incidents, Preliminary 2014

(Number, percent.)

Characteristic	Count	Percent
Total	4,679	100.0
Industry		
Private industry	4,251	90.9
Government	428	9.1
Construction	874	18.7
Transportation and warehousing	735	15.7
Agriculture, forestry, fishing and hunting	568	12.1
Government	428	9.1
Professional and business services	418	8.9
Manufacturing	341	7.3
Retail trade	267	5.7
Leisure and hospitality	207	4.4
Other services (exc. public administration)	174	3.7
Public administration	71	1.5
Wholesale trade	179	3.8
Mining[1]	181	3.9
Educational and health services	144	3.1
Financial activities	114	2.4
Information	1	0.0
Utilities	17	0.4
Occupation		
Fishers and related fishing workers	22	0.5
Logging workers	77	1.6
Aircraft pilots and flight engineers	71	1.5
Farmers, ranchers, and other agricultural managers	263	5.6
Extraction workers	87	1.9
Roofers	81	1.7
Refuse and recyclable material collectors	27	0.6
Driver/sales workers and truck drivers	835	17.8
Industrial machinery installation, repair, and maintenance workers	43	0.9
Police and sheriff's patrol officers	96	2.1

1 CFOI has used several versions of the Standard Occupation Classification (SOC) system since 2003 to define occupation. For more information on the version of SOC used in this year, see the definitions page at http://www.bls.gov/iif/oshcfdef.htm.

Table 2-25. Number of Fatal Work Injuries, by State, 2013 and Preliminary 2014

(Number.)

State	2013	2014[1]	Net change
Total	4,585	4,383	202
Alabama	78	70	8
Alaska	32	30	2
Arizona	95	86	9
Arkansas	63	67	4
California	396	334	62
Colorado	65	83	18
Connecticut	29	33	4
Delaware	11	11	0
District of Columbia	25	11	14
Florida	239	221	18
Georgia	117	148	31
Hawaii	11	31	20
Idaho	30	34	4
Illinois	176	163	13
Indiana	127	127	0
Iowa	72	90	18
Kansas	55	69	14
Kentucky	86	82	4
Louisiana	114	120	6
Maine	19	18	1
Maryland	79	73	6
Massachusetts	57	51	6
Michigan	135	138	3
Minnesota	69	62	7
Mississippi	68	71	3
Missouri	118	106	12
Montana	28	27	1
Nebraska	39	54	15
Nevada	42	40	2
New Hampshire	14	17	3
New Jersey	102	85	17
New Mexico	54	50	4
New York	178	203	25
North Carolina	109	128	19
North Dakota	56	38	18
Ohio	149	184	35
Oklahoma	92	91	1
Oregon	49	69	20
Pennsylvania	183	175	8
Rhode Island	10	10	0
South Carolina	75	62	13
South Dakota	20	28	8
Tennessee	95	124	29
Texas	508	524	16
Utah	37	54	17
Vermont	7	8	1
Virginia	128	116	12
Washington	56	86	30
West Virginia	61	38	23
Wisconsin	97	97	0
Wyoming	26	37	11

1 Preliminary data.

Table 2-26. Years of Potential Life Lost Before Age 75 for Selected Causes of Death, by Sex, Race, and Hispanic Origin, Selected Years, 1980–2013

(Years lost before 75 per 100,000 population.)

Sex, race, Hispanic origin, and cause of death[1]	Crude 2013[3]	Age-adjusted[2] 1980[2]	1990[2]	1995[2]	2000[3]	2005[3]	2010[3]	2011[3]	2012[3]	2013[3]
ALL PERSONS										
All causes	7,002.7	10,448.4	9,085.5	8,626.2	7,578.1	7,315.7	6,642.9	6,635.2	6,588.0	6,593.1
Diseases of heart	1,070.9	2,238.7	1,617.7	1,475.4	1,253.0	1,107.5	972.4	962.4	951.9	952.3
Ischemic heart disease	630.4	1,729.3	1,153.6	1,013.2	841.8	698.9	577.3	567.0	558.4	546.1
Cerebrovascular diseases	177.2	357.5	259.6	246.5	223.3	192.9	169.3	164.0	161.6	158.1
Malignant neoplasms	1,527.1	2,108.8	2,003.8	1,841.6	1,674.1	1,519.8	1,395.8	1,370.9	1,356.2	1,328.6
Trachea, bronchus, and lung	362.1	548.5	561.4	497.3	443.1	390.5	331.3	318.7	309.9	298.2
Colorectal	139.2	190.0	164.7	152.0	141.9	124.3	125.0	124.1	123.0	123.5
Prostate[4]	57.6	84.9	96.8	83.5	63.6	54.4	52.2	48.5	48.1	47.5
Breast[5]	278.5	463.2	451.6	398.6	332.6	295.4	262.4	259.4	256.0	250.0
Chronic lower respiratory diseases	211.1	169.1	187.4	190.4	188.1	180.1	172.4	174.7	171.6	176.6
Influenza and pneumonia	88.8	160.2	141.5	126.9	87.1	83.6	71.4	81.8	67.4	82.3
Chronic liver disease and cirrhosis	192.0	300.3	196.9	173.7	164.1	152.5	163.9	169.1	173.3	176.9
Diabetes mellitus[6]	189.3	134.4	155.9	174.7	178.4	179.4	158.2	167.6	164.3	168.3
Alzheimer's disease	14.0	V	V	V	10.9	11.7	11.7	11.5	11.0	11.1
Human immunodeficiency virus (HIV) disease	57.7	X	383.8	595.3	174.6	134.5	76.6	68.0	61.8	58.1
Unintentional injuries	1,027.8	1,543.5	1,162.1	1,057.2	1,026.5	1,137.2	1,025.2	1,056.8	1,046.1	1,051.2
Motor vehicle-related injuries	378.6	912.9	716.4	616.3	574.3	565.9	400.6	394.8	402.4	386.6
Poisoning	417.1	68.0	81.2	123.1	163.6	289.1	379.7	414.8	408.8	430.9
Nephritis, nephrotic syndrome and nephrosis[6]	74.4	NA	50.4	47.5	70.7	74.2	73.1	65.0	65.2	65.7
Suicide[7]	394.4	392.0	393.1	384.7	334.5	348.9	385.2	395.6	402.1	401.6
Homicide[7]	222.1	425.5	417.4	378.6	266.5	278.2	239.0	236.2	240.9	229.8
MALE										
All causes	8,678.3	13,777.2	11,973.5	11,289.2	9,572.2	9,244.2	8,329.5	8,304.1	8,249.1	8,249.5
Diseases of heart	1,473.5	3,352.1	2,356.0	2,117.4	1,766.0	1,559.0	1,370.8	1,351.1	1,336.6	1,338.2
Ischemic heart disease	917.1	2,715.1	1,766.3	1,531.5	1,255.4	1,040.6	864.8	848.6	831.8	816.2
Cerebrovascular diseases	200.3	396.7	286.6	276.9	244.6	213.3	190.7	185.3	183.7	182.1
Malignant neoplasms	1,609.9	2,360.8	2,214.6	2,008.5	1,810.8	1,632.9	1,500.8	1,467.6	1,450.9	1,415.9
Trachea, bronchus, and lung	408.5	821.1	764.8	645.6	554.9	472.8	390.5	374.0	361.1	345.1
Colorectal	162.4	214.9	194.3	179.4	167.3	145.7	148.0	146.0	144.4	146.8
Prostate	57.6	84.9	96.8	83.5	63.6	54.4	52.2	48.5	48.1	47.5
Chronic lower respiratory diseases	215.0	235.1	224.8	213.1	206.0	194.3	182.8	185.5	179.7	185.2
Influenza and pneumonia	100.5	202.5	180.0	155.7	102.8	98.0	82.6	93.5	77.5	94.1
Chronic liver disease and cirrhosis	260.0	415.0	283.9	254.8	236.9	216.4	226.9	228.9	237.2	242.1
Diabetes mellitus[6]	229.4	140.4	170.4	194.6	203.8	216.1	194.8	206.4	203.5	208.6
Alzheimer's disease	12.1	V	V	V	10.6	10.8	10.7	10.6	10.2	10.2
Human immunodeficiency virus (HIV) disease	83.8	X	686.2	991.2	258.9	194.0	109.5	94.8	87.0	84.3
Unintentional injuries	1,441.8	2,342.7	1,715.1	1,531.6	1,475.6	1,622.6	1,432.1	1,472.5	1,459.7	1,463.5
Motor vehicle-related injuries	546.7	1,359.7	1,018.4	851.1	796.4	802.0	569.2	563.5	574.3	552.2
Poisoning	557.4	96.4	123.6	193.1	242.1	400.4	503.8	550.6	541.5	573.1
Nephritis, nephrotic syndrome and nephrosis[6]	83.3	NA	58.9	55.6	81.1	85.8	82.3	75.6	75.3	75.3
Suicide[7]	612.0	605.6	634.8	628.4	539.1	553.4	607.0	618.4	625.9	619.8
Homicide[7]	359.7	675.0	658.0	589.6	410.5	443.6	380.3	373.7	383.6	365.9
FEMALE										
All causes	5,337.8	7,350.3	6,333.1	6,057.5	5,644.6	5,429.0	4,994.0	5,000.3	4,959.6	4,967.9
Diseases of heart	670.8	1,246.0	948.5	883.9	774.6	680.2	593.6	592.5	585.4	584.5
Ischemic heart disease	345.4	852.1	600.3	537.8	457.6	377.2	305.2	300.2	299.3	290.0
Cerebrovascular diseases	154.2	324.0	235.9	218.7	203.9	173.9	149.1	143.9	140.7	135.4
Malignant neoplasms	1,444.9	1,896.8	1,826.6	1,698.9	1,555.3	1,419.0	1,301.0	1,284.0	1,271.0	1,250.3
Trachea, bronchus, and lung	315.9	310.4	382.2	365.2	342.1	315.2	276.9	267.9	262.8	255.1
Colorectal	116.2	168.7	138.7	127.5	118.7	104.5	103.4	103.5	102.8	101.5
Breast	278.5	463.2	451.6	398.6	332.6	295.4	262.4	259.4	256.0	250.0
Chronic lower respiratory diseases	207.2	114.0	155.9	171.0	172.3	167.2	162.8	164.7	164.1	168.7
Influenza and pneumonia	77.1	122.0	106.2	100.2	72.3	69.9	60.7	70.7	57.8	70.9
Chronic liver disease and cirrhosis	124.3	194.5	115.1	96.6	94.5	91.4	103.5	111.9	111.9	114.4
Diabetes mellitus[6]	149.5	128.5	142.3	155.9	154.4	144.5	123.5	130.8	127.0	129.8
Alzheimer's disease	15.8	V	V	V	11.1	12.5	12.6	12.4	11.8	12.0
Human immunodeficiency virus (HIV) disease	31.8	X	87.8	205.7	92.0	76.4	44.4	41.9	37.2	32.5
Unintentional injuries	616.4	755.3	607.4	580.1	573.2	647.9	616.4	638.5	629.6	635.7
Motor vehicle-related injuries	211.5	470.4	411.6	378.4	348.5	326.4	230.5	224.4	228.7	219.0
Poisoning	277.7	40.2	39.1	53.6	85.0	177.3	255.1	278.0	275.1	287.7
Nephritis, nephrotic syndrome and nephrosis[6]	65.5	NA	42.4	40.0	60.8	63.3	64.6	55.0	55.6	56.6
Suicide[7]	178.3	184.2	153.3	140.8	129.1	144.1	163.7	172.3	177.6	182.5
Homicide[7]	85.4	181.3	174.3	163.2	118.9	108.8	94.9	95.5	94.9	90.4
WHITE[8]										
All causes	6,864.3	9,554.1	8,159.5	7,744.9	6,949.5	6,823.2	6,342.8	6,365.7	6,321.6	6,338.2
Diseases of heart	1,032.2	2,100.8	1,490.3	1,353.0	1,149.4	1,012.4	900.9	895.3	882.5	881.8
Ischemic heart disease	640.1	1,682.7	1,113.4	975.2	805.3	671.4	563.7	553.3	544.8	532.0
Cerebrovascular diseases	157.7	300.7	213.1	205.2	187.1	160.5	142.7	139.5	138.7	135.1
Malignant neoplasms	1,572.4	2,035.9	1,929.3	1,780.5	1,627.8	1,485.8	1,375.8	1,351.9	1,340.7	1,317.7

Table 2-26. Years of Potential Life Lost Before Age 75 for Selected Causes of Death, by Sex, Race, and Hispanic Origin, Selected Years, 1980–2013— continued

(Years lost before 75 per 100,000 population.)

Sex, race, Hispanic origin, and cause of death[1]	Crude 2013[3]	Age-adjusted[2] 1980[2]	1990[2]	1995[2]	2000[3]	2005[3]	2010[3]	2011[3]	2012[3]	2013[3]
Trachea, bronchus, and lung	383.0	529.9	544.2	487.1	436.3	388.1	332.8	320.5	311.4	300.4
Colorectal	138.5	186.8	157.8	145.0	134.1	117.3	118.4	117.9	117.9	118.6
Prostate[4]	53.9	74.8	86.6	73.0	54.3	46.6	45.3	41.7	42.1	41.9
Breast[5]	272.0	460.2	441.7	381.5	315.6	275.2	245.0	241.6	239.3	236.0
Chronic lower respiratory diseases	228.7	165.4	182.3	185.7	185.3	181.5	176.1	178.3	175.3	180.1
Influenza and pneumonia	86.7	130.8	116.9	108.3	77.7	76.7	66.7	77.1	63.2	78.4
Chronic liver disease and cirrhosis	210.6	257.3	175.8	164.6	162.7	157.2	173.5	179.6	185.9	189.3
Diabetes mellitus[6]	174.3	115.7	133.7	149.4	155.6	156.3	139.0	148.7	145.4	149.2
Alzheimer's disease	15.8	V	V	V	11.4	12.3	12.4	12.3	11.7	11.8
Human immunodeficiency virus (HIV) disease	31.6	X	309.0	422.6	94.7	70.5	39.9	36.1	32.8	31.5
Unintentional injuries	1,089.1	1,520.4	1,139.7	1,040.9	1,031.8	1,183.1	1,098.6	1,134.9	1,119.7	1,125.2
Motor vehicle-related injuries	387.4	939.9	726.7	623.6	586.1	591.1	419.0	413.1	420.1	401.2
Poisoning	472.2	64.9	74.4	115.4	167.2	314.4	435.4	475.3	467.6	493.0
Nephritis, nephrotic syndrome and nephrosis[6]	62.1	NA	37.0	36.1	52.5	56.5	57.4	50.9	51.1	52.7
Suicide[7]	440.3	414.5	417.7	411.6	362.0	385.1	430.8	444.8	450.8	451.2
Homicide[7]	120.6	271.7	234.9	220.2	156.6	161.7	138.7	135.5	135.9	127.7
BLACK OR AFRICAN AMERICAN [8]										
All causes	9,508.1	17,873.4	16,593.0	15,809.7	12,897.1	11,788.4	9,832.5	9,659.5	9,555.7	9,528.5
Diseases of heart	1,597.4	3,619.9	2,891.8	2,681.8	2,275.2	2,011.1	1,691.1	1,647.8	1,645.0	1,647.0
Ischemic heart disease	757.2	2,305.1	1,676.1	1,510.2	1,300.1	1,058.3	818.8	803.3	792.0	776.7
Cerebrovascular diseases	309.9	883.2	656.4	583.6	507.0	434.1	358.1	338.0	326.5	319.2
Malignant neoplasms	1,645.8	2,946.1	2,894.8	2,597.1	2,294.7	2,030.4	1,796.7	1,770.5	1,724.1	1,666.7
Trachea, bronchus, and lung	363.6	776.0	811.3	683.0	593.0	500.4	405.6	387.2	377.5	362.4
Colorectal	169.2	232.3	241.8	226.9	222.4	195.7	188.6	185.3	177.0	174.2
Prostate[4]	100.7	200.3	223.5	210.0	171.0	139.6	127.3	120.1	113.6	109.9
Breast[5]	384.2	524.2	592.9	577.4	500.0	480.1	420.8	420.2	406.2	389.8
Chronic lower respiratory diseases	198.2	203.7	240.6	244.0	232.7	207.4	187.7	192.7	192.8	200.1
Influenza and pneumonia	121.4	384.9	330.8	269.8	161.2	143.7	109.8	123.4	106.2	122.9
Chronic liver disease and cirrhosis	120.5	644.0	371.8	250.3	185.6	136.0	120.2	123.1	116.2	122.4
Diabetes mellitus[6]	314.4	305.3	361.5	400.8	383.4	373.1	316.4	324.1	316.6	323.8
Alzheimer's disease	8.9	V	V	V	8.3	10.9	10.0	10.0	9.3	9.8
Human immunodeficiency virus (HIV) disease	224.4	X	1,014.7	1,945.4	763.3	590.3	329.5	287.8	259.0	238.4
Unintentional injuries	955.2	1,751.5	1,392.7	1,272.1	1,152.8	1,129.7	896.7	918.4	925.8	953.0
Motor vehicle-related injuries	408.4	750.2	699.5	621.8	580.8	530.4	393.4	386.6	404.0	402.6
Poisoning	253.2	99.4	144.3	209.6	196.6	252.2	218.9	240.8	242.1	265.6
Nephritis, nephrotic syndrome and nephrosis[6]	161.1	NA	160.9	140.0	216.9	214.8	193.2	174.3	172.4	165.7
Suicide[7]	208.7	238.0	261.4	254.2	208.7	193.6	196.4	202.3	210.4	207.0
Homicide[7]	847.5	1,580.8	1,612.9	1,352.8	941.6	967.5	821.2	813.0	842.9	813.5
AMERICAN INDIAN OR ALASKA NATIVE [8]										
All causes	6,359.5	13,390.9	9,506.2	9,332.5	7,758.2	7,705.7	6,771.3	6,712.5	6,842.6	6,698.8
Diseases of heart	708.1	1,819.9	1,391.0	1,296.3	1,030.1	945.6	820.6	796.0	797.4	807.4
Ischemic heart disease	419.3	1,208.2	901.8	877.3	709.3	591.1	487.6	484.2	486.4	484.4
Cerebrovascular diseases	107.6	269.3	223.3	255.3	198.1	195.8	129.7	144.3	121.5	124.1
Malignant neoplasms	755.5	1,101.3	1,141.1	1,099.5	995.7	1,021.4	929.5	836.0	856.9	852.4
Trachea, bronchus, and lung	141.6	181.1	268.1	267.7	227.8	255.5	211.0	185.1	188.5	166.0
Colorectal	91.4	78.8	82.4	103.5	93.8	102.9	95.8	104.5	90.0	103.3
Prostate[4]	26.3	66.7	42.0	51.1	44.5	36.3	36.8	30.8	36.7	32.6
Breast[5]	97.7	205.5	213.4	195.9	174.1	139.2	145.0	121.7	120.0	108.5
Chronic lower respiratory diseases	116.0	89.3	129.0	145.3	151.8	146.8	154.5	137.6	133.2	135.6
Influenza and pneumonia	99.6	307.9	206.3	199.7	124.0	102.5	99.3	100.5	80.8	109.0
Chronic liver disease and cirrhosis	497.9	1,190.3	535.1	604.8	519.4	459.3	510.8	518.8	553.3	562.2
Diabetes mellitus[6]	248.2	305.5	292.3	360.6	305.6	327.7	267.6	297.1	286.4	281.7
Alzheimer's disease	4.5	V	V	V	*	*	8.8	7.7	6.2	5.7
Human immunodeficiency virus (HIV) disease	30.2	X	70.1	246.9	68.4	81.4	46.1	32.1	32.1	33.8
Unintentional injuries	1,389.5	3,541.0	2,183.9	1,980.9	1,700.1	1,670.0	1,377.7	1,437.1	1,505.2	1,388.2
Motor vehicle-related injuries	603.5	2,102.4	1,301.5	1,210.3	1,032.2	894.0	570.6	614.2	637.0	575.7
Poisoning	464.0	92.9	119.5	161.5	180.1	302.0	449.6	479.1	514.1	487.3
Nephritis, nephrotic syndrome and nephrosis[6]	65.3	NA	88.5	70.3	102.0	94.6	81.7	68.3	67.5	73.7
Suicide[7]	480.9	515.0	495.9	445.2	403.1	446.5	437.9	423.4	437.6	463.0
Homicide[7]	234.9	628.9	434.2	432.7	278.5	298.4	256.4	234.4	244.5	227.8
ASIAN OR PACIFIC ISLANDER [8]										
All causes	3,061.9	5,378.4	4,705.2	4,333.2	3,811.1	3,433.5	3,061.2	3,014.4	3,049.4	3,050.9
Diseases of heart	421.9	952.8	702.2	664.9	567.9	505.8	400.1	403.8	404.0	413.1
Ischemic heart disease	256.3	697.7	486.6	440.6	381.1	322.5	250.6	255.7	248.3	250.4
Cerebrovascular diseases	135.1	266.9	233.5	220.0	199.4	160.5	148.3	136.5	136.0	134.3
Malignant neoplasms	848.3	1,218.6	1,166.4	1,122.1	1,033.8	931.0	874.7	853.6	855.5	830.7
Trachea, bronchus, and lung	139.8	238.2	204.7	197.0	185.8	167.1	148.2	146.6	145.2	136.7
Colorectal	89.6	115.9	105.1	99.5	91.6	77.7	87.6	84.5	85.6	87.0
Prostate[4]	13.7	17.0	32.4	25.3	18.8	20.3	17.0	18.2	14.7	14.4
Breast[5]	154.2	222.2	216.5	237.8	200.8	175.0	156.9	156.5	161.7	146.5
Chronic lower respiratory diseases	35.1	56.4	72.8	65.8	56.5	35.4	33.2	34.2	30.6	35.0

Table 2-26. Years of Potential Life Lost Before Age 75 for Selected Causes of Death, by Sex, Race, and Hispanic Origin, Selected Years, 1980–2013— continued

(Years lost before 75 per 100,000 population.)

Sex, race, Hispanic origin, and cause of death[1]	Crude 2013[3]	1980[2]	1990[2]	1995[2]	2000[3]	2005[3]	2010[3]	2011[3]	2012[3]	2013[3]
Influenza and pneumonia	36.6	79.3	74.0	64.3	48.6	39.3	38.4	43.3	33.5	36.4
Chronic liver disease and cirrhosis	44.1	85.6	72.4	48.4	44.8	43.2	41.7	40.9	37.8	42.9
Diabetes mellitus[6]	75.8	83.1	74.0	83.5	77.0	77.1	69.5	72.3	77.0	74.0
Alzheimer's disease	3.4	V	V	V	3.5	3.1	3.2	2.7	3.8	3.6
Human immunodeficiency virus (HIV) disease	11.6	X	77.0	110.4	19.9	16.6	10.7	10.0	9.9	11.2
Unintentional injuries	314.5	742.7	636.6	525.7	425.7	393.5	303.0	306.6	311.8	308.5
Motor vehicle-related injuries	139.5	472.6	445.5	351.9	263.4	228.9	147.9	138.5	135.9	136.5
Poisoning	75.3	*	17.6	24.5	25.9	40.6	46.5	62.9	64.9	71.5
Nephritis, nephrotic syndrome and nephrosis[6]	31.5	NA	26.7	23.8	33.6	31.5	38.1	26.7	29.9	31.1
Suicide[7]	214.7	217.1	200.6	211.1	168.6	158.0	199.7	190.2	207.6	206.0
Homicide[7]	65.5	201.1	205.8	202.3	113.1	123.3	68.8	78.0	68.3	64.4
HISPANIC OR LATINO [8,9]										
All causes	4,297.8	NA	7,963.3	7,426.7	6,037.6	5,701.1	4,795.1	4,681.7	4,678.4	4,668.1
Diseases of heart	447.7	NA	1,082.0	962.0	821.3	726.9	598.1	585.0	570.7	571.0
Ischemic heart disease	254.3	NA	756.6	665.8	564.6	483.5	366.6	351.7	341.7	340.0
Cerebrovascular diseases	116.4	NA	238.0	232.0	207.8	184.8	150.4	149.0	144.3	145.5
Malignant neoplasms	746.9	NA	1,232.2	1,172.0	1,098.2	1,016.7	951.2	925.6	947.3	927.9
Trachea, bronchus, and lung	74.6	NA	193.7	173.9	152.1	138.2	115.0	108.6	107.3	102.9
Colorectal	72.2	NA	100.2	97.9	101.4	86.5	94.0	88.7	86.7	92.8
Prostate[4]	22.6	NA	47.7	60.8	42.9	42.1	38.2	38.1	37.0	35.9
Breast[5]	148.3	NA	299.3	257.7	230.7	194.9	180.0	176.2	192.5	181.2
Chronic lower respiratory diseases	43.7	NA	78.8	82.1	68.5	62.2	59.6	54.3	53.2	56.2
Influenza and pneumonia	55.3	NA	130.1	108.5	76.0	69.1	57.5	59.3	53.1	64.3
Chronic liver disease and cirrhosis	165.1	NA	329.1	281.4	252.1	210.7	201.6	209.3	209.5	206.1
Diabetes mellitus[6]	123.7	NA	177.8	228.8	215.6	202.4	158.5	160.2	160.0	161.6
Alzheimer's disease	5.2	NA	V	V	6.9	7.8	8.4	8.2	7.7	8.5
Human immunodeficiency virus (HIV) disease	45.7	X	600.1	865.0	209.4	140.2	74.9	69.5	55.2	52.5
Unintentional injuries	752.6	NA	1,190.6	1,017.9	920.1	966.1	708.7	727.9	719.5	735.9
Motor vehicle-related injuries	365.5	NA	740.8	593.0	540.2	558.0	340.3	334.3	346.0	344.8
Poisoning	217.0	NA	121.9	173.9	145.9	179.5	191.2	213.1	207.7	224.3
Nephritis, nephrotic syndrome and nephrosis[6]	45.4	NA	54.4	35.3	62.0	65.9	67.7	56.3	57.1	57.5
Suicide[7]	201.3	NA	256.2	245.1	188.5	190.9	193.6	195.0	198.1	195.6
Homicide[7]	217.6	NA	720.8	575.4	335.1	336.2	238.0	221.5	215.4	199.3
WHITE, NOT HISPANIC OR LATINO [9]										
All causes	7,403.1	NA	8,022.5	7,607.5	6,960.5	6,903.8	6,545.3	6,614.9	6,560.4	6,593.2
Diseases of heart	1,166.6	NA	1,504.0	1,368.2	1,175.1	1,045.9	943.2	939.9	929.3	930.5
Ischemic heart disease	729.0	NA	1,127.2	988.7	824.7	692.9	590.8	582.3	574.7	560.9
Cerebrovascular diseases	165.0	NA	210.1	199.6	183.0	155.5	139.1	135.5	135.2	130.3
Malignant neoplasms	1,760.9	NA	1,974.1	1,814.2	1,668.4	1,532.2	1,421.5	1,400.2	1,383.3	1,362.2
Trachea, bronchus, and lung	458.9	NA	566.8	507.0	460.3	414.5	359.1	347.4	337.7	327.2
Colorectal	153.2	NA	162.1	147.8	136.2	120.6	121.2	122.2	122.4	122.1
Prostate[4]	61.4	NA	89.2	73.6	54.9	46.8	45.9	41.9	42.4	42.3
Breast[5]	298.9	NA	451.5	389.3	322.3	283.8	252.6	249.0	243.5	242.3
Chronic lower respiratory diseases	274.0	NA	188.1	190.6	193.8	192.9	189.1	193.4	190.0	195.9
Influenza and pneumonia	93.0	NA	112.3	105.8	76.4	77.1	67.8	79.8	64.5	80.5
Chronic liver disease and cirrhosis	217.1	NA	162.4	151.4	150.9	148.0	166.9	172.6	179.6	183.9
Diabetes mellitus[6]	183.5	NA	131.2	142.8	150.2	151.4	136.7	147.4	143.0	147.0
Alzheimer's disease	18.4	NA	V	V	11.7	12.6	12.7	12.6	12.1	12.1
Human immunodeficiency virus (HIV) disease	26.8	X	271.2	362.1	76.0	57.0	31.3	27.8	26.9	25.7
Unintentional injuries	1,155.5	NA	1,114.7	1,026.1	1,041.4	1,214.1	1,183.0	1,227.3	1,210.5	1,214.6
Motor vehicle-related injuries	383.9	NA	715.7	618.0	588.8	586.9	430.6	426.3	431.0	407.4
Poisoning	530.7	NA	68.3	105.4	169.4	342.2	494.0	540.8	533.1	561.8
Nephritis, nephrotic syndrome and nephrosis[6]	65.2	NA	34.5	35.7	51.1	54.9	55.3	49.5	49.8	51.2
Suicide[7]	495.8	NA	433.0	427.7	389.2	421.2	483.8	502.5	510.2	512.9
Homicide[7]	91.8	NA	162.0	148.6	113.2	110.7	103.4	103.4	106.6	100.6

NA = Not available.   V = Data for Alzheimer's disease are only presented for data years 1999 and beyond due to large differences in death rates caused by changes in the coding of the causes of death between ICD-9 and ICD-10.   X = Not applicable.   * = Figure does not meet standards of reliability or precision.   1 Underlying cause of death code was coded according to the 9th Revision of the International Classification of Diseases (ICD) in 1980-1998.   2 Age-adjusted rates are calculated using the year 2000 standard population. Prior to 2001, age-adjusted rates were calculated using standard million proportions based on rounded population numbers. Starting with 2001 data, unrounded population numbers are used to calculate age-adjusted rates.   3 Starting with 1999 data, cause of death is coded according to ICD-10.   4 Rate for male population only.   5 Rate for female population only.   6 Starting with 2011 data, the rules for selecting renal failure as the underlying cause of death were changed, affecting the number of deaths in the nephritis, nephrotic syndrome and nephrosis and Diabetes categories. These changes directly affect deaths with mention of renal failure and other associated conditions, such as Diabetes mellitus with renal complications. The result is a decrease in the number of deaths for nephritis, nephrotic syndrome and nephrosis and an increase in the number of deaths for diabetes mellitus. Therefore, trend data for these two causes of death should be interpreted with caution.   7 Figures for 2001 include September 11th-related deaths for which death certificates were filed as of October 24, 2002.   8 The race groups, White, Black, Asian or Pacific Islander, and American Indian or Alaska Native, include persons of Hispanic and non-Hispanic origin. Persons of Hispanic origin may be of any race. Death rates for the American Indian or Alaska Native, Asian or Pacific Islander, and Hispanic populations are known to be underestimated.   9 Prior to 1997, excludes data from states lacking an Hispanic origin item on the death certificate.

Table 2-27A. Number of Deaths, Death Rates, and Age-Adjusted Death Rates for Major Causes of Death, by State and Territory, 2013

(Number, rates per 100,000 population, age–adjusted rates per 100,000 U.S. standard population.)

State and territory	All causes			Human immunodeficiency virus (HIV) disease (B20–B24)			Malignant neoplasms (C00–C97)			Diabetes mellitus (E10–E14)		
	Number	Rate	Age-adjusted rate[1]	Number	Rate	Age-adjusted rate[1]	Number	Rate	Age-adjusted rate[1]	Number	Rate	Age-adjusted rate[1]
United States [2]	2,596,993	821.5	731.9	6,955	2.2	2.1	584,881	185.0	163.2	75,578	23.9	21.2
Alabama	50,189	1,038.3	925.2	122	2.5	2.5	10,328	213.7	182.2	1,349	27.9	24.3
Alaska	3,997	543.7	724.4	7	*	*	1,016	138.2	171.9	112	15.2	20.1
Arizona	50,534	762.6	674.2	97	1.5	1.5	11,347	171.2	147.0	1,786	27.0	23.5
Arkansas	30,437	1,028.5	893.8	68	2.3	2.6	6,688	226.0	190.0	835	28.2	24.2
California	248,359	647.9	630.1	696	1.8	1.8	57,714	150.6	147.0	8,057	21.0	20.6
Colorado	33,712	639.9	655.4	58	1.1	1.0	7,357	139.6	139.2	788	15.0	15.0
Connecticut	29,632	824.0	646.3	67	1.9	1.6	6,619	184.1	148.4	664	18.5	14.8
Delaware	7,967	860.6	726.8	36	3.9	3.4	1,905	205.8	167.6	218	23.5	19.4
District of Columbia	4,719	730.0	752.0	79	12.2	12.0	1,095	169.4	178.2	108	16.7	17.9
Florida	181,112	926.3	663.4	940	4.8	4.5	42,735	218.6	155.9	5,238	26.8	19.2
Georgia	75,088	751.5	806.2	385	3.9	3.7	16,417	164.3	167.6	2,199	22.0	23.0
Hawaii	10,505	748.2	590.8	8	*	*	2,332	166.1	135.5	271	19.3	15.5
Idaho	12,434	771.3	730.6	7	*	*	2,707	167.9	156.2	404	25.1	23.7
Illinois	103,401	802.7	724.0	188	1.5	1.4	24,491	190.1	171.9	2,798	21.7	19.7
Indiana	60,716	924.0	832.2	77	1.2	1.1	13,258	201.8	179.5	1,943	29.6	26.3
Iowa	28,948	936.7	723.7	18	*	*	6,509	210.6	168.4	747	24.2	19.0
Kansas	25,414	878.2	757.7	29	1.0	1.0	5,379	185.9	163.1	654	22.6	19.8
Kentucky	43,759	995.6	899.9	51	1.2	1.1	10,085	229.4	199.3	1,187	27.0	24.1
Louisiana	43,270	935.5	897.7	214	4.6	4.7	9,419	203.6	188.5	1,329	28.7	26.9
Maine	13,547	1,019.9	754.2	17	*	*	3,227	242.9	175.2	373	28.1	20.4
Maryland	45,689	770.6	710.4	229	3.9	3.5	10,609	178.9	162.9	1,249	21.1	19.1
Massachusetts	54,567	815.3	663.5	86	1.3	1.0	12,858	192.1	159.6	1,142	17.1	14.1
Michigan	92,408	933.8	782.3	125	1.3	1.2	20,367	205.8	170.5	2,825	28.5	23.8
Minnesota	40,987	756.2	651.0	38	0.7	0.7	9,601	177.1	155.4	1,163	21.5	18.8
Mississippi	30,703	1,026.4	959.6	119	4.0	4.0	6,527	218.2	197.0	1,071	35.8	32.9
Missouri	57,444	950.4	807.7	80	1.3	1.3	12,955	214.3	179.4	1,477	24.4	20.5
Montana	9,511	936.9	761.3	5	*	*	1,997	196.7	154.1	250	24.6	19.7
Nebraska	15,754	843.1	714.7	17	*	*	3,459	185.1	161.3	471	25.2	21.7
Nevada	21,468	769.4	769.8	71	2.5	2.4	4,817	172.6	164.7	424	15.2	14.8
New Hampshire	10,897	823.4	679.1	7	*	*	2,584	195.2	158.0	310	23.4	18.7
New Jersey	71,403	802.3	676.4	295	3.3	2.8	16,315	183.3	156.2	2,043	23.0	19.4
New Mexico	16,805	805.9	731.8	23	1.1	1.1	3,482	167.0	145.4	646	31.0	27.6
New York	150,919	768.0	649.3	719	3.7	3.3	35,738	181.9	155.8	4,094	20.8	17.8
North Carolina	83,329	846.1	777.6	266	2.7	2.5	18,589	188.8	167.6	2,402	24.4	21.8
North Dakota	6,233	861.6	709.7	2	*	*	1,286	177.8	151.8	197	27.2	22.3
Ohio	113,258	978.8	811.2	139	1.2	1.2	24,986	215.9	177.6	3,563	30.8	25.4
Oklahoma	38,384	996.8	910.7	57	1.5	1.5	8,039	208.8	185.7	1,269	33.0	29.9
Oregon	33,939	863.6	717.5	50	1.3	1.2	7,799	198.4	163.4	1,109	28.2	23.4
Pennsylvania	129,123	1,010.8	761.3	247	1.9	1.8	28,512	223.2	170.6	3,804	29.8	22.6
Rhode Island	9,792	931.2	709.6	17	*	*	2,326	221.2	174.6	258	24.5	18.9
South Carolina	44,582	933.7	837.8	146	3.1	3.0	9,745	204.1	174.0	1,240	26.0	22.5
South Dakota	7,099	840.2	679.3	4	*	*	1,577	186.7	154.5	237	28.1	22.7
Tennessee	63,406	976.1	881.1	153	2.4	2.3	13,953	214.8	185.5	1,827	28.1	24.8
Texas	179,183	677.5	751.6	624	2.4	2.4	38,412	145.2	156.9	5,273	19.9	21.6
Utah	16,366	564.2	710.4	24	0.8	1.0	2,971	102.4	127.6	578	19.9	25.3
Vermont	5,639	899.9	710.6	7	*	*	1,318	210.3	163.4	139	22.2	17.4
Virginia	62,716	759.2	724.8	122	1.5	1.4	14,414	174.5	162.0	1,626	19.7	18.4
Washington	51,264	735.3	679.3	63	0.9	0.8	11,928	171.1	156.1	1,616	23.2	21.3
West Virginia	21,843	1,178.0	923.8	19	*	*	4,718	254.4	190.8	841	45.4	34.1
Wisconsin	50,026	871.1	720.1	35	0.6	0.6	11,425	198.9	165.1	1,285	22.4	18.5
Wyoming	4,516	775.1	731.7	2	*	*	946	162.4	148.2	89	15.3	14.2
Puerto Rico	29,009	802.4	667.8	242	6.7	6.4	5,198	143.8	116.9	3,127	86.5	70.1
Virgin Islands	NA	NA	NA	NA	NA	NA	NA	NA	NA	NA	NA	NA
Guam	873	544.3	767.6	3	*	*	162	101.0	141.6	38	23.7	29.8
American Samoa	262	478.8	1,020.8	-	*	*	40	73.1	122.6	32	58.5	116.5
Northern Marianas	185	361.5	779.0	-	*	*	38	74.3	144.6	11	*	*

Table 2-27B. Number of Deaths, Death Rates, and Age-Adjusted Death Rates for Major Causes of Death, by State and Territory, 2013

(Number, rates per 100,000 population, age–adjusted rates per 100,000 U.S. standard population.)

State and territory	Parkinson's disease (G20–G21)			Alzheimer's disease (G30)			Disease of the heart (I00–I09, I11, I13, I20–I51)			Essential hypertension and hypertensive renal disease (I10, I12, I15)		
	Number	Rate	Age-adjusted rate	Number	Rate	Age-adjusted rate	Number	Rate	Age-adjusted rate	Number	Rate	Age-adjusted rate
United States [2]	25,196	8.0	7.3	84,767	26.8	23.5	611,105	193.3	169.8	30,770	9.7	8.5
Alabama	425	8.8	8.1	1,398	28.9	26.7	12,472	258.0	228.4	585	12.1	10.6
Alaska	36	4.9	8.9	72	9.8	18.9	706	96.0	135.0	35	4.8	6.9
Arizona	584	8.8	7.8	2,383	36.0	31.7	10,755	162.3	141.1	775	11.7	10.2
Arkansas	196	6.6	5.8	918	31.0	27.2	7,377	249.3	214.1	276	9.3	8.1
California	2,543	6.6	6.7	11,891	31.0	30.0	60,299	157.3	151.8	4,720	12.3	11.9
Colorado	372	7.1	7.8	1,316	25.0	27.2	6,456	122.5	125.7	260	4.9	5.2
Connecticut	279	7.8	6.0	824	22.9	16.2	7,090	197.2	148.9	374	10.4	7.8
Delaware	81	8.7	7.4	192	20.7	17.6	1,861	201.0	168.0	69	7.5	6.2
District of Columbia	34	5.3	5.8	130	20.1	19.8	1,340	207.3	213.5	56	8.7	9.0
Florida	1,947	10.0	6.7	5,093	26.0	16.9	42,656	218.2	149.8	2,147	11.0	7.5
Georgia	631	6.3	7.6	2,048	20.5	25.0	16,550	165.6	178.7	1,084	10.8	11.8
Hawaii	98	7.0	5.2	260	18.5	12.6	2,521	179.6	139.0	112	8.0	6.0
Idaho	142	8.8	8.8	347	21.5	21.0	2,495	154.8	145.4	135	8.4	8.0
Illinois	1,044	8.1	7.5	2,919	22.7	19.8	24,839	192.8	170.9	1,049	8.1	7.2
Indiana	555	8.4	7.8	2,104	32.0	28.5	13,773	209.6	186.2	651	9.9	8.7
Iowa	359	11.6	8.8	1,252	40.5	28.2	6,995	226.3	168.8	324	10.5	7.7
Kansas	307	10.6	9.3	742	25.6	20.8	5,364	185.4	156.1	218	7.5	6.4
Kentucky	337	7.7	7.2	1,462	33.3	31.4	9,971	226.9	203.4	319	7.3	6.6
Louisiana	284	6.1	6.2	1,505	32.5	32.9	10,346	223.7	214.1	454	9.8	9.4
Maine	177	13.3	9.8	401	30.2	21.6	2,807	211.3	152.3	97	7.3	5.3
Maryland	457	7.7	7.6	919	15.5	14.3	11,244	189.7	172.7	452	7.6	7.0
Massachusetts	549	8.2	6.8	1,699	25.4	19.4	12,023	179.6	141.5	488	7.3	5.6
Michigan	926	9.4	8.0	3,220	32.5	26.4	24,156	244.1	199.8	1,034	10.4	8.4
Minnesota	572	10.6	9.1	1,427	26.3	21.5	7,714	142.3	119.6	555	10.2	8.4
Mississippi	204	6.8	6.7	925	30.9	30.0	7,715	257.9	240.0	502	16.8	15.6
Missouri	554	9.2	7.8	2,026	33.5	27.5	14,095	233.2	194.7	442	7.3	6.1
Montana	101	9.9	8.3	267	26.3	20.7	2,004	197.4	154.3	70	6.9	5.4
Nebraska	198	10.6	8.8	557	29.8	23.6	3,381	180.9	147.9	221	11.8	9.3
Nevada	170	6.1	6.6	448	16.1	18.4	5,434	194.8	195.1	179	6.4	6.8
New Hampshire	106	8.0	6.9	351	26.5	21.5	2,434	183.9	148.9	92	7.0	5.5
New Jersey	703	7.9	6.7	1,812	20.4	16.2	18,460	207.4	170.1	846	9.5	7.8
New Mexico	174	8.3	7.9	339	16.3	14.9	3,425	164.2	147.1	169	8.1	7.4
New York	1,208	6.1	5.2	2,556	13.0	10.4	44,039	224.1	184.8	2,269	11.5	9.5
North Carolina	752	7.6	7.2	2,872	29.2	27.7	17,830	181.1	165.3	856	8.7	7.9
North Dakota	59	8.2	6.6	363	50.2	36.6	1,382	191.0	150.7	86	11.9	8.5
Ohio	1,088	9.4	7.9	3,798	32.8	26.0	26,878	232.3	187.9	1,317	11.4	9.1
Oklahoma	324	8.4	7.9	1,145	29.7	27.6	9,721	252.5	228.5	396	10.3	9.3
Oregon	390	9.9	8.5	1,312	33.4	27.2	6,523	166.0	135.1	526	13.4	10.7
Pennsylvania	1,298	10.2	7.5	3,271	25.6	17.4	31,629	247.6	179.0	1,165	9.1	6.5
Rhode Island	100	9.5	7.6	346	32.9	22.3	2,364	224.8	163.4	76	7.2	5.2
South Carolina	391	8.2	7.7	1,623	34.0	32.4	9,648	202.1	180.0	422	8.8	7.9
South Dakota	77	9.1	7.2	418	49.5	34.9	1,630	192.9	150.1	74	8.8	6.6
Tennessee	482	7.4	7.0	2,536	39.0	36.9	14,803	227.9	204.1	688	10.6	9.6
Texas	1,710	6.5	7.9	5,293	20.0	24.3	40,203	152.0	170.7	1,961	7.4	8.5
Utah	188	6.5	8.9	412	14.2	19.4	3,323	114.6	149.0	138	4.8	6.2
Vermont	73	11.6	9.3	269	42.9	32.9	1,220	194.7	149.6	69	11.0	8.4
Virginia	551	6.7	6.8	1,642	19.9	19.7	13,663	165.4	157.2	627	7.6	7.2
Washington	589	8.4	8.3	3,277	47.0	43.6	10,524	151.0	138.2	570	8.2	7.6
West Virginia	158	8.5	6.5	590	31.8	24.6	4,666	251.6	193.7	282	15.2	11.7
Wisconsin	578	10.1	8.4	1,671	29.1	22.7	11,362	197.9	159.3	427	7.4	5.9
Wyoming	35	6.0	6.0	126	21.6	21.0	939	161.2	152.4	31	5.3	5.0
Puerto Rico	168	4.6	3.8	1,822	50.4	40.8	5,061	140.0	113.5	565	15.6	12.8
Virgin Islands	NA	NA	NA	NA	NA	NA	NA	NA	NA	NA	NA	NA
Guam	5	*	*	2	*	*	283	176.5	270.5	7	*	*
American Samoa	-	*	*	1	*	*	34	62.1	123.6	8	*	*
Northern Marianas	1	*	*	-	*	*	38	74.3	182.2	5	*	*

Table 2-27C. Number of Deaths, Death Rates, and Age-Adjusted Death Rates for Major Causes of Death, by State and Territory, 2013

(Number, rates per 100,000 population, age–adjusted rates per 100,000 U.S. standard population.)

State and territory	Cerebrovascular disease (I60–I69)			Influenza and pneumonia (J09–J18)			Chronic lower respiratory disease (J40–J47)			Chronic liver disease and cirrhosis (K70,K73–K74)		
	Number	Rate	Age-adjusted rate	Number	Rate	Age-adjusted rate	Number	Rate	Age-adjusted rate	Number	Rate	Age-adjusted rate
United States [2]	128,978	40.8	36.2	56,979	18.0	15.9	149,205	47.2	42.1	36,427	11.5	10.2
Alabama	2,604	53.9	48.1	1,035	21.4	19.2	3,043	63.0	54.8	577	11.9	10.1
Alaska	189	25.7	40.7	66	9.0	14.1	197	26.8	37.9	82	11.2	11.3
Arizona	2,162	32.6	28.6	776	11.7	10.4	3,345	50.5	43.5	1,069	16.1	14.7
Arkansas	1,637	55.3	47.6	794	26.8	23.2	2,090	70.6	60.1	338	11.4	9.8
California	13,698	35.7	34.9	6,551	17.1	16.6	13,598	35.5	35.3	4,824	12.6	11.8
Colorado	1,588	30.1	32.0	606	11.5	12.0	2,297	43.6	45.9	712	13.5	12.6
Connecticut	1,348	37.5	28.3	604	16.8	12.2	1,348	37.5	29.7	336	9.3	7.7
Delaware	409	44.2	37.0	150	16.2	13.6	482	52.1	43.5	82	8.9	7.2
District of Columbia	187	28.9	30.1	83	12.8	13.2	150	23.2	25.0	51	7.9	8.1
Florida	8,698	44.5	30.6	2,662	13.6	9.5	11,379	58.2	39.9	2,668	13.6	10.7
Georgia	3,694	37.0	41.4	1,494	15.0	16.8	4,172	41.8	45.4	898	9.0	8.5
Hawaii	634	45.2	34.8	457	32.5	24.1	279	19.9	15.6	112	8.0	6.9
Idaho	598	37.1	35.4	259	16.1	15.1	808	50.1	46.7	207	12.8	11.7
Illinois	5,294	41.1	36.7	2,441	18.9	16.8	5,532	42.9	39.3	1,279	9.9	9.0
Indiana	2,996	45.6	40.7	1,132	17.2	15.3	4,266	64.9	58.4	752	11.4	10.1
Iowa	1,409	45.6	33.9	761	24.6	17.8	1,892	61.2	47.8	308	10.0	8.4
Kansas	1,320	45.6	38.1	715	24.7	20.1	1,673	57.8	50.3	248	8.6	7.8
Kentucky	1,990	45.3	41.7	919	20.9	19.1	3,187	72.5	64.6	558	12.7	10.8
Louisiana	2,098	45.4	44.0	892	19.3	18.6	2,274	49.2	47.3	503	10.9	9.7
Maine	620	46.7	33.4	258	19.4	14.0	902	67.9	49.1	151	11.4	8.4
Maryland	2,315	39.0	36.1	1,103	18.6	17.2	2,051	34.6	32.5	455	7.7	6.8
Massachusetts	2,354	35.2	27.7	1,551	23.2	18.0	2,572	38.4	31.7	597	8.9	7.5
Michigan	4,373	44.2	36.3	1,896	19.2	15.8	5,539	56.0	46.7	1,171	11.8	10.0
Minnesota	2,073	38.2	32.0	751	13.9	11.6	2,287	42.2	37.1	517	9.5	8.3
Mississippi	1,500	50.1	47.2	769	25.7	24.3	1,755	58.7	54.3	327	10.9	9.7
Missouri	2,935	48.6	40.6	1,352	22.4	18.7	3,798	62.8	52.9	598	9.9	8.4
Montana	480	47.3	37.6	210	20.7	16.4	647	63.7	50.7	150	14.8	13.0
Nebraska	820	43.9	36.4	343	18.4	14.5	1,032	55.2	47.7	181	9.7	8.9
Nevada	905	32.4	33.3	513	18.4	18.6	1,482	53.1	54.1	402	14.4	12.9
New Hampshire	441	33.3	27.6	226	17.1	13.9	668	50.5	42.0	147	11.1	8.7
New Jersey	3,456	38.8	32.4	1,356	15.2	12.6	3,245	36.5	31.1	795	8.9	7.5
New Mexico	689	33.0	30.0	337	16.2	14.8	1,052	50.4	44.7	452	21.7	19.7
New York	6,176	31.4	26.3	4,892	24.9	20.5	7,110	36.2	30.7	1,559	7.9	6.9
North Carolina	4,503	45.7	42.4	1,931	19.6	18.3	4,987	50.6	46.3	1,154	11.7	10.2
North Dakota	306	42.3	32.4	134	18.5	14.6	331	45.8	38.2	90	12.4	12.1
Ohio	5,690	49.2	39.9	2,374	20.5	16.6	7,007	60.6	49.7	1,396	12.1	10.1
Oklahoma	1,880	48.8	44.5	759	19.7	18.0	2,680	69.6	62.4	582	15.1	13.8
Oregon	1,775	45.2	37.3	496	12.6	10.4	2,029	51.6	43.0	547	13.9	11.7
Pennsylvania	6,604	51.7	37.2	2,884	22.6	16.2	6,716	52.6	39.3	1,265	9.9	8.0
Rhode Island	397	37.8	27.7	195	18.5	12.9	476	45.3	34.7	124	11.8	9.9
South Carolina	2,508	52.5	47.6	747	15.6	14.2	2,756	57.7	50.8	681	14.3	12.1
South Dakota	418	49.5	38.0	184	21.8	16.2	416	49.2	39.3	122	14.4	13.4
Tennessee	3,157	48.6	44.4	1,564	24.1	22.1	3,904	60.1	53.2	867	13.3	11.6
Texas	9,283	35.1	40.2	3,339	12.6	14.4	9,800	37.1	42.4	3,412	12.9	12.9
Utah	836	28.8	38.2	413	14.2	18.6	718	24.8	32.0	193	6.7	7.7
Vermont	260	41.5	31.7	77	12.3	9.3	353	56.3	44.1	75	12.0	9.5
Virginia	3,287	39.8	38.6	1,442	17.5	17.0	3,181	38.5	37.3	843	10.2	9.0
Washington	2,652	38.0	35.5	768	11.0	10.1	2,933	42.1	39.4	966	13.9	12.2
West Virginia	983	53.0	40.7	481	25.9	20.2	1,590	85.7	64.5	294	15.9	12.5
Wisconsin	2,536	44.2	36.0	1,125	19.6	15.5	2,789	48.6	40.3	618	10.8	9.1
Wyoming	213	36.6	35.1	112	19.2	18.4	387	66.4	63.1	92	15.8	14.3
Puerto Rico	1,342	37.1	29.9	747	20.7	17.0	998	27.6	22.3	219	6.1	5.1
Virgin Islands	NA	NA	NA	NA	NA	NA	NA	NA	NA	NA	NA	NA
Guam	71	44.3	64.5	16	*	*	27	16.8	28.7	23	14.3	16.7
American Samoa	18	*	*	6	*	*	9	*	*	5	*	*
Northern Marianas	17	*	*	8	*	*	4	*	*	2	*	*

Table 2-27D. Number of Deaths, Death Rates, and Age-Adjusted Death Rates for Major Causes of Death, by State and Territory, 2013

(Number, rates per 100,000 population, age–adjusted rates per 100,000 U.S. standard population.)

State and territory	Nephritis, nephrotic syndrome, and nephrosis (N00–N07, N–17–N19, N–25–N27)			Accidents (V01–X59, Y85–Y86)			Motor vehicle accidents[3]			Intentional self-harm (suicide) (*U03, X60–X84, Y87.0)		
	Number	Rate	Age-adjusted rate	Number	Rate	Age-adjusted rate	Number	Rate	Age-adjusted rate	Number	Rate	Age-adjusted rate
United States [2]	47,112	14.9	13.2	130,557	41.3	39.4	35,369	11.2	10.9	41,149	13.0	12.6
Alabama	1,057	21.9	19.3	2,329	48.2	47.2	909	18.8	18.8	721	14.9	14.4
Alaska	49	6.7	10.1	353	48.0	52.5	66	9.0	8.6	171	23.3	23.2
Arizona	374	5.6	4.9	3,349	50.5	48.6	859	13.0	12.7	1,163	17.6	17.5
Arkansas	762	25.7	22.0	1,373	46.4	44.8	537	18.1	18.3	516	17.4	17.3
California	2,840	7.4	7.2	11,538	30.1	29.2	3,375	8.8	8.6	4,025	10.5	10.2
Colorado	450	8.5	9.0	2,422	46.0	46.4	510	9.7	9.5	1,007	19.1	18.6
Connecticut	565	15.7	11.9	1,582	44.0	39.3	300	8.3	8.3	330	9.2	8.7
Delaware	178	19.2	16.0	412	44.5	42.9	115	12.4	12.0	122	13.2	12.5
District of Columbia	54	8.4	8.8	216	33.4	33.6	30	4.6	4.7	38	5.9	5.7
Florida	3,130	16.0	11.1	8,736	44.7	39.1	2,437	12.5	12.0	2,928	15.0	13.8
Georgia	1,652	16.5	18.1	3,727	37.3	38.3	1,268	12.7	12.7	1,212	12.1	12.0
Hawaii	209	14.9	11.3	467	33.3	30.1	112	8.0	7.8	171	12.2	11.8
Idaho	148	9.2	8.8	776	48.1	47.7	261	16.2	16.0	308	19.1	19.2
Illinois	2,444	19.0	17.1	4,511	35.0	33.6	1,118	8.7	8.5	1,321	10.3	9.9
Indiana	1,352	20.6	18.4	2,898	44.1	43.1	828	12.6	12.4	944	14.4	14.2
Iowa	369	11.9	8.8	1,422	46.0	40.0	346	11.2	10.7	447	14.5	14.4
Kansas	594	20.5	17.3	1,359	47.0	44.4	378	13.1	12.9	425	14.7	14.7
Kentucky	991	22.5	20.5	2,513	57.2	55.7	696	15.8	15.3	701	15.9	15.5
Louisiana	1,108	24.0	23.1	2,333	50.4	50.5	761	16.5	16.4	583	12.6	12.4
Maine	252	19.0	13.6	644	48.5	42.6	168	12.6	12.0	245	18.4	17.4
Maryland	737	12.4	11.4	1,732	29.2	27.9	531	9.0	8.7	569	9.6	9.2
Massachusetts	1,261	18.8	15.1	2,393	35.8	32.5	375	5.6	5.2	572	8.5	8.2
Michigan	1,660	16.8	13.9	4,225	42.7	40.1	1,053	10.6	10.3	1,295	13.1	12.9
Minnesota	653	12.0	10.2	2,405	44.4	40.1	466	8.6	8.3	678	12.5	12.1
Mississippi	731	24.4	22.8	1,692	56.6	55.6	681	22.8	22.6	388	13.0	13.0
Missouri	1,305	21.6	18.0	2,981	49.3	47.0	779	12.9	12.7	960	15.9	15.6
Montana	130	12.8	10.3	623	61.4	57.7	237	23.3	23.3	243	23.9	23.7
Nebraska	222	11.9	10.0	703	37.6	34.9	237	12.7	12.5	220	11.8	11.6
Nevada	370	13.3	13.3	1,184	42.4	41.9	278	10.0	9.9	541	19.4	18.6
New Hampshire	175	13.2	10.9	619	46.8	42.5	138	10.4	10.0	185	14.0	12.8
New Jersey	1,400	15.7	13.1	3,028	34.0	31.8	564	6.3	6.1	757	8.5	8.0
New Mexico	302	14.5	13.2	1,245	59.7	59.0	326	15.6	15.7	431	20.7	20.3
New York	2,285	11.6	9.7	5,927	30.2	27.7	1,316	6.7	6.3	1,687	8.6	8.1
North Carolina	1,780	18.1	16.6	4,324	43.9	42.7	1,359	13.8	13.5	1,284	13.0	12.6
North Dakota	117	16.2	12.9	326	45.1	41.7	124	17.1	17.7	128	17.7	17.3
Ohio	1,985	17.2	14.0	5,497	47.5	45.0	1,135	9.8	9.5	1,526	13.2	12.9
Oklahoma	606	15.7	14.4	2,474	64.3	62.7	727	18.9	18.7	665	17.3	17.2
Oregon	327	8.3	6.8	1,755	44.7	40.1	361	9.2	8.8	698	17.8	16.8
Pennsylvania	2,767	21.7	15.7	6,359	49.8	44.9	1,334	10.4	10.0	1,788	14.0	13.4
Rhode Island	149	14.2	10.4	537	51.1	45.3	77	7.3	6.7	132	12.6	12.2
South Carolina	869	18.2	16.0	2,287	47.9	46.6	786	16.5	16.2	696	14.6	14.0
South Dakota	64	7.6	5.9	425	50.3	46.7	145	17.2	17.0	147	17.4	18.0
Tennessee	1,068	16.4	14.8	3,540	54.5	52.7	1,019	15.7	15.5	1,030	15.9	15.4
Texas	3,722	14.1	15.9	9,395	35.5	37.0	3,612	13.7	13.8	3,059	11.6	11.7
Utah	312	10.8	14.1	1,103	38.0	43.4	230	7.9	8.6	579	20.0	21.4
Vermont	30	4.8	3.8	352	56.2	49.6	74	11.8	11.4	112	17.9	16.8
Virginia	1,547	18.7	18.0	2,951	35.7	34.9	775	9.4	9.1	1,072	13.0	12.5
Washington	461	6.6	6.1	2,826	40.5	38.7	537	7.7	7.5	1,027	14.7	14.0
West Virginia	450	24.3	18.6	1,395	75.2	71.7	330	17.8	17.5	323	17.4	16.4
Wisconsin	993	17.3	14.0	2,969	51.7	46.8	598	10.4	10.2	850	14.8	14.4
Wyoming	56	9.6	9.4	325	55.8	55.2	91	15.6	15.9	129	22.1	21.5
Puerto Rico	890	24.6	20.0	1,028	28.4	25.8	354	9.8	9.4	241	6.7	6.3
Virgin Islands	NA	NA	NA	NA	NA	NA	NA	NA	NA	NA	NA	NA
Guam	21	13.1	19.3	41	25.6	28.1	18	*	*	25	15.6	15.3
American Samoa	6	*	*	14	*	*	1	*	*	1	*	*
Northern Marianas	12	*	*	8	*	*	2	*	*	1	*	*

Table 2-27E. Number of Deaths, Death Rates, and Age-Adjusted Death Rates for Major Causes of Death, by State and Territory, 2013

(Number, rates per 100,000 population, age–adjusted rates per 100,000 U.S. standard population.)

State and territory	Assault (homicide) (*U01–*U02,X85–Y09, Y87.1) Number	Rate	Age-adjusted rate[1]	Alcohol–induced causes[4] Number	Rate	Age-adjusted rate[1]	Drug–induced causes[5] Number	Rate	Age-adjusted rate[1]	Injury by firearms[6] Number	Rate	Age-adjusted rate[1]
United States [2]	16,121	5.1	5.2	29,001	9.2	8.2	46,471	14.7	14.6	33,636	10.6	10.4
Alabama	417	8.6	8.9	259	5.4	4.7	648	13.4	13.8	860	17.8	17.6
Alaska	43	5.8	5.6	126	17.1	16.7	110	15.0	15.1	144	19.6	19.8
Arizona	389	5.9	6.0	1,138	17.2	16.0	1,304	19.7	19.9	941	14.2	14.1
Arkansas	212	7.2	7.5	189	6.4	5.9	343	11.6	11.8	501	16.9	16.8
California	1,890	4.9	4.9	4,560	11.9	11.2	4,747	12.4	11.9	3,026	7.9	7.7
Colorado	184	3.5	3.5	788	15.0	13.8	864	16.4	15.9	619	11.7	11.5
Connecticut	100	2.8	2.9	281	7.8	6.8	600	16.7	16.4	161	4.5	4.4
Delaware	52	5.6	5.8	63	6.8	6.0	170	18.4	19.1	100	10.8	10.3
District of Columbia	90	13.9	12.1	65	10.1	9.9	113	17.5	16.6	71	11.0	8.9
Florida	1,150	5.9	6.2	2,070	10.6	8.8	2,603	13.3	13.2	2,442	12.5	11.9
Georgia	641	6.4	6.4	673	6.7	6.2	1,160	11.6	11.4	1,262	12.6	12.6
Hawaii	33	2.4	2.4	70	5.0	4.5	167	11.9	11.5	38	2.7	2.6
Idaho	31	1.9	2.0	215	13.3	11.9	217	13.5	13.9	227	14.1	14.1
Illinois	792	6.1	6.2	813	6.3	5.8	1,607	12.5	12.3	1,117	8.7	8.6
Indiana	400	6.1	6.2	533	8.1	7.3	1,122	17.1	17.5	857	13.0	13.0
Iowa	60	1.9	2.1	313	10.1	9.0	287	9.3	9.7	253	8.2	8.0
Kansas	117	4.0	4.2	212	7.3	6.8	356	12.3	12.8	331	11.4	11.4
Kentucky	202	4.6	4.7	331	7.5	6.6	1,049	23.9	24.3	622	14.2	13.7
Louisiana	552	11.9	12.2	299	6.5	5.8	836	18.1	18.4	886	19.2	19.3
Maine	30	2.3	2.2	144	10.8	8.5	183	13.8	13.9	158	11.9	10.9
Maryland	421	7.1	7.2	322	5.4	4.8	908	15.3	14.9	578	9.7	9.7
Massachusetts	144	2.2	2.2	484	7.2	6.2	1,200	17.9	17.7	213	3.2	3.1
Michigan	635	6.4	6.7	884	8.9	7.8	1,812	18.3	18.5	1,190	12.0	12.0
Minnesota	131	2.4	2.5	527	9.7	8.7	579	10.7	10.5	427	7.9	7.6
Mississippi	291	9.7	10.0	176	5.9	5.3	327	10.9	11.2	525	17.6	17.8
Missouri	392	6.5	6.7	450	7.4	6.5	1,041	17.2	17.7	880	14.6	14.4
Montana	33	3.3	3.7	194	19.1	16.8	156	15.4	16.2	172	16.9	16.7
Nebraska	75	4.0	4.1	181	9.7	9.1	137	7.3	7.5	168	9.0	9.0
Nevada	151	5.4	5.4	368	13.2	11.8	622	22.3	21.4	395	14.2	13.8
New Hampshire	22	1.7	1.7	174	13.1	10.3	217	16.4	16.1	93	7.0	6.4
New Jersey	419	4.7	4.9	551	6.2	5.4	1,331	15.0	14.9	506	5.7	5.7
New Mexico	135	6.5	6.7	491	23.5	22.7	471	22.6	23.3	326	15.6	15.5
New York	686	3.5	3.5	1,480	7.5	6.7	2,483	12.6	12.1	863	4.4	4.2
North Carolina	563	5.7	5.8	855	8.7	7.6	1,308	13.3	13.4	1,223	12.4	12.1
North Dakota	13	*	*	100	13.8	13.5	27	3.7	3.8	86	11.9	11.8
Ohio	648	5.6	5.9	899	7.8	6.8	2,450	21.2	21.6	1,289	11.1	11.0
Oklahoma	258	6.7	7.0	466	12.1	11.4	800	20.8	20.9	632	16.4	16.5
Oregon	90	2.3	2.3	719	18.3	15.5	545	13.9	13.3	462	11.8	11.0
Pennsylvania	634	5.0	5.3	790	6.2	5.2	2,525	19.8	20.1	1,451	11.4	11.2
Rhode Island	31	2.9	2.8	120	11.4	10.1	252	24.0	23.3	56	5.3	5.3
South Carolina	318	6.7	6.8	416	8.7	7.4	648	13.6	13.5	745	15.6	15.2
South Dakota	20	2.4	2.5	123	14.6	13.7	57	6.7	7.1	80	9.5	10.0
Tennessee	405	6.2	6.3	618	9.5	8.3	1,284	19.8	19.5	1,030	15.9	15.4
Texas	1,354	5.1	5.1	1,769	6.7	6.5	2,606	9.9	9.9	2,778	10.5	10.6
Utah	53	1.8	1.9	215	7.4	8.4	612	21.1	22.8	339	11.7	12.6
Vermont	10	*	*	100	16.0	12.7	99	15.8	15.9	65	10.4	9.2
Virginia	333	4.0	4.0	496	6.0	5.2	890	10.8	10.6	864	10.5	10.2
Washington	204	2.9	2.9	1,042	14.9	13.3	1,042	14.9	14.5	632	9.1	8.7
West Virginia	74	4.0	4.2	160	8.6	7.3	583	31.4	32.9	280	15.1	14.3
Wisconsin	176	3.1	3.2	584	10.2	8.9	874	15.2	15.3	570	9.9	9.7
Wyoming	17	*	*	105	18.0	16.3	99	17.0	17.4	102	17.5	16.7
Puerto Rico	865	23.9	25.1	214	5.9	4.9	73	2.0	2.0	856	23.7	24.8
Virgin Islands	NA	NA	NA	NA	NA	NA	NA	NA	NA	NA	NA	NA
Guam	6	*	*	4	*	*	2	*	*	6	*	*
American Samoa	1	*	*	2	*	*	-	*	*	-	*	*
Northern Marianas	-	*	*	1	*	*	1	*	*	1	*	*

- = Quantity zero.   * = Figure does not meet standards of reliability or precision.   NA = Not available.   1 Death rates are affected by the population composition of the area. Age-adjusted death rates should be used for comparisons between areas.   2 Excludes data for Puerto Rico, Virgin Islands, Guam, American Samoa and Northern Marianas.   3 ICD–10 codes for Motor vehicle accidents are V02–V04, V09.0, V09.2, V12–V14, V19.0–V19.2, V19.4–V19.6, V20–V79, V80.3–V80.5, V81.0–V81.1, V82.0–V82.1, V83–V86, V87.0–V87.8, V88.0–V88.8, V89.0, and V89.   4 Causes of death attributable to alcohol-induced mortality include ICD–10 codes E24.4, F10, G31.2, G62.1, G72.1, I42.6, K29.2, K70, K85.2, K86.0, R78.0, X45, X65, and Y15.   5 Causes of death attributable to drug-induced mortality include ICD–10 codes D52.1, D59.0, D59.2, D61.1, D64.2, E06.4, E16.0, E23.1, E24.2, E27.3, E66.1, F11.1-F11.5, F11.7-F11.9, F12.1-F12.5, F12.7-F12.9, F13.1-F13.5, F13.7-F13.9, F14.1-F14.5, F14.7-F14.9, F15.1-F15.5, F15.7-F15.9, F16.1-F16.5, F16.7-F16.9, F17.3-F17.5, F17.7-F17.9, F18.1-F18.5, F18.7-F18.9, F19.1-F19.5, F19.7-F19.9, G21.1, G24.0, G25.1, G25.4, G25.6, G44.4, G62.0, G72.0, I95.2, J70.2-J70.4, K85.3, L10.5, L27.0-L27.1, M10.2, M32.0, M80.4, M81.4, M83.5, M87.1, R50.2, R78.1-R78.5, X40-X44, X60-X64, X85, and Y10-Y14.   6 ICD–10 codes for Injury by firearms are *U01.4, W32-W34, X72-X74, X93-X95, Y22-Y24, and Y35.0.

Table 2-28. Death Rates for All Causes, by Sex, Race, Hispanic Origin, and Age, Selected Years 1950–2013

(Deaths per 100,000 resident population.)

Sex, race, Hispanic origin, and age	1950[1]	1960[1]	1970	1980	1990	2000	2010	2011	2012	2013
All Persons										
All ages, age-adjusted[2]	1,446.0	1,339.2	1,222.6	1,039.1	938.7	869.0	747.0	741.3	732.8	731.9
All ages, crude	963.8	954.7	945.3	878.3	863.8	854.0	799.5	807.3	810.2	821.5
Under 1 year	3,299.2	2,696.4	2,142.4	1,288.3	971.9	736.7	623.4	600.1	599.3	594.7
1 to 4 years	139.4	109.1	84.5	63.9	46.8	32.4	26.5	26.3	26.3	25.5
5 to 14 years	60.1	46.6	41.3	30.6	24.0	18.0	12.9	13.2	12.6	13.0
15 to 24 years	128.1	106.3	127.7	115.4	99.2	79.9	67.7	67.7	66.4	64.8
25 to 34 years	178.7	146.4	157.4	135.5	139.2	101.4	102.9	104.7	105.4	106.1
35 to 44 years	358.7	299.4	314.5	227.9	223.2	198.9	170.5	172.0	170.7	172.0
45 to 54 years	853.9	756.0	730.0	584.0	473.4	425.6	407.1	409.8	405.4	406.1
55 to 64 years	1,901.0	1,735.1	1,658.8	1,346.3	1,196.9	992.2	851.9	849.4	854.2	860.0
65 to 74 years	4,104.3	3,822.1	3,582.7	2,994.9	2,648.6	2,399.1	1,875.1	1,846.2	1,802.5	1,802.1
75 to 84 years	9,331.1	8,745.2	8,004.4	6,692.6	6,007.2	5,666.5	4,790.2	4,753.0	4,674.5	4,648.1
85 years and over	20,196.9	19,857.5	16,344.9	15,980.3	15,327.4	15,524.4	13,934.3	13,779.3	13,678.6	13,660.4
Male										
All ages, age-adjusted[2]	1,674.2	1,609.0	1,542.1	1,348.1	1,202.8	1,053.8	887.1	875.3	865.1	863.6
All ages, crude	1,106.1	1,104.5	1,090.3	976.9	918.4	853.0	812.0	818.7	824.5	839.1
Under 1 year	3,728.0	3,059.3	2,410.0	1,428.5	1,082.8	806.5	680.2	652.1	651.5	650.5
1 to 4 years	151.7	119.5	93.2	72.6	52.4	35.9	29.6	29.1	29.2	28.6
5 to 14 years	70.9	55.7	50.5	36.7	28.5	20.9	14.6	15.2	14.4	14.6
15 to 24 years	167.9	152.1	188.5	172.3	147.4	114.9	97.6	97.7	95.3	92.6
25 to 34 years	216.5	187.9	215.3	196.1	204.3	138.6	141.5	143.0	144.3	145.4
35 to 44 years	428.8	372.8	402.6	299.2	310.4	255.2	212.5	213.7	212.8	213.8
45 to 54 years	1,067.1	992.2	958.5	767.3	610.3	542.8	505.9	507.3	500.8	500.7
55 to 64 years	2,395.3	2,309.5	2,282.7	1,815.1	1,553.4	1,230.7	1,075.5	1,071.1	1,080.2	1,088.4
65 to 74 years	4,931.4	4,914.4	4,873.8	4,105.2	3,491.5	2,979.6	2,275.1	2,236.2	2,186.4	2,186.0
75 to 84 years	10,426.0	10,178.4	10,010.2	8,816.7	7,888.6	6,972.6	5,693.7	5,610.8	5,500.6	5,474.2
85 years and over	21,636.0	21,186.3	17,821.5	18,801.1	18,056.6	17,501.4	15,414.3	15,069.8	14,974.4	14,911.6
Female										
All ages, age-adjusted[2]	1,236.0	1,105.3	971.4	817.9	750.9	731.4	634.9	632.4	624.7	623.5
All ages, crude	823.5	809.2	807.8	785.3	812.0	855.0	787.4	796.3	796.4	804.4
Under 1 year	2,854.6	2,321.3	1,863.7	1,141.7	855.7	663.4	564.0	545.8	544.6	536.1
1 to 4 years	126.7	98.4	75.4	54.7	41.0	28.7	23.3	23.3	23.2	22.4
5 to 14 years	48.9	37.3	31.8	24.2	19.3	15.0	11.1	11.1	10.8	11.2
15 to 24 years	89.1	61.3	68.1	57.5	49.0	43.1	36.4	36.2	36.0	35.6
25 to 34 years	142.7	106.6	101.6	75.9	74.2	63.5	64.0	65.9	65.8	66.0
35 to 44 years	290.3	229.4	231.1	159.3	137.9	143.2	128.9	130.7	129.0	130.5
45 to 54 years	641.5	526.7	517.2	412.9	342.7	312.5	311.4	315.2	312.7	314.1
55 to 64 years	1,404.8	1,196.4	1,098.9	934.3	878.8	772.2	643.5	642.9	643.8	647.4
65 to 74 years	3,333.2	2,871.8	2,579.7	2,144.7	1,991.2	1,921.2	1,527.5	1,505.8	1,466.1	1,464.6
75 to 84 years	8,399.6	7,633.1	6,677.6	5,440.1	4,883.1	4,814.7	4,137.7	4,124.2	4,062.5	4,029.1
85 years and over	19,194.7	19,008.4	15,518.0	14,746.9	14,274.3	14,719.2	13,219.2	13,143.4	13,030.0	13,021.6
White Male [3]										
All ages, age-adjusted[2]	1,642.5	1,586.0	1,513.7	1,317.6	1,165.9	1,029.4	878.5	870.2	860.0	859.2
All ages, crude	1,089.5	1,098.5	1,086.7	983.3	930.9	887.8	866.1	876.4	882.8	899.1
Under 1 year	3,400.5	2,694.1	2,113.2	1,230.3	896.1	667.6	584.3	560.6	558.5	566.4
1 to 4 years	135.5	104.9	83.6	66.1	45.9	32.6	27.4	27.2	27.3	26.2
5 to 14 years	67.2	52.7	48.0	35.0	26.4	19.8	13.8	14.5	13.3	13.9
15 to 24 years	152.4	143.7	170.8	167.0	131.3	105.8	91.8	92.5	89.7	87.1
25 to 34 years	185.3	163.2	176.6	171.3	176.1	124.1	135.6	138.0	139.3	139.8
35 to 44 years	380.9	332.6	343.5	257.4	268.2	233.6	206.6	208.9	207.2	208.0
45 to 54 years	984.5	932.2	882.9	698.9	548.7	496.9	491.9	495.1	489.0	491.7
55 to 64 years	2,304.4	2,225.2	2,202.6	1,728.5	1,467.2	1,163.3	1,033.0	1,033.3	1,043.5	1,050.7
65 to 74 years	4,864.9	4,848.4	4,810.1	4,035.7	3,397.7	2,905.7	2,232.4	2,199.7	2,150.5	2,152.0
75 to 84 years	10,526.3	10,299.6	10,098.8	8,829.8	7,844.9	6,933.1	5,703.6	5,650.4	5,529.5	5,507.2
85 years and over	22,116.3	21,750.0	18,551.7	19,097.3	18,268.3	17,716.4	15,640.3	15,335.7	15,271.5	15,220.4
Black or African American Male [3]										
All ages, age-adjusted[2]	1,909.1	1,811.1	1,873.9	1,697.8	1,644.5	1,403.5	1,104.0	1,067.1	1,058.6	1,052.8
All ages, crude	1,257.7	1,181.7	1,186.6	1,034.1	1,008.0	834.1	725.4	719.4	728.0	739.3
Under 1 year	NA	5,306.8	4,298.9	2,586.7	2,112.4	1,567.6	1,206.5	1,149.9	1,147.3	1,120.1
1 to 4 years[4]	1,412.6	208.5	150.5	110.5	85.8	54.5	42.9	42.7	41.6	40.6
5 to 14 years	95.1	75.1	67.1	47.4	41.2	28.2	19.6	20.5	21.3	19.6
15 to 24 years	289.7	212.0	320.6	209.1	252.2	181.4	142.8	140.3	138.7	135.5
25 to 34 years	503.5	402.5	559.5	407.3	430.8	261.0	216.7	212.2	212.8	218.6
35 to 44 years	878.1	762.0	956.6	689.8	699.6	453.0	307.5	304.8	306.1	312.4

Table 2-28. Death Rates for All Causes, by Sex, Race, Hispanic Origin, and Age, Selected Years 1950–2013— continued

(Deaths per 100,000 resident population.)

Sex, race, Hispanic origin, and age	1950[1]	1960[1]	1970	1980	1990	2000	2010	2011	2012	2013
45 to 54 years	1,905.0	1,624.8	1,777.5	1,479.9	1,261.0	1,017.7	716.3	706.3	696.3	678.8
55 to 64 years	3,773.2	3,316.4	3,256.9	2,873.0	2,618.4	2,080.1	1,662.1	1,623.4	1,615.8	1,628.0
65 to 74 years	5,310.3	5,798.7	5,803.2	5,131.1	4,946.1	4,253.5	3,205.6	3,127.2	3,077.9	3,064.4
75 to 84 years[5]	10,101.9	8,605.1	9,454.9	9,231.6	9,129.5	8,486.0	6,721.5	6,358.9	6,416.8	6,362.4
85 years and over	NA	14,844.8	12,222.3	16,098.8	16,954.9	16,791.0	14,715.3	14,159.4	13,775.7	13,657.1
American Indian or Alaska Native Male[3]										
All ages, age-adjusted[2]	NA	NA	NA	1,111.5	916.2	841.5	730.2	691.7	690.5	689.2
All ages, crude	NA	NA	NA	597.1	476.4	415.6	397.5	395.1	410.2	416.5
Under 1 year	NA	NA	NA	1,598.1	1,056.6	700.2	542.5	486.5	528.4	493.4
1 to 4 years	NA	NA	NA	82.7	77.4	44.9	34.3	28.8	34.2	41.5
5 to 14 years	NA	NA	NA	43.7	33.4	20.2	18.1	13.1	16.8	12.1
15 to 24 years	NA	NA	NA	311.1	219.8	136.2	116.4	107.0	107.9	98.0
25 to 34 years	NA	NA	NA	360.6	256.1	179.1	156.2	161.9	175.3	172.7
35 to 44 years	NA	NA	NA	556.8	365.4	295.2	258.2	250.9	248.6	244.4
45 to 54 years	NA	NA	NA	871.3	619.9	520.0	496.1	500.6	500.8	506.4
55 to 64 years	NA	NA	NA	1,547.5	1,211.3	1,090.4	951.2	894.8	939.2	937.8
65 to 74 years	NA	NA	NA	2,968.4	2,461.7	2,478.3	1,971.0	1,908.1	1,948.9	1,845.9
75 to 84 years	NA	NA	NA	5,607.0	5,389.2	5,351.2	4,451.8	4,240.5	4,190.2	4,224.5
85 years and over	NA	NA	NA	12,635.2	11,243.9	10,725.8	10,268.1	9,169.4	8,618.1	9,034.3
Asian or Pacific Islander Male[3]										
All ages, age-adjusted[2]	NA	NA	NA	786.5	716.4	624.2	512.1	490.7	484.1	487.8
All ages, crude	NA	NA	NA	375.3	334.3	332.9	327.0	328.6	332.8	347.4
Under 1 year	NA	NA	NA	816.5	605.3	529.4	434.4	410.0	430.9	408.9
1 to 4 years	NA	NA	NA	50.9	45.0	23.3	19.3	15.4	16.3	19.3
5 to 14 years	NA	NA	NA	23.4	20.7	12.9	8.4	9.2	9.0	11.1
15 to 24 years	NA	NA	NA	80.8	76.0	55.2	43.0	42.5	41.5	42.2
25 to 34 years	NA	NA	NA	83.5	79.6	55.0	52.6	53.9	54.9	54.2
35 to 44 years	NA	NA	NA	128.3	130.8	104.9	83.5	84.2	92.0	88.5
45 to 54 years	NA	NA	NA	342.3	287.1	249.7	213.7	216.8	216.5	220.4
55 to 64 years	NA	NA	NA	881.1	789.1	642.4	519.0	502.8	505.9	517.6
65 to 74 years	NA	NA	NA	2,236.1	2,041.4	1,661.0	1,226.0	1,167.1	1,109.2	1,126.4
75 to 84 years	NA	NA	NA	5,389.5	5,008.6	4,328.2	3,438.7	3,311.2	3,218.0	3,239.9
85 years and over	NA	NA	NA	13,753.6	12,446.3	12,125.3	10,824.5	10,143.4	10,116.5	10,142.8
Hispanic or Latino Male[3,6]										
All ages, age-adjusted[2]	NA	NA	NA	NA	886.4	818.1	677.7	647.3	643.9	639.8
All ages, crude	NA	NA	NA	NA	411.6	331.3	310.8	309.7	316.5	323.7
Under 1 year	NA	NA	NA	NA	921.8	637.1	556.8	487.6	509.1	501.1
1 to 4 years	NA	NA	NA	NA	53.8	31.5	25.0	25.5	23.5	23.1
5 to 14 years	NA	NA	NA	NA	26.0	17.9	11.4	12.5	12.3	11.7
15 to 24 years	NA	NA	NA	NA	159.3	107.7	79.4	78.5	76.4	72.9
25 to 34 years	NA	NA	NA	NA	234.0	120.2	100.9	98.5	100.0	99.9
35 to 44 years	NA	NA	NA	NA	341.8	211.0	146.2	142.4	142.7	143.3
45 to 54 years	NA	NA	NA	NA	533.9	439.0	351.9	357.3	342.7	348.0
55 to 64 years	NA	NA	NA	NA	1,123.7	965.7	815.1	791.0	816.3	797.4
65 to 74 years	NA	NA	NA	NA	2,368.2	2,287.9	1,775.0	1,722.4	1,679.1	1,710.4
75 to 84 years	NA	NA	NA	NA	5,369.1	5,395.3	4,461.9	4,303.5	4,250.9	4,218.1
85 years and over	NA	NA	NA	NA	12,272.1	13,086.2	11,779.8	10,707.8	10,799.6	10,596.0
White, not Hispanic or Latino Male[6]										
All ages, age-adjusted[2]	NA	NA	NA	NA	1,170.9	1,035.4	892.5	887.2	876.2	876.8
All ages, crude	NA	NA	NA	NA	985.9	978.5	987.5	1,004.1	1,011.2	1,032.1
Under 1 year	NA	NA	NA	NA	865.4	658.7	575.9	572.6	558.2	571.5
1 to 4 years	NA	NA	NA	NA	43.8	32.4	27.5	27.0	27.9	26.9
5 to 14 years	NA	NA	NA	NA	25.7	20.0	14.3	14.8	13.3	14.4
15 to 24 years	NA	NA	NA	NA	123.4	103.5	93.4	94.8	92.0	89.6
25 to 34 years	NA	NA	NA	NA	165.3	123.0	143.6	147.9	149.0	149.9
35 to 44 years	NA	NA	NA	NA	257.1	233.9	219.1	223.8	221.7	223.1
45 to 54 years	NA	NA	NA	NA	544.5	497.7	508.1	512.3	508.0	511.5
55 to 64 years	NA	NA	NA	NA	1,479.7	1,170.9	1,046.2	1,050.0	1,058.0	1,069.0
65 to 74 years	NA	NA	NA	NA	3,434.5	2,930.5	2,256.9	2,227.4	2,175.8	2,174.3
75 to 84 years	NA	NA	NA	NA	7,920.4	6,977.8	5,770.3	5,727.3	5,599.2	5,582.7
85 years and over	NA	NA	NA	NA	18,505.4	17,853.2	15,816.6	15,568.2	15,504.4	15,485.9
White Female[3]										
All ages, age-adjusted[2]	1,198.0	1,074.4	944.0	796.1	728.8	715.3	630.8	630.3	623.8	623.6
All ages, crude	803.3	800.9	812.6	806.1	846.9	912.3	857.3	868.9	869.9	879.4

Table 2-28. Death Rates for All Causes, by Sex, Race, Hispanic Origin, and Age, Selected Years 1950–2013— continued

(Deaths per 100,000 resident population.)

Sex, race, Hispanic origin, and age	1950[1]	1960[1]	1970	1980	1990	2000	2010	2011	2012	2013
Under 1 year	2,566.8	2,007.7	1,614.6	962.5	690.0	550.5	488.0	469.8	471.5	456.8
1 to 4 years	112.2	85.2	66.1	49.3	36.1	25.5	21.6	21.7	21.7	20.1
5 to 14 years	45.1	34.7	29.9	22.9	17.9	14.1	10.6	10.5	10.4	10.6
15 to 24 years	71.5	54.9	61.6	55.5	45.9	41.1	36.2	36.0	35.5	35.5
25 to 34 years	112.8	85.0	84.1	65.4	61.5	55.1	61.4	63.6	64.6	64.6
35 to 44 years	235.8	191.1	193.3	138.2	117.4	125.7	122.8	124.9	124.1	126.8
45 to 54 years	546.4	458.8	462.9	372.7	309.3	281.4	295.1	301.8	300.1	303.4
55 to 64 years	1,293.8	1,078.9	1,014.9	876.2	822.7	730.9	617.8	619.2	620.5	623.4
65 to 74 years	3,242.8	2,779.3	2,470.7	2,066.6	1,923.5	1,868.3	1,504.9	1,491.2	1,450.9	1,453.2
75 to 84 years	8,481.5	7,696.6	6,698.7	5,401.7	4,839.1	4,785.3	4,165.4	4,158.2	4,110.6	4,072.0
85 years and over	19,679.5	19,477.7	15,980.2	14,979.6	14,400.6	14,890.7	13,419.3	13,380.8	13,281.9	13,316.1
Black or African American Female [3]										
All ages, age-adjusted[2]	1,545.5	1,369.7	1,228.7	1,033.3	975.1	927.6	752.5	739.8	723.9	720.6
All ages, crude	1,002.0	905.0	829.2	733.3	747.9	733.0	642.7	643.4	642.3	651.1
Under 1 year	NA	4,162.2	3,368.8	2,123.7	1,735.5	1,279.8	994.4	962.3	944.4	980.7
1 to 4 years[4]	1,139.3	173.3	129.4	84.4	67.6	45.3	33.2	33.8	33.0	33.4
5 to 14 years	72.8	53.8	43.8	30.5	27.5	20.0	14.5	14.6	14.0	14.8
15 to 24 years	213.1	107.5	111.9	70.5	68.7	58.3	43.3	43.5	43.6	41.2
25 to 34 years	393.3	273.2	231.0	150.0	159.5	121.8	92.9	94.9	89.5	91.0
35 to 44 years	758.1	568.5	533.0	323.9	298.6	271.9	199.3	198.5	192.9	187.9
45 to 54 years	1,576.4	1,177.0	1,043.9	768.2	639.4	588.3	481.0	467.6	461.5	454.4
55 to 64 years	3,089.4	2,510.9	1,986.2	1,561.0	1,452.6	1,227.2	972.2	952.3	950.4	962.2
65 to 74 years	4,000.2	4,064.2	3,860.9	3,057.4	2,865.7	2,689.6	2,021.2	1,969.2	1,918.7	1,909.2
75 to 84 years[5]	8,347.0	6,730.0	6,691.5	6,212.1	5,688.3	5,696.5	4,580.9	4,535.3	4,396.0	4,418.0
85 years and over	NA	13,052.6	10,706.6	12,367.2	13,309.5	13,941.3	12,589.9	12,364.2	12,149.6	11,929.2
American Indian or Alaska Native Female [3]										
All ages, age-adjusted[2]	NA	NA	NA	662.4	561.8	604.5	541.7	522.5	512.3	508.3
All ages, crude	NA	NA	NA	380.1	330.4	346.1	332.4	338.1	340.9	348.2
Under 1 year	NA	NA	NA	1,352.6	688.7	492.2	366.4	411.6	425.9	305.9
1 to 4 years	NA	NA	NA	87.5	37.8	39.8	24.4	25.1	22.7	25.5
5 to 14 years	NA	NA	NA	33.5	25.5	17.7	10.5	12.3	9.6	10.9
15 to 24 years	NA	NA	NA	90.3	69.0	58.9	43.6	45.4	47.7	42.8
25 to 34 years	NA	NA	NA	178.5	102.3	84.8	85.6	88.0	98.8	93.5
35 to 44 years	NA	NA	NA	286.0	156.4	171.9	146.6	164.9	162.2	172.4
45 to 54 years	NA	NA	NA	491.4	380.9	284.9	326.2	336.6	329.6	334.5
55 to 64 years	NA	NA	NA	837.1	805.9	772.1	623.8	611.5	587.2	616.6
65 to 74 years	NA	NA	NA	1,765.5	1,679.4	1,899.8	1,481.7	1,376.1	1,390.3	1,314.7
75 to 84 years	NA	NA	NA	3,612.9	3,073.2	3,850.0	3,391.9	3,300.8	3,256.9	3,221.9
85 years and over	NA	NA	NA	8,567.4	8,201.1	9,118.2	9,277.9	8,448.2	7,987.3	8,008.4
Asian or Pacific Islander Female [3]										
All ages, age-adjusted[2]	NA	NA	NA	425.9	469.3	416.8	359.0	349.8	348.8	343.0
All ages, crude	NA	NA	NA	222.5	234.3	262.3	277.3	283.8	292.0	297.4
Under 1 year	NA	NA	NA	755.8	518.2	434.3	341.8	342.5	349.0	329.3
1 to 4 years	NA	NA	NA	35.4	32.0	20.0	16.3	11.8	14.8	18.4
5 to 14 years	NA	NA	NA	21.5	13.0	11.7	7.9	7.9	7.2	8.8
15 to 24 years	NA	NA	NA	32.3	28.8	22.4	17.0	15.9	18.4	17.7
25 to 34 years	NA	NA	NA	45.4	37.5	27.6	27.1	24.6	24.4	25.7
35 to 44 years	NA	NA	NA	89.7	69.9	65.6	49.0	52.5	50.4	51.5
45 to 54 years	NA	NA	NA	214.1	182.7	155.5	127.9	130.2	130.3	128.0
55 to 64 years	NA	NA	NA	440.8	483.4	390.9	298.8	303.7	301.5	287.2
65 to 74 years	NA	NA	NA	1,027.7	1,089.2	996.4	788.7	719.4	731.9	703.9
75 to 84 years	NA	NA	NA	2,833.6	3,127.9	2,882.4	2,445.5	2,446.0	2,330.6	2,346.7
85 years and over	NA	NA	NA	7,923.3	10,254.0	9,052.2	8,590.1	8,251.9	8,469.0	8,240.4
Hispanic or Latina Female [3,6]										
All ages, age-adjusted[2]	NA	NA	NA	NA	537.1	546.0	463.4	452.8	452.5	448.6
All ages, crude	NA	NA	NA	NA	285.4	274.6	260.9	264.6	272.7	279.4
Under 1 year	NA	NA	NA	NA	746.6	553.6	462.9	430.2	428.9	433.7
1 to 4 years	NA	NA	NA	NA	42.1	27.5	20.2	21.3	20.0	18.4
5 to 14 years	NA	NA	NA	NA	17.3	13.4	8.9	9.5	10.0	9.9
15 to 24 years	NA	NA	NA	NA	40.6	31.7	26.3	25.6	25.5	25.6
25 to 34 years	NA	NA	NA	NA	62.9	43.4	38.9	39.2	40.0	41.4
35 to 44 years	NA	NA	NA	NA	109.3	100.5	75.2	74.1	73.6	78.3
45 to 54 years	NA	NA	NA	NA	253.3	223.8	193.9	185.7	192.0	189.6
55 to 64 years	NA	NA	NA	NA	607.5	548.4	450.1	435.9	442.8	437.2
65 to 74 years	NA	NA	NA	NA	1,453.8	1,423.2	1,085.5	1,077.4	1,046.7	1,039.9

Table 2-28. Death Rates for All Causes, by Sex, Race, Hispanic Origin, and Age, Selected Years 1950–2013— continued

(Deaths per 100,000 resident population.)

Sex, race, Hispanic origin, and age	1950[1]	1960[1]	1970	1980	1990	2000	2010	2011	2012	2013
75 to 84 years	NA	NA	NA	NA	3,351.3	3,624.5	3,067.4	3,085.1	3,063.5	3,037.8
85 years and over	NA	NA	NA	NA	10,098.7	11,202.8	10,237.3	9,727.2	9,805.6	9,651.3
White, not Hispanic or Latina Female[4]										
All ages, age-adjusted[2]	NA	NA	NA	NA	734.6	721.5	643.3	644.6	637.6	638.4
All ages, crude	NA	NA	NA	NA	903.6	1,007.3	981.2	998.1	998.8	1,011.5
Under 1 year	NA	NA	NA	NA	655.3	530.9	480.4	468.6	469.2	448.5
1 to 4 years	NA	NA	NA	NA	34.0	24.4	21.8	21.1	21.7	20.4
5 to 14 years	NA	NA	NA	NA	17.6	13.9	10.9	10.6	10.1	10.6
15 to 24 years	NA	NA	NA	NA	46.0	42.6	38.4	38.4	37.8	38.0
25 to 34 years	NA	NA	NA	NA	60.6	56.8	66.8	69.6	70.7	70.2
35 to 44 years	NA	NA	NA	NA	116.8	128.1	133.1	136.6	136.0	138.6
45 to 54 years	NA	NA	NA	NA	312.1	285.0	307.7	317.8	315.2	320.5
55 to 64 years	NA	NA	NA	NA	834.5	742.1	631.5	635.2	635.9	640.5
65 to 74 years	NA	NA	NA	NA	1,940.2	1,891.0	1,535.9	1,522.8	1,480.2	1,483.9
75 to 84 years	NA	NA	NA	NA	4,887.3	4,819.3	4,232.6	4,227.0	4,178.1	4,142.2
85 years and over	NA	NA	NA	NA	14,533.1	14,971.7	13,543.5	13,544.3	13,437.0	13,502.5

NA = Not available.   1 Includes deaths of persons who were not residents of the 50 states and the District of Columbia (DC).   2 Age-adjusted rates are calculated using the year 2000 standard population. Prior to 2001, age-adjusted rates were calculated using standard million proportions based on rounded population numbers. Starting with 2001 data, unrounded population numbers are used to calculate age-adjusted rates.   3 The race groups, White, Black, Asian or Pacific Islander, and American Indian and Alaska Native, include persons of Hispanic and non-Hispanic origin. Persons of Hispanic origin may be of any race. Death rates for the American Indian and Alaska Native, Asian or Pacific Islander, and Hispanic populations are known to be underestimated.   4 In 1950, rate is for the age group under 5 years.   5 In 1950, rate is for the age group 75 years and over.   6Prior to 1997, excludes data from states lacking an Hispanic-origin item on the death certificate.

Table 2-29. Death Rates for Diseases of the Heart, by Sex, Race, Hispanic Origin, and Age, Selected Years, 1950–2013

(Deaths per 100,000 resident population.)

Sex, race, Hispanic origin, and age	1950[1,2]	1960[1,2]	1970[2]	1980[2]	1990[2]	2000[3]	2010[3]	2011[3]	2012[3]	2013[3]
All Persons										
All ages, age-adjusted[4]	588.8	559.0	492.7	412.1	321.8	257.6	179.1	173.7	170.5	169.8
All ages, crude	356.8	369.0	362.0	336.0	289.5	252.6	193.6	191.5	191.0	193.3
Under 1 year	4.1	6.6	13.1	22.8	20.1	13.0	8.3	7.7	8.5	7.8
1 to 4 years	1.6	1.3	1.7	2.6	1.9	1.2	1.0	1.0	1.0	1.1
5 to 14 years	3.9	1.3	0.8	0.9	0.9	0.7	0.5	0.5	0.4	0.4
15 to 24 years	8.2	4.0	3.0	2.9	2.5	2.6	2.4	2.3	2.2	2.1
25 to 34 years	20.9	15.6	11.4	8.3	7.6	7.4	7.8	7.9	7.6	7.6
35 to 44 years	88.3	74.6	66.7	44.6	31.4	29.2	25.8	26.2	25.9	25.6
45 to 54 years	309.2	271.8	238.4	180.2	120.5	94.2	81.6	80.7	79.7	80.3
55 to 64 years	804.3	737.9	652.3	494.1	367.3	261.2	186.6	183.2	184.6	184.6
65 to 74 years	1,857.2	1,740.5	1,558.2	1,218.6	894.3	665.6	409.2	399.0	388.3	390.3
75 to 84 years	4,311.0	4,089.4	3,683.8	2,993.1	2,295.7	1,780.3	1,172.0	1,134.7	1,103.7	1,095.1
85 years and over	9,152.5	9,317.8	7,891.3	7,777.1	6,739.9	5,926.1	4,285.2	4,111.6	4,046.1	4,013.9
Male										
All ages, age-adjusted[4]	699.0	687.6	634.0	538.9	412.4	320.0	225.1	218.1	214.7	214.5
All ages, crude	424.7	439.5	422.5	368.6	297.6	249.8	202.5	201.2	202.3	206.5
Under 1 year	4.7	7.8	15.1	25.5	21.9	13.3	9.8	7.9	9.6	8.7
1 to 4 years	1.7	1.4	1.9	2.8	1.9	1.4	1.1	1.0	1.0	1.2
5 to 14 years	3.5	1.4	0.9	1.0	0.9	0.8	0.5	0.5	0.5	0.4
15 to 24 years	8.3	4.2	3.7	3.7	3.1	3.2	3.2	3.0	2.9	2.8
25 to 34 years	24.4	20.1	15.2	11.4	10.3	9.6	10.7	10.5	10.4	10.2
35 to 44 years	120.4	112.7	103.2	68.7	48.1	41.4	36.0	36.6	35.8	35.5
45 to 54 years	441.2	420.4	376.4	282.6	183.0	140.2	117.8	116.7	114.3	115.1
55 to 64 years	1,100.5	1,066.9	987.2	746.8	537.3	371.7	269.5	263.6	266.4	267.3
65 to 74 years	2,310.2	2,291.3	2,170.3	1,728.0	1,250.0	898.3	553.0	540.4	527.7	530.9
75 to 84 years	4,825.8	4,742.4	4,534.8	3,834.3	2,968.2	2,248.1	1,475.7	1,426.6	1,388.1	1,382.4
85 years and over	9,661.4	9,788.9	8,426.2	8,752.7	7,418.4	6,430.0	4,833.6	4,622.7	4,582.7	4,564.2
Female										
All ages, age-adjusted[4]	486.6	447.0	381.6	320.8	257.0	210.9	143.3	138.7	135.5	134.3
All ages, crude	289.7	300.6	304.5	305.1	281.8	255.3	184.9	182.0	180.2	180.6
Under 1 year	3.4	5.4	10.9	20.0	18.3	12.5	6.8	7.5	7.3	6.9
1 to 4 years	1.6	1.1	1.6	2.5	1.9	1.0	0.9	1.0	0.9	0.9
5 to 14 years	4.3	1.2	0.8	0.9	0.8	0.5	0.4	0.5	0.4	0.4
15 to 24 years	8.2	3.7	2.3	2.1	1.8	2.1	1.5	1.5	1.5	1.5
25 to 34 years	17.6	11.3	7.7	5.3	5.0	5.2	4.9	5.3	4.8	4.9
35 to 44 years	57.0	38.2	32.2	21.4	15.1	17.2	15.6	15.9	16.0	15.7
45 to 54 years	177.8	127.5	109.9	84.5	61.0	49.8	46.5	45.9	46.0	46.6
55 to 64 years	507.0	429.4	351.6	272.1	215.7	159.3	109.3	108.4	108.4	107.5
65 to 74 years	1,434.9	1,261.3	1,082.7	828.6	616.8	474.0	284.2	275.7	266.2	266.8
75 to 84 years	3,873.0	3,582.7	3,120.8	2,497.0	1,893.8	1,475.1	952.7	920.7	893.0	879.8
85 years and over	8,798.1	9,016.8	7,591.8	7,350.5	6,478.1	5,720.9	4,020.3	3,859.7	3,777.5	3,732.9
White Male [5]										
All ages, age-adjusted[4]	701.4	694.5	640.2	539.6	409.2	316.7	222.9	216.9	213.1	213.1
All ages, crude	434.2	454.6	438.3	384.0	312.7	265.8	217.8	217.1	218.0	222.6
45 to 54 years	424.1	413.2	365.7	269.8	170.6	130.7	111.2	110.8	108.3	109.8
55 to 64 years	1,082.6	1,056.0	979.3	730.6	516.7	351.8	257.0	251.7	253.2	254.0
65 to 74 years	2,309.4	2,297.9	2,177.2	1,729.7	1,230.5	877.8	536.3	524.9	513.5	516.0
75 to 84 years	4,908.0	4,839.9	4,617.6	3,883.2	2,983.4	2,247.0	1,475.1	1,434.2	1,392.6	1,389.0
85 years and over	9,952.3	10,135.8	8,818.0	8,958.0	7,558.7	6,560.8	4,943.1	4,754.6	4,712.4	4,701.6
Black or African American Male [5]										
All ages, age-adjusted[4]	641.5	615.2	607.3	561.4	485.4	392.5	280.6	266.1	265.3	262.8
All ages, crude	348.4	330.6	330.3	301.0	256.8	211.1	174.6	171.0	174.7	177.2
45 to 54 years	624.1	514.0	512.8	433.4	328.9	247.2	190.9	184.1	182.4	178.3
55 to 64 years	1,434.0	1,236.8	1,135.4	987.2	824.0	631.2	437.8	425.2	435.9	430.0
65 to 74 years	2,140.1	2,281.4	2,237.8	1,847.2	1,632.9	1,268.8	847.8	825.5	805.5	807.5
75 to 84 years[6]	4,107.9	3,533.6	3,783.4	3,578.8	3,107.1	2,597.6	1,807.1	1,680.2	1,677.7	1,660.0
85 years and over	NA	6,037.9	5,367.6	6,819.5	6,479.6	5,633.5	4,202.7	3,846.9	3,822.1	3,754.5
American Indian or Alaska Native Male [5]										
All ages, age-adjusted[4]	NA	NA	NA	320.5	264.1	222.2	158.7	153.4	152.5	152.3
All ages, crude	NA	NA	NA	130.6	108.0	90.1	75.0	76.9	78.3	82.3
45 to 54 years	NA	NA	NA	238.1	173.8	108.5	98.0	91.8	87.4	101.6
55 to 64 years	NA	NA	NA	496.3	411.0	285.0	217.2	210.6	198.5	206.2
65 to 74 years	NA	NA	NA	1,009.4	839.1	748.2	425.1	470.4	451.5	465.2

Table 2-29. Death Rates for Diseases of the Heart, by Sex, Race, Hispanic Origin, and Age, Selected Years, 1950–2013 — continued

(Deaths per 100,000 resident population.)

Sex, race, Hispanic origin, and age	1950[1,2]	1960[1,2]	1970[2]	1980[2]	1990[2]	2000[3]	2010[3]	2011[3]	2012[3]	2013[3]
75 to 84 years	NA	NA	NA	2,062.2	1,788.8	1,655.7	1,042.6	1,068.8	1,138.9	1,071.8
85 years and over	NA	NA	NA	4,413.7	3,860.3	3,318.3	2,833.1	2,395.7	2,278.2	2,269.1
Asian or Pacific Islander Male [5]										
All ages, age-adjusted[4]	NA	NA	NA	286.9	220.7	185.5	127.2	115.1	116.1	118.4
All ages, crude	NA	NA	NA	119.8	88.7	90.6	77.0	74.2	76.8	81.9
45 to 54 years	NA	NA	NA	112.0	70.4	61.1	49.2	52.7	51.8	50.9
55 to 64 years	NA	NA	NA	306.7	226.1	182.6	119.3	112.9	118.4	133.3
65 to 74 years	NA	NA	NA	852.4	623.5	482.5	294.4	270.3	255.1	274.9
75 to 84 years	NA	NA	NA	2,010.9	1,642.2	1,354.7	855.5	772.1	748.7	754.6
85 years and over	NA	NA	NA	5,923.0	4,617.8	4,154.2	3,132.9	2,695.9	2,842.2	2,848.5
Hispanic or Latino Male [5,7]										
All ages, age-adjusted[4]	NA	NA	NA	NA	270.0	238.2	165.1	152.2	151.6	151.5
All ages, crude	NA	NA	NA	NA	91.0	74.7	64.1	62.5	64.3	66.9
45 to 54 years	NA	NA	NA	NA	116.4	84.3	66.1	66.0	61.7	63.5
55 to 64 years	NA	NA	NA	NA	363.0	264.8	185.9	172.3	177.5	178.0
65 to 74 years	NA	NA	NA	NA	829.9	684.8	424.5	412.9	406.1	416.6
75 to 84 years	NA	NA	NA	NA	1,971.3	1,733.2	1,160.9	1,092.7	1,069.1	1,057.5
85 years and over	NA	NA	NA	NA	4,711.9	4,897.5	3,577.9	3,076.1	3,147.0	3,106.2
White, Not Hispanic or Latino Male[7]										
All ages, age-adjusted[4]	NA	NA	NA	NA	413.6	319.9	226.9	221.6	217.7	217.9
All ages, crude	NA	NA	NA	NA	336.5	297.5	251.8	252.4	253.2	259.0
45 to 54 years	NA	NA	NA	NA	172.8	134.3	117.2	117.1	115.2	117.2
55 to 64 years	NA	NA	NA	NA	521.3	356.3	261.9	258.0	259.1	260.2
65 to 74 years	NA	NA	NA	NA	1,243.4	885.1	542.2	530.9	518.3	520.2
75 to 84 years	NA	NA	NA	NA	3,007.7	2,261.9	1,491.4	1,452.9	1,409.6	1,408.1
85 years and over	NA	NA	NA	NA	7,663.4	6,606.6	5,006.6	4,841.0	4,796.1	4,794.2
White Female [5]										
All ages, age-adjusted[4]	479.2	441.7	376.7	315.9	250.9	205.6	140.4	136.5	133.4	132.0
All ages, crude	290.5	306.5	313.8	319.2	298.4	274.5	201.5	198.8	196.7	196.8
45 to 54 years	142.4	103.4	91.4	71.2	50.2	40.9	40.7	40.5	40.7	41.0
55 to 64 years	460.7	383.0	317.7	248.1	192.4	141.3	98.2	98.0	97.8	95.9
65 to 74 years	1,401.6	1,229.8	1,044.0	796.7	583.6	445.2	268.4	261.3	251.7	252.5
75 to 84 years	3,926.2	3,629.7	3,143.5	2,493.6	1,874.3	1,452.4	941.6	912.8	888.1	871.8
85 years and over	9,086.9	9,280.8	7,839.9	7,501.6	6,563.4	5,801.4	4,086.7	3,938.3	3,855.8	3,821.0
Black or African American Female [5]										
All ages, age-adjusted[4]	538.9	488.9	435.6	378.6	327.5	277.6	185.3	176.2	172.7	172.1
All ages, crude	289.9	268.5	261.0	249.7	237.0	212.6	154.8	150.3	150.9	153.4
45 to 54 years	526.8	360.7	290.9	202.4	155.3	125.0	96.6	91.6	92.6	94.2
55 to 64 years	1,210.7	952.3	710.5	530.1	442.0	332.8	218.6	209.2	211.1	213.0
65 to 74 years	1,659.4	1,680.5	1,553.2	1,210.3	1,017.5	815.2	475.9	461.6	449.3	450.8
75 to 84 years[6]	3,499.3	2,926.9	2,964.1	2,707.2	2,250.9	1,913.1	1,227.2	1,158.4	1,114.8	1,122.2
85 years and over	NA	5,650.0	5,003.8	5,796.5	5,766.1	5,298.7	3,783.8	3,559.7	3,513.5	3,425.3
American Indian or Alaska Native Female [5]										
All ages, age-adjusted[4]	NA	NA	NA	175.4	153.1	143.6	103.5	99.4	92.9	93.9
All ages, crude	NA	NA	NA	80.3	77.5	71.9	55.9	57.3	55.7	58.4
45 to 54 years	NA	NA	NA	65.2	62.0	40.2	37.7	40.9	39.4	37.3
55 to 64 years	NA	NA	NA	193.5	197.0	149.4	89.0	99.3	83.9	100.5
65 to 74 years	NA	NA	NA	577.2	492.8	391.8	248.1	225.8	245.0	220.1
75 to 84 years	NA	NA	NA	1,364.3	1,050.3	1,044.1	684.7	715.5	698.2	664.6
85 years and over	NA	NA	NA	2,893.3	2,868.7	3,146.3	2,614.1	2,259.3	1,874.7	2,089.2
Asian or Pacific Islander Female [5]										
All ages, age-adjusted[4]	NA	NA	NA	132.3	149.2	115.7	81.2	76.2	74.0	73.3
All ages, crude	NA	NA	NA	57.0	62.0	65.0	59.0	59.1	59.6	61.8
45 to 54 years	NA	NA	NA	28.6	17.5	15.9	10.6	12.0	10.5	12.5
55 to 64 years	NA	NA	NA	92.9	99.0	68.8	40.6	42.1	40.9	41.7
65 to 74 years	NA	NA	NA	313.3	323.9	229.6	141.6	125.4	126.8	124.7
75 to 84 years	NA	NA	NA	1,053.2	1,130.9	866.2	574.3	551.7	505.2	521.0
85 years and over	NA	NA	NA	3,211.0	4,161.2	3,367.2	2,581.8	2,364.5	2,381.5	2,272.4
Hispanic or Latina Female [5,7]										
All ages, age-adjusted[4]	NA	NA	NA	NA	177.2	163.7	107.8	101.2	98.6	97.0
All ages, crude	NA	NA	NA	NA	79.4	71.5	54.6	54.1	54.7	55.9
45 to 54 years	NA	NA	NA	NA	43.5	28.2	24.5	22.3	21.9	22.2

Table 2-29. Death Rates for Diseases of the Heart, by Sex, Race, Hispanic Origin, and Age, Selected Years, 1950–2013 — continued

(Deaths per 100,000 resident population.)

Sex, race, Hispanic origin, and age	1950[1,2]	1960[1,2]	1970[2]	1980[2]	1990[2]	2000[3]	2010[3]	2011[3]	2012[3]	2013[3]
55 to 64 years	NA	NA	NA	NA	153.2	111.2	72.3	71.3	71.9	63.1
65 to 74 years	NA	NA	NA	NA	460.4	366.3	212.2	202.2	192.3	195.8
75 to 84 years	NA	NA	NA	NA	1,259.7	1,169.4	756.0	720.3	711.9	702.3
85 years and over	NA	NA	NA	NA	4,440.3	4,605.8	3,140.3	2,868.0	2,781.3	2,738.8
White, not Hispanic or Latina Female[7]										
All ages, age-adjusted[4]	NA	NA	NA	NA	252.6	206.8	142.5	138.8	135.8	134.6
All ages, crude	NA	NA	NA	NA	320.0	304.9	232.2	230.0	227.5	228.0
45 to 54 years	NA	NA	NA	NA	50.2	41.9	42.9	43.1	43.5	44.0
55 to 64 years	NA	NA	NA	NA	193.6	142.9	100.3	100.2	99.9	99.0
65 to 74 years	NA	NA	NA	NA	584.7	448.5	271.9	265.3	255.5	256.3
75 to 84 years	NA	NA	NA	NA	1,890.2	1,458.9	951.5	923.8	898.1	881.3
85 years and over	NA	NA	NA	NA	6,615.2	5,822.7	4,122.8	3,985.5	3,903.8	3,876.5

NA = Not available.   1 Includes deaths of persons who were not residents of the 50 states and the District of Columbia.   2 Underlying cause of death was coded according to the 6th Revision of the International Classification of Diseases (ICD) in 1950, 7th Revision in 1960, 8th Revision in 1970, and 9th Revision in 1980-1998.   3 Starting with 1999 data, cause of death is coded according to ICD-10.   4 Age-adjusted rates are calculated using the year 2000 standard population. Prior to 2001, age-adjusted rates were calculated using standard million proportions based on rounded population numbers. Starting with 2001 data, unrounded population numbers are used to calculate age-adjusted rates.   5 The race groups, White, Black, Asian or Pacific Islander, and American Indian or Alaska Native, include persons of Hispanic and non-Hispanic origin. Persons of Hispanic origin may be of any race. Death rates for the American Indian or Alaska Native, Asian or Pacific Islander, and Hispanic populations are known to be underestimated.   6 In 1950, rate is for the age group 75 years and over.   7 Prior to 1997, excludes data from states lacking an Hispanic-origin item on the death certificate.

Table 2-30. Death Rates for Cerebrovascular Diseases, by Sex, Race, Hispanic Origin, and Age, Selected Years, 1950–2013

(Deaths per 100,000 resident population.)

Sex, race, Hispanic origin, and age	1950[1,2]	1960[1,2]	1970[2]	1980[2]	1990[2]	2000[3]	2010[3]	2011[3]	2012[3]	2013[3]
All Persons										
All ages, age-adjusted[4]	180.7	177.9	147.7	96.2	65.3	60.9	39.1	37.9	36.9	36.2
All ages, crude	104.0	108.0	101.9	75.0	57.8	59.6	41.9	41.4	40.9	40.8
Under 1 year	5.1	4.1	5.0	4.4	3.8	3.3	3.3	3.4	2.6	2.7
1 to 4 years	0.9	0.8	1.0	0.5	0.3	0.3	0.3	0.3	0.3	0.2
5 to 14 years	0.5	0.7	0.7	0.3	0.2	0.2	0.2	0.2	0.2	0.2
15 to 24 years	1.6	1.8	1.6	1.0	0.6	0.5	0.4	0.4	0.4	0.3
25 to 34 years	4.2	4.7	4.5	2.6	2.2	1.5	1.3	1.3	1.3	1.2
35 to 44 years	18.7	14.7	15.6	8.5	6.4	5.8	4.6	4.2	4.3	4.2
45 to 54 years	70.4	49.2	41.6	25.2	18.7	16.0	13.1	12.8	12.8	12.4
55 to 64 years	194.2	147.3	115.8	65.1	47.9	41.0	29.3	29.4	28.7	28.9
65 to 74 years	554.7	469.2	384.1	219.0	144.2	128.6	81.7	78.2	75.7	74.2
75 to 84 years	1,499.6	1,491.3	1,254.2	786.9	498.0	461.3	288.3	285.4	272.2	268.9
85 years and over	2,990.1	3,680.5	3,014.3	2,283.7	1,628.9	1,589.2	993.8	943.7	931.2	906.0
Male										
All ages, age-adjusted[4]	186.4	186.1	157.4	102.2	68.5	62.4	39.3	37.9	37.1	36.7
All ages, crude	102.5	104.5	94.5	63.4	46.7	46.9	34.5	34.1	34.1	34.5
Under 1 year	6.4	5.0	5.8	5.0	4.4	3.8	3.2	3.6	2.6	3.0
1 to 4 years	1.1	0.9	1.2	0.4	0.3	*	0.3	0.4	0.4	0.3
5 to 14 years	0.5	0.7	0.8	0.3	0.2	0.2	0.3	0.2	0.2	0.2
15 to 24 years	1.8	1.9	1.8	1.1	0.7	0.5	0.5	0.5	0.5	0.4
25 to 34 years	4.2	4.5	4.4	2.6	2.1	1.5	1.3	1.3	1.4	1.3
35 to 44 years	17.5	14.6	15.7	8.7	6.8	5.8	5.0	4.5	4.8	4.7
45 to 54 years	67.9	52.2	44.4	27.2	20.5	17.5	14.9	14.5	14.2	14.2
55 to 64 years	205.2	163.8	138.7	74.6	54.3	47.2	34.7	34.9	34.5	35.1
65 to 74 years	589.6	530.7	449.5	258.6	166.6	145.0	92.0	88.1	85.7	85.0
75 to 84 years	1,543.6	1,555.9	1,361.6	866.3	551.1	490.8	295.2	289.7	277.7	277.9
85 years and over	3,048.6	3,643.1	2,895.2	2,193.6	1,528.5	1,484.3	892.0	840.0	832.1	808.4
Female										
All ages, age-adjusted[4]	175.8	170.7	140.0	91.7	62.6	59.1	38.3	37.2	36.1	35.2
All ages, crude	105.6	111.4	109.0	85.9	68.4	71.8	49.1	48.4	47.6	46.9
Under 1 year	3.7	3.2	4.0	3.8	3.1	2.7	3.4	3.1	2.6	2.5
1 to 4 years	0.7	0.7	0.7	0.5	0.3	0.4	0.3	*	0.3	*
5 to 14 years	0.4	0.6	0.6	0.3	0.2	0.2	0.2	0.2	0.2	0.2
15 to 24 years	1.5	1.6	1.4	0.8	0.6	0.5	0.4	0.4	0.3	0.3
25 to 34 years	4.3	4.9	4.7	2.6	2.2	1.5	1.2	1.2	1.1	1.1
35 to 44 years	19.9	14.8	15.6	8.4	6.1	5.7	4.2	4.0	3.8	3.7
45 to 54 years	72.9	46.3	39.0	23.3	17.0	14.5	11.4	11.0	11.4	10.6
55 to 64 years	183.1	131.8	95.3	56.8	42.2	35.3	24.3	24.4	23.3	23.1
65 to 74 years	522.1	415.7	333.3	188.7	126.7	115.1	72.8	69.6	67.0	64.8
75 to 84 years	1,462.2	1,441.1	1,183.1	740.1	466.2	442.1	283.4	282.1	268.2	262.1
85 years and over	2,949.4	3,704.4	3,081.0	2,323.1	1,667.6	1,632.0	1,043.0	994.9	980.9	955.8
White Male [5]										
All ages, age-adjusted[4]	182.1	181.6	153.7	98.7	65.5	59.8	37.6	36.2	35.4	35.0
All ages, crude	100.5	102.7	93.5	63.1	46.9	48.4	35.8	35.4	35.3	35.8
45 to 54 years	53.7	40.9	35.6	21.7	15.4	13.6	12.2	11.8	11.4	11.7
55 to 64 years	182.2	139.0	119.9	64.0	45.7	39.7	29.0	29.3	29.4	29.9
65 to 74 years	569.7	501.0	420.0	239.8	152.9	133.8	83.3	80.3	78.1	77.6
75 to 84 years	1,556.3	1,564.8	1,361.6	852.7	539.2	480.0	288.3	283.4	270.9	271.1
85 years and over	3,127.1	3,734.8	3,018.1	2,230.8	1,545.4	1,490.7	903.2	846.2	838.2	815.2
Black or African American Male [5]										
All ages, age-adjusted[4]	228.8	238.5	206.4	142.0	102.2	89.6	56.6	55.3	53.8	54.1
All ages, crude	122.0	122.9	108.8	73.0	53.0	46.1	34.5	34.5	34.1	35.1
45 to 54 years	211.9	166.1	136.1	82.1	68.4	49.5	33.6	33.9	33.4	30.7
55 to 64 years	522.8	439.9	343.4	189.7	141.7	115.4	83.2	81.4	76.0	78.1
65 to 74 years	783.6	899.2	780.1	472.3	326.9	268.5	182.6	172.0	164.9	165.0
75 to 84 years[6]	1,504.9	1,475.2	1,445.7	1,066.3	721.5	659.2	398.0	384.7	385.0	387.4
85 years and over	NA	2,700.0	1,963.1	1,873.2	1,421.5	1,458.8	804.5	826.7	796.8	814.1
American Indian or Alaska Native Male [5]										
All ages, age-adjusted[4]	NA	NA	NA	66.4	44.3	46.1	29.8	25.8	25.5	22.7
All ages, crude	NA	NA	NA	23.1	16.0	16.8	12.0	11.8	12.0	11.3
45 to 54 years	NA	NA	NA	*	*	13.3	11.7	10.4	10.7	9.2
55 to 64 years	NA	NA	NA	72.0	39.8	48.6	22.1	29.0	26.9	23.8
65 to 74 years	NA	NA	NA	170.5	120.3	144.7	68.0	66.8	84.4	72.5

Table 2-30. Death Rates for Cerebrovascular Diseases, by Sex, Race, Hispanic Origin, and Age, Selected Years, 1950–2013— continued

(Deaths per 100,000 resident population.)

Sex, race, Hispanic origin, and age	1950[1,2]	1960[1,2]	1970[2]	1980[2]	1990[2]	2000[3]	2010[3]	2011[3]	2012[3]	2013[3]
75 to 84 years	NA	NA	NA	523.9	325.9	373.3	267.5	226.3	172.2	191.0
85 years and over	NA	NA	NA	1,384.7	949.8	834.9	580.4	425.6	506.3	348.3
Asian or Pacific Islander Male [5]										
All ages, age-adjusted[4]	NA	NA	NA	71.4	59.1	58.0	35.2	33.5	33.2	31.2
All ages, crude	NA	NA	NA	28.7	23.3	27.2	21.5	21.2	21.7	21.3
45 to 54 years	NA	NA	NA	17.0	15.6	15.0	14.7	12.9	13.2	15.7
55 to 64 years	NA	NA	NA	59.9	51.8	49.3	31.7	31.4	30.0	27.7
65 to 74 years	NA	NA	NA	197.9	167.9	135.6	84.9	75.6	78.1	73.0
75 to 84 years	NA	NA	NA	619.5	483.9	438.7	260.0	258.2	239.3	230.5
85 years and over	NA	NA	NA	1,399.0	1,196.6	1,415.6	778.7	746.2	776.0	686.7
Hispanic or Latino Male [5,7]										
All ages, age-adjusted[4]	NA	NA	NA	NA	46.5	50.5	33.9	32.6	32.0	31.8
All ages, crude	NA	NA	NA	NA	15.6	15.8	13.2	13.3	13.5	14.0
45 to 54 years	NA	NA	NA	NA	20.0	18.1	14.3	13.9	13.5	13.8
55 to 64 years	NA	NA	NA	NA	49.2	48.8	31.9	35.2	33.3	33.9
65 to 74 years	NA	NA	NA	NA	126.4	136.1	84.4	80.4	75.5	82.1
75 to 84 years	NA	NA	NA	NA	356.6	392.9	266.5	245.4	248.1	242.1
85 years and over	NA	NA	NA	NA	866.3	1,029.9	679.1	665.4	644.9	620.6
White, Not Hispanic or Latino Male										
All ages, age-adjusted[4]	NA	NA	NA	NA	66.3	59.9	37.5	36.1	35.3	34.9
All ages, crude	NA	NA	NA	NA	50.6	53.9	40.7	40.3	40.3	40.8
45 to 54 years	NA	NA	NA	NA	14.9	13.0	11.6	11.2	10.8	11.0
55 to 64 years	NA	NA	NA	NA	45.1	38.7	28.4	28.3	28.5	29.0
65 to 74 years	NA	NA	NA	NA	154.5	133.1	82.6	79.8	77.7	76.6
75 to 84 years	NA	NA	NA	NA	547.3	482.3	288.6	284.9	271.2	272.0
85 years and over	NA	NA	NA	NA	1,578.7	1,505.9	913.2	854.8	848.0	825.6
White Female [5]										
All ages, age-adjusted[4]	169.7	165.0	135.5	89.0	60.3	57.3	37.2	36.2	35.2	34.2
All ages, crude	103.3	110.1	109.8	88.6	71.6	76.9	53.0	52.3	51.5	50.6
45 to 54 years	55.0	33.8	30.5	18.6	13.5	11.2	9.1	9.0	9.3	9.0
55 to 64 years	156.9	103.0	78.1	48.6	35.8	30.2	20.6	21.1	19.8	19.8
65 to 74 years	498.1	383.3	303.2	172.5	116.1	107.3	66.8	64.6	62.3	60.0
75 to 84 years	1,471.3	1,444.7	1,176.8	728.8	456.5	434.2	280.2	278.0	265.4	257.7
85 years and over	3,017.9	3,795.7	3,167.6	2,362.7	1,685.9	1,646.7	1,052.8	1,008.1	994.7	970.4
Black or African American Female [5]										
All ages, age-adjusted[4]	238.4	232.5	189.3	119.6	84.0	76.2	49.6	47.0	45.4	44.7
All ages, crude	128.3	127.7	112.2	77.8	60.7	58.3	41.1	39.6	39.2	39.2
45 to 54 years	248.9	166.2	119.4	61.8	44.1	38.1	26.7	23.6	25.0	21.1
55 to 64 years	567.7	452.0	272.4	138.4	96.9	76.4	51.3	48.2	48.8	47.7
65 to 74 years	754.4	830.5	673.5	361.7	236.7	190.9	126.2	116.7	111.2	109.1
75 to 84 years[6]	1,496.7	1,413.1	1,338.3	917.5	595.0	549.2	347.2	342.0	321.6	333.0
85 years and over	NA	2,578.9	2,210.5	1,891.6	1,495.2	1,556.5	1,001.5	948.1	927.2	894.1
American Indian or Alaska Native Female [5]										
All ages, age-adjusted[4]	NA	NA	NA	51.2	38.4	43.7	26.5	27.9	24.8	25.5
All ages, crude	NA	NA	NA	22.0	19.3	21.5	14.2	15.9	14.4	15.4
45 to 54 years	NA	NA	NA	*	*	14.4	10.6	11.2	7.2	9.0
55 to 64 years	NA	NA	NA	*	40.7	37.9	22.4	19.2	20.0	19.1
65 to 74 years	NA	NA	NA	128.3	100.5	79.5	59.4	64.2	58.8	60.6
75 to 84 years	NA	NA	NA	404.2	282.0	391.1	173.6	237.7	205.5	187.2
85 years and over	NA	NA	NA	1,095.5	776.2	931.5	700.0	550.3	531.3	593.6
Asian or Pacific Islander Female [5]										
All ages, age-adjusted[4]	NA	NA	NA	60.8	54.9	49.1	31.4	30.0	28.9	27.9
All ages, crude	NA	NA	NA	26.4	24.3	28.7	23.5	23.7	23.7	23.8
45 to 54 years	NA	NA	NA	20.3	19.7	13.3	7.9	9.1	9.2	8.6
55 to 64 years	NA	NA	NA	43.7	42.1	33.3	22.1	22.5	20.0	18.2
65 to 74 years	NA	NA	NA	136.1	124.0	102.8	65.6	55.8	56.3	54.0
75 to 84 years	NA	NA	NA	446.6	396.6	386.0	218.4	237.2	213.4	203.0
85 years and over	NA	NA	NA	1,545.2	1,395.0	1,246.6	872.8	758.7	770.1	754.6
Hispanic or Latina Female [5,7]										
All ages, age-adjusted[4]	NA	NA	NA	NA	43.7	43.0	30.2	29.0	28.2	27.6
All ages, crude	NA	NA	NA	NA	20.1	19.4	15.7	15.7	15.8	16.1
45 to 54 years	NA	NA	NA	NA	15.2	12.4	9.2	9.5	8.8	9.1

Table 2-30. Death Rates for Cerebrovascular Diseases, by Sex, Race, Hispanic Origin, and Age, Selected Years, 1950–2013— continued

(Deaths per 100,000 resident population.)

Sex, race, Hispanic origin, and age	1950[1,2]	1960[1,2]	1970[2]	1980[2]	1990[2]	2000[3]	2010[3]	2011[3]	2012[3]	2013[3]
55 to 64 years	NA	NA	NA	NA	38.5	31.9	22.1	21.0	19.9	19.7
65 to 74 years	NA	NA	NA	NA	102.6	95.2	60.6	59.2	59.3	53.6
75 to 84 years	NA	NA	NA	NA	308.5	311.3	221.6	233.9	217.6	211.4
85 years and over	NA	NA	NA	NA	1,055.3	1,108.9	799.3	692.5	705.9	698.4
White, not Hispanic or Latina Female[7]										
All ages, age-adjusted[4]	NA	NA	NA	NA	61.0	57.6	37.4	36.5	35.5	34.5
All ages, crude	NA	NA	NA	NA	77.2	85.5	60.8	60.2	59.2	58.3
45 to 54 years	NA	NA	NA	NA	13.2	10.9	9.0	8.8	9.2	8.8
55 to 64 years	NA	NA	NA	NA	35.7	29.9	20.3	20.9	19.6	19.6
65 to 74 years	NA	NA	NA	NA	116.9	107.6	66.9	64.8	62.1	60.2
75 to 84 years	NA	NA	NA	NA	461.9	438.3	283.4	280.6	268.1	260.3
85 years and over	NA	NA	NA	NA	1,714.7	1,661.6	1,063.0	1,022.8	1,008.1	984.3

NA = Not available.   * = Rates based on fewer than 20 deaths are considered unreliable and are not shown.   1 Includes deaths of persons who were not residents of the 50 states and the District of Columbia.   2 Underlying cause of death was coded according to the 6th Revision of the International Classification of Diseases (ICD) in 1950, 7th Revision in 1960, 8th Revision in 1970, and 9th Revision in 1980-1998.   3 Starting with 1999 data, cause of death is coded according to ICD-10.   4 Age-adjusted rates are calculated using the year 2000 standard population. Prior to 2001, age-adjusted rates were calculated using standard million proportions based on rounded population numbers. Starting with 2001 data, unrounded population numbers are used to calculate age-adjusted rates.   5 The race groups, White, Black, Asian or Pacific Islander, and American Indian or Alaska Native, include persons of Hispanic and non-Hispanic origin. Persons of Hispanic origin may be of any race. Death rates for the American Indian or Alaska Native, Asian or Pacific Islander, and Hispanic populations are known to be underestimated.   6 In 1950, rate is for the age group 75 years and over.   7 Prior to 1997, excludes data from states lacking an Hispanic-origin item on the death certificate.

Figure 2-8. Age-Adjusted Death Rate for Heart Diseases, by Race and Sex, 1950–2013

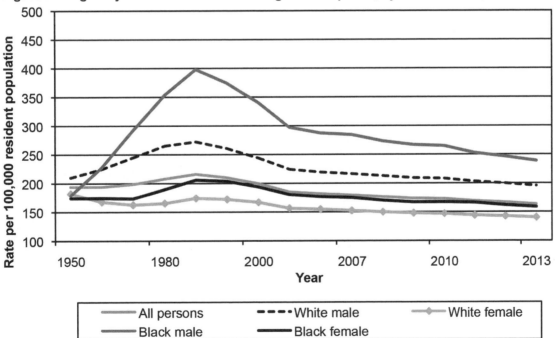

Figure 2-9. Age-Adjusted Death Rate for Malignant Neoplasm, by Race and Sex, 1950–2013

Table 2-31. Death Rates for Malignant Neoplasms, by Sex, Race, Hispanic Origin, and Age, Selected Years, 1950–2013

(Deaths per 100,000 resident population.)

Sex, race, Hispanic origin, and age	1950[1,2]	1960[1,2]	1970[2]	1980[2]	1990[2]	2000[3]	2010[3]	2011[3]	2012[3]	2013[3]
All Persons										
All ages, age-adjusted[4]	193.9	193.9	198.6	207.9	216.0	199.6	172.8	169.0	166.5	163.2
All ages, crude	139.8	149.2	162.8	183.9	203.2	196.5	186.2	185.1	185.6	185.0
Under 1 year	8.7	7.2	4.7	3.2	2.3	2.4	1.6	1.8	1.6	1.6
1 to 4 years	11.7	10.9	7.5	4.5	3.5	2.7	2.1	2.2	2.4	2.1
5 to 14 years	6.7	6.8	6.0	4.3	3.1	2.5	2.2	2.1	2.2	2.2
15 to 24 years	8.6	8.3	8.3	6.3	4.9	4.4	3.7	3.7	3.6	3.4
25 to 34 years	20.0	19.5	16.5	13.7	12.6	9.8	8.8	8.4	8.7	8.6
35 to 44 years	62.7	59.7	59.5	48.6	43.3	36.6	28.8	28.8	28.0	28.1
45 to 54 years	175.1	177.0	182.5	180.0	158.9	127.5	111.6	109.3	108.5	105.5
55 to 64 years	390.7	396.8	423.0	436.1	449.6	366.7	300.1	295.8	293.2	288.2
65 to 74 years	698.8	713.9	754.2	817.9	872.3	816.3	666.1	647.6	632.2	616.9
75 to 84 years	1,153.3	1,127.4	1,169.2	1,232.3	1,348.5	1,335.6	1,202.2	1,179.1	1,161.7	1,139.4
85 years and over	1,451.0	1,450.0	1,320.7	1,594.6	1,752.9	1,819.4	1,729.5	1,676.2	1,658.9	1,635.4
Male										
All ages, age-adjusted[4]	208.1	225.1	247.6	271.2	280.4	248.9	209.9	204.0	200.3	196.0
All ages, crude	142.9	162.5	182.1	205.3	221.3	207.2	198.3	197.2	197.9	197.6
Under 1 year	9.7	7.7	4.4	3.7	2.4	2.6	1.5	1.9	1.7	1.5
1 to 4 years	12.5	12.4	8.3	5.2	3.7	3.0	2.4	2.2	2.7	2.2
5 to 14 years	7.4	7.6	6.7	4.9	3.5	2.7	2.3	2.3	2.4	2.2
15 to 24 years	9.7	10.2	10.4	7.8	5.7	5.1	4.5	4.3	4.1	3.8
25 to 34 years	17.7	18.8	16.3	13.4	12.6	9.2	8.6	8.1	8.4	8.6
35 to 44 years	45.6	48.9	53.0	44.0	38.5	32.7	25.2	24.9	24.0	24.0
45 to 54 years	156.2	170.8	183.5	188.7	162.5	130.9	113.8	110.7	110.1	106.5
55 to 64 years	413.1	459.9	511.8	520.8	532.9	415.8	344.9	340.4	336.9	331.3
65 to 74 years	791.5	890.5	1,006.8	1,093.2	1,122.2	1,001.9	789.2	765.8	746.7	726.2
75 to 84 years	1,332.6	1,389.4	1,588.3	1,790.5	1,914.4	1,760.6	1,514.2	1,478.5	1,447.6	1,414.5
85 years and over	1,668.3	1,741.2	1,720.8	2,369.5	2,739.9	2,710.7	2,452.6	2,339.8	2,303.1	2,272.6
Female										
All ages, age-adjusted[4]	182.3	168.7	163.2	166.7	175.7	167.6	146.7	144.0	142.1	139.5
All ages, crude	136.8	136.4	144.4	163.6	186.0	186.2	174.4	173.4	173.7	172.8
Under 1 year	7.6	6.8	5.0	2.7	2.2	2.3	1.6	1.6	1.5	1.8
1 to 4 years	10.8	9.3	6.7	3.7	3.2	2.5	1.9	2.1	2.2	1.9
5 to 14 years	6.0	6.0	5.2	3.6	2.8	2.2	2.2	1.9	2.0	2.1
15 to 24 years	7.6	6.5	6.2	4.8	4.1	3.6	2.8	3.0	3.0	3.0
25 to 34 years	22.2	20.1	16.7	14.0	12.6	10.4	9.0	8.6	8.9	8.6
35 to 44 years	79.3	70.0	65.6	53.1	48.1	40.4	32.3	32.8	31.9	32.1
45 to 54 years	194.0	183.0	181.5	171.8	155.5	124.2	109.4	108.0	107.0	104.6
55 to 64 years	368.2	337.7	343.2	361.7	375.2	321.3	258.5	254.1	252.5	248.1
65 to 74 years	612.3	560.2	557.9	607.1	677.4	663.6	559.1	544.5	531.9	520.8
75 to 84 years	1,000.7	924.1	891.9	903.1	1,010.3	1,058.5	977.0	959.6	950.0	933.3
85 years and over	1,299.7	1,263.9	1,096.7	1,255.7	1,372.1	1,456.4	1,380.1	1,349.1	1,336.4	1,310.1
White Male [5]										
All ages, age-adjusted[4]	210.0	224.7	244.8	265.1	272.2	243.9	208.2	203.1	199.7	195.5
All ages, crude	147.2	166.1	185.1	208.7	227.7	218.1	212.7	212.0	213.1	213.0
25 to 34 years	17.7	18.8	16.2	13.6	12.3	9.2	8.8	8.1	8.5	8.5
35 to 44 years	44.5	46.3	50.1	41.1	35.8	30.9	25.2	25.2	24.2	23.9
45 to 54 years	150.8	164.1	172.0	175.4	149.9	123.5	111.6	108.6	108.2	105.7
55 to 64 years	409.4	450.9	498.1	497.4	508.2	401.9	334.9	332.4	329.4	323.1
65 to 74 years	798.7	887.3	997.0	1,070.7	1,090.7	984.3	782.8	759.5	742.8	723.3
75 to 84 years	1,367.6	1,413.7	1,592.7	1,779.7	1,883.2	1,736.0	1,511.6	1,485.2	1,453.0	1,421.7
85 years and over	1,732.7	1,791.4	1,772.2	2,375.6	2,715.1	2,693.7	2,453.5	2,347.1	2,318.7	2,290.7
Black or African American Male [5]										
All ages, age-adjusted[4]	178.9	227.6	291.9	353.4	397.9	340.3	264.8	252.6	246.1	238.7
All ages, crude	106.6	136.7	171.6	205.5	221.9	188.5	169.0	166.4	166.4	165.6
25 to 34 years	18.0	18.4	18.8	14.1	15.7	10.1	9.2	9.2	9.1	10.2
35 to 44 years	55.7	72.9	81.3	73.8	64.3	48.4	30.1	28.9	26.6	27.3
45 to 54 years	211.7	244.7	311.2	333.0	302.6	214.2	150.9	145.6	145.0	132.4
55 to 64 years	490.8	579.7	689.2	812.5	859.2	626.4	496.7	478.4	468.8	464.0
65 to 74 years	636.5	938.5	1,168.9	1,417.2	1,613.9	1,363.8	1,027.8	1,004.1	970.2	941.5
75 to 84 years	853.5	1,053.3	1,624.8	2,029.6	2,478.3	2,351.8	1,826.8	1,705.6	1,685.7	1,633.2
85 years and over	NA	1,155.2	1,387.0	2,393.9	3,238.3	3,264.8	2,854.6	2,675.3	2,540.2	2,465.6

Table 2-31. Death Rates for Malignant Neoplasms, by Sex, Race, Hispanic Origin, and Age, Selected Years, 1950–2013— continued

(Deaths per 100,000 resident population.)

Sex, race, Hispanic origin, and age	1950[1,2]	1960[1,2]	1970[2]	1980[2]	1990[2]	2000[3]	2010[3]	2011[3]	2012[3]	2013[3]
American Indian or Alaska Native Male[5]										
All ages, age-adjusted[4]	NA	NA	NA	140.5	145.8	155.8	151.0	132.7	127.9	132.3
All ages, crude	NA	NA	NA	58.1	61.4	67.0	74.1	68.0	70.5	73.6
25 to 34 years	NA	NA	NA	*	*	*	7.4	*	*	6.2
35 to 44 years	NA	NA	NA	*	22.8	21.4	13.4	11.3	14.2	13.1
45 to 54 years	NA	NA	NA	86.9	86.9	70.3	70.0	70.6	65.9	61.9
55 to 64 years	NA	NA	NA	213.4	246.2	255.6	249.5	197.2	216.2	233.5
65 to 74 years	NA	NA	NA	613.0	530.6	648.0	597.7	523.8	558.4	477.8
75 to 84 years	NA	NA	NA	936.4	1,038.4	1,152.5	1,104.4	1,018.5	885.2	1,009.1
85 years and over	NA	NA	NA	1,471.2	1,654.4	1,584.2	1,741.3	1,459.3	1,288.7	1,488.1
Asian or Pacific Islander Male[5]										
All ages, age-adjusted[4]	NA	NA	NA	165.2	172.5	150.8	131.0	125.7	123.1	120.9
All ages, crude	NA	NA	NA	81.9	82.7	85.2	88.6	89.0	89.0	90.5
25 to 34 years	NA	NA	NA	6.3	9.2	7.4	6.5	6.8	7.4	6.5
35 to 44 years	NA	NA	NA	29.4	27.7	26.1	18.2	16.1	19.4	20.3
45 to 54 years	NA	NA	NA	108.2	92.6	78.5	67.4	67.6	65.9	67.6
55 to 64 years	NA	NA	NA	298.5	274.6	229.2	195.2	193.7	186.7	186.4
65 to 74 years	NA	NA	NA	581.2	687.2	559.4	446.2	436.6	396.5	387.5
75 to 84 years	NA	NA	NA	1,147.6	1,229.9	1,086.1	980.4	917.6	936.3	899.5
85 years and over	NA	NA	NA	1,798.7	1,837.0	1,823.2	1,707.2	1,626.3	1,577.7	1,575.3
Hispanic or Latino Male[5,6]										
All ages, age-adjusted[4]	NA	NA	NA	NA	174.7	171.7	149.4	144.9	141.9	138.8
All ages, crude	NA	NA	NA	NA	65.5	61.3	64.2	65.0	66.3	66.9
25 to 34 years	NA	NA	NA	NA	8.0	6.9	7.2	6.7	7.6	7.8
35 to 44 years	NA	NA	NA	NA	22.5	20.1	16.5	16.4	17.3	16.4
45 to 54 years	NA	NA	NA	NA	96.6	79.4	69.7	69.2	67.6	66.4
55 to 64 years	NA	NA	NA	NA	294.0	253.1	225.4	224.3	224.8	217.4
65 to 74 years	NA	NA	NA	NA	655.5	651.2	552.0	528.2	524.3	515.6
75 to 84 years	NA	NA	NA	NA	1,233.4	1,306.4	1,118.7	1,104.5	1,068.1	1,051.3
85 years and over	NA	NA	NA	NA	2,019.4	2,049.7	1,861.2	1,728.5	1,652.6	1,606.6
White, Not Hispanic or Latino Male[6]										
All ages, age-adjusted[4]	NA	NA	NA	NA	276.7	247.7	212.6	207.6	204.0	200.0
All ages, crude	NA	NA	NA	NA	246.2	244.4	245.8	245.6	247.0	247.3
25 to 34 years	NA	NA	NA	NA	12.8	9.7	9.1	8.4	8.5	8.5
35 to 44 years	NA	NA	NA	NA	36.8	32.3	27.0	27.2	25.7	25.6
45 to 54 years	NA	NA	NA	NA	153.9	127.2	117.2	114.4	114.2	111.9
55 to 64 years	NA	NA	NA	NA	520.6	412.0	344.2	341.8	338.6	332.9
65 to 74 years	NA	NA	NA	NA	1,109.0	1,002.1	798.5	775.7	757.4	737.2
75 to 84 years	NA	NA	NA	NA	1,906.6	1,750.2	1,534.4	1,508.2	1,475.9	1,444.8
85 years and over	NA	NA	NA	NA	2,744.4	2,714.1	2,480.8	2,377.1	2,353.6	2,330.5
White Female[5]										
All ages, age-adjusted[4]	182.0	167.7	162.5	165.2	174.0	166.9	146.9	144.0	142.5	140.2
All ages, crude	139.9	139.8	149.4	170.3	196.1	199.4	188.2	186.8	187.5	186.8
25 to 34 years	20.9	18.8	16.3	13.5	11.9	10.1	8.8	8.3	8.7	8.5
35 to 44 years	74.5	66.6	62.4	50.9	46.2	38.2	31.3	31.4	31.0	31.8
45 to 54 years	185.8	175.7	177.3	166.4	150.9	120.1	106.5	105.0	104.5	103.0
55 to 64 years	362.5	329.0	338.6	355.5	368.5	319.7	255.3	250.6	249.7	245.4
65 to 74 years	616.5	562.1	554.7	605.2	675.1	665.6	563.7	549.2	535.5	526.4
75 to 84 years	1,026.6	939.3	903.5	905.4	1,011.8	1,063.4	988.6	970.1	962.1	945.4
85 years and over	1,348.3	1,304.9	1,126.6	1,266.8	1,372.3	1,459.1	1,389.8	1,359.9	1,351.4	1,326.5
Black or African American Female[5]										
All ages, age-adjusted[4]	174.1	174.3	173.4	189.5	205.9	193.8	167.1	166.1	161.7	158.5
All ages, crude	111.8	113.8	117.3	136.5	156.1	151.8	145.5	147.5	146.3	146.2
25 to 34 years	34.3	31.0	20.9	18.3	18.7	13.5	10.8	12.2	12.1	10.4
35 to 44 years	119.8	102.4	94.6	73.5	67.4	58.9	44.5	46.4	42.5	40.7
45 to 54 years	277.0	254.8	228.6	230.2	209.9	173.9	146.4	144.9	140.2	134.8
55 to 64 years	484.6	442.7	404.8	450.4	482.4	391.0	331.1	327.6	320.9	320.0
65 to 74 years	477.3	541.6	615.8	662.4	773.2	753.1	631.0	623.1	617.8	593.4
75 to 84 years	605.3	696.3	763.3	923.9	1,059.9	1,124.0	1,008.2	1,010.4	985.6	984.3
85 years and over	NA	728.9	791.5	1,159.9	1,431.3	1,527.7	1,418.6	1,390.9	1,318.4	1,306.5

Table 2-31. Death Rates for Malignant Neoplasms, by Sex, Race, Hispanic Origin, and Age, Selected Years, 1950–2013— continued

(Deaths per 100,000 resident population.)

Sex, race, Hispanic origin, and age	1950[1,2]	1960[1,2]	1970[2]	1980[2]	1990[2]	2000[3]	2010[3]	2011[3]	2012[3]	2013[3]
American Indian or Alaska Native Female [5]										
All ages, age-adjusted[4]	NA	NA	NA	94.0	106.9	108.3	102.0	92.6	99.1	94.3
All ages, crude	NA	NA	NA	50.4	62.1	61.3	64.8	61.3	66.7	65.8
25 to 34 years	NA	NA	NA	*	*	*	6.3	*	*	6.4
35 to 44 years	NA	NA	NA	36.9	31.0	23.7	14.2	16.2	16.1	18.8
45 to 54 years	NA	NA	NA	96.9	104.5	59.7	68.7	68.4	62.5	69.1
55 to 64 years	NA	NA	NA	198.4	213.3	200.9	185.9	160.7	176.2	155.1
65 to 74 years	NA	NA	NA	350.8	438.9	458.3	432.2	375.6	394.4	373.0
75 to 84 years	NA	NA	NA	446.4	554.3	714.0	682.3	621.8	753.5	656.2
85 years and over	NA	NA	NA	786.5	843.7	983.2	885.7	828.6	763.3	844.8
Asian or Pacific Islander Female [5]										
All ages, age-adjusted[4]	NA	NA	NA	93.0	103.0	100.7	93.5	91.5	90.9	86.0
All ages, crude	NA	NA	NA	54.1	60.5	72.1	78.5	79.8	80.9	78.6
25 to 34 years	NA	NA	NA	9.5	7.3	8.1	7.1	5.1	5.6	6.4
35 to 44 years	NA	NA	NA	38.7	29.8	28.9	21.7	23.3	23.2	22.1
45 to 54 years	NA	NA	NA	99.8	93.9	78.2	69.5	69.9	71.2	63.6
55 to 64 years	NA	NA	NA	174.7	196.2	176.5	152.6	155.9	149.9	139.7
65 to 74 years	NA	NA	NA	301.9	346.2	357.4	314.4	299.6	290.3	280.7
75 to 84 years	NA	NA	NA	522.1	641.4	650.1	654.5	640.9	626.5	601.5
85 years and over	NA	NA	NA	800.0	971.7	988.5	994.4	957.6	1,012.6	925.7
Hispanic or Latina Female [5,6]										
All ages, age-adjusted[4]	NA	NA	NA	NA	111.9	110.8	99.4	97.5	99.3	97.3
All ages, crude	NA	NA	NA	NA	60.7	58.5	59.0	59.4	62.4	63.0
25 to 34 years	NA	NA	NA	NA	9.7	7.8	8.4	7.2	8.1	8.8
35 to 44 years	NA	NA	NA	NA	34.8	30.7	23.5	24.0	24.4	25.4
45 to 54 years	NA	NA	NA	NA	100.5	84.7	74.0	66.2	73.2	69.1
55 to 64 years	NA	NA	NA	NA	205.4	192.5	165.9	161.6	165.1	164.7
65 to 74 years	NA	NA	NA	NA	404.8	410.0	355.2	348.2	342.8	342.0
75 to 84 years	NA	NA	NA	NA	663.0	716.5	657.6	672.0	662.9	656.7
85 years and over	NA	NA	NA	NA	1,022.7	1,056.5	1,043.4	1,006.5	1,073.7	996.6
White, not Hispanic or Latina Female [6]										
All ages, age-adjusted[4]	NA	NA	NA	NA	177.5	170.0	150.6	147.9	146.0	143.9
All ages, crude	NA	NA	NA	NA	210.6	220.6	215.0	213.9	214.4	214.0
25 to 34 years	NA	NA	NA	NA	11.9	10.5	8.8	8.4	8.6	8.1
35 to 44 years	NA	NA	NA	NA	47.0	38.9	32.8	32.8	32.3	32.9
45 to 54 years	NA	NA	NA	NA	154.9	123.0	110.5	110.4	108.8	108.0
55 to 64 years	NA	NA	NA	NA	379.5	328.9	263.4	259.0	257.9	253.3
65 to 74 years	NA	NA	NA	NA	688.5	681.0	580.4	566.0	551.1	541.4
75 to 84 years	NA	NA	NA	NA	1,027.2	1,075.3	1,010.4	990.3	983.0	966.6
85 years and over	NA	NA	NA	NA	1,385.7	1,468.7	1,403.8	1,375.6	1,362.4	1,343.5

NA = Not available.   * = Rates based on fewer than 20 deaths are considered unreliable and are not shown.   1 Includes deaths of persons who were not residents of the 50 states and the District of Columbia. 2 Underlying cause of death was coded according to the 6th Revision of the International Classification of Diseases (ICD) in 1950, 7th Revision in 1960, 8th Revision in 1970, and 9th Revision in 1980-1998.   3 Starting with 1999 data, cause of death is coded according to ICD-10.   4 Age-adjusted rates are calculated using the year 2000 standard population. Prior to 2001, age-adjusted rates were calculated using standard million proportions based on rounded population numbers. Starting with 2001 data, unrounded population numbers are used to calculate age-adjusted rates.   5 The race groups, White, Black, Asian or Pacific Islander, and American Indian or Alaska Native, include persons of Hispanic and non-Hispanic origin. Persons of Hispanic origin may be of any race. Death rates for the American Indian or Alaska Native, Asian or Pacific Islander, and Hispanic populations are known to be underestimated.   6 Prior to 1997, excludes data from states lacking an Hispanic-origin item on the death certificate.

Table 2-32. Death Rates for Malignant Neoplasm of Breast Among Females, by Race, Hispanic Origin, and Age, Selected Years, 1950–2013

(Deaths per 100,000 resident population.)

Sex, race, Hispanic origin, and age	1950[1,2]	1960[1,2]	1970[2]	1980[2]	1990[2]	2000[3]	2010[3]	2011[3]	2012[3]	2013[3]
All Females										
All ages, age-adjusted[4]	31.9	31.7	32.1	31.9	33.3	26.8	22.1	21.6	21.3	20.8
All ages, crude	24.7	26.1	28.4	30.6	34.0	29.2	26.1	25.9	25.8	25.5
Under 25 years	*	*	*	*	*	*	*	*	*	*
25 to 34 years	3.8	3.8	3.9	3.3	2.9	2.3	1.6	1.7	1.7	1.6
35 to 44 years	20.8	20.2	20.4	17.9	17.8	12.4	9.8	9.9	9.7	9.6
45 to 54 years	46.9	51.4	52.6	48.1	45.4	33.0	25.7	25.2	25.2	24.6
55 to 64 years	69.9	70.8	77.6	80.5	78.6	59.3	47.7	46.2	45.4	44.1
65 to 74 years	95.0	90.0	93.8	101.1	111.7	88.3	73.9	72.5	70.0	68.4
75 to 84 years	139.8	129.9	127.4	126.4	146.3	128.9	109.1	108.2	106.9	104.4
85 years and over	195.5	191.9	157.1	169.3	196.8	205.7	185.8	176.5	177.3	173.0
White[5]										
All ages, age-adjusted[4]	32.4	32.0	32.5	32.1	33.2	26.3	21.5	21.0	20.8	20.4
All ages, crude	25.7	27.2	29.9	32.3	35.9	30.7	27.3	26.9	26.9	26.7
35 to 44 years	20.8	19.7	20.2	17.3	17.1	11.3	8.8	8.9	8.8	8.8
45 to 54 years	47.1	51.2	53.0	48.1	44.3	31.2	23.9	23.4	23.5	23.0
55 to 64 years	70.9	71.8	79.3	81.3	78.5	57.9	45.9	44.1	43.5	42.5
65 to 74 years	96.3	91.6	95.9	103.7	113.3	89.3	73.3	71.9	69.6	68.4
75 to 84 years	143.6	132.8	129.6	128.4	148.2	130.2	110.2	108.8	107.8	105.0
85 years and over	204.2	199.7	161.9	171.7	198.0	205.5	186.8	178.3	178.8	174.9
Black or African American[5]										
All ages, age-adjusted[4]	25.3	27.9	28.9	31.7	38.1	34.5	30.3	30.2	29.4	28.3
All ages, crude	16.4	18.7	19.7	22.9	29.0	27.9	27.5	27.8	27.5	26.7
35 to 44 years	21.0	24.8	24.4	24.1	25.8	20.9	18.3	17.6	16.8	16.3
45 to 54 years	46.5	54.4	52.0	52.7	60.5	51.5	40.9	41.0	40.1	39.2
55 to 64 years	64.3	63.2	64.7	79.9	93.1	80.9	70.5	69.7	67.6	63.7
65 to 74 years	67.0	72.3	77.3	84.3	112.2	98.6	97.4	95.8	89.7	86.6
75 to 84 years[6]	81.0	87.5	101.8	114.1	140.5	139.8	123.2	130.4	129.7	126.1
85 years and over	NA	92.1	112.1	149.9	201.5	238.7	214.6	199.2	204.4	193.1
American Indian or Alaska Native[5]										
All ages, age-adjusted[4]	NA	NA	NA	10.8	13.7	13.6	11.5	10.8	10.8	10.1
All ages, crude	NA	NA	NA	6.1	8.6	8.7	8.0	7.6	7.9	7.5
35 to 44 years	NA	NA	NA	*	*	*	*	*	*	*
45 to 54 years	NA	NA	NA	*	23.9	14.4	13.2	11.2	10.8	11.2
55 to 64 years	NA	NA	NA	*	*	40.0	25.2	21.8	22.5	20.6
65 to 74 years	NA	NA	NA	*	*	42.5	34.3	38.5	46.8	38.2
75 to 84 years	NA	NA	NA	*	*	71.8	61.1	59.4	64.1	50.5
85 years and over	NA	NA	NA	*	*	*	*	*	*	*
Asian or Pacific Islander[5]										
All ages, age-adjusted[4]	NA	NA	NA	11.9	13.7	12.3	11.9	11.3	11.3	11.1
All ages, crude	NA	NA	NA	8.2	9.3	10.2	10.8	10.7	10.9	10.8
35 to 44 years	NA	NA	NA	10.4	8.4	8.1	5.4	6.4	6.4	5.7
45 to 54 years	NA	NA	NA	23.4	26.4	22.3	17.0	15.7	16.7	15.6
55 to 64 years	NA	NA	NA	35.7	33.8	31.3	28.4	29.3	27.8	27.2
65 to 74 years	NA	NA	NA	*	38.5	34.7	37.9	34.6	37.1	32.7
75 to 84 years	NA	NA	NA	*	48.0	37.5	53.2	46.7	40.3	48.6
85 years and over	NA	NA	NA	*	*	68.2	77.5	71.4	77.4	82.8
Hispanic or Latina[5,7]										
All ages, age-adjusted[4]	NA	NA	NA	NA	19.5	16.9	14.4	14.1	14.7	14.6
All ages, crude	NA	NA	NA	NA	11.5	9.7	9.2	9.3	10.0	10.0
35 to 44 years	NA	NA	NA	NA	11.7	8.7	6.2	7.0	7.2	7.2
45 to 54 years	NA	NA	NA	NA	32.8	23.9	18.6	17.3	20.3	18.0
55 to 64 years	NA	NA	NA	NA	45.8	39.1	32.7	29.6	31.8	31.2
65 to 74 years	NA	NA	NA	NA	64.8	54.9	49.0	46.3	45.7	46.3
75 to 84 years	NA	NA	NA	NA	67.2	74.9	61.8	68.5	63.9	73.3
85 years and over	NA	NA	NA	NA	102.8	105.8	117.8	108.7	121.8	112.0

White, not Hispanic or Latina[7]

Table 2-32. Death Rates for Malignant Neoplasm of Breast Among Females, by Race, Hispanic Origin, and Age, Selected Years, 1950–2013— continued

(Deaths per 100,000 resident population.)

Sex, race, Hispanic origin, and age	1950[1,2]	1960[1,2]	1970[2]	1980[2]	1990[2]	2000[3]	2010[3]	2011[3]	2012[3]	2013[3]
All ages, age-adjusted[4]	NA	NA	NA	NA	33.9	26.8	22.1	21.6	21.3	20.9
All ages, crude	NA	NA	NA	NA	38.5	33.8	31.0	30.7	30.6	30.3
35 to 44 years	NA	NA	NA	NA	17.5	11.6	9.3	9.3	9.0	9.1
45 to 54 years	NA	NA	NA	NA	45.2	31.7	24.5	24.2	23.8	23.6
55 to 64 years	NA	NA	NA	NA	80.6	59.2	47.1	45.4	44.6	43.5
65 to 74 years	NA	NA	NA	NA	115.7	91.4	75.1	74.1	71.6	70.1
75 to 84 years	NA	NA	NA	NA	151.4	132.2	113.6	111.6	111.1	107.3
85 years and over	NA	NA	NA	NA	201.5	208.3	189.9	181.7	181.8	178.5

NA = Not available.   * = Rates based on fewer than 20 deaths are considered unreliable and are not shown.   1 Includes deaths of persons who were not residents of the 50 states and the District of Columbia.   2 Underlying cause of death was coded according to the 6th Revision of the International Classification of Diseases (ICD) in 1950, 7th Revision in 1960, 8th Revision in 1970, and 9th Revision in 1980-1998.   3 Starting with 1999 data, cause of death is coded according to ICD-10.   4 Age-adjusted rates are calculated using the year 2000 standard population. Prior to 2001, age-adjusted rates were calculated using standard million proportions based on rounded population numbers. Starting with 2001 data, unrounded population numbers are used to calculate age-adjusted rates.   5 The race groups, White, Black, Asian or Pacific Islander, and American Indian or Alaska Native, include persons of Hispanic and non-Hispanic origin. Persons of Hispanic origin may be of any race. Death rates for the American Indian or Alaska Native, Asian or Pacific Islander, and Hispanic populations are known to be underestimated.   6 In 1950, rate is for the age group 75 years and over.   7 Prior to 1997, excludes data from states lacking an Hispanic-origin item on the death certificate.

Table 2-33. Death Rates for Malignant Neoplasms of the Trachea, Bronchus, and Lung, by Sex, Race, Hispanic Origin, and Age, Selected Years, 1950–2012

(Deaths per 100,000 resident population.)

Sex, race, Hispanic origin, and age	1950[1,2]	1960[1,2]	1970[2]	1980[2]	1990[2]	2000[3]	2010[3]	2011[3]	2012[3]
All Persons									
All ages, age-adjusted[4]	15.0	24.1	37.1	49.9	59.3	56.1	47.6	46.0	44.9
All ages, crude	12.2	20.3	32.1	45.8	56.8	55.3	51.3	50.4	50.2
Under 25 years	0.1	0.0	0.1	0.0	0.0	0.0	0.0	0.0	0.0
25 to 34 years	0.8	1.0	0.9	0.6	0.7	0.5	0.4	0.3	0.4
35 to 44 years	4.5	6.8	11.0	9.2	6.8	6.1	3.3	3.1	2.9
45 to 54 years	20.4	29.6	43.4	54.1	46.8	31.6	26.9	25.7	25.1
55 to 64 years	48.7	75.3	109.1	138.2	160.6	122.4	85.4	83.5	81.5
65 to 74 years	59.7	108.1	164.5	233.3	288.4	284.2	223.9	214.3	206.1
75 to 84 years	55.8	91.5	163.2	240.5	333.3	370.8	357.2	345.9	339.6
85 years and over	42.3	65.6	101.7	176.0	242.5	302.1	332.4	323.7	323.7
Male									
All ages, age-adjusted[4]	24.6	43.6	67.5	85.2	91.1	76.7	60.3	57.7	56.1
All ages, crude	19.9	35.4	53.4	68.6	75.1	65.5	57.8	56.6	56.1
Under 25 years	0.0	0.0	0.1	0.1	0.0	*	*	0.0	0.0
25 to 34 years	1.1	1.4	1.3	0.8	0.9	0.5	0.4	0.3	0.5
35 to 44 years	7.1	10.5	16.1	11.9	8.5	6.9	3.2	3.1	2.9
45 to 54 years	35.0	50.6	67.5	76.0	59.7	38.5	30.0	28.1	27.7
55 to 64 years	83.8	139.3	189.7	213.6	222.9	154.0	104.9	102.5	98.3
65 to 74 years	98.7	204.3	320.8	403.9	430.4	377.9	274.9	262.8	250.0
75 to 84 years	82.6	167.1	330.8	488.8	572.9	532.2	461.9	442.4	432.0
85 years and over	62.5	107.7	194.0	368.1	513.2	521.2	492.3	467.3	473.4
Female									
All ages, age-adjusted[4]	5.8	7.5	13.1	24.4	37.1	41.3	38.1	37.1	36.4
All ages, crude	4.5	6.4	11.9	24.3	39.4	45.4	45.0	44.4	44.4
Under 25 years	0.1	0.0	0.0	*	*	*	0.0	*	*
25 to 34 years	0.5	0.5	0.5	0.5	0.5	0.5	0.4	0.3	0.3
35 to 44 years	1.9	3.2	6.1	6.5	5.2	5.3	3.3	3.1	2.9
45 to 54 years	5.8	9.2	21.0	33.7	34.5	25.0	23.8	23.3	22.6
55 to 64 years	13.6	15.4	36.8	72.0	105.0	93.3	67.2	65.7	65.9
65 to 74 years	23.3	24.4	43.1	102.7	177.6	206.9	179.5	171.9	167.5
75 to 84 years	32.9	32.8	52.4	94.1	190.1	265.6	281.7	275.3	271.1
85 years and over	28.2	38.8	50.0	91.9	138.1	212.8	255.2	252.9	248.7
White Male [5]									
All ages, age-adjusted[4]	25.1	43.6	67.1	83.8	89.0	75.7	60.1	57.7	56.0
All ages, crude	20.8	36.4	54.6	70.2	77.8	69.4	62.3	61.2	60.6
45 to 54 years	35.1	49.2	63.3	70.9	55.2	35.7	28.8	27.4	26.9
55 to 64 years	85.4	139.2	186.8	205.6	213.7	150.8	101.8	100.7	96.4
65 to 74 years	101.5	207.5	325.0	401.0	422.1	374.9	275.7	262.9	250.8
75 to 84 years	85.5	170.4	336.7	493.5	572.2	529.9	465.5	446.7	434.4
85 years and over	67.4	109.4	199.6	374.1	516.3	522.4	495.0	471.0	475.7
Black or African American Male [5]									
All ages, age-adjusted[4]	17.8	42.6	75.4	107.6	125.4	101.1	73.7	69.6	68.6
All ages, crude	12.1	28.1	47.7	66.6	73.7	58.3	48.7	47.2	47.3
45 to 54 years	34.4	68.4	115.4	133.8	114.9	70.7	45.2	40.4	40.6
55 to 64 years	68.3	146.8	234.3	321.1	358.6	223.5	155.4	145.4	138.4
65 to 74 years	53.8	168.3	300.5	472.3	585.4	488.8	341.3	333.1	312.8
75 to 84 years	36.2	107.3	271.6	472.9	645.4	642.5	509.1	479.7	494.6
85 years and over	NA	82.8	137.0	311.3	499.5	562.8	521.8	473.9	485.0
American Indian or Alaska Native Male [5]									
All ages, age-adjusted[4]	NA	NA	NA	31.7	47.5	42.9	41.6	38.1	35.9
All ages, crude	NA	NA	NA	14.2	20.0	18.1	20.8	18.9	19.4
45 to 54 years	NA	NA	NA	*	26.6	14.5	19.7	16.4	13.0
55 to 64 years	NA	NA	NA	72.0	97.8	86.0	67.6	52.9	59.7
65 to 74 years	NA	NA	NA	202.8	194.3	184.8	213.2	164.1	185.8
75 to 84 years	NA	NA	NA	*	356.2	367.9	325.8	333.2	259.8
85 years and over	NA	NA	NA	*	*	*	276.4	328.3	310.7
Asian or Pacific Islander Male [5]									
All ages, age-adjusted[4]	NA	NA	NA	43.3	44.2	40.9	33.8	32.9	32.7
All ages, crude	NA	NA	NA	22.1	20.7	22.7	22.5	22.7	22.9
45 to 54 years	NA	NA	NA	33.3	18.8	17.2	13.8	12.2	13.0

Table 2-33. Death Rates for Malignant Neoplasms of the Trachea, Bronchus, and Lung, by Sex, Race, Hispanic Origin, and Age, Selected Years, 1950–2012— continued

(Deaths per 100,000 resident population.)

Sex, race, Hispanic origin, and age	1950[1,2]	1960[1,2]	1970[2]	1980[2]	1990[2]	2000[3]	2010[3]	2011[3]	2012[3]
55 to 64 years	NA	NA	NA	94.4	74.4	61.4	51.1	45.0	45.3
65 to 74 years	NA	NA	NA	174.3	215.8	183.2	127.0	131.3	114.8
75 to 84 years	NA	NA	NA	301.3	307.5	323.2	286.4	276.1	279.4
85 years and over	NA	NA	NA	*	421.3	378.0	382.0	370.7	411.4
Hispanic or Latino Male [5,6]									
All ages, age-adjusted[4]	NA	NA	NA	NA	44.1	39.0	29.6	28.7	26.8
All ages, crude	NA	NA	NA	NA	16.2	13.3	11.9	12.0	11.7
45 to 54 years	NA	NA	NA	NA	21.5	14.8	9.0	8.3	8.5
55 to 64 years	NA	NA	NA	NA	80.7	58.6	40.1	39.4	35.6
65 to 74 years	NA	NA	NA	NA	195.5	167.3	126.2	120.2	116.4
75 to 84 years	NA	NA	NA	NA	313.4	327.5	256.3	240.6	237.3
85 years and over	NA	NA	NA	NA	420.7	368.8	307.9	330.3	258.0
White, Not Hispanic or Latino Male [5]									
All ages, age-adjusted[4]	NA	NA	NA	NA	91.1	77.9	62.7	60.3	58.5
All ages, crude	NA	NA	NA	NA	84.7	78.9	73.8	72.7	72.2
45 to 54 years	NA	NA	NA	NA	57.8	37.7	31.8	30.6	29.9
55 to 64 years	NA	NA	NA	NA	221.0	157.7	107.8	106.9	102.8
65 to 74 years	NA	NA	NA	NA	431.4	387.3	287.3	274.4	261.3
75 to 84 years	NA	NA	NA	NA	580.4	537.7	479.3	461.0	448.1
85 years and over	NA	NA	NA	NA	520.9	527.3	504.4	478.2	488.3
White Female [5]									
All ages, age-adjusted[4]	5.9	6.8	13.1	24.5	37.6	42.3	39.3	38.3	37.6
All ages, crude	4.7	5.9	12.3	25.6	42.4	49.9	50.0	49.3	49.4
45 to 54 years	5.7	9.0	20.9	33.0	34.6	24.8	24.3	23.9	23.0
55 to 64 years	13.7	15.1	37.2	71.9	105.7	96.1	68.9	67.2	68.0
65 to 74 years	23.7	24.8	42.9	104.6	181.3	213.2	187.4	179.6	174.3
75 to 84 years	34.0	32.7	52.6	95.2	194.6	272.7	290.5	284.9	280.7
85 years and over	29.3	39.1	50.6	92.4	138.3	215.9	258.3	256.3	254.5
Black or African American Female [5]									
All ages, age-adjusted[4]	4.5	6.8	13.7	24.8	36.8	39.8	36.5	35.4	34.7
All ages, crude	2.8	4.3	9.4	18.3	28.1	30.8	31.4	31.2	31.1
45 to 54 years	7.5	11.3	23.9	43.4	41.3	32.9	27.7	26.8	25.9
55 to 64 years	12.9	17.9	33.5	79.9	117.9	95.3	74.0	73.3	71.0
65 to 74 years	14.0	18.1	46.1	88.0	164.3	194.1	163.1	156.9	158.2
75 to 84 years	*	31.3	49.1	79.4	148.1	224.3	249.2	240.5	239.8
85 years and over	NA	34.2	44.8	85.8	134.9	185.9	249.3	236.8	211.2
American Indian or Alaska Native Female [5]									
All ages, age-adjusted[4]	NA	NA	NA	11.7	19.3	24.8	26.3	23.9	25.6
All ages, crude	NA	NA	NA	6.0	11.2	14.0	16.0	15.3	16.9
45 to 54 years	NA	NA	NA	*	22.9	12.1	13.2	13.8	13.0
55 to 64 years	NA	NA	NA	*	53.7	52.6	40.3	39.5	44.9
65 to 74 years	NA	NA	NA	*	78.5	151.5	141.8	110.2	116.5
75 to 84 years	NA	NA	NA	*	111.8	136.3	185.9	189.7	203.3
85 years and over	NA	NA	NA	*	*	*	200.0	168.3	183.2
Asian or Pacific Islander Female [5]									
All ages, age-adjusted[4]	NA	NA	NA	15.4	18.9	18.4	18.3	18.6	17.8
All ages, crude	NA	NA	NA	8.4	10.5	12.6	14.9	15.8	15.5
45 to 54 years	NA	NA	NA	13.5	11.3	9.9	8.8	8.5	10.9
55 to 64 years	NA	NA	NA	24.6	38.3	30.4	28.0	29.0	25.1
65 to 74 years	NA	NA	NA	62.4	71.6	77.0	67.0	70.6	68.6
75 to 84 years	NA	NA	NA	117.7	137.9	135.0	160.3	149.1	142.8
85 years and over	NA	NA	NA	*	172.9	175.3	171.1	200.8	181.7
Hispanic or Latina Female [5,6]									
All ages, age-adjusted[4]	NA	NA	NA	NA	14.1	14.7	13.8	13.3	13.6
All ages, crude	NA	NA	NA	NA	7.2	7.2	7.7	7.6	8.0
45 to 54 years	NA	NA	NA	NA	8.7	7.1	7.1	5.7	6.0
55 to 64 years	NA	NA	NA	NA	25.1	22.2	19.3	18.5	20.5
65 to 74 years	NA	NA	NA	NA	66.8	66.0	51.7	54.2	51.7
75 to 84 years	NA	NA	NA	NA	94.3	112.3	117.3	108.6	110.8
85 years and over	NA	NA	NA	NA	118.2	137.5	143.4	144.8	152.4

Table 2-33. Death Rates for Malignant Neoplasms of the Trachea, Bronchus, and Lung, by Sex, Race, Hispanic Origin, and Age, Selected Years, 1950–2012— continued

(Deaths per 100,000 resident population.)

Sex, race, Hispanic origin, and age	1950[1,2]	1960[1,2]	1970[2]	1980[2]	1990[2]	2000[3]	2010[3]	2011[3]	2012[3]
White, not Hispanic or Latina Female[6]									
All ages, age-adjusted[4]	NA	NA	NA	NA	39.0	44.1	41.7	40.7	39.9
All ages, crude	NA	NA	NA	NA	46.2	56.4	59.0	58.5	58.6
45 to 54 years	NA	NA	NA	NA	36.6	26.4	26.9	26.8	25.8
55 to 64 years	NA	NA	NA	NA	111.3	102.2	74.0	72.4	73.3
65 to 74 years	NA	NA	NA	NA	186.4	222.9	199.5	191.3	185.5
75 to 84 years	NA	NA	NA	NA	199.1	279.2	303.0	298.7	294.2
85 years and over	NA	NA	NA	NA	139.0	218.0	263.8	261.9	259.6

NA = Not available.   * = Rates based on fewer than 20 deaths are considered unreliable and are not shown.   0.0 = Quantity more than zero but less than 0.05.   1 Includes deaths of persons who were not residents of the 50 states and the District of Columbia.   2 Underlying cause of death was coded according to the 6th Revision of the International Classification of Diseases (ICD) in 1950, 7th Revision in 1960, 8th Revision in 1970, and 9th Revision in 1980-1998.   3 Starting with 1999 data, cause of death is coded according to ICD-10.   4 Age-adjusted rates are calculated using the year 2000 standard population. Prior to 2001, age-adjusted rates were calculated using standard million proportions based on rounded population numbers. Starting with 2001 data, unrounded population numbers are used to calculate age-adjusted rates.   5 The race groups, White, Black, Asian or Pacific Islander, and American Indian or Alaska Native, include persons of Hispanic and non-Hispanic origin. Persons of Hispanic origin may be of any race. Death rates for the American Indian or Alaska Native, Asian or Pacific Islander, and Hispanic populations are known to be underestimated.   6 Prior to 1997, excludes data from states lacking an Hispanic-origin item on the death certificate.

Table 2-34. Death Rates for Human Immunodeficiency Virus (HIV) Disease, by Sex, Race, Hispanic Origin, and Age, Selected Years, 1987–2013

(Deaths per 100,000 resident population.)

Sex, race, Hispanic origin, and age[1]	1987[2]	1990[2]	2000[3]	2010[3]	2011[3]	2012[3]	2013[3]
All Persons							
All ages, age-adjusted[4]	5.6	10.2	5.2	2.6	2.4	2.2	2.1
All ages, crude	5.6	10.1	5.1	2.7	2.5	2.3	2.2
Under 1 year	2.3	2.7	*	*	*	*	*
1 to 4 years	0.7	0.8	*	*	*	*	*
5 to 14 years	0.1	0.2	0.1	*	*	*	*
15 to 24 years	1.3	1.5	0.5	0.3	0.3	0.3	0.2
25 to 34 years	11.7	19.7	6.1	1.8	1.6	1.5	1.5
35 to 44 years	14.0	27.4	13.1	4.6	4.0	3.3	3.1
45 to 54 years	8.0	15.2	11.0	6.9	6.2	5.8	5.4
55 to 64 years	3.5	6.2	5.1	5.0	4.7	4.6	4.6
65 to 74 years	1.3	2.0	2.2	2.2	2.3	2.3	2.3
75 to 84 years	0.8	0.7	0.7	0.9	1.1	1.0	1.2
85 years and over	*	*	*	0.4	0.4	0.4	*
Male							
All ages, age-adjusted[4]	10.4	18.5	7.9	3.8	3.4	3.2	3.1
All ages, crude	10.2	18.5	7.9	4.0	3.6	3.4	3.3
Under 1 year	2.2	2.4	*	*	*	*	*
1 to 4 years	0.7	0.8	*	*	*	*	*
5 to 14 years	0.2	0.3	0.1	*	*	*	*
15 to 24 years	2.2	2.2	0.5	0.4	0.4	0.3	0.4
25 to 34 years	20.7	34.5	8.0	2.3	2.0	2.1	2.1
35 to 44 years	26.3	50.2	19.8	6.3	5.2	4.2	4.2
45 to 54 years	15.5	29.1	17.8	10.6	9.3	8.7	8.2
55 to 64 years	6.8	12.0	8.7	7.9	7.4	7.4	7.2
65 to 74 years	2.4	3.7	3.8	3.8	3.9	4.1	3.8
75 to 84 years	1.2	1.1	1.3	1.7	1.9	2.0	2.2
85 years and over	*	*	*	*	*	*	*
Female							
All ages, age-adjusted[4]	1.1	2.2	2.5	1.4	1.3	1.2	1.1
All ages, crude	1.1	2.2	2.5	1.4	1.4	1.2	1.2
Under 1 year	2.5	3.0	*	*	*	*	*
1 to 4 years	0.7	0.8	*	*	*	*	*
5 to 14 years	*	0.2	0.1	*	*	*	*
15 to 24 years	0.3	0.7	0.4	0.2	0.3	0.2	0.1
25 to 34 years	2.8	4.9	4.2	1.3	1.1	0.9	0.8
35 to 44 years	2.1	5.2	6.5	2.9	2.7	2.4	2.0
45 to 54 years	0.8	1.9	4.4	3.4	3.2	3.1	2.8
55 to 64 years	0.5	1.1	1.8	2.3	2.2	2.1	2.2
65 to 74 years	0.5	0.8	0.8	0.9	0.9	0.8	1.1
75 to 84 years	0.5	0.4	0.3	0.4	0.5	0.3	0.5
85 years and over	*	*	*	*	*	*	*
All Ages, Age-Adjusted [4]							
White male	8.7	15.7	4.6	2.3	2.0	2.0	1.9
Black or African American male	26.2	46.3	35.1	16.5	14.5	13.3	12.7
American Indian or Alaska Native male	*	3.3	3.5	2.6	2.0	1.5	2.1
Asian or Pacific Islander male	2.5	4.3	1.2	0.7	0.7	0.6	0.7
Hispanic or Latino male[5]	18.8	28.8	10.6	4.6	4.2	3.5	3.4
White, not Hispanic or Latino male[5]	10.7	14.1	3.8	1.8	1.6	1.7	1.6
White female	0.6	1.1	1.0	0.5	0.5	0.4	0.4
Black or African American female	4.6	10.1	13.2	7.5	6.8	6.3	5.7
American Indian or Alaska Native female	*	*	1.0	*	*	*	*
Asian or Pacific Islander female	*	*	0.2	*	*	*	*
Hispanic or Latina female[5]	2.1	3.8	2.9	1.1	1.3	1.0	0.9
White, not Hispanic or Latina female[5]	0.5	0.7	0.7	0.4	0.4	0.3	0.3

Table 2-34. Death Rates for Human Immunodeficiency Virus (HIV) Disease, by Sex, Race, Hispanic Origin, and Age, Selected Years, 1987–2013— continued

(Deaths per 100,000 resident population.)

Sex, race, Hispanic origin, and age[1]	1987[2]	1990[2]	2000[3]	2010[3]	2011[3]	2012[3]	2013[3]
Age 25 to 44 Years							
All persons	12.7	23.2	9.8	3.2	2.8	2.4	2.3
White male	19.2	35.0	8.8	2.5	2.2	1.9	1.9
Black or African American male	60.2	102.0	55.4	17.1	13.8	11.9	11.7
American Indian or Alaska Native male	*	7.7	5.5	*	*	*	*
Asian or Pacific Islander male	4.1	8.1	1.9	*	*	0.8	0.9
Hispanic or Latino male[5]	36.8	59.3	14.3	4.1	3.7	2.7	2.8
White, not Hispanic or Latino male[5]	23.3	31.6	7.4	1.9	1.6	1.6	1.5
White female	1.2	2.3	2.1	0.7	0.7	0.5	0.5
Black or African American female	11.6	23.6	26.7	10.3	9.4	8.5	6.7
American Indian or Alaska Native female	*	*	*	*	*	*	*
Asian or Pacific Islander female	*	*	*	*	*	*	*
Hispanic or Latina female[5]	4.9	8.9	4.6	1.2	1.1	0.8	0.7
White, not Hispanic or Latina female[5]	1.0	1.5	1.6	0.6	0.6	0.4	0.4
Age 45 to 64 Years							
All persons	5.8	11.1	8.7	6.1	5.5	5.3	5.1
White male	9.9	18.6	8.1	5.6	5.0	5.1	4.8
Black or African American male	27.3	53.0	71.6	39.8	36.2	32.4	30.8
American Indian or Alaska Native male	*	*	*	7.0	*	*	6.0
Asian or Pacific Islander male	*	6.5	2.1	1.9	1.5	1.2	1.2
Hispanic or Latino male[5]	25.8	37.9	23.3	11.5	10.1	8.9	8.5
White, not Hispanic or Latino male[5]	12.6	16.9	6.5	4.7	4.2	4.4	4.1
White female	0.5	0.9	1.3	1.0	1.1	1.0	1.0
Black or African American female	2.6	7.5	19.6	16.3	14.2	13.6	12.6
American Indian or Alaska Native female	*	*	*	*	*	*	*
Asian or Pacific Islander female	*	*	*	*	*	*	*
Hispanic or Latina female[5]	*	3.1	5.8	2.5	3.3	2.5	2.1
White, not Hispanic or Latina female[5]	0.5	0.7	0.9	0.8	0.8	0.8	0.9

* = Rates based on fewer than 20 deaths are considered unreliable and are not shown.   1 The race groups, White, Black, Asian or Pacific Islander, and American Indian or Alaska Native, include persons of Hispanic and non-Hispanic origin. Persons of Hispanic origin may be of any race. Death rates for the American Indian or Alaska Native, Asian or Pacific Islander, and Hispanic populations are known to be underestimated.   2 Categories for the coding and classification of human immunodeficiency virus (HIV) disease were introduced in the United States in 1987.   3 Starting with 1999 data, cause of death is coded according to ICD-10.   4 Age-adjusted rates are calculated using the year 2000 standard population. Prior to 2001, age-adjusted rates were calculated using standard million proportions based on rounded population numbers. Starting with 2001 data, unrounded population numbers are used to calculate age-adjusted rates.   5 Prior to 1997, excludes data from states lacking an Hispanic-origin item on the death certificate.

Table 2-35. Death Rates for Motor Vehicle–Related Injuries, by Sex, Race, Hispanic Origin, and Age, Selected Years, 1950–2013

(Deaths per 100,000 resident population.)

Sex, race, Hispanic origin, and age	1950[1,2]	1960[1,2]	1970[2]	1980[2]	1990[2]	2000[3]	2010[3]	2011[3]	2012[3]	2013[3]
All Persons										
All ages, age-adjusted[4]	24.6	23.1	27.6	22.3	18.5	15.4	11.3	11.1	11.4	10.9
All ages, crude	23.1	21.3	26.9	23.5	18.8	15.4	11.4	11.3	11.6	11.2
Under 1 year	8.4	8.1	9.8	7.0	4.9	4.4	2.0	2.4	1.8	1.7
1 to 14 years	9.8	8.6	10.5	8.2	6.0	4.3	2.3	2.3	2.2	2.2
1 to 4 years	11.5	10.0	11.5	9.2	6.3	4.2	2.8	2.6	2.9	2.7
5 to 14 years	8.8	7.9	10.2	7.9	5.9	4.3	2.2	2.1	2.0	2.1
15 to 24 years	34.4	38.0	47.2	44.8	34.1	26.9	16.6	16.2	16.1	15.2
15 to 19 years	29.6	33.9	43.6	43.0	33.1	26.0	13.6	13.2	12.6	11.4
20 to 24 years	38.8	42.9	51.3	46.6	35.0	28.0	19.7	19.1	19.3	18.8
25 to 34 years	24.6	24.3	30.9	29.1	23.6	17.3	14.0	13.7	14.5	13.9
35 to 44 years	20.3	19.3	24.9	20.9	16.9	15.3	11.6	11.3	11.8	11.4
45 to 64 years	25.2	23.0	26.5	18.0	15.7	14.3	11.9	11.9	12.4	12.1
45 to 54 years	22.2	21.4	25.5	18.6	15.6	14.2	12.0	12.3	12.6	12.2
55 to 64 years	29.0	25.1	27.9	17.4	15.9	14.4	11.9	11.5	12.2	11.9
65 years and over	43.1	34.7	36.2	22.5	23.1	21.4	16.0	15.9	15.7	15.1
65 to 74 years	39.1	31.4	32.8	19.2	18.6	16.5	12.3	13.0	13.0	12.2
75 to 84 years	52.7	41.8	43.5	28.1	29.1	25.7	18.8	18.3	17.9	17.8
85 years and over	45.1	37.9	34.2	27.6	31.2	30.4	23.8	21.8	22.1	21.0
Male										
All ages, age-adjusted[4]	38.5	35.4	41.5	33.6	26.5	21.7	16.2	16.1	16.5	15.9
All ages, crude	35.4	31.8	39.7	35.3	26.7	21.3	16.3	16.3	16.6	16.1
Under 1 year	9.1	8.6	9.3	7.3	5.0	4.6	2.2	2.8	1.9	1.7
1 to 14 years	12.3	10.7	13.0	10.0	7.0	4.9	2.7	2.5	2.5	2.5
1 to 4 years	13.0	11.5	12.9	10.2	6.9	4.7	3.0	2.7	3.1	3.0
5 to 14 years	11.9	10.4	13.1	9.9	7.0	5.0	2.5	2.5	2.3	2.4
15 to 24 years	56.7	61.2	73.2	68.4	49.5	37.4	23.1	22.8	22.5	21.2
15 to 19 years	46.3	51.7	64.1	62.6	45.5	33.9	17.8	17.2	16.2	14.7
20 to 24 years	66.7	73.2	84.4	74.3	53.3	41.2	28.5	28.2	28.4	27.3
25 to 34 years	40.8	40.1	49.4	46.3	35.7	25.5	21.0	20.4	21.5	20.8
35 to 44 years	32.5	29.9	37.7	31.7	24.7	22.0	16.9	16.7	17.6	16.9
45 to 64 years	37.7	33.3	38.9	26.5	21.9	20.2	17.9	18.2	18.6	18.2
45 to 54 years	33.6	31.6	37.2	27.6	22.0	20.4	17.9	18.6	18.8	18.3
55 to 64 years	43.1	35.6	40.9	25.4	21.7	19.8	17.8	17.7	18.5	18.1
65 years and over	66.6	52.1	54.4	33.9	32.1	29.5	22.2	22.3	22.1	21.5
65 to 74 years	59.1	45.8	47.3	27.3	24.2	21.7	17.1	18.2	18.5	17.5
75 to 84 years	85.0	66.0	68.2	44.3	41.2	35.6	25.9	25.7	24.8	24.9
85 years and over	78.1	62.7	63.1	56.1	64.5	57.5	40.2	35.4	35.3	35.3
Female										
All ages, age-adjusted[4]	11.5	11.7	14.9	11.8	11.0	9.5	6.5	6.3	6.5	6.2
All ages, crude	10.9	11.0	14.7	12.3	11.3	9.7	6.8	6.5	6.7	6.4
Under 1 year	7.6	7.5	10.4	6.7	4.9	4.2	1.8	1.9	1.8	1.8
1 to 14 years	7.2	6.3	7.9	6.3	4.9	3.7	2.0	2.0	1.9	1.9
1 to 4 years	10.0	8.4	10.0	8.1	5.6	3.8	2.5	2.6	2.6	2.3
5 to 14 years	5.7	5.4	7.2	5.7	4.7	3.6	1.8	1.8	1.7	1.8
15 to 24 years	12.6	15.1	21.6	20.8	17.9	15.9	9.9	9.4	9.3	8.9
15 to 19 years	12.9	16.0	22.7	22.8	20.0	17.5	9.2	9.0	8.9	7.9
20 to 24 years	12.2	14.0	20.4	18.9	16.0	14.2	10.5	9.7	9.8	9.9
25 to 34 years	9.3	9.2	13.0	12.2	11.5	8.8	6.9	7.0	7.4	6.9
35 to 44 years	8.5	9.1	12.9	10.4	9.2	8.8	6.2	6.0	6.2	5.9
45 to 64 years	12.6	13.1	15.3	10.3	10.1	8.7	6.3	5.9	6.4	6.3
45 to 54 years	10.9	11.6	14.5	10.2	9.6	8.2	6.3	6.1	6.5	6.3
55 to 64 years	14.9	15.2	16.2	10.5	10.8	9.5	6.3	5.7	6.4	6.2
65 years and over	21.9	20.3	23.1	15.0	17.2	15.8	11.3	10.9	10.8	10.0
65 to 74 years	20.6	19.0	21.6	13.0	14.1	12.3	8.2	8.4	8.2	7.5
75 to 84 years	25.2	23.0	27.2	18.5	21.9	19.2	13.7	12.8	12.9	12.5
85 years and over	22.1	22.0	18.0	15.2	18.3	19.3	15.9	15.1	15.5	13.7
White Male [5]										
All ages, age-adjusted[4]	37.9	34.8	40.4	33.8	26.3	21.8	16.7	16.6	17.0	16.3
All ages, crude	35.1	31.5	39.1	35.9	26.7	21.6	17.0	16.9	17.3	16.7
Under 1 year	9.1	8.8	9.1	7.0	4.8	4.2	2.0	2.5	1.9	1.7
1 to 14 years	12.4	10.6	12.5	9.8	6.6	4.8	2.7	2.6	2.4	2.4
15 to 24 years	58.3	62.7	75.2	73.8	52.5	39.6	24.6	24.6	24.5	22.9
25 to 34 years	39.1	38.6	47.0	46.6	35.4	25.1	21.4	20.9	22.0	21.1
35 to 44 years	30.9	28.4	35.2	30.7	23.7	21.8	17.4	17.0	18.0	17.3

Table 2-35. Death Rates for Motor Vehicle–Related Injuries, by Sex, Race, Hispanic Origin, and Age, Selected Years, 1950–2013—continued

(Deaths per 100,000 resident population.)

Sex, race, Hispanic origin, and age	1950[1,2]	1960[1,2]	1970[2]	1980[2]	1990[2]	2000[3]	2010[3]	2011[3]	2012[3]	2013[3]
45 to 64 years	36.2	31.7	36.5	25.2	20.6	19.7	18.3	18.5	19.0	18.5
65 years and over	67.1	52.1	54.2	32.7	31.4	29.4	22.7	22.8	22.6	22.1
Black or African American Male [5]										
All ages, age-adjusted[4]	34.8	39.6	51.0	34.2	29.9	24.4	16.7	16.7	17.4	17.0
All ages, crude	37.2	33.1	44.3	31.1	28.1	22.5	15.9	15.8	16.6	16.4
Under 1 year	NA	*	10.6	7.8	*	6.7	*	*	*	*
1 to 14 years[6]	10.4	11.2	16.3	11.4	8.9	5.5	3.0	2.7	3.2	3.3
15 to 24 years	42.5	46.4	58.1	34.9	36.1	30.2	19.4	17.7	17.5	17.6
25 to 34 years	54.4	51.0	70.4	44.9	39.5	32.6	24.9	22.4	25.6	25.1
35 to 44 years	46.7	43.6	59.5	41.2	33.5	27.2	19.4	20.8	20.8	20.5
45 to 64 years	54.6	47.8	61.7	39.5	33.3	27.1	19.1	20.2	20.8	21.1
65 years and over	52.6	48.2	53.4	42.4	36.3	32.1	20.0	21.3	21.8	18.5
American Indian or Alaska Native Male [5]										
All ages, age-adjusted[4]	NA	NA	NA	78.9	48.3	35.8	21.1	22.5	22.2	20.0
All ages, crude	NA	NA	NA	74.6	47.6	33.6	19.8	21.8	22.2	19.0
1 to 14 years	NA	NA	NA	15.1	11.6	7.8	*	*	6.8	3.9
15 to 24 years	NA	NA	NA	126.1	75.2	56.8	31.9	30.9	27.3	26.8
25 to 34 years	NA	NA	NA	107.0	78.2	49.8	23.8	34.8	32.0	30.3
35 to 44 years	NA	NA	NA	82.8	57.0	36.3	24.5	21.9	30.4	19.8
45 to 64 years	NA	NA	NA	77.4	45.9	32.0	23.2	27.4	27.0	20.4
65 years and over	NA	NA	NA	97.0	43.0	48.5	26.6	23.7	*	25.8
Asian or Pacific Islander Male [5]										
All ages, age-adjusted[4]	NA	NA	NA	19.0	17.9	10.6	6.5	6.6	5.9	6.4
All ages, crude	NA	NA	NA	17.1	15.8	9.8	6.2	6.2	5.6	5.9
1 to 14 years	NA	NA	NA	8.2	6.3	2.5	*	*	*	1.5
15 to 24 years	NA	NA	NA	27.2	25.7	17.0	9.6	9.3	8.9	8.1
25 to 34 years	NA	NA	NA	18.8	17.0	10.4	7.8	6.6	5.8	5.9
35 to 44 years	NA	NA	NA	13.1	12.2	6.9	4.1	4.8	3.5	5.3
45 to 64 years	NA	NA	NA	13.7	15.1	10.1	6.0	6.5	6.3	5.9
65 years and over	NA	NA	NA	37.3	33.6	21.1	14.6	14.9	12.5	14.3
Hispanic or Latino Male [5,7]										
All ages, age-adjusted[4]	NA	NA	NA	NA	29.5	21.3	14.0	13.7	13.9	14.2
All ages, crude	NA	NA	NA	NA	29.2	20.1	12.8	12.9	13.1	13.3
1 to 14 years	NA	NA	NA	NA	7.2	4.4	2.5	2.3	2.5	2.5
15 to 24 years	NA	NA	NA	NA	48.2	34.7	20.2	20.7	20.3	20.5
25 to 34 years	NA	NA	NA	NA	41.0	24.9	18.0	17.4	19.9	18.2
35 to 44 years	NA	NA	NA	NA	28.0	21.6	13.9	13.9	13.9	14.5
45 to 64 years	NA	NA	NA	NA	28.9	21.7	14.3	15.2	14.7	15.9
65 years and over	NA	NA	NA	NA	35.3	28.9	20.7	18.0	17.5	18.8
White, Not Hispanic or Latino Male										
All ages, age-adjusted[4]	NA	NA	NA	NA	25.7	21.7	17.1	17.0	17.3	16.5
All ages, crude	NA	NA	NA	NA	26.0	21.5	17.6	17.6	18.0	17.2
1 to 14 years	NA	NA	NA	NA	6.4	4.9	2.7	2.7	2.2	2.3
15 to 24 years	NA	NA	NA	NA	52.3	40.3	25.4	25.3	25.3	23.0
25 to 34 years	NA	NA	NA	NA	34.0	24.7	21.9	21.5	22.0	21.4
35 to 44 years	NA	NA	NA	NA	23.1	21.6	18.0	17.5	18.9	17.8
45 to 64 years	NA	NA	NA	NA	19.8	19.3	18.6	18.7	19.3	18.6
65 years and over	NA	NA	NA	NA	31.1	29.3	22.7	23.0	22.9	22.3
White Female [5]										
All ages, age-adjusted[4]	11.4	11.7	14.9	12.2	11.2	9.8	6.8	6.6	6.8	6.4
All ages, crude	10.9	11.2	14.8	12.8	11.6	10.0	7.1	6.9	7.1	6.7
Under 1 year	7.8	7.5	10.2	7.1	4.7	3.5	1.9	1.4	1.6	1.7
1 to 14 years	7.2	6.2	7.5	6.2	4.8	3.7	2.1	2.0	1.9	1.8
15 to 24 years	12.6	15.6	22.7	23.0	19.5	17.1	10.8	10.1	10.0	9.5
25 to 34 years	9.0	9.0	12.7	12.2	11.6	8.9	7.1	7.3	7.6	7.1
35 to 44 years	8.1	8.9	12.3	10.6	9.2	8.9	6.5	6.4	6.6	6.1
45 to 64 years	12.7	13.1	15.1	10.4	9.9	8.7	6.4	6.1	6.5	6.4
65 years and over	22.2	20.8	23.7	15.3	17.4	16.2	11.5	11.3	11.3	10.4
Black or African American Female [5]										
All ages, age-adjusted[4]	9.3	10.4	14.1	8.5	9.6	8.4	5.9	5.7	5.9	5.7
All ages, crude	10.2	9.7	13.4	8.3	9.4	8.2	5.8	5.7	5.9	5.7

Table 2-35. Death Rates for Motor Vehicle–Related Injuries, by Sex, Race, Hispanic Origin, and Age, Selected Years, 1950–2013—continued

(Deaths per 100,000 resident population.)

Sex, race, Hispanic origin, and age	1950[1,2]	1960[1,2]	1970[2]	1980[2]	1990[2]	2000[3]	2010[3]	2011[3]	2012[3]	2013[3]
Under 1 year	NA	8.1	11.9	*	7.0	*	*	*	*	*
1 to 14 years[6]	7.2	6.9	10.2	6.3	5.3	3.9	2.0	2.3	2.4	2.3
15 to 24 years	11.6	9.9	13.4	8.0	9.9	11.7	7.8	7.6	7.7	7.7
25 to 34 years	10.8	9.8	13.3	10.6	11.1	9.4	6.8	7.1	7.4	7.2
35 to 44 years	11.1	11.0	16.1	8.3	9.4	8.2	5.8	5.4	5.7	6.4
45 to 64 years	11.8	12.7	16.7	9.2	10.7	9.0	6.3	5.9	6.5	6.2
65 years and over	14.3	13.2	15.7	9.5	13.5	10.4	8.6	7.6	7.7	5.9
American Indian or Alaska Native Female [5]										
All ages, age-adjusted[4]	NA	NA	NA	32.0	17.5	19.5	10.6	10.8	10.2	11.0
All ages, crude	NA	NA	NA	32.0	17.3	18.6	10.0	10.5	10.1	10.7
1 to 14 years	NA	NA	NA	15.0	8.1	6.5	*	*	*	4.9
15 to 24 years	NA	NA	NA	42.3	31.4	30.3	13.4	14.7	16.2	13.6
25 to 34 years	NA	NA	NA	52.5	18.8	22.3	17.7	18.0	15.1	17.0
35 to 44 years	NA	NA	NA	38.1	18.2	22.0	13.1	11.3	11.6	14.2
45 to 64 years	NA	NA	NA	32.6	17.6	17.8	8.4	8.7	10.5	8.7
65 years and over	NA	NA	NA	*	*	24.0	14.8	14.4	*	*
Asian or Pacific Islander Female [5]										
All ages, age-adjusted[4]	NA	NA	NA	9.3	10.4	6.7	3.9	3.3	3.3	3.4
All ages, crude	NA	NA	NA	8.2	9.0	5.9	3.6	3.1	3.3	3.4
1 to 14 years	NA	NA	NA	7.4	3.6	2.3	*	*	*	*
15 to 24 years	NA	NA	NA	7.4	11.4	6.0	3.3	3.7	3.0	3.0
25 to 34 years	NA	NA	NA	7.3	7.3	4.5	3.1	1.9	2.8	2.5
35 to 44 years	NA	NA	NA	8.6	7.5	4.9	2.0	2.3	1.7	*
45 to 64 years	NA	NA	NA	8.5	11.8	6.4	4.3	3.0	4.2	4.1
65 years and over	NA	NA	NA	18.6	24.3	18.5	12.2	10.2	8.7	10.8
Hispanic or Latina Female [5,7]										
All ages, age-adjusted[4]	NA	NA	NA	NA	9.6	7.9	5.3	4.8	5.3	5.2
All ages, crude	NA	NA	NA	NA	8.9	7.2	4.9	4.5	4.9	4.8
1 to 14 years	NA	NA	NA	NA	4.8	3.9	2.0	1.7	1.9	1.7
15 to 24 years	NA	NA	NA	NA	11.6	10.6	7.7	6.3	7.2	7.4
25 to 34 years	NA	NA	NA	NA	9.4	6.5	5.0	5.1	5.4	5.1
35 to 44 years	NA	NA	NA	NA	8.0	7.3	4.5	4.6	4.5	4.7
45 to 64 years	NA	NA	NA	NA	11.4	8.3	5.6	4.8	5.6	5.3
65 years and over	NA	NA	NA	NA	14.9	13.4	9.4	8.6	9.2	9.0
White, not Hispanic or Latina Female										
All ages, age-adjusted[4]	NA	NA	NA	NA	11.3	10.0	7.0	6.9	7.0	6.6
All ages, crude	NA	NA	NA	NA	11.7	10.3	7.5	7.3	7.5	7.1
1 to 14 years	NA	NA	NA	NA	4.7	3.5	2.0	2.1	1.8	1.8
15 to 24 years	NA	NA	NA	NA	20.4	18.4	11.4	11.0	10.7	10.0
25 to 34 years	NA	NA	NA	NA	11.7	9.3	7.6	7.7	8.2	7.5
35 to 44 years	NA	NA	NA	NA	9.3	9.0	6.9	6.7	7.0	6.4
45 to 64 years	NA	NA	NA	NA	9.7	8.7	6.4	6.2	6.6	6.5
65 years and over	NA	NA	NA	NA	17.5	16.3	11.6	11.5	11.4	10.5

NA = Not available.   * = Rates based on fewer than 20 deaths are considered unreliable and are not shown.   1 Includes deaths of persons who were not residents of the 50 states and the District of Columbia.   2 Underlying cause of death was coded according to the 6th Revision of the International Classification of Diseases (ICD) in 1950, 7th Revision in 1960, 8th Revision in 1970, and 9th Revision in 1980-1998.   3 Starting with 1999 data, cause of death is coded according to ICD-10.   4 Age-adjusted rates are calculated using the year 2000 standard population. Prior to 2001, age-adjusted rates were calculated using standard million proportions based on rounded population numbers. Starting with 2001 data, unrounded population numbers are used to calculate age-adjusted rates.   5 The race groups, White, Black, Asian or Pacific Islander, and American Indian or Alaska Native, include persons of Hispanic and non-Hispanic origin. Persons of Hispanic origin may be of any race. Death rates for the American Indian or Alaska Native, Asian or Pacific Islander, and Hispanic populations are known to be underestimated.   6 In 1950, rate is for the age group under 15 years.   7 Prior to 1997, excludes data from states lacking an Hispanic-origin item on the death certificate.

Table 2-36. Occupant and Alcohol-Impaired Driving Deaths, by State, 2003–2012

(Number.)

State	Alcohol-impaired driving deaths	Occupant deaths
United States	119,100	277,245
Alabama	3,190	8,264
Alaska	222	506
Arizona	2,912	6,481
Arkansas	1,769	4,933
California	10,327	23,125
Colorado	1,702	3,879
Connecticut	1,039	1,893
Delaware	427	852
District of Columbia	124	175
Florida	8,476	17,862
Georgia	3,699	11,355
Hawaii	484	671
Idaho	712	1,883
Illinois	3,866	8,138
Indiana	2,210	6,292
Iowa	968	3,162
Kansas	1,214	3,473
Kentucky	2,041	6,749
Louisiana	3,046	6,533
Maine	491	1,339
Maryland	1,716	3,829
Massachusetts	1,370	2,661
Michigan	2,912	7,348
Minnesota	1,442	3,685
Mississippi	2,560	6,687
Missouri	3,314	8,073
Montana	932	1,890
Nebraska	682	2,034
Nevada	1,025	2,213
New Hampshire	399	919
New Jersey	1,816	4,185
New Mexico	1,254	3,066
New York	3,752	7,717
North Carolina	4,102	10,804
North Dakota	502	1,003
Ohio	3,637	8,759
Oklahoma	2,205	5,871
Oregon	1,232	3,035
Pennsylvania	4,663	10,355
Rhode Island	308	507
South Carolina	3,870	7,195
South Dakota	537	1,228
Tennessee	3,423	9,004
Texas	13,138	25,017
Utah	469	2,059
Vermont	212	587
Virginia	2,613	6,796
Washington	1,921	3,819
West Virginia	2,577	5,099
Wisconsin	1,092	2,953
Wyoming	506	1,282

Note: Alcohol-Impaired Driving Fatalities 2003-2012; All persons killed in crashes involving a driver with BAC >= .08 g/dL. Occupant Fatalities 2003-2012; All occupants killed where body type = 1-79. Source: Fatality Analysis Reporting System (FARS) 2003-2011 and 2012 ARF.

Table 2-37. Death Rates for Drug Poisoning and Drug Poisoning Involving Opioid Analgesics, by Sex, Race, Hispanic Origin, and Age, Selected Years, 1999–2013

(Deaths per 100,000 resident population.)

Sex, race, Hispanic origin, and age	1999	2000	2005	2010	2011	2012	2013
Drug poisoning deaths per 100,000 resident population[1]							
All Persons							
All ages, age-adjusted[2]	6.1	6.2	10.1	12.3	13.2	13.1	13.8
All ages, crude	6.0	6.2	10.1	12.4	13.3	13.2	13.9
Under 15 years	0.1	0.1	0.2	0.2	0.2	0.2	0.2
15 to 24 years	3.2	3.7	6.9	8.2	8.6	8.0	8.3
25 to 34 years	8.1	7.9	13.6	18.4	20.2	20.1	20.9
35 to 44 years	14.0	14.3	19.6	20.8	22.5	22.1	23.0
45 to 54 years	11.1	11.6	21.1	25.1	26.7	26.9	27.5
55 to 64 years	4.2	4.2	9.0	15.0	15.9	16.6	19.2
65 to 74 years	2.4	2.0	3.2	4.7	5.4	5.8	6.4
75 to 84 years	2.8	2.4	3.1	3.4	3.4	3.4	3.6
85 years and over	3.8	4.4	4.1	4.7	4.2	4.3	4.3
Male							
All ages, age-adjusted[2]	8.2	8.3	12.8	15.0	16.1	16.1	17.0
All ages, crude	8.2	8.4	12.9	15.2	16.3	16.3	17.2
Under 15 years	0.1	0.2	0.2	0.3	0.2	0.2	0.2
15 to 24 years	4.5	5.3	10.0	11.6	12.4	11.4	11.7
25 to 34 years	11.5	11.3	18.7	25.0	27.5	27.0	28.6
35 to 44 years	19.2	19.5	24.4	24.9	26.8	27.1	28.1
45 to 54 years	15.2	15.7	25.8	28.5	30.4	30.4	31.5
55 to 64 years	4.9	4.4	10.6	17.3	18.5	19.4	22.7
65 to 74 years	2.7	2.1	3.3	4.5	5.4	6.2	6.9
75 to 84 years	2.5	2.5	3.4	3.6	3.4	3.2	3.7
85 years and over	4.4	5.9	5.2	5.1	4.3	5.3	5.9
Female							
All ages, age-adjusted[2]	3.9	4.1	7.3	9.6	10.2	10.2	10.6
All ages, crude	3.9	4.1	7.4	9.8	10.3	10.3	10.7
Under 15 years	0.1	0.1	0.2	0.2	0.2	0.2	0.2
15 to 24 years	1.8	1.9	3.5	4.6	4.6	4.4	4.8
25 to 34 years	4.6	4.6	8.5	11.9	12.8	13.1	13.0
35 to 44 years	8.7	9.2	14.8	16.8	18.2	17.1	18.0
45 to 54 years	7.2	7.7	16.5	21.8	23.1	23.4	23.6
55 to 64 years	3.5	3.9	7.5	12.9	13.5	14.0	15.9
65 to 74 years	2.1	2.0	3.1	4.8	5.3	5.5	5.9
75 to 84 years	3.0	2.3	2.9	3.3	3.4	3.5	3.4
85 years and over	3.5	3.9	3.7	4.5	4.2	3.8	3.5
All Ages, Age-Adjusted [2,3]							
White male	8.1	8.4	13.6	16.8	18.1	18.1	19.0
Black or African American male	11.5	10.8	12.8	10.1	11.0	11.3	12.9
American Indian or Alaska Native male	5.7	6.1	10.8	11.8	12.9	12.8	12.9
Asian or Pacific Islander male	1.5	1.4	2.2	2.5	3.2	3.1	3.2
Hispanic or Latino male	8.6	7.1	8.4	7.6	8.1	8.5	9.2
White, not Hispanic or Latino male	8.0	8.6	14.7	19.0	20.5	20.4	21.4
White female	4.0	4.3	8.0	10.9	11.7	11.6	12.1
Black or African American female	3.9	4.1	6.0	5.7	5.9	6.0	6.3
American Indian or Alaska Native female	4.6	3.7	8.6	9.7	10.7	12.2	11.6
Asian or Pacific Islander female	1.0	0.8	1.3	1.5	1.6	1.4	1.5
Hispanic or Latina female	2.2	2.0	3.0	3.6	4.0	4.0	4.1
White, not Hispanic or Latina female	4.3	4.5	8.8	12.5	13.3	13.2	13.8
All Persons							
All ages, age-adjusted[2]	1.4	1.5	3.7	5.4	5.4	5.1	5.1
All ages, crude	1.4	1.6	3.7	5.4	5.4	5.1	5.1
Under 15 years	*	0.0	0.1	0.1	0.1	0.1	0.1
15 to 24 years	0.7	0.8	2.7	3.9	3.6	2.8	2.6
25 to 34 years	1.9	1.9	5.3	8.5	8.5	7.7	7.5
35 to 44 years	3.5	3.7	6.9	9.1	9.3	8.8	8.6
45 to 54 years	2.9	3.2	7.9	10.9	11.2	10.6	10.6
55 to 64 years	1.0	1.1	3.1	6.2	6.3	6.6	7.5
65 to 74 years	0.4	0.4	1.0	1.5	1.8	2.0	2.3
75 to 84 years	0.3	0.2	0.6	0.7	0.7	0.9	0.8
85 years and over	*	*	0.9	1.1	0.8	0.8	0.9

Table 2-37. Death Rates for Drug Poisoning and Drug Poisoning Involving Opioid Analgesics, by Sex, Race, Hispanic Origin, and Age, Selected Years, 1999–2013 — continued

(Deaths per 100,000 resident population.)

Sex, race, Hispanic origin, and age	1999	2000	2005	2010	2011	2012	2013
Male							
All ages, age-adjusted[2]	2.0	2.0	4.6	6.5	6.5	6.0	5.9
All ages, crude	2.0	2.1	4.6	6.6	6.5	6.0	5.9
Under 15 years	*	*	0.1	0.2	0.1	0.1	0.1
15 to 24 years	1.0	1.2	4.2	5.6	5.3	4.2	3.9
25 to 34 years	2.7	2.7	7.2	11.7	11.4	10.0	10.0
35 to 44 years	5.0	4.9	8.3	10.9	10.9	10.3	9.6
45 to 54 years	3.9	4.3	9.4	12.0	12.1	11.1	11.1
55 to 64 years	1.1	1.0	3.5	7.0	6.9	7.3	8.0
65 to 74 years	0.5	0.3	0.7	1.2	1.7	2.0	2.2
75 to 84 years	*	*	0.6	0.7	0.7	0.7	0.9
85 years and over	*	*	*	1.3	*	1.0	1.3
Female							
All ages, age-adjusted[2]	0.9	1.1	2.8	4.2	4.3	4.2	4.3
All ages, crude	0.9	1.1	2.8	4.2	4.4	4.2	4.4
Under 15 years	*	*	*	0.1	0.1	0.1	0.1
15 to 24 years	0.3	0.4	1.2	2.1	1.9	1.5	1.4
25 to 34 years	1.1	1.2	3.4	5.3	5.5	5.3	5.0
35 to 44 years	2.1	2.5	5.6	7.3	7.8	7.3	7.6
45 to 54 years	1.9	2.2	6.5	9.8	10.2	10.1	10.1
55 to 64 years	0.8	1.1	2.8	5.5	5.7	6.0	6.9
65 to 74 years	0.3	0.4	1.2	1.7	1.8	2.0	2.4
75 to 84 years	0.4	*	0.6	0.7	0.7	0.9	0.7
85 years and over	*	*	0.8	1.1	0.8	0.7	0.8
All Ages, Age-Adjusted [2,3]							
White male	2.2	2.3	5.3	7.7	7.6	7.0	6.8
Black or African American male	1.2	1.2	2.1	2.2	2.4	2.3	2.7
American Indian or Alaska Native male	*	1.9	4.4	5.3	5.5	5.8	4.8
Asian or Pacific Islander male	*	*	0.5	0.8	1.0	0.7	0.9
Hispanic or Latino male	2.9	1.7	2.2	2.4	2.6	2.5	2.7
White, not Hispanic or Latino male	2.1	2.3	5.9	9.0	8.8	8.1	7.9
White female	1.0	1.2	3.2	4.8	5.1	4.9	5.0
Black or African American female	0.6	0.6	1.4	2.0	2.0	2.0	2.2
American Indian or Alaska Native female	*	*	3.8	4.9	4.6	5.4	5.4
Asian or Pacific Islander female	*	*	0.4	0.5	0.4	0.4	0.3
Hispanic or Latina female	0.5	0.5	1.0	1.3	1.4	1.5	1.5
White, not Hispanic or Latina female	1.1	1.3	3.5	5.6	5.8	5.6	5.8

0.0 = Rate more than zero but less than 0.05.   * = Rates based on fewer than 20 deaths are considered unreliable and are not shown.   1 Drug poisoning was coded using underlying cause of death according to the 10th Revision of the International Classification of Diseases (ICD-10).   2 Age-adjusted rates are calculated using the year 2000 standard population with unrounded population numbers.   3 The race groups, White, Black, Asian or Pacific Islander, and American Indian or Alaska Native, include persons of Hispanic and non-Hispanic origin. Persons of Hispanic origin may be of any race. Death rates for the American Indian or Alaska Native, Asian or Pacific Islander, and Hispanic populations are known to be underestimated.

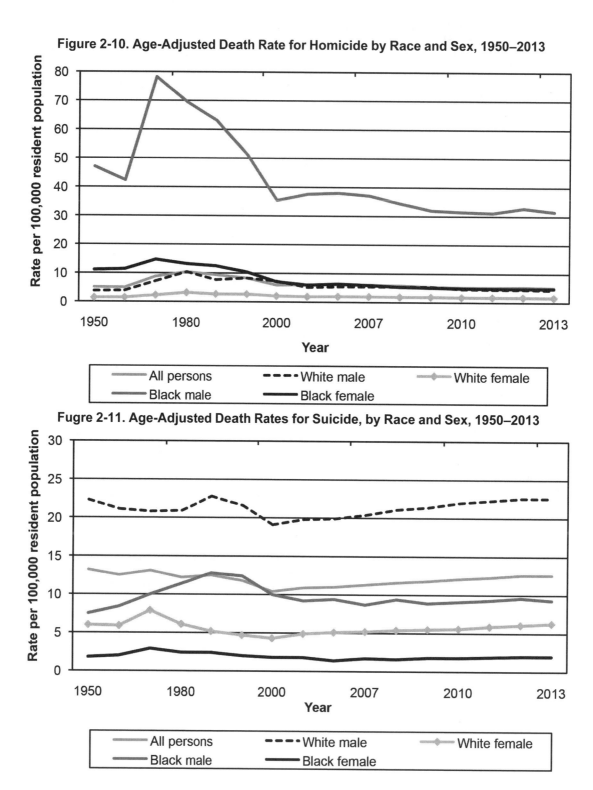

Figure 2-10. Age-Adjusted Death Rate for Homicide by Race and Sex, 1950–2013

Fugre 2-11. Age-Adjusted Death Rates for Suicide, by Race and Sex, 1950–2013

Table 2-38. Death Rates for Homicide, by Sex, Race, Hispanic Origin, and Age, Selected Years, 1950–2013

(Deaths per 100,000 resident population.)

Sex, race, Hispanic origin, and age	1950[1,2]	1960[1,2]	1970[2]	1980[2]	1990[2]	2000[3]	2010[3]	2011[3]	2012[3]	2013[3]
All Persons										
All ages, age-adjusted[4]	5.1	5.0	8.8	10.4	9.4	5.9	5.3	5.3	5.4	5.2
All ages, crude	5.0	4.6	8.1	10.6	9.9	6.0	5.3	5.2	5.3	5.1
Under 1 year	4.4	4.8	4.3	5.9	8.4	9.2	7.9	7.3	7.3	7.2
1 to 14 years	0.6	0.6	1.1	1.5	1.8	1.3	1.1	1.2	1.1	1.1
1 to 4 years	0.6	0.7	1.9	2.5	2.5	2.3	2.4	2.5	2.1	2.1
5 to 14 years	0.5	0.5	0.9	1.2	1.5	0.9	0.6	0.7	0.8	0.7
15 to 24 years	5.8	5.6	11.3	15.4	19.7	12.6	10.7	10.4	10.5	9.8
15 to 19 years	3.9	3.9	7.7	10.5	16.9	9.5	8.3	7.8	7.6	6.6
20 to 24 years	8.5	7.7	15.6	20.2	22.2	16.0	13.2	13.0	13.3	12.8
25 to 44 years	8.9	8.5	14.9	17.5	14.7	8.7	8.2	8.1	8.5	8.2
25 to 34 years	9.3	9.2	16.2	19.3	17.4	10.4	10.4	10.0	10.3	9.9
35 to 44 years	8.4	7.8	13.5	14.9	11.6	7.1	6.0	6.2	6.7	6.4
45 to 64 years	5.0	5.3	8.7	9.0	6.3	4.0	3.8	3.8	3.9	3.8
45 to 54 years	5.9	6.1	10.0	11.0	7.5	4.7	4.4	4.6	4.6	4.5
55 to 64 years	3.9	4.1	7.1	7.0	5.0	3.0	2.9	2.9	3.0	3.0
65 years and over	3.0	2.7	4.6	5.5	4.0	2.4	2.0	2.0	2.0	2.0
65 to 74 years	3.2	2.8	4.9	5.7	3.8	2.4	2.1	2.0	2.1	2.0
75 to 84 years	2.5	2.3	4.0	5.2	4.3	2.4	1.9	2.0	2.0	2.1
85 years and over	2.3	2.4	4.2	5.3	4.6	2.4	2.0	2.2	1.9	1.9
Male										
All ages, age-adjusted[4]	7.9	7.5	14.3	16.6	14.8	9.0	8.4	8.3	8.5	8.2
All ages, crude	7.7	6.8	13.1	17.1	15.9	9.3	8.4	8.3	8.5	8.2
Under 1 year	4.5	4.7	4.5	6.3	8.8	10.4	8.8	8.2	8.1	8.7
1 to 14 years	0.6	0.6	1.2	1.6	2.0	1.5	1.4	1.4	1.3	1.2
1 to 4 years	0.5	0.7	1.9	2.7	2.7	2.5	2.8	2.9	2.4	2.3
5 to 14 years	0.6	0.5	1.0	1.2	1.7	1.1	0.8	0.8	0.9	0.8
15 to 24 years	8.6	8.4	18.2	24.0	32.5	20.9	18.2	17.6	17.7	16.7
15 to 19 years	5.5	5.7	12.1	15.9	27.8	15.5	14.0	13.0	12.8	11.4
20 to 24 years	13.5	11.8	25.6	32.2	36.9	26.7	22.6	22.1	22.4	21.6
25 to 44 years	13.8	12.8	24.4	28.9	23.5	13.3	13.3	13.2	13.9	13.4
25 to 34 years	14.4	13.9	26.8	31.9	27.7	16.7	17.3	16.6	17.1	16.4
35 to 44 years	13.2	11.7	21.7	24.5	18.6	10.3	9.2	9.6	10.6	10.1
45 to 64 years	8.1	8.1	14.8	15.2	10.2	6.0	5.6	5.7	5.8	5.7
45 to 54 years	9.5	9.4	16.8	18.4	11.9	6.9	6.7	6.8	7.0	6.9
55 to 64 years	6.3	6.4	12.1	11.8	8.0	4.6	4.3	4.4	4.4	4.3
65 years and over	4.8	4.3	7.7	8.8	5.8	3.3	2.6	2.7	2.8	2.8
65 to 74 years	5.2	4.6	8.5	9.2	5.8	3.4	2.9	2.7	3.0	2.9
75 to 84 years	3.9	3.7	5.9	8.1	5.7	3.2	2.1	2.7	2.5	2.5
85 years and over	2.5	3.6	7.4	7.5	6.7	3.3	2.2	2.5	2.2	2.9
Female										
All ages, age-adjusted[4]	2.4	2.6	3.7	4.4	4.0	2.8	2.3	2.2	2.2	2.1
All ages, crude	2.4	2.4	3.4	4.5	4.2	2.8	2.2	2.2	2.2	2.1
Under 1 year	4.2	4.9	4.1	5.6	8.0	7.9	6.9	6.2	6.5	5.5
1 to 14 years	0.6	0.5	1.0	1.4	1.6	1.1	0.9	1.0	1.0	0.9
1 to 4 years	0.7	0.7	1.9	2.2	2.3	2.1	1.9	2.2	1.8	2.0
5 to 14 years	0.5	0.4	0.7	1.1	1.2	0.7	0.5	0.5	0.6	0.5
15 to 24 years	3.0	2.8	4.6	6.6	6.2	3.9	2.9	2.9	2.9	2.6
15 to 19 years	2.4	1.9	3.2	4.9	5.4	3.1	2.3	2.2	2.0	1.6
20 to 24 years	3.7	3.8	6.2	8.2	7.0	4.7	3.4	3.5	3.7	3.6
25 to 44 years	4.2	4.3	5.8	6.4	6.0	4.0	3.1	3.1	3.0	3.0
25 to 34 years	4.5	4.6	6.0	6.9	7.1	4.1	3.3	3.3	3.3	3.2
35 to 44 years	3.8	4.0	5.7	5.7	4.8	4.0	2.9	2.8	2.8	2.7
45 to 64 years	1.9	2.5	3.1	3.4	2.8	2.1	2.0	2.0	2.0	2.0
45 to 54 years	2.3	2.9	3.7	4.1	3.2	2.5	2.3	2.4	2.3	2.3
55 to 64 years	1.4	2.0	2.5	2.8	2.3	1.6	1.7	1.5	1.6	1.7
65 years and over	1.4	1.3	2.3	3.3	2.8	1.8	1.6	1.6	1.5	1.4
65 to 74 years	1.3	1.3	2.2	3.0	2.2	1.6	1.4	1.4	1.3	1.3
75 to 84 years	1.4	1.3	2.7	3.5	3.4	2.0	1.8	1.5	1.7	1.7
85 years and over	2.1	1.6	2.5	4.3	3.8	2.0	2.0	2.1	1.7	1.4
White Male[5]										
All ages, age-adjusted[4]	3.8	3.9	7.2	10.4	8.3	5.2	4.7	4.6	4.6	4.4
All ages, crude	3.6	3.6	6.6	10.7	8.8	5.2	4.7	4.6	4.6	4.4
Under 1 year	4.3	3.8	2.9	4.3	6.4	8.2	8.5	6.5	6.4	6.8

Table 2-38. Death Rates for Homicide, by Sex, Race, Hispanic Origin, and Age, Selected Years, 1950–2013 — continued

(Deaths per 100,000 resident population.)

Sex, race, Hispanic origin, and age	1950[1,2]	1960[1,2]	1970[2]	1980[2]	1990[2]	2000[3]	2010[3]	2011[3]	2012[3]	2013[3]
1 to 14 years	0.4	0.5	0.7	1.2	1.3	1.2	1.0	1.1	1.0	0.9
15 to 24 years	3.2	5.0	7.6	15.1	15.2	9.9	8.2	7.6	7.5	7.1
25 to 44 years	5.4	5.5	11.6	17.2	13.0	7.4	6.9	6.8	7.1	6.5
25 to 34 years	4.9	5.7	12.5	18.5	14.7	8.4	8.3	7.9	8.1	7.4
35 to 44 years	6.1	5.2	10.8	15.2	11.1	6.5	5.5	5.6	6.0	5.6
45 to 64 years	4.8	4.6	8.3	9.8	6.9	4.1	4.1	4.1	4.1	4.0
65 years and over	3.8	3.1	5.4	6.7	4.1	2.5	2.1	2.3	2.4	2.4
Black or African American Male [5]										
All ages, age-adjusted[4]	47.0	42.3	78.2	69.4	63.1	35.4	31.5	31.2	32.8	31.6
All ages, crude	44.7	35.0	66.0	65.7	68.5	37.2	33.4	33.0	34.5	33.1
Under 1 year	NA	10.3	14.3	18.6	21.4	23.3	12.3	17.0	17.6	17.9
1 to 14 years[6]	1.8	1.5	4.4	4.1	5.8	3.1	3.4	3.1	3.2	2.6
15 to 24 years	53.8	43.2	98.3	82.6	137.1	85.3	71.0	69.4	70.8	66.6
25 to 44 years	92.8	80.5	140.2	130.0	105.4	55.8	55.9	55.4	59.2	57.9
25 to 34 years	104.3	86.4	154.5	142.9	123.7	73.9	76.1	72.5	73.9	73.2
35 to 44 years	80.0	74.4	124.0	109.3	81.2	38.5	34.5	36.5	42.6	40.4
45 to 64 years	46.0	44.6	82.3	70.6	41.4	21.9	17.6	18.4	18.8	18.4
65 years and over	16.5	17.3	33.3	30.9	25.7	12.8	8.0	6.8	7.5	7.3
American Indian or Alaska Native Male [5]										
All ages, age-adjusted[4]	NA	NA	NA	23.3	16.7	10.7	8.8	8.9	9.0	8.2
All ages, crude	NA	NA	NA	23.1	16.6	10.7	9.5	9.0	9.4	8.3
15 to 24 years	NA	NA	NA	35.4	25.1	17.0	17.6	11.2	12.4	7.1
25 to 44 years	NA	NA	NA	39.2	25.7	17.0	14.8	13.8	15.3	15.4
45 to 64 years	NA	NA	NA	22.1	14.8	*	6.5	10.9	9.7	8.0
Asian or Pacific Islander Male [5]										
All ages, age-adjusted[4]	NA	NA	NA	9.1	7.3	4.3	2.6	2.9	2.5	2.3
All ages, crude	NA	NA	NA	8.3	7.9	4.4	2.7	2.9	2.7	2.3
15 to 24 years	NA	NA	NA	9.3	14.9	7.8	4.0	4.2	3.8	3.5
25 to 44 years	NA	NA	NA	11.3	9.6	4.6	3.3	4.1	3.7	2.7
45 to 64 years	NA	NA	NA	10.4	7.0	6.1	3.1	2.0	2.9	2.5
Hispanic or Latino Male [5,7]										
All ages, age-adjusted[4]	NA	NA	NA	NA	27.4	11.8	8.7	7.9	7.9	7.3
All ages, crude	NA	NA	NA	NA	31.0	13.4	9.5	8.6	8.5	7.8
Under 1 year	NA	NA	NA	NA	8.7	6.6	7.0	5.8	5.0	6.8
1 to 14 years	NA	NA	NA	NA	3.1	1.7	1.1	1.3	0.9	0.9
15 to 24 years	NA	NA	NA	NA	55.4	28.5	19.7	17.6	17.1	15.3
25 to 44 years	NA	NA	NA	NA	46.4	17.2	13.2	12.0	12.3	11.0
25 to 34 years	NA	NA	NA	NA	50.9	19.9	16.8	14.6	14.7	13.3
35 to 44 years	NA	NA	NA	NA	39.3	13.5	8.9	9.0	9.5	8.4
45 to 64 years	NA	NA	NA	NA	20.5	9.1	6.9	5.9	5.9	6.1
65 years and over	NA	NA	NA	NA	9.4	4.4	3.2	3.5	3.3	2.9
White, not Hispanic or Latino Male [7]										
All ages, age-adjusted[4]	NA	NA	NA	NA	5.6	3.6	3.3	3.4	3.5	3.4
All ages, crude	NA	NA	NA	NA	5.8	3.6	3.3	3.4	3.5	3.3
Under 1 year	NA	NA	NA	NA	5.4	8.3	8.7	6.9	6.8	6.5
1 to 14 years	NA	NA	NA	NA	0.9	1.0	0.9	1.0	1.0	0.9
15 to 24 years	NA	NA	NA	NA	7.5	4.7	4.1	3.9	3.9	3.9
25 to 44 years	NA	NA	NA	NA	8.7	5.2	4.7	4.9	5.1	4.9
25 to 34 years	NA	NA	NA	NA	9.3	5.2	5.0	5.4	5.5	5.2
35 to 44 years	NA	NA	NA	NA	8.0	5.2	4.4	4.5	4.8	4.6
45 to 64 years	NA	NA	NA	NA	5.7	3.6	3.6	3.7	3.7	3.6
65 years and over	NA	NA	NA	NA	3.7	2.3	2.0	2.2	2.3	2.3
White Female [4]										
All ages, age-adjusted[4]	1.4	1.5	2.3	3.2	2.7	2.1	1.8	1.8	1.8	1.7
All ages, crude	1.4	1.4	2.1	3.2	2.8	2.1	1.8	1.8	1.8	1.7
Under 1 year	3.9	3.5	2.9	4.3	5.1	5.0	5.8	4.9	5.9	4.3
1 to 14 years	0.4	0.4	0.7	1.1	1.0	0.8	0.7	0.8	0.8	0.7
15 to 24 years	1.3	1.5	2.7	4.7	4.0	2.7	2.0	1.9	1.9	1.8
25 to 44 years	2.0	2.1	3.3	4.2	3.8	2.9	2.4	2.5	2.4	2.3
45 to 64 years	1.5	1.7	2.1	2.6	2.3	1.8	1.7	1.7	1.7	1.7
65 years and over	1.2	1.2	1.9	2.9	2.2	1.6	1.6	1.4	1.4	1.4

Table 2-38. Death Rates for Homicide, by Sex, Race, Hispanic Origin, and Age, Selected Years, 1950–2013 — continued

(Deaths per 100,000 resident population.)

Sex, race, Hispanic origin, and age	1950[1,2]	1960[1,2]	1970[2]	1980[2]	1990[2]	2000[3]	2010[3]	2011[3]	2012[3]	2013[3]
Black or African American Female [4]										
All ages, age-adjusted[4]	11.1	11.4	14.7	13.2	12.5	7.1	5.0	4.9	4.9	4.9
All ages, crude	11.5	10.4	13.2	13.5	13.4	7.2	5.1	5.0	4.9	4.9
Under 1 year	NA	13.8	10.7	12.8	22.8	22.2	13.9	11.9	11.5	12.4
1 to 14 years[6]	1.8	1.2	3.1	3.3	4.7	2.7	2.0	2.2	2.0	2.1
15 to 24 years	16.5	11.9	17.7	18.4	18.9	10.7	7.5	8.1	8.0	6.9
25 to 44 years	22.5	22.7	25.3	22.6	21.0	11.0	7.4	7.0	7.1	7.2
45 to 64 years	6.8	10.3	13.4	10.8	6.5	4.5	4.2	3.9	3.9	4.3
65 years and over	3.6	3.0	7.4	8.0	9.4	3.5	1.8	2.3	2.2	2.0
American Indian or Alaska Native Female [4]										
All ages, age-adjusted[4]	NA	NA	NA	8.1	4.6	3.0	2.5	2.8	2.4	2.4
All ages, crude	NA	NA	NA	7.7	4.8	2.9	2.5	2.7	2.6	2.4
15 to 24 years	NA	NA	NA	*	*	*	*	*	*	*
25 to 44 years	NA	NA	NA	13.7	6.9	5.9	4.7	*	3.6	3.7
45 to 64 years	NA	NA	NA	*	*	*	*	*	*	*
Asian or Pacific Islander Female [5]										
All ages, age-adjusted[4]	NA	NA	NA	3.1	2.8	1.7	1.2	1.3	1.2	0.9
All ages, crude	NA	NA	NA	3.1	2.8	1.7	1.2	1.3	1.2	0.9
15 to 24 years	NA	NA	NA	*	*	*	*	*	*	*
25 to 44 years	NA	NA	NA	4.6	3.8	2.2	1.3	1.5	1.2	1.3
45 to 64 years	NA	NA	NA	*	*	2.0	1.4	1.3	1.6	1.1
Hispanic or Latina Female [5,7]										
All ages, age-adjusted[4]	NA	NA	NA	NA	4.3	2.8	1.8	1.8	1.8	1.6
All ages, crude	NA	NA	NA	NA	4.7	2.8	1.8	1.9	1.8	1.6
Under 1 year	NA	NA	NA	NA	*	7.4	6.6	3.9	4.6	4.0
1 to 14 years	NA	NA	NA	NA	1.9	1.0	0.5	0.9	0.8	0.7
15 to 24 years	NA	NA	NA	NA	8.1	3.7	2.6	2.3	2.2	2.5
25 to 44 years	NA	NA	NA	NA	6.1	3.7	2.5	2.8	2.4	2.4
45 to 64 years	NA	NA	NA	NA	3.3	2.9	1.6	1.5	1.8	1.2
65 years and over	NA	NA	NA	NA	*	2.4	1.3	*	*	*
White, not Hispanic or Latina Female [7]										
All ages, age-adjusted[4]	NA	NA	NA	NA	2.5	1.9	1.8	1.7	1.7	1.7
All ages, crude	NA	NA	NA	NA	2.5	1.9	1.7	1.7	1.7	1.7
Under 1 year	NA	NA	NA	NA	4.4	4.1	5.3	5.0	6.1	4.4
1 to 14 years	NA	NA	NA	NA	0.8	0.8	0.7	0.7	0.8	0.7
15 to 24 years	NA	NA	NA	NA	3.3	2.3	1.8	1.7	1.7	1.6
25 to 44 years	NA	NA	NA	NA	3.5	2.7	2.4	2.3	2.4	2.2
45 to 64 years	NA	NA	NA	NA	2.2	1.6	1.7	1.7	1.7	1.8
65 years and over	NA	NA	NA	NA	2.2	1.6	1.6	1.5	1.4	1.5

NA = Not available.   * = Rates based on fewer than 20 deaths are considered unreliable and are not shown.   1 Includes deaths of persons who were not residents of the 50 states and the District of Columbia.   2 Underlying cause of death was coded according to the 6th Revision of the International Classification of Diseases (ICD) in 1950, 7th Revision in 1960, 8th Revision in 1970, and 9th Revision in 1980-1998.   3 Starting with 1999 data, cause of death is coded according to ICD-10.   4 Age-adjusted rates are calculated using the year 2000 standard population. Prior to 2001, age-adjusted rates were calculated using standard million proportions based on rounded population numbers. Starting with 2001 data, unrounded population numbers are used to calculate age-adjusted rates.   5 The race groups, White, Black, Asian or Pacific Islander, and American Indian or Alaska Native, include persons of Hispanic and non-Hispanic origin. Persons of Hispanic origin may be of any race. Death rates for the American Indian or Alaska Native, Asian or Pacific Islander, and Hispanic populations are known to be underestimated.   6 In 1950, rate is for the age group under 15 years.   7 Prior to 1997, excludes data from states lacking an Hispanic-origin item on the death certificate.

Table 2-39. Death Rates for Suicide, by Sex, Race, Hispanic Origin, and Age, Selected Years, 1950–2013

(Deaths per 100,000 resident population.)

Sex, race, Hispanic origin, and age	1950[1,2]	1960[1,2]	1970[2]	1980[2]	1990[2]	2000[3]	2010[3]	2011[3]	2012[3]	2013[3]
All Persons										
All ages, age-adjusted[4]	13.2	12.5	13.1	12.2	12.5	10.4	12.1	12.3	12.6	12.6
All ages, crude	11.4	10.6	11.6	11.9	12.4	10.4	12.4	12.7	12.9	13.0
Under 1 year	X	X	X	X	X	X	X	X	X	X
1 to 4 years	X	X	X	X	X	X	X	X	X	X
5 to 14 years	0.2	0.3	0.3	0.4	0.8	0.7	0.7	0.7	0.8	1.0
15 to 24 years	4.5	5.2	8.8	12.3	13.2	10.2	10.5	11.0	11.1	11.1
15 to 19 years	2.7	3.6	5.9	8.5	11.1	8.0	7.5	8.3	8.3	8.3
20 to 24 years	6.2	7.1	12.2	16.1	15.1	12.5	13.6	13.6	13.7	13.7
25 to 44 years	11.6	12.2	15.4	15.6	15.2	13.4	15.0	15.4	15.7	15.5
25 to 34 years	9.1	10.0	14.1	16.0	15.2	12.0	14.0	14.6	14.7	14.8
35 to 44 years	14.3	14.2	16.9	15.4	15.3	14.5	16.0	16.2	16.7	16.2
45 to 64 years	23.5	22.0	20.6	15.9	15.3	13.5	18.6	18.6	19.1	19.0
45 to 54 years	20.9	20.7	20.0	15.9	14.8	14.4	19.6	19.8	20.0	19.7
55 to 64 years	26.8	23.7	21.4	15.9	16.0	12.1	17.5	17.1	18.0	18.1
65 years and over	30.0	24.5	20.8	17.6	20.5	15.2	14.9	15.3	15.4	16.1
65 to 74 years	29.6	23.0	20.8	16.9	17.9	12.5	13.7	14.1	14.0	15.0
75 to 84 years	31.1	27.9	21.2	19.1	24.9	17.6	15.7	16.5	16.8	17.1
85 years and over	28.8	26.0	19.0	19.2	22.2	19.6	17.6	16.9	17.8	18.6
Male										
All ages, age-adjusted[4]	21.2	20.0	19.8	19.9	21.5	17.7	19.8	20.0	20.4	20.3
All ages, crude	17.8	16.5	16.8	18.6	20.4	17.1	19.9	20.2	20.6	20.6
Under 1 year	X	X	X	X	X	X	X	X	X	X
1 to 4 years	X	X	X	X	X	X	X	X	X	X
5 to 14 years	0.3	0.4	0.5	0.6	1.1	1.2	0.9	1.0	1.1	1.2
15 to 24 years	6.5	8.2	13.5	20.2	22.0	17.1	16.9	17.6	17.4	17.3
15 to 19 years	3.5	5.6	8.8	13.8	18.1	13.0	11.7	12.9	12.5	12.4
20 to 24 years	9.3	11.5	19.3	26.8	25.7	21.4	22.2	22.3	22.0	21.9
25 to 44 years	17.2	17.9	20.9	24.0	24.4	21.3	23.6	24.0	24.5	24.1
25 to 34 years	13.4	14.7	19.8	25.0	24.8	19.6	22.5	23.1	23.4	23.4
35 to 44 years	21.3	21.0	22.1	22.5	23.9	22.8	24.6	24.9	25.7	24.8
45 to 64 years	37.1	34.4	30.0	23.7	24.3	21.3	29.2	28.9	29.5	29.0
45 to 54 years	32.0	31.6	27.9	22.9	23.2	22.4	30.4	30.1	30.2	29.6
55 to 64 years	43.6	38.1	32.7	24.5	25.7	19.4	27.7	27.3	28.7	28.3
65 years and over	52.8	44.0	38.4	35.0	41.6	31.1	29.0	29.4	29.5	30.9
65 to 74 years	50.5	39.6	36.0	30.4	32.2	22.7	23.9	24.4	24.1	26.0
75 to 84 years	58.3	52.5	42.8	42.3	56.1	38.6	32.3	33.8	34.2	34.7
85 years and over	58.3	57.4	42.4	50.6	65.9	57.5	47.3	44.1	46.9	48.5
Female										
All ages, age-adjusted[4]	5.6	5.6	7.4	5.7	4.8	4.0	5.0	5.2	5.4	5.5
All ages, crude	5.1	4.9	6.6	5.5	4.8	4.0	5.2	5.4	5.5	5.7
Under 1 year	X	X	X	X	X	X	X	X	X	X
1 to 4 years	X	X	X	X	X	X	X	X	X	X
5 to 14 years	0.1	0.1	0.2	0.2	0.4	0.3	0.4	0.4	0.4	0.7
15 to 24 years	2.6	2.2	4.2	4.3	3.9	3.0	3.9	4.0	4.5	4.5
15 to 19 years	1.8	1.6	2.9	3.0	3.7	2.7	3.1	3.5	3.9	3.9
20 to 24 years	3.3	2.9	5.7	5.5	4.1	3.2	4.7	4.5	4.9	5.2
25 to 44 years	6.2	6.6	10.2	7.7	6.2	5.4	6.4	6.8	6.8	6.8
25 to 34 years	4.9	5.5	8.6	7.1	5.6	4.3	5.3	6.0	5.9	6.1
35 to 44 years	7.5	7.7	11.9	8.5	6.8	6.4	7.5	7.6	7.7	7.6
45 to 64 years	9.9	10.2	12.0	8.9	7.1	6.2	8.6	8.8	9.1	9.4
45 to 54 years	9.9	10.2	12.6	9.4	6.9	6.7	9.0	9.8	10.2	10.0
55 to 64 years	9.9	10.2	11.4	8.4	7.3	5.4	8.0	7.6	8.0	8.7
65 years and over	9.4	8.4	8.1	6.1	6.4	4.0	4.2	4.5	4.5	4.6
65 to 74 years	10.1	8.4	9.0	6.5	6.7	4.0	4.8	5.2	5.2	5.4
75 to 84 years	8.1	8.9	7.0	5.5	6.3	4.0	3.7	3.8	3.9	3.9
85 years and over	8.2	6.0	5.9	5.5	5.4	4.2	3.3	3.5	3.2	3.3
White Male [5]										
All ages, age-adjusted[4]	22.3	21.1	20.8	20.9	22.8	19.1	22.0	22.3	22.6	22.6
All ages, crude	19.0	17.6	18.0	19.9	22.0	18.8	22.6	23.0	23.3	23.4
15 to 24 years	6.6	8.6	13.9	21.4	23.2	17.9	18.3	19.3	19.0	18.7
25 to 44 years	17.9	18.5	21.5	24.6	25.4	22.9	26.2	26.8	27.2	26.8
45 to 64 years	39.3	36.5	31.9	25.0	26.0	23.2	33.0	32.8	33.5	33.0
65 years and over	55.8	46.7	41.1	37.2	44.2	33.3	31.7	32.1	32.2	34.1

Table 2-39. Death Rates for Suicide, by Sex, Race, Hispanic Origin, and Age, Selected Years, 1950–2013 — continued

(Deaths per 100,000 resident population.)

Sex, race, Hispanic origin, and age	1950[1,2]	1960[1,2]	1970[2]	1980[2]	1990[2]	2000[3]	2010[3]	2011[3]	2012[3]	2013[3]
65 to 74 years	53.2	42.0	38.7	32.5	34.2	24.3	26.3	26.7	26.4	28.9
75 to 84 years	61.9	55.7	45.5	45.5	60.2	41.1	34.9	36.8	37.0	38.1
85 years and over	61.9	61.3	45.8	52.8	70.3	61.6	50.8	47.0	50.7	52.6
Black or African American Male [5]										
All ages, age-adjusted[4]	7.5	8.4	10.0	11.4	12.8	10.0	9.1	9.3	9.6	9.3
All ages, crude	6.3	6.4	8.0	10.3	12.0	9.4	8.7	9.0	9.2	9.0
15 to 24 years	4.9	4.1	10.5	12.3	15.1	14.2	11.1	11.5	11.4	11.5
25 to 44 years	9.8	12.6	16.1	19.2	19.6	14.3	14.5	14.4	15.3	14.4
45 to 64 years	12.7	13.0	12.4	11.8	13.1	9.9	9.5	9.5	9.6	10.0
65 years and over	9.0	9.9	8.7	11.4	14.9	11.5	8.3	9.4	9.6	8.4
65 to 74 years	10.0	11.3	8.7	11.1	14.7	11.1	7.6	9.1	8.4	7.8
75 to 84 years[6]	*	*	*	10.5	14.4	12.1	9.9	8.4	12.5	9.1
85 years and over	NA	*	*	*	*	*	*	*	*	*
American Indian or Alaska Native Male [5]										
All ages, age-adjusted[4]	NA	NA	NA	19.3	20.1	16.0	15.5	16.4	17.4	18.1
All ages, crude	NA	NA	NA	20.9	20.9	15.9	16.1	16.1	17.5	17.9
15 to 24 years	NA	NA	NA	45.3	49.1	26.2	30.6	27.6	29.3	29.1
25 to 44 years	NA	NA	NA	31.2	27.8	24.5	20.9	24.2	24.3	26.6
45 to 64 years	NA	NA	NA	*	*	15.4	17.8	14.9	19.1	18.3
65 years and over	NA	NA	NA	*	*	*	*	*	*	*
Asian or Pacific Islander Male [5]										
All ages, age-adjusted[4]	NA	NA	NA	10.7	9.6	8.6	9.5	8.7	9.4	9.1
All ages, crude	NA	NA	NA	8.8	8.7	7.9	9.3	8.6	9.3	9.2
15 to 24 years	NA	NA	NA	10.8	13.5	9.1	10.9	9.6	9.7	11.9
25 to 44 years	NA	NA	NA	11.0	10.6	9.9	10.6	10.6	11.8	11.9
45 to 64 years	NA	NA	NA	13.0	9.7	9.7	12.8	11.1	12.3	10.9
65 years and over	NA	NA	NA	18.6	16.8	15.4	14.9	13.3	12.9	10.9
Hispanic or Latino Male [5,7]										
All ages, age-adjusted[4]	NA	NA	NA	NA	13.7	10.3	9.9	9.4	9.5	9.3
All ages, crude	NA	NA	NA	NA	11.4	8.4	8.5	8.4	8.5	8.3
15 to 24 years	NA	NA	NA	NA	14.7	10.9	10.7	10.7	11.5	10.1
25 to 44 years	NA	NA	NA	NA	16.2	11.2	11.2	11.7	11.4	11.5
45 to 64 years	NA	NA	NA	NA	16.1	12.0	12.9	11.6	12.0	11.4
65 years and over	NA	NA	NA	NA	23.4	19.5	15.7	13.7	13.5	14.2
White, not Hispanic or Latino Male [7]										
All ages, age-adjusted[4]	NA	NA	NA	NA	23.5	20.2	24.2	24.8	25.2	25.3
All ages, crude	NA	NA	NA	NA	23.1	20.4	25.7	26.2	26.7	26.9
15 to 24 years	NA	NA	NA	NA	24.4	19.5	20.4	21.9	21.2	21.4
25 to 44 years	NA	NA	NA	NA	26.4	25.1	30.3	31.0	31.7	31.2
45 to 64 years	NA	NA	NA	NA	26.8	24.0	35.4	35.5	36.3	36.1
65 years and over	NA	NA	NA	NA	45.4	33.9	32.7	33.4	33.6	35.6
White Female [5]										
All ages, age-adjusted[4]	6.0	5.9	7.9	6.1	5.2	4.3	5.6	5.9	6.1	6.3
All ages, crude	5.5	5.3	7.1	5.9	5.3	4.4	5.9	6.1	6.3	6.5
15 to 24 years	2.7	2.3	4.2	4.6	4.2	3.1	4.2	4.4	4.6	5.0
25 to 44 years	6.6	7.0	11.0	8.1	6.6	6.0	7.3	7.7	7.8	7.9
45 to 64 years	10.6	10.9	13.0	9.6	7.7	6.9	9.9	10.2	10.6	10.9
65 years and over	9.9	8.8	8.5	6.4	6.8	4.3	4.5	4.8	4.9	5.1
Black or African American Female [5]										
All ages, age-adjusted[4]	1.8	2.0	2.9	2.4	2.4	1.8	1.8	1.9	2.0	2.0
All ages, crude	1.5	1.6	2.6	2.2	2.3	1.7	1.8	1.9	2.0	2.0
15 to 24 years	1.8	*	3.8	2.3	2.3	2.2	2.0	2.3	2.8	2.6
25 to 44 years	2.3	3.0	4.8	4.3	3.8	2.6	2.8	3.1	3.1	2.9
45 to 64 years	2.7	3.1	2.9	2.5	2.9	2.1	2.1	2.0	2.4	2.7
65 years and over	*	*	2.6	*	1.9	1.3	*	1.2	*	*
American Indian or Alaska Native Female [5]										
All ages, age-adjusted[4]	NA	NA	NA	4.7	3.6	3.8	6.1	5.0	4.3	5.3
All ages, crude	NA	NA	NA	4.7	3.7	4.0	5.9	5.0	4.5	5.4
15 to 24 years	NA	NA	NA	*	*	*	10.4	7.1	9.7	9.4
25 to 44 years	NA	NA	NA	10.7	*	7.2	7.4	7.8	6.6	7.5
45 to 64 years	NA	NA	NA	*	*	*	6.2	5.8	*	6.6

Table 2-39. Death Rates for Suicide, by Sex, Race, Hispanic Origin, and Age, Selected Years, 1950–2013 — continued

(Deaths per 100,000 resident population.)

Sex, race, Hispanic origin, and age	1950[1,2]	1960[1,2]	1970[2]	1980[2]	1990[2]	2000[3]	2010[3]	2011[3]	2012[3]	2013[3]
65 years and over	NA	NA	NA	*	*	*	*	*	*	*
Asian or Pacific Islander Female[5]										
All ages, age-adjusted[4]	NA	NA	NA	5.5	4.1	2.8	3.4	3.4	3.6	3.0
All ages, crude	NA	NA	NA	4.7	3.4	2.7	3.4	3.5	3.7	3.1
15 to 24 years	NA	NA	NA	*	3.9	2.7	3.5	3.1	5.5	3.6
25 to 44 years	NA	NA	NA	5.4	3.8	3.3	4.1	4.3	3.9	3.7
45 to 64 years	NA	NA	NA	7.9	5.0	3.2	4.7	4.6	4.3	3.9
65 years and over	NA	NA	NA	*	8.5	5.2	4.3	5.1	5.3	3.3
Hispanic or Latina Female[5,7]										
All ages, age-adjusted[4]	NA	NA	NA	NA	2.3	1.7	2.1	2.0	2.2	2.3
All ages, crude	NA	NA	NA	NA	2.2	1.5	2.0	1.9	2.1	2.2
15 to 24 years	NA	NA	NA	NA	3.1	2.0	3.1	2.9	2.9	3.3
25 to 44 years	NA	NA	NA	NA	3.1	2.1	2.4	2.6	2.7	2.8
45 to 64 years	NA	NA	NA	NA	2.5	2.5	2.8	2.7	3.2	3.2
65 years and over	NA	NA	NA	NA	*	*	2.2	1.6	2.1	1.2
White, not Hispanic or Latina Female[6]										
All ages, age-adjusted[4]	NA	NA	NA	NA	5.4	4.7	6.2	6.7	6.9	7.1
All ages, crude	NA	NA	NA	NA	5.6	4.9	6.7	7.0	7.2	7.5
15 to 24 years	NA	NA	NA	NA	4.3	3.3	4.4	4.8	5.1	5.4
25 to 44 years	NA	NA	NA	NA	7.0	6.7	8.6	9.1	9.2	9.3
45 to 64 years	NA	NA	NA	NA	8.0	7.3	10.7	11.1	11.6	12.0
65 years and over	NA	NA	NA	NA	7.0	4.4	4.7	5.1	5.1	5.4

NA = Not available.   X = Not applicable.   * = Rates based on fewer than 20 deaths are considered unreliable and are not shown.   1 Includes deaths of persons who were not residents of the 50 states and the District of Columbia.   2 Underlying cause of death was coded according to the 6th Revision of the International Classification of Diseases (ICD) in 1950, 7th Revision in 1960, 8th Revision in 1970, and 9th Revision in 1980-1998.   3 Starting with 1999 data, cause of death is coded according to ICD-10.   4 Age-adjusted rates are calculated using the year 2000 standard population. Prior to 2001, age-adjusted rates were calculated using standard million proportions based on rounded population numbers. Starting with 2001 data, unrounded population numbers are used to calculate age-adjusted rates.   5 he race groups, White, Black, Asian or Pacific Islander, and American Indian or Alaska Native, include persons of Hispanic and non-Hispanic origin. Persons of Hispanic origin may be of any race. Death rates for the American Indian or Alaska Native, Asian or Pacific Islander, and Hispanic populations are known to be underestimated.   6 In 1950, rate is for the age group 75 years and over.   7 Prior to 1997, excludes data from states lacking an Hispanic-origin item on the death certificate.

Table 2-40. Death Rates for Firearm-Related Injuries, by Sex, Race, Hispanic Origin, and Age, Selected Years, 1970–2013

(Deaths per 100,000 resident population.)

Sex, race, Hispanic origin, and age	1970[1]	1980[1]	1990[1]	2000[2]	2010[2]	2011[2]	2012[2]	2013[2]
All Persons								
All ages, age-adjusted[3]	14.3	14.8	14.6	10.2	10.1	10.2	10.5	10.4
All ages, crude	13.1	14.9	14.9	10.2	10.3	10.4	10.7	10.6
Under 1 year	*	*	*	*	*	*	*	*
1 to 14 years	1.6	1.4	1.5	0.7	0.6	0.7	0.7	0.7
1 to 4 years	1.0	0.7	0.6	0.3	0.4	0.5	0.4	0.4
5 to 14 years	1.7	1.6	1.9	0.9	0.7	0.8	0.8	0.8
15 to 24 years	15.5	20.6	25.8	16.8	14.2	14.4	14.7	14.1
15 to 19 years	11.4	14.7	23.3	12.9	10.6	10.7	10.7	9.7
20 to 24 years	20.3	26.4	28.1	20.9	17.9	18.0	18.5	18.1
25 to 44 years	20.9	22.5	19.3	13.1	13.3	13.4	13.8	13.9
25 to 34 years	22.2	24.3	21.8	14.5	15.0	15.0	15.3	15.3
35 to 44 years	19.6	20.0	16.3	11.9	11.7	11.7	12.4	12.3
45 to 64 years	17.6	15.2	13.6	10.0	11.6	11.7	12.0	11.9
45 to 54 years	18.1	16.4	13.9	10.5	12.0	12.2	12.4	12.3
55 to 64 years	17.0	13.9	13.3	9.4	11.1	11.0	11.6	11.5
65 years and over	13.8	13.5	16.0	12.2	11.7	12.1	12.2	12.5
65 to 74 years	14.5	13.8	14.4	10.6	10.7	10.9	10.8	11.3
75 to 84 years	13.4	13.4	19.4	13.9	12.7	13.7	14.1	14.1
85 years and over	10.2	11.6	14.7	14.2	13.2	13.1	13.6	13.9
Male								
All ages, age-adjusted[3]	24.8	25.9	26.1	18.1	17.9	18.0	18.5	18.3
All ages, crude	22.2	25.7	26.2	17.8	18.0	18.1	18.7	18.5
Under 1 year	*	*	*	*	*	*	*	*
1 to 14 years	2.3	2.0	2.2	1.1	1.0	1.0	1.0	1.0
1 to 4 years	1.2	0.9	0.7	0.4	0.6	0.6	0.5	0.6
5 to 14 years	2.7	2.5	2.9	1.4	1.1	1.1	1.1	1.2
15 to 24 years	26.4	34.8	44.7	29.4	25.0	25.0	25.6	24.4
15 to 19 years	19.2	24.5	40.1	22.4	18.4	18.4	18.5	17.0
20 to 24 years	35.1	45.2	49.1	37.0	31.8	31.5	32.4	31.2
25 to 44 years	34.1	38.1	32.6	22.0	22.9	22.7	23.6	23.7
25 to 34 years	36.5	41.4	37.0	24.9	26.4	25.9	26.4	26.3
35 to 44 years	31.6	33.2	27.4	19.4	19.3	19.4	20.7	20.8
45 to 64 years	31.0	25.9	23.4	17.1	19.9	19.8	20.5	20.1
45 to 54 years	30.7	27.3	23.2	17.6	20.3	20.1	20.4	20.4
55 to 64 years	31.3	24.5	23.7	16.3	19.3	19.5	20.5	19.8
65 years and over	29.7	29.7	35.3	26.4	24.1	24.8	25.0	25.3
65 to 74 years	29.5	27.8	28.2	20.3	20.0	20.3	20.2	20.9
75 to 84 years	31.0	33.0	46.9	32.2	27.5	29.5	30.1	29.8
85 years and over	26.2	34.9	49.3	44.7	37.4	36.1	37.5	38.3
Female								
All ages, age-adjusted[3]	4.8	4.7	4.2	2.8	2.7	2.9	3.0	3.0
All ages, crude	4.4	4.7	4.3	2.8	2.7	2.9	3.0	3.0
Under 1 year	*	*	*	*	*	*	*	*
1 to 14 years	0.8	0.7	0.8	0.3	0.3	0.4	0.4	0.4
1 to 4 years	0.9	0.5	0.5	*	0.3	0.3	0.3	0.3
5 to 14 years	0.8	0.7	1.0	0.4	0.3	0.4	0.5	0.4
15 to 24 years	4.8	6.1	6.0	3.5	2.9	3.2	3.2	3.2
15 to 19 years	3.5	4.6	5.7	2.9	2.3	2.5	2.4	2.0
20 to 24 years	6.4	7.7	6.3	4.2	3.5	3.8	3.9	4.3
25 to 44 years	8.3	7.4	6.1	4.2	3.8	4.0	4.0	4.0
25 to 34 years	8.4	7.5	6.7	4.0	3.5	3.9	4.0	4.1
35 to 44 years	8.2	7.2	5.4	4.4	4.1	4.0	4.1	4.0
45 to 64 years	5.4	5.4	4.5	3.4	3.7	3.9	4.0	4.1
45 to 54 years	6.4	6.2	4.9	3.6	3.8	4.5	4.6	4.5
55 to 64 years	4.2	4.6	4.0	3.0	3.4	3.1	3.3	3.8
65 years and over	2.4	2.5	3.1	2.2	2.2	2.3	2.3	2.4
65 to 74 years	2.8	3.1	3.6	2.5	2.6	2.7	2.6	2.8
75 to 84 years	1.7	1.7	2.9	2.0	2.1	2.1	2.3	2.3
85 years and over	*	1.3	1.3	1.7	1.5	1.7	1.6	1.5
White Male [4]								
All ages, age-adjusted[3]	19.7	22.1	22.0	15.9	16.1	16.2	16.5	16.5
All ages, crude	17.6	21.8	21.8	15.6	16.5	16.6	17.0	17.1
1 to 14 years	1.8	1.9	1.9	1.0	0.8	0.9	0.9	1.0
15 to 24 years	16.9	28.4	29.5	19.6	16.2	16.5	16.7	16.0
25 to 44 years	24.2	29.5	25.7	18.0	18.6	18.4	18.8	18.9

Table 2-40. Death Rates for Firearm-Related Injuries, by Sex, Race, Hispanic Origin, and Age, Selected Years, 1970–2013 — continued

(Deaths per 100,000 resident population.)

Sex, race, Hispanic origin, and age	1970[1]	1980[1]	1990[1]	2000[2]	2010[2]	2011[2]	2012[2]	2013[2]
25 to 34 years	24.3	31.1	27.8	18.1	19.1	19.1	19.2	19.1
35 to 44 years	24.1	27.1	23.3	17.9	18.0	17.7	18.4	18.8
45 to 64 years	27.4	23.3	22.8	17.4	21.3	21.3	22.0	21.6
65 years and over	29.9	30.1	36.8	28.2	26.5	27.1	27.4	28.0
Black or African American Male [4]								
All ages, age-adjusted[3]	70.8	60.1	56.3	34.2	31.8	31.7	33.4	32.1
All ages, crude	60.8	57.7	61.9	36.1	33.4	33.2	34.8	33.5
1 to 14 years	5.3	3.0	4.4	1.8	1.9	1.4	1.5	1.4
15 to 24 years	97.3	77.9	138.0	89.3	73.2	72.4	74.2	69.9
25 to 44 years	126.2	114.1	90.3	54.1	57.3	57.4	61.1	60.2
25 to 34 years	145.6	128.4	108.6	74.8	78.2	75.5	77.1	76.6
35 to 44 years	104.2	92.3	66.1	34.3	35.2	37.5	43.1	41.5
45 to 64 years	71.1	55.6	34.5	18.4	16.5	16.3	17.0	16.7
65 years and over	30.6	29.7	23.9	13.8	9.4	10.7	11.1	8.8
American Indian or Alaska Native Male [4]								
All ages, age-adjusted[3]	NA	24.0	19.4	13.1	11.7	11.9	13.5	12.9
All ages, crude	NA	27.5	20.5	13.2	12.5	11.7	13.4	12.5
15 to 24 years	NA	55.3	49.1	26.9	26.0	19.0	21.2	18.4
25 to 44 years	NA	43.9	25.4	16.6	16.9	17.1	20.1	18.8
45 to 64 years	NA	*	*	12.2	11.1	11.6	14.3	13.5
65 years and over	NA	*	*	*	*	*	*	*
Asian or Pacific Islander Male [4]								
All ages, age-adjusted[3]	NA	7.8	8.8	6.0	4.2	4.0	4.4	4.1
All ages, crude	NA	8.2	9.4	6.2	4.4	4.1	4.6	4.3
15 to 24 years	NA	10.8	21.0	9.3	6.8	5.7	6.3	5.9
25 to 44 years	NA	12.8	10.9	8.1	6.0	5.7	6.4	6.4
45 to 64 years	NA	10.4	8.1	7.4	4.4	4.4	5.0	4.6
65 years and over	NA	*	*	*	3.9	4.0	4.0	*
Hispanic or Latino Male [4,5]								
All ages, age-adjusted[3]	NA	NA	27.6	13.6	10.5	9.8	10.1	9.4
All ages, crude	NA	NA	29.9	14.2	10.5	9.9	10.1	9.4
1 to 14 years	NA	NA	2.6	1.0	0.6	0.7	0.6	0.5
15 to 24 years	NA	NA	55.5	30.8	20.9	19.2	19.6	17.4
25 to 44 years	NA	NA	42.7	17.3	14.4	13.9	14.4	13.8
25 to 34 years	NA	NA	47.3	20.3	18.0	17.0	17.3	16.2
35 to 44 years	NA	NA	35.4	13.2	10.2	10.2	11.0	11.1
45 to 64 years	NA	NA	21.4	12.0	9.1	8.0	8.2	8.2
65 years and over	NA	NA	19.1	12.2	9.9	9.6	9.7	8.1
White, not Hispanic or Latino Male [5]								
All ages, age-adjusted[3]	NA	NA	20.6	15.5	16.6	16.9	17.2	17.5
All ages, crude	NA	NA	20.4	15.7	17.6	18.0	18.5	18.8
1 to 14 years	NA	NA	1.6	1.0	0.9	1.0	1.0	1.2
15 to 24 years	NA	NA	24.1	16.2	14.2	15.1	15.2	15.1
25 to 44 years	NA	NA	23.3	17.9	19.4	19.4	19.8	20.2
25 to 34 years	NA	NA	24.7	17.2	18.9	19.3	19.3	19.7
35 to 44 years	NA	NA	21.6	18.4	19.9	19.6	20.3	20.8
45 to 64 years	NA	NA	22.7	17.8	22.8	23.0	23.8	23.5
65 years and over	NA	NA	37.4	29.0	27.6	28.4	28.7	29.6
White Female [4]								
All ages, age-adjusted[3]	4.0	4.2	3.8	2.7	2.7	2.9	2.9	3.0
All ages, crude	3.7	4.1	3.8	2.7	2.8	3.0	3.0	3.1
15 to 24 years	3.4	5.1	4.8	2.8	2.3	2.6	2.4	2.7
25 to 44 years	6.9	6.2	5.3	3.9	3.7	3.9	4.0	3.9
45 to 64 years	5.0	5.1	4.5	3.5	4.1	4.3	4.4	4.7
65 years and over	2.2	2.5	3.1	2.4	2.5	2.6	2.5	2.7
Black or African American Female [4]								
All ages, age-adjusted[3]	11.1	8.7	7.3	3.9	3.3	3.3	3.6	3.4
All ages, crude	10.0	8.8	7.8	4.0	3.3	3.4	3.7	3.4
15 to 24 years	15.2	12.3	13.3	7.6	6.4	6.7	7.2	6.1
25 to 44 years	19.4	16.1	12.4	6.5	5.6	5.6	5.8	6.0
45 to 64 years	10.2	8.2	4.8	3.1	2.2	2.2	2.7	2.5

Table 2-40. Death Rates for Firearm-Related Injuries, by Sex, Race, Hispanic Origin, and Age, Selected Years, 1970–2013 — continued

(Deaths per 100,000 resident population.)

Sex, race, Hispanic origin, and age	1970[1]	1980[1]	1990[1]	2000[2]	2010[2]	2011[2]	2012[2]	2013[2]
65 years and over	4.3	3.1	3.1	1.3	*	1.0	1.3	0.9
American Indian or Alaska Native Female [4]								
All ages, age-adjusted[3]	NA	5.8	3.3	2.9	2.6	2.4	1.8	2.0
All ages, crude	NA	5.8	3.4	2.9	2.4	2.3	1.8	2.0
15 to 24 years	NA	*	*	*	*	*	*	*
25 to 44 years	NA	10.2	*	5.5	3.7	3.3	*	*
45 to 64 years	NA	*	*	*	*	*	*	*
65 years and over	NA	*	*	*	*	*	*	*
Asian or Pacific Islander Female [4]								
All ages, age-adjusted[3]	NA	2.0	1.9	1.1	0.6	0.8	0.9	0.9
All ages, crude	NA	2.1	2.1	1.2	0.6	0.9	0.9	0.9
15 to 24 years	NA	*	*	*	*	*	*	*
25 to 44 years	NA	3.2	2.7	1.5	1.1	1.4	1.1	1.5
45 to 64 years	NA	*	*	*	*	1.0	0.9	0.8
65 years and over	NA	*	*	*	*	*	*	*
Hispanic or Latina Female [4,5]								
All ages, age-adjusted[3]	NA	NA	3.3	1.8	1.3	1.3	1.3	1.3
All ages, crude	NA	NA	3.6	1.8	1.3	1.3	1.3	1.3
15 to 24 years	NA	NA	6.9	2.9	2.1	2.1	1.9	2.3
25 to 44 years	NA	NA	5.1	2.5	1.8	2.0	2.0	2.0
45 to 64 years	NA	NA	2.4	2.2	1.5	1.3	1.4	1.2
65 years and over	NA	NA	*	*	*	*	*	*
White, not Hispanic or Latina Female [5]								
All ages, age-adjusted[3]	NA	NA	3.7	2.8	3.0	3.2	3.3	3.3
All ages, crude	NA	NA	3.7	2.9	3.1	3.3	3.4	3.5
15 to 24 years	NA	NA	4.3	2.7	2.3	2.6	2.5	2.8
25 to 44 years	NA	NA	5.1	4.2	4.2	4.4	4.5	4.4
45 to 64 years	NA	NA	4.6	3.6	4.4	4.7	4.9	5.2
65 years and over	NA	NA	3.2	2.4	2.6	2.7	2.7	2.9

NA = Not available.   * = Rates based on fewer than 20 deaths are considered unreliable and are not shown.   1 Underlying cause of death was coded according to the 8th Revision of the International Classification of Diseases (ICD) in 1970 and 9th Revision in 1980–1998.   2 Starting with 1999 data, cause of death is coded according to ICD–10.   3 Age-adjusted rates are calculated using the year 2000 standard population. Prior to 2001, age-adjusted rates were calculated using standard million proportions based on rounded population numbers. Starting with 2001 data, unrounded population numbers are used to calculate age-adjusted rates.   4 The race groups, White, Black, Asian or Pacific Islander, and American Indian or Alaska Native, include persons of Hispanic and non-Hispanic origin. Persons of Hispanic origin may be of any race. Death rates for the American Indian or Alaska Native, Asian or Pacific Islander, and Hispanic populations are known to be underestimated.   5 Prior to 1997, data from states that did not report Hispanic origin on the death certificate were excluded.

Figure 2-12. States with the Highest and Lowest Infant Mortality Rates

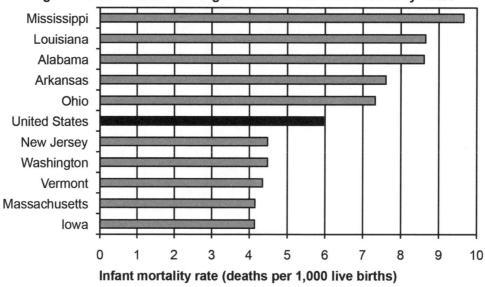

Infant mortality rate (deaths per 1,000 live births)

Table 2-41. Infant, Neonatal, and Postneonatal Mortality Rates, by Race and Sex, Selected Years, 1940–2013

(Rates are infant [under 1 year], neonatal [under 28 days], and postneonatal [28 days to 11 months]; deaths per 1,000 live births in specified group).

Year	All races			White[1]			All other[1]					
							Total[1]			Black[1]		
	Both sexes	Male	Female	Both sexes	Male	Female	Both sexes	Male	Female	Both sexes	Male	Female
INFANT MORTALITY RATE												
Race of Mother [2]												
1980	12.60	13.93	11.21	10.86	12.12	9.52	20.19	21.89	18.43	22.19	24.16	20.15
1981	11.93	13.14	10.66	10.34	11.50	9.12	18.82	20.36	17.24	20.81	22.54	19.03
1982	11.52	12.77	10.21	9.94	11.08	8.73	18.31	20.07	16.49	20.48	22.45	18.44
1983	11.16	12.31	9.96	9.61	10.66	8.49	17.80	19.44	16.11	19.98	21.95	17.96
1984	10.79	11.90	9.62	9.30	10.38	8.17	17.05	18.37	15.69	19.15	20.67	17.58
1985	10.64	11.91	9.32	9.17	10.39	7.88	16.84	18.33	15.28	19.01	20.76	17.22
1986	10.35	11.55	9.10	8.80	9.87	7.67	16.72	18.45	14.91	18.90	20.91	16.81
1987	10.08	11.17	8.94	8.48	9.45	7.45	16.46	18.06	14.80	18.75	20.63	16.83
1988	9.95	10.99	8.86	8.36	9.35	7.31	16.08	17.33	14.79	18.54	20.04	16.99
1989	9.81	10.81	8.77	8.08	9.01	7.10	16.33	17.60	15.02	18.61	20.02	17.15
1990	9.22	10.26	8.13	7.56	8.51	6.56	15.52	16.96	14.03	17.96	19.62	16.25
1991	8.94	10.00	7.84	7.30	8.26	6.30	15.07	16.53	13.57	17.57	19.38	15.71
1992	8.52	9.39	7.61	6.92	7.69	6.12	14.44	15.72	13.10	16.85	18.38	15.26
1993	8.37	9.25	7.43	6.82	7.56	6.05	14.07	15.58	12.52	16.52	18.33	14.67
1994	8.02	8.81	7.20	6.57	7.22	5.89	13.47	14.82	12.08	15.83	17.49	14.12
1995	7.59	8.33	6.81	6.29	6.99	5.55	12.61	13.53	11.65	15.12	16.34	13.86
1996	7.32	8.02	6.59	6.07	6.67	5.44	12.18	13.31	11.01	14.68	16.04	13.27
1997	7.23	7.95	6.47	6.03	6.67	5.36	11.76	12.83	10.65	14.16	15.47	12.82
1998	7.20	7.83	6.54	5.95	6.47	5.41	11.92	13.01	10.79	14.31	15.75	12.82
1999	7.06	7.72	6.36	5.77	6.35	5.15	11.94	12.94	10.90	14.56	15.92	13.16
2000	6.91	7.57	6.21	5.68	6.22	5.11	11.44	12.57	10.26	14.09	15.50	12.63
2001	6.85	7.52	6.14	5.65	6.21	5.06	11.33	12.44	10.18	14.02	15.48	12.52
2002	6.97	7.64	6.27	5.79	6.42	5.13	11.41	12.24	10.55	14.36	15.43	13.25
2003	6.85	7.60	6.07	5.72	6.36	5.05	11.09	12.24	9.90	14.01	15.53	12.43
2004	6.79	7.47	6.09	5.66	6.22	5.07	10.92	12.01	9.77	13.79	15.19	12.33
2005	6.87	7.56	6.15	5.73	6.32	5.11	10.92	11.98	9.82	13.73	15.15	12.27
2006	6.69	7.32	6.03	5.56	6.10	4.99	10.60	11.54	9.61	13.29	14.38	12.16
2007	6.75	7.38	6.09	5.64	6.17	5.08	10.55	11.51	9.54	13.24	14.49	11.94
2008	6.61	7.21	5.97	5.55	6.05	5.02	10.16	11.11	9.18	12.74	13.93	11.50
2009	6.39	7.01	5.75	5.30	5.79	4.78	10.02	11.06	8.94	12.64	14.08	11.15
2010	6.15	6.69	5.57	5.20	5.65	4.73	9.28	10.16	8.36	11.63	12.71	10.51
2011	6.07	6.58	5.52	5.12	5.54	4.67	9.13	9.96	8.27	11.51	12.61	10.37
2012	5.98	6.50	5.43	5.09	5.50	4.65	8.78	9.65	7.88	11.19	12.33	10.01
2013	5.96	6.52	5.38	5.07	5.59	4.52	8.79	9.46	8.08	11.22	12.03	10.39
Race of Child [3]												
1940	47.02	52.45	41.29	43.23	48.32	37.84	73.78	82.21	65.19	72.94	81.07	64.61
1950	29.21	32.75	25.48	26.77	30.21	23.13	44.46	48.87	39.93	43.91	48.27	39.44
1960	26.04	29.33	22.59	22.91	26.01	19.64	43.21	47.88	38.46	44.32	49.12	39.43
1970	20.01	22.37	17.52	17.75	19.95	15.42	30.92	34.20	27.53	32.65	36.18	29.01
1975	16.07	17.86	14.18	14.17	15.94	12.30	24.23	26.24	22.17	26.21	28.32	24.03
1976	15.24	16.82	13.57	13.31	14.81	11.71	23.50	25.51	21.42	25.54	27.83	23.19
1977	14.12	15.75	12.40	12.34	13.90	10.68	21.68	23.71	19.58	23.64	25.91	21.30
1978	13.78	15.26	12.23	12.01	13.37	10.58	21.06	23.15	18.90	23.11	25.39	20.77
1979	13.07	14.50	11.56	11.42	12.82	9.94	19.81	21.47	18.09	21.78	23.66	19.85
1980	12.60	13.93	11.21	11.00	12.27	9.65	19.12	20.73	17.47	21.37	23.27	19.43
NEONATAL MORTALITY RATE												
Race of Mother [2]												
1980	8.48	9.31	7.60	7.39	8.19	6.54	13.21	14.27	12.13	14.62	15.91	13.29
1981	8.02	8.81	7.20	6.99	7.73	6.20	12.51	13.52	11.48	13.98	15.16	12.77
1982	7.70	8.48	6.88	6.69	7.39	5.94	12.04	13.15	10.88	13.62	14.86	12.34
1983	7.28	8.01	6.52	6.31	6.98	5.61	11.41	12.46	10.33	12.93	14.20	11.63
1984	7.00	7.66	6.31	6.09	6.72	5.41	10.87	11.66	10.06	12.32	13.22	11.40
1985	6.96	7.75	6.13	6.00	6.75	5.21	11.00	12.00	9.95	12.62	13.81	11.39
1986	6.71	7.42	5.97	5.72	6.34	5.05	10.79	11.83	9.70	12.31	13.59	10.98
1987	6.46	7.11	5.79	5.40	5.96	4.82	10.68	11.72	9.61	12.30	13.52	11.05
1988	6.32	6.95	5.65	5.27	5.84	4.67	10.33	11.22	9.42	12.05	13.14	10.93
1989	6.23	6.79	5.63	5.15	5.66	4.60	10.30	11.08	9.49	11.92	12.84	10.97
1990	5.85	6.50	5.16	4.79	5.38	4.17	9.86	10.79	8.89	11.55	12.69	10.38

Table 2-41. Infant, Neonatal, and Postneonatal Mortality Rates, by Race and Sex, Selected Years, 1940–2013 — continued

(Rates are infant [under 1 year], neonatal [under 28 days], and postneonatal [28 days to 11 months]; deaths per 1,000 live births in specified group).

Year	All races			White[1]			All other[1]					
							Total[1]			Black[1]		
	Both sexes	Male	Female	Both sexes	Male	Female	Both sexes	Male	Female	Both sexes	Male	Female
1991	5.59	6.17	4.98	4.53	5.01	4.04	9.52	10.54	8.47	11.25	12.56	9.89
1992	5.37	5.84	4.89	4.35	4.72	3.96	9.19	10.02	8.32	10.83	11.83	9.79
1993	5.29	5.75	4.81	4.29	4.64	3.92	9.02	9.90	8.11	10.69	11.76	9.59
1994	5.12	5.58	4.64	4.20	4.55	3.83	8.60	9.51	7.65	10.21	11.32	9.07
1995	4.91	5.36	4.44	4.08	4.50	3.64	8.13	8.71	7.53	9.85	10.63	9.05
1996	4.77	5.18	4.34	3.97	4.31	3.62	7.86	8.59	7.12	9.56	10.45	8.65
1997	4.77	5.20	4.32	3.99	4.37	3.59	7.74	8.36	7.09	9.40	10.12	8.65
1998	4.80	5.21	4.37	3.98	4.31	3.63	7.91	8.63	7.17	9.55	10.51	8.56
1999	4.73	5.11	4.33	3.88	4.19	3.56	7.94	8.60	7.25	9.77	10.72	8.79
2000	4.63	5.06	4.17	3.82	4.16	3.46	7.60	8.39	6.79	9.38	10.39	8.35
2001	4.54	4.97	4.08	3.78	4.15	3.39	7.37	8.06	6.65	9.21	10.15	8.25
2002	4.66	5.06	4.25	3.89	4.27	3.50	7.55	8.03	7.05	9.51	10.13	8.87
2003	4.62	5.08	4.14	3.87	4.26	3.46	7.40	8.14	6.64	9.40	10.40	8.37
2004	4.52	4.94	4.09	3.78	4.14	3.41	7.19	7.82	6.54	9.13	9.95	8.27
2005	4.54	4.93	4.12	3.79	4.10	3.46	7.18	7.88	6.47	9.07	9.96	8.14
2006	4.45	4.84	4.05	3.72	4.05	3.37	7.00	7.58	6.40	8.82	9.49	8.12
2007	4.42	4.79	4.02	3.70	4.01	3.37	6.86	7.49	6.22	8.65	9.48	7.78
2008	4.29	4.67	3.89	3.62	3.94	3.28	6.54	7.14	5.92	8.23	8.99	7.45
2009	4.18	4.53	3.81	3.48	3.76	3.19	6.48	7.10	5.83	8.17	9.04	7.28
2010	4.05	4.37	3.71	3.46	3.73	3.18	6.00	6.51	5.45	7.49	8.08	6.89
2011	4.06	4.36	3.73	3.46	3.71	3.20	5.99	6.49	5.46	7.53	8.17	6.88
2012	4.01	4.34	3.67	3.45	3.71	3.18	5.76	6.31	5.20	7.34	8.04	6.61
2013	4.04	4.37	3.68	3.47	3.79	3.13	5.83	6.22	5.43	7.43	7.93	6.92
Race of Child[3]												
1940	28.75	32.56	24.74	27.20	30.85	23.33	39.71	44.87	34.45	39.90	44.78	34.89
1950	20.50	23.34	17.50	19.37	22.18	16.40	27.54	30.76	24.23	27.80	31.09	24.44
1960	18.73	21.24	16.09	17.24	19.66	14.70	26.86	30.04	23.62	27.83	31.13	24.49
1970	15.08	16.96	13.10	13.77	15.55	11.88	21.43	23.87	18.91	22.76	25.37	20.07
1975	11.58	12.91	10.18	10.38	11.70	8.98	16.78	18.21	15.31	18.32	19.78	16.81
1976	10.92	12.03	9.75	9.66	10.73	8.52	16.31	17.68	14.90	17.92	19.47	16.32
1977	9.88	11.00	8.70	8.75	9.83	7.60	14.66	16.02	13.27	16.08	17.60	14.52
1978	9.49	10.54	8.38	8.39	9.34	7.38	14.01	15.54	12.43	15.47	17.17	13.72
1979	8.87	9.79	7.89	7.88	8.80	6.92	12.89	13.91	11.83	14.31	15.45	13.14
1980	8.48	9.31	7.60	7.48	8.29	6.62	12.52	13.51	11.49	14.08	15.32	12.81
POSTNEONATAL MORTALITY RATE												
Race of Mother[2]												
1980	4.13	4.62	3.61	3.47	3.93	2.98	6.97	7.62	6.30	7.57	8.25	6.87
1981	3.91	4.34	3.46	3.35	3.77	2.92	6.31	6.84	5.76	6.83	7.38	6.26
1982	3.82	4.29	3.33	3.25	3.68	2.79	6.28	6.92	5.61	6.86	7.59	6.10
1983	3.88	4.30	3.44	3.29	3.68	2.88	6.39	6.98	5.78	7.05	7.75	6.32
1984	3.79	4.23	3.31	3.22	3.65	2.76	6.18	6.71	5.63	6.83	7.46	6.18
1985	3.68	4.15	3.19	3.17	3.64	2.67	5.84	6.33	5.33	6.40	6.95	5.83
1986	3.64	4.13	3.13	3.08	3.53	2.62	5.93	6.62	5.21	6.59	7.33	5.83
1987	3.62	4.06	3.15	3.08	3.49	2.64	5.77	6.34	5.18	6.45	7.10	5.77
1988	3.64	4.04	3.21	3.09	3.51	2.65	5.75	6.11	5.37	6.49	6.90	6.07
1989	3.59	4.01	3.14	2.93	3.35	2.49	6.03	6.52	5.53	6.69	7.18	6.19
1990	3.38	3.76	2.97	2.78	3.14	2.39	5.66	6.16	5.13	6.41	6.93	5.87
1991	3.35	3.82	2.86	2.76	3.25	2.26	5.55	5.99	5.10	6.32	6.82	5.81
1992	3.14	3.55	2.72	2.58	2.97	2.16	5.25	5.69	4.78	6.02	6.54	5.47
1993	3.07	3.50	2.62	2.54	2.92	2.13	5.06	5.68	4.42	5.83	6.57	5.08
1994	2.90	3.22	2.56	2.37	2.67	2.06	4.88	5.32	4.42	5.61	6.17	5.04
1995	2.67	2.97	2.37	2.21	2.49	1.91	4.47	4.82	4.11	5.27	5.71	4.81
1996	2.55	2.84	2.24	2.09	2.36	1.81	4.32	4.72	3.90	5.11	5.60	4.62
1997	2.45	2.75	2.14	2.04	2.30	1.77	4.02	4.47	3.56	4.77	5.34	4.17
1998	2.40	2.62	2.16	1.97	2.16	1.78	4.01	4.38	3.62	4.76	5.24	4.26
1999	2.33	2.61	2.03	1.88	2.16	1.60	4.00	4.34	3.64	4.79	5.20	4.36
2000	2.28	2.51	2.04	1.86	2.06	1.66	3.83	4.18	3.47	4.70	5.11	4.28
2001	2.31	2.55	2.06	1.87	2.06	1.67	3.96	4.37	3.53	4.81	5.32	4.27
2002	2.31	2.58	2.03	1.89	2.15	1.63	3.86	4.21	3.50	4.85	5.30	4.38
2003	2.23	2.52	1.94	1.84	2.09	1.58	3.69	4.10	3.26	4.60	5.13	4.06
2004	2.27	2.53	2.00	1.87	2.07	1.66	3.72	4.19	3.23	4.66	5.24	4.06
2005	2.34	2.63	2.03	1.94	2.22	1.65	3.73	4.10	3.36	4.67	5.19	4.13
2006	2.24	2.48	1.98	1.84	2.05	1.62	3.60	3.96	3.22	4.47	4.89	4.04
2007	2.34	2.58	2.07	1.94	2.16	1.71	3.68	4.02	3.32	4.59	5.01	4.16

Table 2-41. Infant, Neonatal, and Postneonatal Mortality Rates, by Race and Sex, Selected Years, 1940–2013 — continued

(Rates are infant [under 1 year], neonatal [under 28 days], and postneonatal [28 days to 11 months]; deaths per 1,000 live births in specified group).

Year	All races			White[1]			All other[1]					
							Total[1]			Black[1]		
	Both sexes	Male	Female	Both sexes	Male	Female	Both sexes	Male	Female	Both sexes	Male	Female
2008	2.32	2.54	2.08	1.93	2.12	1.73	3.62	3.97	3.26	4.50	4.93	4.06
2009	2.10	2.32	1.87	1.74	1.92	1.55	3.29	3.65	2.91	4.14	4.63	3.62
2010	2.22	2.48	1.94	1.82	2.04	1.59	3.55	3.96	3.11	4.47	5.05	3.87
2011	2.01	2.22	1.79	1.66	1.84	1.47	3.15	3.47	2.81	3.98	4.44	3.49
2012	1.97	2.16	1.76	1.63	1.79	1.47	3.02	3.34	2.69	3.85	4.29	3.40
2013	1.93	2.15	1.70	1.60	1.80	1.39	2.95	3.24	2.65	3.79	4.10	3.47
Race of Child [3]												
1940	18.27	19.89	16.55	16.03	17.47	14.50	34.07	37.35	30.74	33.05	36.29	29.72
1950	8.71	9.41	7.98	7.40	8.04	6.73	16.92	18.11	15.70	16.10	17.18	15.00
1960	7.31	8.10	6.49	5.66	6.35	4.94	16.35	17.84	14.84	16.48	17.99	14.95
1970	4.93	5.41	4.42	3.98	4.40	3.54	9.49	10.33	8.62	9.89	10.81	8.94
1975	4.49	4.95	4.00	3.80	4.24	3.33	7.45	8.03	6.86	7.89	8.54	7.22
1976	4.32	4.79	3.83	3.65	4.08	3.19	7.19	7.83	6.52	7.63	8.36	6.88
1977	4.24	4.75	3.71	3.59	4.07	3.08	7.01	7.69	6.31	7.56	8.32	6.78
1978	4.30	4.72	3.85	3.63	4.03	3.20	7.05	7.60	6.48	7.64	8.22	7.05
1979	4.20	4.71	3.67	3.54	4.02	3.03	6.92	7.57	6.25	7.47	8.21	6.71
1980	4.13	4.62	3.61	3.52	3.98	3.02	6.61	7.22	5.97	7.29	7.95	6.62

1 Multiple-race data were reported by 42 states and the District of Columbia in 2012 and 2013, by 38 states and the District of Columbia in 2011, by 37 states and the District of Columbia in 2010, by 34 states and the District of Columbia in 2008 and 2009, bby 27 states and the District of Columbia in 2007, by 25 states and the District of Columbia in 2006, by 21 states and the District of Columbia in 2005, by 15 states in 2004, and by 7 states in 2003. Multiple-race data were reported for births by 38 states and the District of Columbia in 2010, by 32 states and the District of Columbia in 2009, by 30 areas in 2008, by 27 areas in 2007, by 23 areas in 2006, by 19 areas in 2005, by 15 areas in 2004, and by 6 areas in 2003. The multiple-race data for these reporting areas were bridged to the single-race categories of the 1977 OMB standards for comparability with other reporting areas.   2 Infant deaths are based on race of child as stated on the death certificate; live births are based on race of mother as stated on the birth certificate.   3 Infant deaths are based on race of child as stated on the death certificate; live births are based on race of parents as stated on the birth certificate.

Table 2-42. Number of Infant Deaths and Infant Mortality Rates, by Selected Cause and Race, 2013

(Infant deaths [under 1 year] per 100,000 live births in specified group. Infant deaths based on race of decedent; live births based on race of mother.)

Cause of death (based on ICD–10, 2004)	Number			Rate		
	All races[1]	White[2]	Black[2]	White[2]	White	Black[2]
All causes	23,440	15,125	7,123	596.1	506.6	1,122.2
Certain infectious and parasitic diseases (A00-B99)	516	316	169	13.1	10.6	26.6
Certain intestinal infectious diseases (A00-A08)	6	3	3	*	*	*
Diarrhea and gastroenteritis of infectious origin (A09)	223	126	76	5.7	4.2	12.0
Tuberculosis (A16-A19)	1	1	-	*	*	*
Tetanus (A33,A35)	-	-	-	*	*	*
Diphtheria (A36)	-	-	-	*	*	*
Whooping cough (A37)	10	8	1	*	*	*
Meningococcal infection (A39)	6	5	-	*	*	*
Septicemia (A40-A41)	152	92	55	3.9	3.1	8.7
Congenital syphilis (A50)	2	2	-	*	*	*
Gonococcal infection (A54)	-	-	-	*	*	*
Viral diseases (A80-B34)	94	65	27	2.4	2.2	4.3
Acute poliomyelitis (A80)	-	-	-	*	*	*
Varicella (chickenpox) (B01)	-	-	-	*	*	*
Measles (B05)	-	-	-	*	*	*
Human immunodeficiency virus (HIV) disease (B20-B24)	-	-	-	*	*	*
Mumps (B26)	-	-	-	*	*	*
Other and unspecified viral diseases (A81-B00,B02-B04,B06-B19,B25,B27-B34)	94	65	27	2.4	2.2	4.3
Candidiasis (B37)	3	2	1	*	*	*
Malaria (B50-B54)	-	-	-	*	*	*
Pneumocystosis (B59)	-	-	-	*	*	*
All other and unspecified infectious and parasitic diseases(A20-A32,A38,A42-A49,A51-A53,A55-A79,B35-B36,B38-B49,B55-B58,B60-B99)	19	12	6	*	*	*
Neoplasms (C00-D48)	116	97	14	3.0	3.2	*
Malignant neoplasms (C00-C97)	64	52	9	1.6	1.7	*
Hodgkin's disease and non-Hodgkin's lymphomas (C81-C85)	-	-	-	*	*	*
Leukemia (C91-C95)	21	16	4	0.5	*	*
Other and unspecified malignant neoplasms (C00-C80,C88,C90,C96-C97)	43	36	5	1.1	1.2	*
In situ neoplasms, benign neoplasms and neoplasms of uncertain or unknown behavior (D00-D48)	52	45	5	1.3	1.5	*
Diseases of the blood and blood-forming organs and certain disorders involving the immune mechanism (D50-D89)	86	53	20	2.2	1.8	3.2
Anemias (D50-D64)	15	6	3	*	*	*
Hemorrhagic conditions and other diseases of blood and blood-forming organs (D65-D76)	51	31	14	1.3	1.0	*
Certain disorders involving the immune mechanism (D80-D89)	20	16	3	0.5	*	*
Endocrine, nutritional and metabolic diseases (E00-E88)	181	116	41	4.6	3.9	6.5
Short stature, not elsewhere classified (E34.3)	2	2	-	*	*	*
Nutritional deficiencies (E40-E64)	5	1	4	*	*	*
Cystic fibrosis (E84)	4	3	1	*	*	*
Volume depletion, disorders of fluid, electrolyte and acid-base balance (E86-E87)	47	30	13	1.2	1.0	*
All other endocrine, nutritional and metabolic diseases (E00-E32,E34.0-E34.2,E34.4-E34.9,E65-E83,E85,E88)	123	80	23	3.1	2.7	3.6
Diseases of the nervous system (G00-G98)	334	253	59	8.5	8.5	9.3
Meningitis (G00,G03)	52	31	17	1.3	1.0	*
Infantile spinal muscular atrophy, type I (Werdnig-Hoffman) (G12.0)	5	5	-	*	*	*
Infantile cerebral palsy (G80)	3	2	1	*	*	*
Anoxic brain damage, not elsewhere classified (G93.1)	36	29	4	0.9	1.0	*
Other diseases of nervous system(G04,G06-G11,G12.1-G12.9,G20-G72,G81-G92,G93.0,G93.2-G93.9,G95-G98)	238	186	37	6.1	6.2	5.8
Diseases of the ear and mastoid process (H60-H93)	1	-	1	*	*	*
Diseases of the circulatory system (I00-I99)	458	286	146	11.6	9.6	23.0
Pulmonary heart disease and diseases of pulmonary circulation (I26-I28)	82	52	26	2.1	1.7	4.1
Pericarditis, endocarditis and myocarditis (I30,I33,I40)	13	8	3	*	*	*
Cardiomyopathy (I42)	96	66	24	2.4	2.2	3.8
Cardiac arrest (I46)	21	14	6	0.5	*	*
Cerebrovascular diseases (I60-I69)	108	63	38	2.7	2.1	6.0
All other diseases of circulatory system (I00-I25,I31,I34-I38,I44-I45,I47-I51,I70-I99)	138	83	49	3.5	2.8	7.7
Diseases of the respiratory system (J00-J98,U04)	521	306	190	13.2	10.2	29.9
Acute upper respiratory infections (J00-J06)	15	9	5	*	*	*
Influenza and pneumonia (J09-J18)	178	101	69	4.5	3.4	10.9
Influenza (J09-J11)	20	13	5	0.5	*	*
Pneumonia (J12-J18)	158	88	64	4.0	2.9	10.1
Acute bronchitis and acute bronchiolitis (J20-J21)	29	17	12	0.7	*	*
Bronchitis, chronic and unspecified (J40-J42)	20	10	9	0.5	*	*
Asthma (J45-J46)	2	1	1	*	*	*
Pneumonitis due to solids and liquids (J69)	16	11	5	*	*	*
Other and unspecified diseases of respiratory system (J22,J30-J39,J43-J44,J47-J68,J70-J98,U04)	261	157	89	6.6	5.3	14.0
Diseases of the digestive system (K00-K92)	174	110	49	4.4	3.7	7.7
Gastritis, duodenitis, and noninfective enteritis and colitis (K29,K50-K55)	40	25	13	1.0	0.8	*
Hernia of abdominal cavity and intestinal obstruction without hernia (K40-K46,K56)	42	27	9	1.1	0.9	*
All other and unspecified diseases of digestive system (K00-K28,K30-K38,K57-K92)	92	58	27	2.3	1.9	4.3
Diseases of the genitourinary system (N00-N95)	100	67	30	2.5	2.2	4.7
Renal failure and other disorders of kidney (N17-N19,N25,N27)	81	57	22	2.1	1.9	3.5
Other and unspecified diseases of genitourinary system (N00-N15,N20-N23,N26,N28-N95)	19	10	8	*	*	*
Certain conditions originating in the perinatal period (P00-P96)	11,952	7,346	4,021	304.0	246.0	633.5
Newborn affected by maternal factors and by complications of pregnancy, labor and delivery (P00-P04)	2,873	1,801	932	73.1	60.3	146.8
Newborn affected by maternal hypertensive disorders (P00.0)	69	42	24	1.8	1.4	3.8
Newborn affected by other maternal conditions which may be unrelated to present pregnancy (P00.1-P00.9)	85	54	27	2.2	1.8	4.3
Newborn affected by maternal complications of pregnancy (P01)	1,595	972	540	40.6	32.6	85.1

Table 2-42. Number of Infant Deaths and Infant Mortality Rates, by Selected Cause and Race, 2013— continued

(Infant deaths [under 1 year] per 100,000 live births in specified group. Infant deaths based on race of decedent; live births based on race of mother.)

Cause of death (based on ICD–10, 2004)	Number			Rate		
	All races[1]	White[2]	Black[2]	White[2]	White	Black[2]
Newborn affected by incompetent cervix (P01.0)	502	269	199	12.8	9.0	31.4
Newborn affected by premature rupture of membranes (P01.1)	784	473	270	19.9	15.8	42.5
Newborn affected by multiple pregnancy (P01.5)	128	104	22	3.3	3.5	3.5
Newborn affected by other maternal complications of pregnancy (P01.2-P01.4,P01.6-P01.9)	181	126	49	4.6	4.2	7.7
Newborn affected by complications of placenta, cord and membranes (P02)	953	616	293	24.2	20.6	46.2
Newborn affected by complications involving placenta (P02.0-P02.3)	446	314	110	11.3	10.5	17.3
Newborn affected by complications involving cord (P02.4-P02.6)	33	23	8	0.8	0.8	*
Newborn affected by chorioamnionitis (P02.7)	471	277	175	12.0	9.3	27.6
Newborn affected by other and unspecified abnormalities of membranes (P02.8-P02.9)	3	2	-	*	*	*
Newborn affected by other complications of labor and delivery (P03)	128	83	40	3.3	2.8	6.3
Newborn affected by noxious influences transmitted via placenta or breast milk (P04)	43	34	8	1.1	1.1	*
Disorders related to length of gestation and fetal malnutrition (P05-P08)	4,313	2,459	1,663	109.7	82.4	262.0
Slow fetal growth and fetal malnutrition (P05)	111	55	50	2.8	1.8	7.9
Disorders related to short gestation and low birth weight, not elsewhere classified (P07)	4,202	2,404	1,613	106.9	80.5	254.1
Extremely low birth weight or extreme immaturity (P07.0,P07.2)	3,202	1,833	1,231	81.4	61.4	193.9
Other low birth weight or preterm (P07.1,P07.3)	1,000	571	382	25.4	19.1	60.2
Disorders related to long gestation and high birth weight (P08)	-	-	-	*	*	*
Birth trauma (P10-P15)	8	5	2	*	*	*
Intrauterine hypoxia and birth asphyxia (P20-P21)	319	226	83	8.1	7.6	13.1
Intrauterine hypoxia (P20)	144	95	46	3.7	3.2	7.2
Birth asphyxia (P21)	175	131	37	4.5	4.4	5.8
Respiratory distress of newborn (P22)	522	342	159	13.3	11.5	25.0
Other respiratory conditions originating in the perinatal period (P23-P28)	784	515	227	19.9	17.2	35.8
Congenital pneumonia (P23)	55	39	15	1.4	1.3	*
Neonatal aspiration syndromes (P24)	42	24	11	1.1	0.8	*
Interstitial emphysema and related conditions originating in the perinatal period (P25)	96	67	24	2.4	2.2	3.8
Pulmonary hemorrhage originating in the perinatal period (P26)	156	99	50	4.0	3.3	7.9
Chronic respiratory disease originating in the perinatal period (P27)	103	69	28	2.6	2.3	4.4
Atelectasis (P28.0-P28.1)	253	168	73	6.4	5.6	11.5
All other respiratory conditions originating in the perinatal period (P28.2-P28.9)	79	49	26	2.0	1.6	4.1
Infections specific to the perinatal period (P35-P39)	740	451	251	18.8	15.1	39.5
Bacterial sepsis of newborn (P36)	578	349	200	14.7	11.7	31.5
Omphalitis of newborn with or without mild hemorrhage (P38)	1	1	-	*	*	*
All other infections specific to the perinatal period (P35,P37,P39)	161	101	51	4.1	3.4	8.0
Hemorrhagic and hematological disorders of newborn (P50-P61)	492	337	137	12.5	11.3	21.6
Neonatal hemorrhage (P50-P52,P54)	389	266	111	9.9	8.9	17.5
Hemorrhagic disease of newborn (P53)	1	1	-	*	*	*
Hemolytic disease of newborn due to isoimmunization and other perinatal jaundice (P55-P59)	15	12	1	*	*	*
Hematological disorders (P60-P61)	87	58	25	2.2	1.9	3.9
Syndrome of infant of a diabetic mother and neonatal diabetes mellitus (P70.0-P70.2)	8	7	1	*	*	*
Necrotizing enterocolitis of newborn (P77)	355	210	129	9.0	7.0	20.3
Hydrops fetalis not due to hemolytic disease (P83.2)	187	135	31	4.8	4.5	4.9
Other perinatal conditions (P29,P70.3-P70.9,P71-P76,P78-P81,P83.0-P83.1,P83.3- P83.9,P90-P96)	1,351	858	406	34.4	28.7	64.0
Congenital malformations, deformations and chromosomal abnormalities (Q00-Q99)	4,758	3,561	942	121.0	119.3	148.4
Anencephaly and similar malformations (Q00)	294	255	31	7.5	8.5	4.9
Congenital hydrocephalus (Q03)	62	47	14	1.6	1.6	*
Spina bifida (Q05)	13	9	2	*	*	*
Other congenital malformations of nervous system (Q01-Q02,Q04,Q06-Q07)	294	211	61	7.5	7.1	9.6
Congenital malformations of heart (Q20-Q24)	1,141	842	240	29.0	28.2	37.8
Other congenital malformations of circulatory system (Q25-Q28)	160	116	30	4.1	3.9	4.7
Congenital malformations of respiratory system (Q30-Q34)	369	264	86	9.4	8.8	13.5
Congenital malformations of digestive system (Q35-Q45)	73	44	20	1.9	1.5	3.2
Congenital malformations of genitourinary system (Q50-Q64)	428	339	75	10.9	11.4	11.8
Congenital malformations and deformations of musculoskeletal system, limbs and integument (Q65-Q85)	549	421	94	14.0	14.1	14.8
Down's syndrome (Q90)	50	32	11	1.3	1.1	*
Edward's syndrome (Q91.0-Q91.3)	455	330	107	11.6	11.1	16.9
Patau's syndrome (Q91.4-Q91.7)	250	184	54	6.4	6.2	8.5
Other congenital malformations and deformations (Q10-Q18,Q86-Q89)	516	389	92	13.1	13.0	14.5
Other chromosomal abnormalities, not elsewhere classified (Q92-Q99)	104	78	25	2.6	2.6	3.9
Symptoms, signs and abnormal clinical and laboratory findings, not elsewhere classified (R00-R99)	2,671	1,674	865	67.9	56.1	136.3
Sudden infant death syndrome (R95)	1,563	996	494	39.7	33.4	77.8
Other symptoms, signs and abnormal clinical and laboratory findings, not elsewhere classified (R00-R53,R55-R94,R96-R99)	1,108	678	371	28.2	22.7	58.4
All other diseases (residual)	20	11	8	0.5	*	*
External causes of mortality (*U01,V01-Y84)	1,552	929	568	39.5	31.1	89.5
Accidents (unintentional injuries) (V01-X59)	1,156	694	427	29.4	23.2	67.3
Transport accidents (V01-V99)	72	52	14	1.8	1.7	*
Motor vehicle accidents (V02-V04,V09.0,V09.2,V12-V14,V19.0-V19.2,V19.4-V19.6, V20-V79,V80.3-V80.5,V81.0-V81.1,V82.0-V82.1,V83-V86,V87.0-V87.8,V88.0- V88.8,V89.0,V89.2)	68	49	14	1.7	1.6	*
Other and unspecified transport accidents (V01,V05-V06,V09.1,V09.3-V09.9,V10- V11,V15-V18,V19.3,V19.8-V19.9,V80.0-V80.2,V80.6-V80.9,V81.2-V81.9,V82.2- V82.9,V87.9,V88.9,V89.1,V89.3,V89.9,V90-V99)	4	3	-	*	*	*
Falls (W00-W19)	15	13	2	*	*	*
Accidental discharge of firearms (W32-W34)	3	1	1	*	*	*
Accidental drowning and submersion (W65-W74)	23	16	6	0.6	*	*
Accidental suffocation and strangulation in bed (W75)	819	472	324	20.8	15.8	51.0
Other accidental suffocation and strangulation (W76-W77,W81-W84)	115	72	42	2.9	2.4	6.6
Accidental inhalation and ingestion of food or other objects causing obstruction of respiratory tract (W78-W80)	45	28	16	1.1	0.9	*
Accidents caused by exposure to smoke, fire and flames (X00-X09)	17	9	8	*	*	*
Accidental poisoning and exposure to noxious substances (X40-X49)	6	2	3	*	*	*

Table 2-42. Number of Infant Deaths and Infant Mortality Rates, by Selected Cause and Race, 2013— continued

(Infant deaths [under 1 year] per 100,000 live births in specified group. Infant deaths based on race of decedent; live births based on race of mother.)

Cause of death (based on ICD–10, 2004)	Number			Rate		
	All races[1]	White[2]	Black[2]	White[2]	White	Black[2]
Other and unspecified accidents (W20-W31,W35-W64,W85-W99,X10-X39,X50-X59)	41	29	11	1.0	1.0	*
Assault (homicide) (*U01,X85-Y09)	282	165	103	7.2	5.5	16.2
Assault (homicide) by hanging, strangulation and suffocation (X91)	22	14	6	0.6	*	*
Assault (homicide) by discharge of firearms (*U01.4,X93-X95)	12	9	2	*	*	*
Neglect, abandonment and other maltreatment syndromes (Y06-Y07)	74	46	24	1.9	1.5	3.8
Assault (homicide) by other and unspecified means(*U01.0-*U01.3,*U01.5-*U01.9,X85-X90,X92,X96-X99,Y00-Y05,Y08-Y09)	174	96	71	4.4	3.2	11.2
Complications of medical and surgical care (Y40-Y84)	11	6	5	*	*	*
Other external causes (Y10-Y36)	103	64	33	2.6	2.1	5.2

- = Quantity zero.   * = Figure does not meet standards of reliability or precision.   1 Includes races other than White and Black.   2 Race categories are consistent with the 1977 Office of Management and Budget (OMB) standards. In 2013, multiple-race data were reported by 42 states and the District of Columbia for deaths and by 44 states and the District of Columbia for birth. The multiple-race data for these reporting areas were bridged to the single-race categories of the 1977 OMB standards for comparability with other reporting areas.

Table 2-43. Number of Infant and Neonatal Deaths and Mortality Rates, by Race, Sex, State, and Territory, 2013

(Infant [under 1 year] and neonatal [under 28 days] deaths per 1,000 live births in specified group. Infant and neonatal deaths are based on race of decedent; live births are based on race of mother.)

Sex, state, and territory	Infant deaths						Neonatal deaths					
	All races[1]		White[2]		Black[2]		All races[1]		White[2]		Black[2]	
	Number	Rate	Number	Rate	Number	Rate	Number	Rate	Number	Rate	Number	Rate
United States [3]	23,440	5.96	15,125	5.07	7,123	11.22	15,867	4.04	10,348	3.47	4,717	7.43
Male	13,119	6.52	8,548	5.59	3,878	12.03	8,800	4.37	5,796	3.79	2,555	7.93
Female	10,321	5.38	6,577	4.52	3,245	10.39	7,067	3.68	4,552	3.13	2,162	6.92
Alabama	501	8.61	271	6.95	228	12.66	322	5.54	165	4.23	155	8.60
Alaska	64	5.59	33	4.46	3	*	29	2.53	17	*	3	*
Arizona	451	5.27	331	4.63	70	14.37	292	3.41	220	3.08	45	9.24
Arkansas	288	7.61	193	6.63	83	11.29	168	4.44	116	3.99	48	6.53
California	2,353	4.76	1,774	4.64	351	10.98	1,649	3.33	1,275	3.33	220	6.88
Colorado	331	5.09	281	4.88	37	9.84	239	3.68	204	3.54	25	6.65
Connecticut	169	4.68	122	4.29	44	8.62	115	3.19	91	3.20	24	4.70
Delaware	68	6.28	33	4.58	35	11.43	47	4.34	21	2.92	26	8.49
District of Columbia	63	6.78	12	*	50	9.77	45	4.84	10	*	34	6.64
Florida	1,326	6.16	744	4.81	557	10.52	865	4.02	482	3.11	365	6.89
Georgia	894	6.94	410	5.46	467	9.85	611	4.75	278	3.70	319	6.73
Hawaii	124	6.53	33	5.46	17	*	87	4.58	21	3.47	15	*
Idaho	126	5.63	117	5.51	3	*	82	3.66	76	3.58	2	*
Illinois	942	6.00	534	4.48	363	13.11	639	4.07	383	3.21	220	7.94
Indiana	600	7.22	419	5.97	165	15.80	381	4.58	266	3.79	105	10.05
Iowa	162	4.14	129	3.66	25	11.20	105	2.69	84	2.38	15	*
Kansas	250	6.44	185	5.41	54	18.20	168	4.33	122	3.57	38	12.81
Kentucky	355	6.38	294	6.01	60	10.99	218	3.91	186	3.80	32	5.86
Louisiana	547	8.65	212	5.79	327	13.25	322	5.09	117	3.19	198	8.02
Maine	90	7.04	86	7.20	4	*	54	4.23	50	4.18	4	*
Maryland	477	6.63	206	4.97	252	10.18	327	4.54	139	3.35	176	7.11
Massachusetts	298	4.15	211	3.77	71	7.74	221	3.08	159	2.84	51	5.56
Michigan	799	7.04	490	5.70	290	12.81	545	4.80	342	3.98	186	8.21
Minnesota	349	5.05	229	4.19	81	10.59	248	3.59	164	3.00	55	7.19
Mississippi	373	9.65	156	7.49	214	12.57	227	5.88	92	4.42	133	7.81
Missouri	491	6.52	343	5.61	138	11.77	327	4.34	223	3.65	95	8.10
Montana	70	5.66	49	4.62	1	*	36	2.91	30	2.83	1	*
Nebraska	139	5.33	118	5.21	16	*	96	3.68	85	3.75	9	*
Nevada	191	5.45	130	4.76	49	11.63	128	3.65	90	3.30	31	7.35
New Hampshire	70	5.65	66	5.70	4	*	50	4.03	47	4.06	3	*
New Jersey	460	4.48	255	3.56	177	9.25	327	3.19	189	2.63	118	6.17
New Mexico	144	5.46	118	5.53	5	*	106	4.02	86	4.03	5	*
New York	1,167	4.92	733	4.49	363	7.61	832	3.51	531	3.26	244	5.12
North Carolina	832	6.99	429	5.39	365	11.37	598	5.03	305	3.83	268	8.35
North Dakota	65	6.13	48	5.37	2	*	51	4.81	39	4.36	1	*
Ohio	1,018	7.33	666	6.07	340	13.63	723	5.20	468	4.26	245	9.82
Oklahoma	364	6.82	243	5.98	77	15.12	217	4.07	152	3.74	41	8.05
Oregon	224	4.96	197	4.90	15	*	155	3.43	136	3.38	10	*
Pennsylvania	938	6.66	622	5.71	298	12.03	679	4.82	450	4.13	213	8.60
Rhode Island	70	6.48	59	6.80	9	*	46	4.26	43	4.96	3	*
South Carolina	389	6.85	195	5.30	192	10.33	263	4.63	135	3.67	127	6.83
South Dakota	80	6.53	49	5.14	5	*	48	3.92	32	3.36	4	*
Tennessee	544	6.80	336	5.62	198	11.09	334	4.18	202	3.38	127	7.11
Texas	2,264	5.84	1,639	5.15	556	11.34	1,516	3.91	1,096	3.44	370	7.55
Utah	263	5.16	233	4.89	8	*	183	3.59	170	3.57	5	*
Vermont	26	4.35	24	4.21	1	*	19	*	18	*	-	*
Virginia	634	6.21	341	4.79	267	11.64	450	4.41	239	3.36	189	8.24
Washington	388	4.48	283	4.08	49	9.35	262	3.03	190	2.74	31	5.91
West Virginia	158	7.59	138	6.96	19	*	94	4.51	83	4.19	10	*
Wisconsin	416	6.24	273	4.92	118	16.96	299	4.49	208	3.75	73	10.49
Wyoming	35	4.58	33	4.65	-	*	22	2.88	21	2.96	-	*
Puerto Rico	261	7.15	254	7.93	7	*	176	4.82	172	5.37	4	*
Virgin Islands	NA	NA	NA	NA	NA	NA	NA	NA	NA	NA	NA	NA
Guam	31	9.44	1	*	1	*	18	*	1	*	1	*
American Samoa	10	*	-	*	-	*	6	*	-	*	-	*
Northern Marianas	8	*	-	*	-	*	6	*	-	*	-	*

- = Quantity zero.   * = Figure does not meet standards of reliability or precision.   NA = Not available.   1 Includes races other than White and Black.   2 Race categories are consistent with the 1977 Office of Management and Budget (OMB) standards. In 2013, multiple-race data were reported by 42 states and the District of Columbia for deaths and by 44 states and the District of Columbia for births.   3 Excludes data for Puerto Rico, Virgin Islands, Guam, American Samoa, and Northern Marianas.

Table 2-44. Selected Characteristics of Discharged Hospice Care Patients, 2007

(Percent.)

Characteristic	Percent
Age	
Under 65 years	16.9
65 years and over	83.1
65 to 74 years	15.4
75 to 84 years	29.5
85 years and over	38.2
Sex	
Male	44.9
Female	55.1
Race and Hispanic Origin	
Hispanic or Latino (of any race)	4.1
Not Hispanic or Latino	
White	86.6
Black or African American	7.6
Marital Status	
Married or living with partner	45.4
Single, divorced, or separated	14.2
Widowed	40.4
Vital Status at Discharge	
Deceased	84.4
Alive	15.6
Medicare Beneficiary	
Yes	84.3
No	15.7
Place of Care on First Day	
Private home	55.3
Nursing home/skilled nursing facility	21.1
Other place	23.6

NOTES AND DEFINITIONS

SOURCES OF DATA

Several different publications were used to obtain the mortality data. A significant amount of notes and information is derived from Murphy SL, Xu JQ, Kochanek KD. *Deaths: Final Data for 2010.* National Vital Statistics Reports; vol. 61, no. 14 Hyattsville, MD: National Center for Health Statistics. 2013. In these tables, the asterisks (*) preceding the cause-of-death codes indicate that they are not part of the *International Classification of Diseases, Tenth Revision (ICD–10), Second Edition.* Updated tables containing data through 2013 were accessed via http://www.cdc.gov/nchs/data/nvsr/nvsr64/nvsr64_02.pdf.

Tables 2-16, 2-17, 2-19 through 2-22, 2-26, 2-28 through 2-35, and 2-37 through 2-40 are from National Center for Health Statistics. *Health, United States, 2013: With Special Feature on Prescription Drugs.* Hyattsville, MD, 2014, an annual report on trends in health statistics compiled by the National Center of Health Statistics (NCHS), a component of the Centers for Disease Control and Prevention (CDC). Updated tables for this publication can be found at http://www.cdc.gov/nchs/hus/contents2014.htm.

Tables 2-23 through 2-25 come from the Census of Fatal Occupational Injuries, which can be found on the Web site of the U.S. Department of Commerce's Bureau of Labor Statistics.

Table 2-36 can be found at https://data.cdc.gov/Motor-Vehicle/Occupant-and-Alcohol-Impaired-Driving-Deaths-in-St/haed-k2ka.

NOTES ON THE DATA

Final data in Part B are based on information from all resident death certificates filed in the 50 states and the District of Columbia. It is believed that more than 99 percent of all deaths that occur in the United States are registered.

Data shown for geographic areas are by place of residence. Beginning with 1970, mortality statistics for the United States exclude deaths of nonresidents of the United States. All data exclude fetal deaths. Mortality statistics for Puerto Rico, Virgin Islands, American Samoa, and Northern Marianas exclude deaths of nonresidents for each area. For Guam, however, mortality statistics exclude deaths that occurred to a resident of any place other than Guam or the United States.

Race and Hispanic origin are reported separately on the death certificate. Therefore, data shown by race include persons of Hispanic and non-Hispanic origin, and data for Hispanic origin include persons of any race. Unless otherwise specified, deaths of Hispanic origin are included in the totals for each race group—White, Black, American Indian or Alaska Native (AIAN), and Asian or Pacific Islander (API)—according to the decedent's race as reported on the death certificate. Data shown for Hispanic persons include all persons of Hispanic origin of any race.

Age-adjusted rates are used to compare relative mortality risks among groups and over time. However, they should be viewed as relative indexes rather than as actual measures of mortality risk. They were computed by the direct method—that is, by applying age-specific death rates to the U.S. standard population age distribution. Beginning with the 1999 data year, NCHS adopted a new population standard for use in age-adjusting death rates. Based on the projected year 2000 population of the United States, the new standard replaced the 1940 standard population that had been used for more than 50 years. The new population standard affects levels of mortality and, to some extent, trends and group comparisons. Of particular note are the effects on race mortality comparisons. Beginning with 2003 data, the traditional standard million population along with corresponding standard weights to six decimal places were replaced by the projected year 2000 population age distribution. The effect of the change is negligible and does not significantly affect comparability with age-adjusted rates calculated using the previous method. All age-adjusted rates shown in this report are based on the 2000 U.S. standard population.

Infant mortality rates are the most commonly used index for measuring the risk of dying during the first year of life. The rates presented in this report are calculated by dividing the number of infant deaths in a calendar year by the number of live births registered for the same period, and are presented as rates per 1,000 or per 100,000 live births. For final birth figures used in the denominator for infant mortality rates, see the CDC's *Births: Final Data for 2010* report. In contrast to infant mortality rates based on live births, infant death rates are based on the estimated population under age 1 year. Infant death rates that appear in tabulations of age-specific death rates in this report are calculated by dividing the number of infant deaths by the April 1, 2010, population estimate of persons under age 1, based on 2010 census populations. These rates are presented per 100,000 population in this age group. Because of differences in the denominators, infant death rates may differ from infant mortality rates.

Race and Hispanic origin are reported separately on the death certificate. Therefore, data shown by race include persons of Hispanic and non-Hispanic origin, and data for Hispanic origin include persons of any race. In this report, unless otherwise specified, deaths of persons of Hispanic origin are included in the totals for each race group (White, Black, American Indian and Alaska Native, and Asian or Pacific Islander) according to the decedent's race as reported on the death certificate. Mortality data for the Hispanic-origin population are based on deaths of residents of all 50 states and the District of Columbia. Death rates for Hispanic, American Indian and Alaska Native, and Asian or Pacific Islander persons should be interpreted with caution because of inconsistencies in reporting Hispanic origin or race on the death certificate compared with censuses, surveys, and birth certificates. Studies have shown underreporting on death certificates of American Indian and Alaska Native, Asian or Pacific Islander, and Hispanic decedents, as well as undercounts of these groups in censuses.

Cause of death statistics are in accordance with the *International Classification of Diseases, Tenth Revision (ICD-10)*.

CONCEPTS AND DEFINITIONS

Age-adjusted death rate—the death rate used to make comparisons of relative mortality risks across groups and over time. This rate should be viewed as a construct or an index rather than as a direct or actual measure of mortality risk. Statistically, it is a weighted average of the age-specific death rates, where the weights represent the fixed population proportions by age.

Age-specific death rate—deaths per 100,000 population in a specified age group, such as 1–4 years or 5–9 years for a specified period.

Cause of death—for the purpose of national mortality statistics, every death is attributed to one underlying condition, based on information reported on the death certificate and using the international rules for selecting the underlying cause of death from the conditions stated on the death certificate. The underlying cause is defined by the World Health Organization as the disease or injury that initiated the train of events leading directly to death, or the circumstances of the accident or violence that produced the fatal injury. Generally more medical information is reported on death certificates than is directly reflected in the underlying cause of death. The conditions that are not selected as underlying cause of death constitute the nonunderlying causes of death, also known as multiple cause of death.

Cause-of-death ranking—selected causes of death of public health and medical importance comprise tabulation lists and are ranked according to the number of deaths assigned to these causes. The top-ranking causes determine the leading causes of death. Certain causes on the tabulation lists are not ranked if, for example, the category title represents a group title (such as major cardiovascular diseases and symptoms, signs, and abnormal clinical and laboratory findings, not elsewhere classified); or the category title begins with the words "other" and "all other". In addition, when one of the titles that represents a subtotal (such as malignant neoplasms) is ranked, its component parts are not ranked.

Crude death rate—total deaths per 100,000 population for a specified period. The crude death rate represents the average chance of dying during a specified period for persons in the entire population.

Fetal death rate—the number of fetal deaths with stated or presumed gestation of 20 weeks or more, divided by the sum of live births plus fetal deaths, per 1,000 live births plus fetal deaths.

Infant deaths—deaths of infants under 1 year of age.

International Classification of Diseases (ICD) —used to code and classify cause-of-death data. It is developed collaboratively by the World Health Organization and 10 international centers, one of which is housed at NCHS. The purpose of it is to promote international comparability in the collection, classification, processing, and presentation of health statistics. Since 1900, it has been modified about once every 10 years, except for the 20-year interval between the ninth and tenth editions. The purpose of the revisions is to stay abreast with advances in medical science. New revisions usually introduce major disruptions in time series of mortality statistics.

Hispanic origin—includes persons of Mexican, Puerto Rican, Cuban, Central and South American, and other or unknown Latin American or Spanish origins. Persons of Hispanic origin may be of any race.

Late fetal death rate—the number of fetal deaths with stated or presumed gestation of 28 weeks or more, divided by the sum of live births plus late fetal deaths per 1,000 live births plus late fetal deaths.

Life expectancy—the average number of years of life remaining to a person at a particular age and is based on a given set of age-specific death rates, generally the mortality conditions existing in the period mentioned.

Maternal mortality rate—the number of maternal deaths per 100,000 live births. The maternal mortality rate is the measure of the likelihood that a pregnant woman will die from maternal causes.

Neonatal deaths—deaths of infants aged 0–27 days.

Perinatal mortality rate—the sum of late fetal deaths plus infant deaths within 7 days of birth divided by the sum of live births plus late fetal deaths, per 1,000 live births plus late fetal deaths.

Perinatal mortality ratio—the sum of late fetal deaths plus infant deaths within 7 days of birth divided by the number of live births, per 1,000 live births.

Postneonatal deaths—deaths of infants aged 28 days–1 year old.

Years of potential life lost (YPLL) —a measure of premature mortality. YPLL is presented for persons under 75 years of age because the average life expectancy in the United States is over 75 years. YPLL-75 is calculated using the following eight age groups: under 1 year, 1–14 years, 15–24 years, 25–34 years, 35–44 years, 45–54 years, 55–64 years, and 65–74 years. The number of deaths for each age group is multiplied by years of life lost, calculated as the difference between age 75 years and the midpoint of the age group. For the eight age groups, the midpoints are 0.5, 7.5, 19.5, 29.5, 39.5, 49.5, 59.5, and 69.5. For example, the death of a person 15–24 years of age counts as 55.5 years of life lost. Years of potential life lost is derived by summing years of life lost over all age groups.

PART 3

HEALTH

DETERMINANTS AND MEASURES OF HEALTH

Figure 3-1. Age-Adjusted Prevalence of Heart Disease, Cancer, and Stroke Among Person 18 Years and Over, Selected Years 1997–1998 and 2012–2013

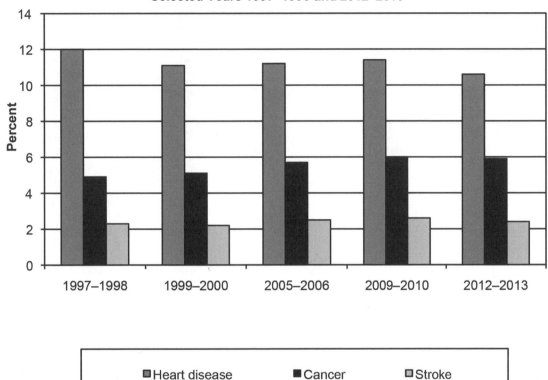

HIGHLIGHTS

- In 2012–2013, according to age-adjusted data, 10.6 percent of people suffered from heart disease, a decline from 12.0 percent in 1997–1998. Although the percent of people with heart disease declined, the percent of people suffering from cancer increased from 4.9 percent to 5.9 percent, while the percentage of people suffering from a stroke increased from 2.3 percent to 2.5 percent in the same time period. (Table 3-4A)

- In 2013, 9.5 percent of adults age 18 years and over had five or more drinks in one day on at least 12 days in the past year. This percentage was down from 21.1 percent in 1997. (Table 3-21)

- Approximately 26.6 percent of American Indian or Alaska Natives and Blacks or African Americans had no usual source of health care in 2013, compared to 19.2 percent of Whites. (Table 3-27)

- The mean annual wage for healthcare practitioners and technical occupations in May 2014 was $76,010. Anesthesiologists earned the most at $246,320, while home health aides earned the least at $22,400. (Table 3-54)

- In 2013, 16.7 percent of people in the United States did not have health insurance. Massachusetts had the highest percentage of insured residents, with only 4.4 percent lacking insurance, while Texas had the highest percentage of uninsured residents at 24.5 percent. (Table 3-71)

Table 3-1. Selected Notifiable Disease Rates and Number of New Cases, Selected Years, 1950–2012

(Cases per 100,000 population; number.)

Disease	1950	1960	1970	1980	1990	2000	2010	2011	2012
Rate									
Diphtheria	3.83	0.51	0.21	0.00	0.00	0.00	-	-	0.00
Haemophilus influenzae, invasive	NA	NA	NA	NA	NA	0.51	1.03	1.15	1.10
Hepatitis A	NA	NA	27.87	12.84	12.64	4.91	0.54	0.45	0.50
Hepatitis B	NA	NA	4.08	8.39	8.48	2.95	1.10	0.94	0.93
Lyme disease[1]	NA	NA	NA	NA	NA	6.53	9.86	10.78	9.96
Meningococcal disease	NA	NA	1.23	1.25	0.99	0.83	0.27	0.25	0.18
Mumps	NA	NA	55.55	3.86	2.17	0.13	0.85	0.13	0.07
Pertussis (whooping cough)	79.82	8.23	2.08	0.76	1.84	2.88	8.97	6.06	15.49
Poliomyelitis, paralytic[2]	NA	1.40	0.02	0.00	0.00	-	-	-	-
Rocky Mountain spotted fever[3]	NA	NA	0.19	0.52	0.26	0.18	0.65	0.91	1.44
Rubella (German measles)	NA	NA	27.75	1.72	0.45	0.06	0.00	0.00	0.00
Rubeola (measles)	211.01	245.42	23.23	5.96	11.17	0.03	0.02	0.06	0.02
Salmonellosis, excluding typhoid fever	NA	3.85	10.84	14.88	19.54	14.51	17.73	16.79	17.27
Shigellosis	15.45	6.94	6.79	8.41	10.89	8.41	4.82	4.32	4.90
Tuberculosis[4]	NA	30.83	18.28	12.25	10.33	6.01	3.64	3.41	3.19
Sexually transmitted diseases[5]									
Syphilis[6]	146.02	68.78	44.80	30.30	54.32	11.20	14.93	14.91	16.02
Primary and secondary	16.73	9.06	10.80	12.00	20.26	2.12	4.49	4.52	5.03
Early latent	39.71	10.11	8.00	8.90	22.19	3.35	4.43	4.25	4.65
Late and late latent[7]	70.22	45.91	24.70	9.20	10.32	5.53	5.89	6.02	6.23
Congenital[8]	368.30	103.70	52.30	7.70	92.95	14.29	8.73	8.48	7.80
Chlamydia[9]	NA	NA	NA	NA	160.19	251.38	426.01	457.59	456.68
Gonorrhea[10]	192.50	145.40	294.20	442.10	276.43	128.67	100.76	104.24	107.46
Chancroid	3.34	0.94	0.70	0.30	1.69	0.03	0.01	0.00	0.00
Number									
Diphtheria	5,796	918	435	3	4	1	-	-	1
Haemophilus influenzae, invasive	NA	NA	NA	NA	NA	1,398	3,151	3,539	3,418
Hepatitis A	NA	NA	56,797	29,087	31,441	13,397	1,670	1,398	1,562
Hepatitis B	NA	NA	8,310	19,015	21,102	8,036	3,374	2,903	2,895
Lyme disease[1]	NA	NA	NA	NA	NA	17,730	30,158	33,097	30,831
Meningococcal disease	NA	NA	2,505	2,840	2,451	2,256	833	759	551
Mumps	NA	NA	104,953	8,576	5,292	338	2,612	404	229
Pertussis (whooping cough)	120,718	14,809	4,249	1,730	4,570	7,867	27,550	18,719	48,277
Poliomyelitis, paralytic[2]	NA	2,525	31	4	6	-	-	-	-
Rocky Mountain spotted fever[3]	464	NA	380	1,163	651	495	1,985	2,802	4,470
Rubella (German measles)	NA	NA	56,552	3,904	1,125	176	5	4	9
Rubeola (measles)	319,124	441,703	47,351	13,506	27,786	86	63	220	55
Salmonellosis, excluding typhoid fever	NA	6,929	22,096	33,715	48,603	39,574	54,424	51,887	53,800
Shigellosis	23,367	12,487	13,845	19,041	27,077	22,922	14,786	13,352	15,283
Tuberculosis[4]	NA	55,494	37,137	27,749	25,701	16,377	11,182	10,528	9,945
Sexually transmitted diseases[5]									
Syphilis[6]	217,558	122,538	91,382	68,832	135,590	31,618	45,844	46,040	49,903
Primary and secondary	23,939	16,145	21,982	27,204	50,578	5,979	13,774	13,970	15,667
Early latent	59,256	18,017	16,311	20,297	55,397	9,465	13,604	13,136	14,503
Late and late latent[7]	113,569	81,798	50,348	20,979	25,750	15,594	18,079	18,576	19,411
Congenital[8]	13,377	4,416	1,953	277	3,865	580	387	358	322
Chlamydia[9]	NA	NA	NA	NA	323,663	709,452	1,307,893	1,412,791	1,422,976
Gonorrhea[10]	286,746	258,933	600,072	1,004,029	690,042	363,136	309,341	321,849	334,826
Chancroid	4,977	1,680	1,416	788	4,212	78	24	8	15

NOTE: The total resident population was used to calculate all rates except sexually transmitted diseases (STDs), which used the civilian resident population prior to 1991.   NA = Not available.   - = Quantity zero.   0.00 = Rate more than zero but less than 0.005.   1 National surveillance case definition revised in 2008; probable cases not previously reported.   2 Cases of vaccine-associated paralytic poliomyelitis caused by polio vaccine virus.   3 Starting with 2010 data, cases of Rocky Mountain spotted fever were reported as Spotted fever rickettsiosis.   4 Case reporting for tuberculosis began in 1953. Data prior to 1975 are not comparable with subsequent years because of changes in reporting criteria effective in 1975. Data from 1993 to 2009 were updated through the Division of Tuberculosis Elimination, National Center for HIV/AIDS, Viral Hepatitis, STD, and TB Prevention (NCHHSTP), as of May 14, 2010.   5 For 1950, data for Alaska and Hawaii were not included. Starting with 1991, data include both civilian and military cases. Adjustments to the number of cases reported from state health departments were made for hardcopy forms and for electronic data submissions through June 9, 2010. Cases and rates shown do not include U.S. outlying areas of Guam, Puerto Rico, and the Virgin Islands.   6 Includes stage of syphilis not stated.   7 Includes cases of unknown duration.   8 Rates include all cases of congenitally acquired syphilis per 100,000 live births. Cases of congenitally acquired syphilis were reported through 1994; starting with 1995 data, only congenital syphilis for cases less than 1 year of age were reported.   9 Prior to 1994, chlamydia was not notifiable. In 1994-1999, cases for New York were exclusively reported by New York City. Starting with 2000 data, includes for New York were exclusively reported by New York City. Starting with 2000 data, includes cases for the entire state.   10 Data for 1994 do not include cases from Georgia.

Table 3-2. Age-Adjusted Cancer Incidence Rates for Selected Cancer Sites, by Sex, Race, and Hispanic Origin, Selected Geographic Areas, Selected Years, 1990–2011

(Number of new cases per 100,000 population. 1)

Site, sex, race, and Hispanic origin	1990	1995	2000	2005	2010	2011	1990–2011 APC[2]
All Sites							
All persons	475.8	471.2	474.8	460.2	447.1	438.1	^-0.4
White	483.4	477.9	486.3	473.2	458.6	448.7	^-0.3
Black or African American	513.5	536.0	520.8	500.3	476.5	466.3	^-0.6
American Indian or Alaska Native[3]	347.0	369.1	362.9	402.9	395.7	370.5	0.3
Asian or Pacific Islander	334.3	337.6	337.4	326.9	317.4	314.0	^-0.4
Hispanic or Latino[4]	355.6	359.3	360.8	364.2	344.1	345.6	^-0.2
White, not Hispanic or Latino[4]	495.4	491.7	504.2	491.3	479.4	468.3	^-0.2
Male	584.0	564.5	565.1	534.1	508.0	491.8	^-0.9
White	591.2	563.9	570.3	543.5	514.9	498.0	^-0.8
Black or African American	686.4	738.0	700.7	630.2	586.6	557.2	^-1.3
American Indian or Alaska Native[3]	393.8	423.0	372.5	425.0	440.6	393.4	-0.1
Asian or Pacific Islander	385.3	396.0	395.2	366.2	339.7	334.3	^-0.9
Hispanic or Latino[4]	416.9	439.9	435.0	426.0	392.7	385.6	^-0.6
White, not Hispanic or Latino[4]	606.8	577.8	589.4	561.6	535.8	518.1	^-0.8
Female	411.5	410.5	413.8	409.2	404.0	400.8	-0.1
White	421.5	423.7	430.6	425.1	419.0	414.9	0.0
Black or African American	405.1	400.9	399.8	412.7	400.2	403.9	0.0
American Indian or Alaska Native[3]	315.6	334.7	362.4	387.9	370.7	359.1	^0.7
Asian or Pacific Islander	294.3	294.8	297.5	302.2	305.9	303.5	0.1
Hispanic or Latina[4]	322.3	310.1	316.9	325.6	314.6	322.5	0.1
White, not Hispanic or Latina[4]	430.8	437.2	446.6	442.7	438.9	433.5	0.1
Lung and Bronchus							
Male	95.0	86.9	77.8	71.5	62.7	60.1	^-2.0
White	94.2	85.1	76.4	70.9	62.5	59.6	^-2.0
Black or African American	133.9	136.7	110.8	97.7	81.5	81.4	^-2.5
American Indian or Alaska Native[3]	74.8	82.8	62.6	67.4	63.1	52.3	-0.9
Asian or Pacific Islander	64.2	60.0	63.3	57.6	50.0	48.7	^-1.2
Hispanic or Latino[4]	59.4	52.4	45.2	44.0	34.1	35.2	^-2.0
White, not Hispanic or Latino[4]	97.4	88.4	80.3	74.7	66.9	63.5	^-1.8
Female	47.2	49.3	48.6	49.9	45.7	44.4	-0.2
White	48.5	51.7	50.8	52.0	47.8	46.1	-0.1
Black or African American	52.9	49.8	54.7	57.9	52.1	48.7	0.0
American Indian or Alaska Native[3]	30.4	46.1	38.5	45.5	36.4	41.5	1.2
Asian or Pacific Islander	28.3	27.2	27.1	30.5	28.8	30.6	^0.3
Hispanic or Latina[4]	26.2	25.1	24.2	22.9	24.3	23.4	^-0.4
White, not Hispanic or Latina[4]	50.8	54.9	54.4	56.5	51.7	50.2	0.0
Colon and Rectum							
Male	72.3	63.2	62.6	54.6	46.7	45.1	^-2.0
White	73.0	62.5	62.2	54.2	45.2	43.3	^-2.2
Black or African American	72.7	74.8	72.7	66.5	57.4	55.5	^-1.2
American Indian or Alaska Native[3]	61.9	66.2	48.0	65.6	63.7	63.3	-0.2
Asian or Pacific Islander	60.8	58.2	57.4	46.9	45.0	44.7	^-1.5
Hispanic or Latino[4]	47.6	46.0	50.5	47.3	42.0	42.6	^-0.6
White, not Hispanic or Latino[4]	75.1	64.0	63.5	54.9	45.8	43.4	^-2.2
Female	50.2	45.9	46.1	41.4	35.8	34.4	^-1.5
White	49.7	45.5	45.6	40.3	34.4	33.4	^-1.6
Black or African American	61.1	54.7	58.0	53.9	45.6	41.5	^-1.1
American Indian or Alaska Native[3]	45.8	47.9	39.1	48.3	41.0	45.7	-0.2
Asian or Pacific Islander	37.6	38.5	37.3	36.7	33.8	31.1	^-1.0
Hispanic or Latina[4]	34.4	31.9	34.0	33.5	30.3	28.8	^-0.5
White, not Hispanic or Latina[4]	50.9	46.8	46.8	41.3	34.9	34.2	^-1.6
Prostate							
Male	166.9	166.5	178.9	153.9	141.7	135.4	^-1.6
White	168.5	161.4	175.1	149.9	137.2	129.6	^-1.7
Black or African American	218.9	277.2	288.8	240.1	214.9	202.7	^-1.6
American Indian or Alaska Native[3]	99.5	92.5	69.6	93.8	83.0	63.9	^-1.7
Asian or Pacific Islander	88.3	103.9	106.7	94.2	76.8	77.1	^-1.5
Hispanic or Latino[4]	118.8	140.8	149.9	132.3	115.4	108.1	^-1.2
White, not Hispanic or Latino[4]	172.3	163.8	178.8	152.6	141.3	134.0	^-1.6
Breast							
Female	129.4	130.9	134.2	124.3	122.9	126.2	^-0.3
White	134.3	136.5	140.9	129.9	127.0	130.0	^-0.3
Black or African American	116.9	122.1	120.9	118.3	122.1	127.3	^0.2
American Indian or Alaska Native[3]	69.6	94.2	99.1	105.6	91.1	104.0	0.5
Asian or Pacific Islander	87.7	87.0	93.7	92.9	98.5	100.8	^0.6
Hispanic or Latina[4]	90.8	89.2	96.7	92.9	86.0	95.0	0.0
White, not Hispanic or Latina[4]	138.7	142.0	147.3	136.6	135.4	137.0	-0.2
Cervix Uteri							
Female	11.9	9.9	8.9	7.9	7.2	7.0	^-2.5
White	11.2	9.2	8.9	7.8	7.2	7.2	^-2.0
Black or African American	16.5	14.8	10.6	9.2	8.4	7.7	^-3.7
American Indian or Alaska Native[3]	14.7	*	*	10.7	8.3	9.5	^-2.0

Table 3-2. Age-Adjusted Cancer Incidence Rates for Selected Cancer Sites, by Sex, Race, and Hispanic Origin, Selected Geographic Areas, Selected Years, 1990–2011— continued

(Number of new cases per 100,000 population. [1])

Site, sex, race, and Hispanic origin	1990	1995	2000	2005	2010	2011	1990–2011 APC[2]
Asian or Pacific Islander	12.1	11.1	7.9	7.8	6.4	5.3	^-4.0
Hispanic or Latina[4]	21.3	17.4	17.0	13.7	10.4	9.3	^-3.8
White, not Hispanic or Latina[4]	9.7	7.8	7.1	6.4	6.2	6.5	^-1.9
Corpus and Uterus, Not Otherwise Specified							
Female	24.7	24.9	23.9	24.1	26.6	26.5	^0.3
White	26.4	26.5	25.6	25.5	27.5	27.1	0.1
Black or African American	17.0	17.8	17.2	21.4	24.5	27.7	^2.3
American Indian or Alaska Native[3]	19.3	*	18.5	14.4	27.5	19.1	*
Asian or Pacific Islander	13.5	17.8	16.5	18.6	22.1	21.5	^1.7
Hispanic or Latina[4]	17.7	16.5	15.8	19.2	20.2	22.0	^1.2
White, not Hispanic or Latina[4]	27.1	27.5	26.9	26.2	28.5	27.6	0.1
Ovary							
Female	15.6	14.5	14.2	13.1	12.4	12.0	^-1.1
White	16.4	15.4	15.1	13.9	13.3	12.8	^-1.0
Black or African American	11.3	10.8	10.7	10.7	9.3	9.7	-0.5
American Indian or Alaska Native[3]	21.9	*	18.9	12.2	11.8	10.7	*
Asian or Pacific Islander	11.2	10.4	10.2	10.8	9.5	9.3	^-0.5
Hispanic or Latina[4]	12.2	11.7	10.6	11.8	11.7	10.9	-0.4
White, not Hispanic or Latina[4]	16.7	15.9	15.7	14.1	13.3	13.0	^-1.0
Oral Cavity and Pharynx							
Male	18.5	16.5	15.8	15.1	15.4	15.8	^-0.8
White	18.0	16.3	15.7	15.5	16.0	16.7	^-0.4
Black or African American	25.4	22.3	19.3	15.7	13.4	13.6	^-2.9
American Indian or Alaska Native[3]	*	*	*	10.4	21.1	15.9	*
Asian or Pacific Islander	14.9	11.8	13.2	11.3	11.6	10.5	^-1.1
Hispanic or Latino[4]	10.7	12.3	9.0	9.7	8.7	10.5	-0.7
White, not Hispanic or Latino[4]	18.8	16.9	16.7	16.4	17.4	17.9	-0.2
Female	7.3	7.0	6.2	6.2	6.1	6.1	^-0.9
White	7.4	7.1	6.2	6.0	6.3	6.3	^-0.9
Black or African American	6.4	6.6	5.4	6.9	5.2	5.1	^-1.3
American Indian or Alaska Native[3]	*	*	*	*	*	*	*
Asian or Pacific Islander	6.1	5.2	6.2	5.8	5.1	4.7	^-1.1
Hispanic or Latina[4]	3.9	3.7	3.7	3.5	4.1	3.7	-0.4
White, not Hispanic or Latina[4]	7.8	7.6	6.6	6.5	6.7	6.9	^-0.7
Stomach							
Male	14.6	13.5	12.6	11.4	10.4	10.4	^-1.7
White	12.8	11.9	10.7	9.6	9.3	9.5	^-1.6
Black or African American	21.4	18.6	18.4	17.4	13.3	13.6	^-2.2
American Indian or Alaska Native[3]	*	24.1	20.2	20.8	18.4	20.0	-0.5
Asian or Pacific Islander	26.8	24.5	22.8	20.1	15.0	13.8	^-3.0
Hispanic or Latino[4]	20.2	19.3	16.1	15.5	14.8	14.0	^-1.6
White, not Hispanic or Latino[4]	12.1	11.1	10.0	8.7	8.2	8.4	^-1.9
Female	6.7	6.2	6.1	5.7	5.6	5.6	^-0.9
White	5.7	5.1	5.0	4.7	4.7	4.7	^-0.9
Black or African American	9.9	9.8	8.6	8.1	8.5	9.3	^-0.9
American Indian or Alaska Native[3]	*	*	*	*	13.0	*	*
Asian or Pacific Islander	15.4	13.0	12.9	10.3	8.8	7.7	^-2.8
Hispanic or Latina[4]	10.8	11.2	10.6	10.2	9.4	8.7	^-1.1
White, not Hispanic or Latina[4]	5.1	4.4	4.2	3.8	3.6	3.8	^-1.6
Pancreas							
Male	13.0	12.7	12.8	13.6	13.6	14.0	^0.5
White	12.7	12.4	12.6	13.4	13.5	14.0	^0.7
Black or African American	19.3	19.1	18.1	18.1	18.5	16.7	-0.3
American Indian or Alaska Native[3]	*	*	*	21.2	17.2	17.4	*
Asian or Pacific Islander	11.0	10.3	10.7	11.7	11.2	12.1	0.1
Hispanic or Latino[4]	10.7	12.0	12.2	12.3	11.5	13.5	^1.1
White, not Hispanic or Latino[4]	12.8	12.4	12.7	13.6	13.7	14.1	^0.7
Female	10.0	9.9	9.9	10.8	11.2	10.4	^0.5
White	9.7	9.6	9.6	10.6	10.8	10.2	^0.6
Black or African American	12.9	15.5	12.7	16.4	15.0	14.9	0.0
American Indian or Alaska Native[3]	*	*	20.4	12.4	12.9	*	*
Asian or Pacific Islander	9.9	8.1	9.2	8.0	10.3	9.0	^0.9
Hispanic or Latina[4]	9.9	9.0	9.1	11.1	9.9	9.6	0.0
White, not Hispanic or Latina[4]	9.7	9.7	9.6	10.6	11.0	10.3	^0.7
Urinary Bladder							
Male	37.2	35.4	36.8	37.0	35.7	33.5	^-0.2
White	40.7	38.9	40.8	41.0	39.8	37.5	-0.1
Black or African American	19.5	19.3	20.2	22.9	22.0	20.3	0.4
American Indian or Alaska Native[3]	*	*	*	16.8	16.0	16.5	*
Asian or Pacific Islander	15.4	16.7	16.6	17.0	17.0	14.5	0.5
Hispanic or Latino[4]	22.4	17.8	20.4	20.0	18.5	19.7	-0.3
White, not Hispanic or Latino[4]	42.4	41.0	43.2	43.7	43.0	40.3	0.0
Female	9.5	9.3	9.1	9.0	8.6	8.2	^-0.5

Table 3-2. Age-Adjusted Cancer Incidence Rates for Selected Cancer Sites, by Sex, Race, and Hispanic Origin, Selected Geographic Areas, Selected Years, 1990–2011— continued

(Number of new cases per 100,000 population. 1)

Site, sex, race, and Hispanic origin	1990	1995	2000	2005	2010	2011	1990–2011 APC[2]
White	10.0	10.1	10.0	9.7	9.4	9.1	^-0.4
Black or African American	8.6	7.2	7.7	7.8	6.9	7.0	-0.4
American Indian or Alaska Native[3]	*	*	*	*	*	*	*
Asian or Pacific Islander	5.3	4.4	4.1	5.1	4.6	4.1	-0.2
Hispanic or Latina[4]	5.8	5.3	5.8	6.0	4.6	5.5	-0.3
White, not Hispanic or Latina[4]	10.3	10.6	10.5	10.3	10.2	9.7	^-0.2
Non-Hodgkin's Lymphoma							
Male	22.6	25.1	23.5	24.7	25.2	23.5	^0.2
White	23.6	26.2	25.0	25.9	26.4	24.8	^0.3
Black or African American	17.4	21.5	17.5	19.5	21.1	17.1	0.1
American Indian or Alaska Native[3]	*	*	15.3	23.2	18.2	10.7	*
Asian or Pacific Islander	16.7	16.5	15.9	17.9	17.2	17.4	0.2
Hispanic or Latino[4]	17.3	21.0	20.4	19.9	22.8	19.8	^0.5
White, not Hispanic or Latino[4]	24.3	26.7	25.5	26.9	27.0	25.5	^0.4
Female	14.5	15.2	16.0	16.5	16.9	15.7	^0.7
White	15.4	16.0	16.9	17.7	18.0	16.3	^0.7
Black or African American	10.3	10.2	11.8	13.2	12.6	12.8	^1.4
American Indian or Alaska Native[3]	*	*	13.5	13.1	12.9	15.0	*
Asian or Pacific Islander	9.1	11.8	11.4	9.5	11.7	11.9	0.6
Hispanic or Latina[4]	13.7	13.1	13.8	15.0	15.4	14.3	^0.9
White, not Hispanic or Latina[4]	15.6	16.2	17.3	18.1	18.3	16.7	^0.8
Leukemia							
Male	17.2	17.6	17.1	17.3	17.4	16.9	0.0
White	18.0	19.0	18.2	18.8	18.8	18.0	0.1
Black or African American	16.0	13.4	14.1	12.6	13.2	13.9	0.0
American Indian or Alaska Native[3]	*	*	*	12.3	*	9.7	*
Asian or Pacific Islander	8.5	10.0	10.4	9.1	9.8	10.0	-0.2
Hispanic or Latino[4]	12.2	14.6	13.1	13.2	12.6	12.9	0.3
White, not Hispanic or Latino[4]	18.3	19.3	18.7	19.2	19.3	18.6	0.1
Female	9.9	10.2	10.4	10.0	10.4	10.0	0.2
White	10.3	10.9	11.0	10.5	11.1	10.8	^0.3
Black or African American	8.5	8.2	9.7	9.4	8.7	8.6	-0.2
American Indian or Alaska Native[3]	*	*	*	*	7.7	*	*
Asian or Pacific Islander	5.7	6.4	6.3	6.3	5.8	6.0	-0.1
Hispanic or Latina[4]	8.5	8.2	7.8	8.2	8.6	8.4	0.3
White, not Hispanic or Latina[4]	10.3	11.1	11.0	10.6	11.4	11.0	^0.4

NOTE: Estimates are based on 13 SEER areas, November 2011 submission and differ from published estimates based on 9 SEER areas or other submission dates. The site variable distinguishes Kaposi Sarcoma and Mesothelioma as individual cancer sites. As a result, Kaposi Sarcoma and Mesothelioma cases do not contribute to other cancer sites.   ^ =Annual percent change (APC) is significantly different from 0 (p<0.05).   0.0 = APC is greater than -0.05 but less than 0.05.   *Estimates are considered unreliable. Data not shown if the rate is based on fewer than 16 cases for the time interval.   1 Age adjusted by 5-year age groups to the year 2000 U.S. standard population. Age-adjusted rates are based on at least 16 cases.   2 APC has been calculated by fitting a linear regression model to the natural logarithm of the yearly rates from 1990–2011.   3 Estimates for the American Indian or Alaska Native populations are based on the Contract Health Service Delivery Area (CHSDA) counties within SEER areas.   4 Hispanic data exclude cases from Alaska. The race groups White, Black, Asian or Pacific Islander, and American Indian or Alaska Native, include persons of Hispanic and non-Hispanic origin. Persons of Hispanic origin may be of any race. The North American Association of Central Cancer Registries (NAACCR) Hispanic Identification Algorithm was used on a combination of variables to classify cases as Hispanic for analytic purposes.

Table 3-3. Five-Year Relative Cancer Survival Rates for Selected Cancer Sites, by Sex and Selected Race, Selected Geographic Areas, Selected Years 1975–1977 through 2004–2010

(Percent of patients.)

Sex and site	White					Black or African American				
	1975–1977	1984–1986	1996–1998	1999–2003	2004–2010	1975–1977	1984–1986	1996–1998	1999–2003	2004–2010
Both Sexes										
All sites	49.8	53.6	64.4	67.7	69.4	39.0	40.1	55.1	58.4	61.5
Oral cavity and pharynx	54.0	56.3	59.9	63.5	67.4	35.8	35.1	36.0	45.0	44.9
Esophagus	5.5	10.2	14.2	18.7	21.0	3.5	8.7	10.2	12.0	13.2
Stomach	14.1	16.8	20.4	23.7	28.1	16.1	19.1	22.4	24.8	28.2
Colon	50.9	59.0	62.9	66.3	66.5	44.7	49.1	53.5	54.1	55.8
Rectum	48.2	57.0	63.6	67.8	68.0	44.4	45.8	54.8	60.2	63.2
Pancreas	2.5	2.6	4.1	5.3	7.2	2.3	4.7	3.4	4.5	6.7
Lung and bronchus	12.2	13.0	14.8	15.8	18.2	11.3	11.1	12.3	12.7	14.9
Urinary bladder	73.3	77.2	79.8	81.0	79.8	50.3	59.4	62.1	65.9	64.0
Non-Hodgkin's lymphoma	46.8	52.0	59.5	67.4	72.5	48.4	46.7	54.2	59.0	63.0
Leukemia	34.6	41.6	49.4	54.1	61.0	33.2	32.7	38.2	45.4	54.0
Male										
All sites	42.7	48.6	64.1	68.1	70.0	32.7	35.4	57.8	61.9	64.9
Oral cavity and pharynx	53.7	54.8	59.1	63.5	67.4	29.7	29.5	31.1	39.8	42.3
Esophagus	4.8	9.0	14.0	18.7	20.9	2.0	8.2	8.5	9.5	12.8
Stomach	13.1	14.4	18.6	22.0	26.7	16.1	16.9	20.2	24.0	23.0
Colon	50.5	59.6	62.9	66.9	67.3	44.0	48.9	55.4	54.2	55.4
Rectum	47.3	56.4	62.9	67.9	68.3	41.4	43.1	53.2	60.1	58.1
Pancreas	2.7	2.1	4.7	5.6	6.9	2.5	3.9	3.1	3.0	7.6
Lung and bronchus	11.1	11.3	13.0	13.7	15.8	10.6	10.3	10.7	11.3	13.0
Prostate gland	68.5	76.4	97.9	99.8	99.8	60.7	65.6	94.8	97.5	97.9
Urinary bladder	74.3	78.4	81.1	81.9	81.4	56.5	62.3	65.3	71.0	68.0
Non-Hodgkin's lymphoma	46.3	50.6	57.6	65.7	71.5	42.6	44.5	52.7	54.0	58.8
Leukemia	33.6	41.3	49.3	54.6	61.9	30.0	31.5	38.8	46.3	58.1
Female										
All sites	56.5	58.5	64.7	67.2	68.7	46.2	45.5	51.9	54.3	57.7
Colon	51.3	58.5	62.9	65.6	65.8	45.3	49.2	51.9	54.0	56.1
Rectum	49.4	57.7	64.5	67.8	67.5	46.8	48.2	56.2	60.0	68.3
Pancreas	2.3	3.1	3.6	5.1	7.4	1.9	5.3	3.5	5.8	5.9
Lung and bronchus	15.4	16.3	17.0	18.3	20.7	13.8	12.8	14.8	14.5	17.1
Melanoma of skin	86.2	90.9	92.7	95.0	95.0	*	*	78.6	71.4	81.2
Breast	75.6	80.0	89.4	91.2	91.8	62.0	65.0	76.1	78.1	80.0
Cervix uteri	69.7	68.8	73.6	72.6	71.0	64.6	57.8	64.7	64.5	62.0
Corpus uteri, not otherwise specified	88.0	84.0	85.2	85.9	85.3	60.2	56.2	61.5	60.5	64.7
Ovary	35.3	37.5	43.2	43.3	44.3	41.8	39.4	39.1	35.7	36.4
Non-Hodgkin's lymphoma	47.3	53.6	61.6	69.4	73.6	54.8	49.6	56.4	64.9	67.7

NOTE: Rates are based on follow-up of patients through 2009. The rate is the ratio of the observed survival rate for the patient group to the expected survival rate for persons in the general population similar to the patient group with respect to age, sex, race, and calendar year of observation. It estimates the chance of surviving the effects of cancer. The site variable distinguishes Kaposi Sarcoma and Mesothelioma as individual cancer sites. As a result, Kaposi Sarcoma and Mesothelioma cases are excluded from each of the sites shown except all sites combined. The race groups White and Black include persons of Hispanic and non-Hispanic origin. Due to death certificate race-ethnicity classification and other methodological issues related to developing life tables, survival rates for race-ethnicity groups other than White and Black are not calculated.   *Data for population groups with fewer than 25 cases are not shown because estimates are considered unreliable.

Table 3-4A. Respondent-Reported Prevalence of Heart Disease[1], Cancer[2], and Stroke[3] Among Adults 18 Years of Age and Over, by Selected Characteristics, Selected Years, 1999–2000 through 2012–2013

(Percent.)

Characteristic	Heart disease[1]										
	1999–2000	2000–2001	2001–2002	2003–2004	2005–2006	2007–2008	2008–2009	2009–2010	2010–2011	2011–2012	2012–2013
18 years and over, age adjusted[4,5]	11.1	11.5	11.5	11.3	11.2	11.3	11.5	11.4	11.1	10.8	10.6
18 years and over, crude[5]	10.9	11.3	11.3	11.3	11.4	11.6	11.8	11.8	11.6	11.4	11.4
Age											
18 to 44 years	4.3	4.4	4.3	4.1	4.0	4.4	4.5	4.4	4.0	3.7	3.8
18 to 24 years	3.3	3.4	3.3	3.0	3.2	3.1	3.3	3.4	3.0	2.6	2.6
25 to 44 years	4.6	4.7	4.6	4.5	4.2	4.8	4.9	4.8	4.4	4.0	4.2
45 to 64 years	12.6	12.9	12.9	12.5	12.9	12.2	12.7	13.1	13.0	12.5	12.1
45 to 54 years	10.0	10.2	10.0	9.4	9.4	8.8	9.5	10.1	9.6	9.2	8.9
55 to 64 years	16.6	17.1	17.4	17.0	17.8	16.8	16.8	17.0	17.1	16.2	15.8
65 years and over	29.6	30.9	31.3	31.8	31.2	31.8	31.7	30.4	30.5	30.3	29.8
65 to 74 years	25.8	26.6	26.6	27.3	26.5	26.9	26.2	25.1	25.6	25.5	25.0
75 years and over	34.3	36.0	36.8	36.8	36.6	37.5	38.0	37.0	36.5	36.4	36.3
Sex [4]											
Male	11.9	12.3	12.4	12.3	12.2	12.5	12.8	12.8	12.4	12.1	11.9
Female	10.5	10.9	10.8	10.7	10.5	10.5	10.5	10.3	10.2	9.7	9.6
Sex and Age											
Male											
18 to 44 years	3.6	3.6	3.6	3.6	3.3	3.8	4.4	4.3	3.7	3.6	3.8
45 to 54 years	10.0	10.2	10.1	8.7	9.8	9.2	10.0	10.4	9.5	9.6	9.8
55 to 64 years	19.7	19.4	19.9	20.4	20.5	18.3	18.8	19.0	19.1	18.5	17.9
65 to 74 years	30.4	31.4	31.9	33.1	31.6	32.0	30.5	30.8	31.3	30.7	30.1
75 years and over	39.2	42.7	43.6	42.6	43.1	46.5	46.6	45.3	44.7	43.5	41.7
Female											
18 to 44 years	4.9	5.1	4.9	4.7	4.7	4.9	4.7	4.5	4.3	3.8	3.7
45 to 54 years	9.9	10.1	9.9	10.1	9.1	8.4	9.0	9.8	9.6	8.9	8.1
55 to 64 years	13.8	14.9	15.2	13.9	15.4	15.4	14.9	15.1	15.3	14.1	13.8
65 to 74 years	22.0	22.7	22.2	22.5	22.2	22.5	22.6	20.2	20.6	21.0	20.5
75 years and over	31.2	31.9	32.6	33.1	32.4	31.7	32.3	31.3	30.9	31.5	32.6
Race [4,6]											
White only	11.3	11.7	11.7	11.6	11.5	11.7	11.9	11.6	11.2	10.8	10.8
Black or African American only	10.6	10.9	10.6	9.8	10.1	10.2	10.7	11.0	10.7	10.7	10.5
American Indian or Alaska Native only	14.7	14.2	11.4	12.8	15.9	11.1	10.2	10.3	12.5	12.1	10.1
Asian only	6.3	7.3	8.8	6.3	6.8	6.0	5.7	6.7	7.2	7.0	6.4
Native Hawaiian or Other Pacific Islander only	*	*	*	*	*	*	*	*	*	*	*
Two or more races	17.0	16.8	16.5	12.5	14.7	16.9	15.2	15.5	16.7	16.8	15.5
Hispanic Origin and Race [4,6]											
Hispanic or Latino	8.0	8.0	8.0	8.5	8.0	8.5	8.4	8.3	8.4	8.2	8.0
Mexican	7.4	7.5	7.8	8.9	7.5	8.3	8.4	8.4	8.4	8.1	8.0
Not Hispanic or Latino	11.4	11.8	11.8	11.6	11.6	11.7	11.9	11.8	11.4	11.1	11.0
White only	11.6	12.0	12.1	12.0	12.0	12.1	12.4	12.1	11.7	11.3	11.3
Black or African American only	10.5	10.9	10.5	9.8	10.2	10.2	10.8	11.1	10.8	10.8	10.5
Education [7,8]											
No high school diploma or GED	13.8	14.3	14.3	14.3	14.2	14.9	14.5	14.5	14.6	13.9	13.7
High school diploma or GED	11.9	12.3	12.4	12.3	12.6	11.9	12.7	12.7	12.4	11.9	12.1
Some college or more	12.0	12.5	12.4	12.2	11.9	12.4	12.4	12.2	11.9	11.6	11.3
Percent of Poverty Level [4,9]											
Below 100 percent	13.6	14.7	14.4	14.3	14.6	14.0	14.1	14.5	13.9	13.3	13.8
100 percent to 199 percent	12.0	12.5	12.4	12.8	12.5	13.0	13.2	12.8	12.3	11.9	12.0
200 percent to 399 percent	11.0	11.3	11.3	11.4	11.0	11.7	11.6	11.3	11.3	10.7	10.5
400 percent or more	10.2	10.6	10.9	10.0	10.1	10.0	10.1	10.0	9.8	9.5	9.3
Hispanic Origin and Race and Percent of Poverty Level [4,8,9]											
Hispanic or Latino											
Below 100 percent	9.7	8.8	8.7	11.3	11.0	11.0	10.3	10.3	9.4	9.4	10.0
100 percent to 199 percent	8.4	8.9	9.0	8.0	8.1	9.6	8.8	7.9	8.3	8.5	8.4
200 percent to 399 percent	8.2	7.3	6.5	8.2	6.9	7.1	7.7	8.4	8.5	7.9	7.0
400 percent or more	5.6	6.6	6.9	5.4	5.1	8.0	7.1	7.2	7.5	7.3	7.2

Table 3-4A. Respondent-Reported Prevalence of Heart Disease[1], Cancer[2], and Stroke[3] Among Adults 18 Years of Age and Over, by Selected Characteristics, Selected Years, 1999–2000 through 2012–2013— continued

(Percent.)

Characteristic	Heart disease[1]											
	1999–2000	2000–2001	2001–2002	2003–2004	2005–2006	2007–2008	2008–2009	2009–2010	2010–2011	2011–2012	2012–2013
Not Hispanic or Latino											
White only											
Below 100 percent	15.2	16.9	16.5	15.9	16.9	16.0	15.9	16.3	15.8	15.1	16.1
100 percent to 199 percent	12.8	13.6	13.5	14.8	14.3	14.7	15.6	15.1	13.8	13.3	13.7
200 percent to 399 percent	11.6	12.0	12.1	12.3	11.9	12.9	12.8	12.1	11.8	11.3	11.1
400 percent or more	10.6	11.0	11.3	10.3	10.6	10.5	10.6	10.5	10.2	9.9	9.7
Black or African American only											
Below 100 percent	13.0	14.5	14.1	14.1	13.2	13.2	15.2	15.7	14.7	14.3	14.0
100 percent to 199 percent	11.2	11.9	12.3	10.5	10.7	11.3	10.9	10.5	11.2	11.8	11.0
200 percent to 399 percent	10.2	9.8	9.0	8.0	9.1	9.3	9.3	10.2	10.5	9.4	9.6
400 percent or more	8.9	8.1	8.0	7.7	8.5	7.7	8.9	8.7	7.3	8.7	8.4
Geographic Region [4]											
Northeast	10.6	10.8	10.9	10.8	11.0	10.9	11.1	10.8	10.1	9.8	9.7
Midwest	11.4	12.2	12.1	11.8	12.3	12.4	12.4	12.1	11.5	11.2	11.8
South	11.5	11.9	11.7	11.7	11.5	11.7	12.3	12.3	12.1	11.7	11.2
West	10.4	10.5	10.9	10.5	9.8	9.9	9.7	9.8	9.9	9.5	9.3
Location of Residence											
Within MSA[10]	10.7	11.1	11.2	10.9	10.9	10.8	11.2	11.2	10.8	10.4	10.3
Outside MSA[10]	12.5	12.9	12.7	13.0	13.0	14.1	13.1	12.5	13.0	12.7	12.5

Table 3-4B. Respondent-Reported Prevalence of Cancer Among Adults 18 Years of Age and Over, by Selected Characteristics, Selected Years, 1999–2000 through 2012–2013

(Percent.)

Characteristic	Cancer[2]										
	1999–2000	2000–2001	2001–2002	2003–2004	2005–2006	2007–2008	2008–2009	2009–2010	2010–2011	2011–2012	2012–2013
18 years and over, age adjusted[4,5]	5.1	5.1	5.3	5.2	5.7	5.6	5.9	6.0	6.0	5.9	5.9
18 years and over, crude[5]	4.9	5.0	5.2	5.2	5.7	5.8	6.1	6.3	6.3	6.2	6.4
Age											
18 to 44 years	1.7	1.7	1.7	1.5	1.8	1.7	1.6	1.6	1.7	1.6	1.6
18 to 24 years	1.0	0.8	0.8	0.7	0.9	0.8	0.8	0.7	0.7	*0.7	*0.5
25 to 44 years	1.9	2.0	2.1	1.7	2.2	2.0	1.9	2.0	2.0	1.9	1.9
45 to 64 years	5.2	5.3	5.7	5.8	6.0	6.3	6.7	7.1	6.9	6.5	6.7
45 to 54 years	4.0	4.1	4.2	4.2	4.4	4.6	4.9	5.3	4.9	4.4	4.4
55 to 64 years	7.2	7.3	7.9	8.1	8.2	8.6	9.2	9.3	9.3	8.9	9.3
65 years and over	15.2	15.2	15.6	15.9	17.1	17.0	17.7	18.1	18.5	18.5	18.4
65 to 74 years	13.1	13.1	13.9	13.8	14.3	14.6	15.8	16.1	15.9	16.2	16.2
75 years and over	17.7	17.8	17.6	18.3	20.2	19.8	20.0	20.5	21.7	21.5	21.4
Sex [4]											
Male	4.4	4.4	4.7	4.7	5.1	4.8	5.0	5.5	5.5	5.3	5.4
Female	5.8	5.8	6.0	5.9	6.4	6.5	6.8	6.6	6.6	6.5	6.5
Sex and Age											
Male											
18 to 44 years	0.8	0.8	0.7	0.7	0.8	0.8	0.7	0.8	0.9	0.8	0.7
45 to 54 years	2.0	2.0	2.2	2.7	2.6	2.6	2.9	3.3	3.1	2.9	2.9
55 to 64 years	5.9	5.7	6.5	6.7	6.8	7.2	7.0	7.8	7.5	7.0	8.2
65 to 74 years	13.9	14.0	16.1	14.3	15.5	14.3	16.2	17.6	16.9	17.3	17.3
75 years and over	20.3	21.6	20.8	22.1	24.3	21.9	22.2	24.8	26.1	24.7	24.6
Female											
18 to 44 years	2.5	2.6	2.7	2.3	2.9	2.5	2.5	2.4	2.5	2.3	2.4
45 to 54 years	5.9	6.0	6.1	5.7	6.2	6.4	6.8	7.3	6.6	5.8	5.9
55 to 64 years	8.4	8.7	9.1	9.5	9.5	10.0	11.2	10.7	10.9	10.7	10.4
65 to 74 years	12.5	12.3	12.1	13.4	13.3	14.8	15.6	14.9	15.0	15.2	15.2
75 years and over	16.1	15.4	15.5	15.9	17.6	18.5	18.5	17.6	18.7	19.3	19.2
Race [4,6]											
White only	5.4	5.4	5.6	5.5	6.0	6.0	6.2	6.3	6.3	6.1	6.2
Black or African American only	3.5	3.4	3.3	4.0	3.9	4.4	4.3	4.7	5.1	4.9	4.8
American Indian or Alaska Native only	*5.7	*	*	7.0	*7.4	*4.3	*5.4	7.0	6.5	*	*4.3
Asian only	*2.3	*2.0	*1.6	3.0	2.9	3.1	3.0	2.9	3.0	3.7	3.4
Native Hawaiian or Other Pacific Islander only	*	*	*	*	*	*	*	*	*	*	*
Two or more races	*4.7	*4.5	7.1	*3.4	7.8	5.8	9.1	9.8	7.9	7.5	8.9
Hispanic Origin and Race [4,6]											
Hispanic or Latino	3.0	2.9	2.9	3.0	3.5	3.7	3.6	3.4	3.4	3.3	3.6
Mexican	2.8	2.6	2.9	2.6	3.1	3.6	3.3	3.2	3.2	2.9	3.3
Not Hispanic or Latino	5.2	5.3	5.5	5.5	5.9	5.9	6.1	6.3	6.3	6.2	6.2
White only	5.5	5.7	5.9	5.8	6.3	6.3	6.5	6.7	6.7	6.5	6.6
Black or African American only	3.6	3.4	3.3	3.9	3.9	4.3	4.2	4.7	5.1	4.8	4.8
Education [7,8]											
No high school diploma or GED	5.5	5.2	5.4	5.6	5.7	5.8	6.1	5.9	5.8	5.4	5.3
High school diploma or GED	5.8	6.1	6.3	5.7	6.4	6.1	6.4	6.7	6.8	6.8	7.0
Some college or more	5.9	6.0	6.2	6.4	6.9	6.9	7.1	7.4	7.4	7.0	7.0
Percent of Poverty Level [4,9]											
Below 100 percent	4.9	5.4	5.4	5.6	5.3	6.2	6.2	5.4	5.3	5.8	5.8
100 percent to 199 percent	5.3	5.0	5.0	5.6	5.7	5.8	6.0	6.1	5.9	5.3	5.5
200 percent to 399 percent	5.1	5.3	5.6	5.2	5.5	5.4	5.5	5.9	6.2	5.9	5.9
400 percent or more	5.1	5.1	5.2	5.0	6.1	5.8	6.0	6.3	6.2	6.2	6.2
Hispanic Origin and Race and Percent of Poverty Level [4,6,9]											
Hispanic or Latino											
Below 100 percent	2.3	2.7	2.9	2.9	3.5	5.0	3.8	2.8	2.9	3.4	3.8
100 percent to 199 percent	3.2	2.2	2.3	3.7	3.3	3.2	3.2	2.5	2.6	2.7	2.8
200 percent to 399 percent	2.7	*3.5	3.5	2.8	3.6	3.2	3.3	4.3	4.7	3.9	4.2
400 percent or more	*4.5	*	*3.1	*1.9	*3.4	3.6	4.2	4.2	3.3	3.5	4.0
Not Hispanic or Latino											
White only											
Below 100 percent	6.2	7.1	7.2	6.9	6.9	8.0	8.1	6.9	6.8	7.5	7.4
100 percent to 199 percent	6.2	6.0	5.9	6.6	6.7	7.4	7.4	7.3	7.3	6.5	6.9
200 percent to 399 percent	5.5	5.8	6.1	5.7	6.0	6.0	6.1	6.5	6.8	6.3	6.3
400 percent or more	5.3	5.3	5.5	5.3	6.5	6.0	6.2	6.6	6.6	6.6	6.6

Table 3-4B. Respondent-Reported Prevalence of Cancer Among Adults 18 Years of Age and Over, by Selected Characteristics, Selected Years, 1999–2000 through 2012–2013— continued

(Percent.)

Characteristic	Cancer[2]										
	1999–2000	2000–2001	2001–2002	2003–2004	2005–2006	2007–2008	2008–2009	2009–2010	2010–2011	2011–2012	2012–2013
Black or African American only											
Below 100 percent	4.0	3.8	3.2	4.6	3.6	4.6	4.9	4.9	4.5	4.3	4.1
100 percent to 199 percent	3.2	3.6	3.2	4.1	4.3	3.5	3.6	4.9	5.2	4.5	4.3
200 percent to 399 percent	3.7	3.0	3.6	3.5	4.2	4.4	4.0	4.3	5.3	5.5	5.7
400 percent or more	4.3	*3.7	*3.3	4.5	3.6	5.4	5.0	5.2	5.6	5.0	4.7
Geographic Region [4]											
Northeast	5.0	4.9	5.0	5.3	5.6	6.1	6.2	5.9	5.6	5.7	6.1
Midwest	5.2	5.2	5.7	5.3	5.7	5.5	5.8	6.4	6.7	6.4	6.4
South	5.0	5.2	5.3	5.2	5.6	5.8	5.9	6.1	6.2	5.8	5.8
West	5.0	5.0	5.1	5.2	5.7	5.3	5.6	5.6	5.5	5.6	5.5
Location of Residence [4]											
Within MSA[10]	5.0	5.0	5.1	5.1	5.6	5.6	5.7	5.9	5.9	5.7	5.8
Outside MSA[10]	5.5	5.5	6.0	5.7	6.0	6.2	7.0	6.8	6.7	6.8	6.7

Table 3-4C. Respondent-Reported Prevalence of Stroke Among Adults 18 Years of Age and Over, by Selected Characteristics, Selected Years, 1999–2000 through 2012–2013

(Percent.)

Characteristic	Stroke[3]										
	1999–2000	2000–2001	2001–2002	2003–2004	2005–2006	2007–2008	2008–2009	2009–2010	2010–2011	2011–2012	2012–2013
18 years and over, age adjusted[4,5]	2.2	2.3	2.4	2.5	2.5	2.6	2.7	2.6	2.6	2.5	2.5
18 years and over, crude[5]	2.1	2.3	2.4	2.5	2.5	2.7	2.8	2.7	2.7	2.7	2.7
Age											
18 to 44 years	0.4	0.4	0.4	0.4	0.4	0.5	0.6	0.6	0.6	0.5	0.5
18 to 24 years	*	*	*	*	*	*	*	*	*	*	*
25 to 44 years	0.5	0.5	0.5	0.5	0.5	0.6	0.7	0.7	0.7	0.7	0.6
45 to 64 years	2.0	2.2	2.4	2.4	2.3	2.9	2.7	2.8	2.9	2.8	2.8
45 to 54 years	1.3	1.5	1.8	1.5	1.5	2.0	1.8	1.9	2.1	2.1	2.0
55 to 64 years	3.1	3.3	3.3	3.7	3.5	4.0	3.8	3.8	3.9	3.7	3.8
65 years and over	8.1	8.6	8.8	9.2	9.2	8.8	9.2	8.6	8.2	8.3	8.4
65 to 74 years	6.2	6.7	6.6	7.1	6.9	6.3	6.3	6.3	6.3	6.4	6.4
75 years and over	10.3	10.9	11.2	11.6	11.8	11.8	12.5	11.4	10.6	10.6	11.1
Sex [4]											
Male	2.4	2.5	2.6	2.7	2.6	2.5	2.7	2.7	2.6	2.5	2.6
Female	2.1	2.2	2.3	2.4	2.4	2.6	2.7	2.6	2.6	2.6	2.5
Sex and Age											
Male											
18 to 44 years	0.3	0.3	0.4	0.4	0.4	*0.3	0.5	0.5	0.5	0.6	0.5
45 to 54 years	1.3	1.6	1.9	1.5	1.5	2.0	1.6	1.6	1.9	1.9	2.0
55 to 64 years	3.7	3.6	3.5	4.2	3.9	4.2	4.4	4.1	4.0	3.5	3.8
65 to 74 years	6.7	7.2	7.2	8.3	7.7	7.0	6.7	6.9	6.6	6.4	7.0
75 years and over	11.3	12.0	12.6	12.5	12.5	11.1	12.8	12.1	10.6	10.3	11.6
Female											
18 to 44 years	0.4	0.5	0.5	0.5	0.5	0.6	0.8	0.6	0.6	0.5	0.6
45 to 54 years	1.4	1.4	1.6	1.5	1.4	2.1	2.1	2.3	2.2	2.3	1.9
55 to 64 years	2.6	2.9	3.2	3.3	3.1	3.8	3.3	3.5	3.9	3.8	3.7
65 to 74 years	5.8	6.2	6.1	6.1	6.3	5.7	6.0	5.7	6.1	6.4	6.0
75 years and over	9.6	10.3	10.4	11.0	11.5	12.2	12.3	10.9	10.6	10.8	10.7
Race [4,6]											
White only	2.1	2.2	2.3	2.4	2.3	2.5	2.6	2.5	2.3	2.3	2.4
Black or African American only	3.5	3.4	3.3	3.4	4.0	3.6	3.7	3.9	4.1	4.1	3.7
American Indian or Alaska Native only	*5.4	*2.6	*	*	*	*	*	*	*4.7	*4.3	*3.3
Asian only	*1.2	*2.7	*3.1	*2.2	1.9	2.1	1.5	1.6	2.4	2.3	1.8
Native Hawaiian or Other Pacific Islander only	*	*	*	*	*	*	*	*	*	*	*
Two or more races	*4.0	*4.4	*4.9	4.0	*4.6	*4.1	*3.5	*3.3	*3.9	5.1	4.7
Hispanic Origin and Race [4,6]											
Hispanic or Latino	1.9	2.5	2.5	2.6	2.1	2.6	2.3	2.3	2.7	2.7	2.6
Mexican	2.0	2.8	2.7	2.9	2.5	2.5	2.5	2.4	2.6	2.7	2.7
Not Hispanic or Latino	2.2	2.3	2.4	2.5	2.5	2.6	2.7	2.6	2.6	2.5	2.6
White only	2.1	2.2	2.3	2.4	2.3	2.4	2.7	2.5	2.3	2.2	2.4
Black or African American only	3.5	3.5	3.3	3.4	4.1	3.6	3.7	3.9	4.2	4.2	3.7
Education [7,8]											
No high school diploma or GED	3.8	3.7	3.8	4.4	4.1	4.4	4.5	4.2	4.4	4.5	4.5
High school diploma or GED	2.5	2.7	2.9	2.8	2.9	3.2	3.3	3.2	3.4	3.2	3.1
Some college or more	1.9	2.2	2.3	2.3	2.3	2.3	2.5	2.5	2.3	2.3	2.4
Percent of Poverty Level [4,9]											
Below 100 percent	3.7	3.6	3.7	4.4	4.1	4.4	4.4	4.4	4.6	4.6	4.7
100 percent to 199 percent	3.2	3.4	3.3	3.5	3.2	3.9	3.6	3.5	3.7	3.6	3.4
200 percent to 399 percent	2.1	2.2	2.4	2.3	2.4	2.5	2.7	2.6	2.5	2.4	2 ¯
400 percent or more	1.5	1.7	1.9	1.8	1.8	1.6	1.8	1.7	1.5	1.5	ʒ
Hispanic Origin and Race and Percent of Poverty Level [4,6,9]											
Hispanic or Latino											
Below 100 percent	2.0	2.3	2.7	3.9	3.1	3.8	2.6	2.9	3.4	3.6	3.8
100 percent to 199 percent	2.2	3.0	3.2	2.8	1.8	2.6	2.6	2.3	3.2	3.4	2.6
200 percent to 399 percent	*2.3	*2.6	2.0	*2.0	*2.0	*2.2	2.4	2.0	2.2	2.4	2.5
400 percent or more	*	*	*	*	*	*2.7	*	*2.6	*2.1	*	*
Not Hispanic or Latino											
White only											
Below 100 percent	3.8	3.5	3.6	4.3	4.1	4.3	4.4	4.4	4.4	4.3	5.0
100 percent to 199 percent	3.0	3.3	3.2	3.5	3.2	4.1	4.0	3.9	3.6	3.4	3.6
200 percent to 399 percent	2.1	2.2	2.3	2.3	2.3	2.6	2.8	2.5	2.3	2.3	2.4
400 percent or more	1.5	1.7	1.8	1.8	1.8	1.5	1.8	1.7	1.4	1.5	1.5
Black or African American only											

Table 3-4C. Respondent-Reported Prevalence of Stroke Among Adults 18 Years of Age and Over, by Selected Characteristics, Selected Years, 1999–2000 through 2012–2013— continued

(Percent.)

Characteristic	Stroke[3]										
	1999–2000	2000–2001	2001–2002	2003–2004	2005–2006	2007–2008	2008–2009	2009–2010	2010–2011	2011–2012	2012–2013
Below 100 percent	4.5	4.5	4.8	5.6	5.3	5.5	6.4	6.2	6.2	6.5	5.4
100 percent to 199 percent	5.1	4.6	3.9	3.8	4.6	4.7	4.0	3.9	4.6	4.6	3.9
200 percent to 399 percent	2.7	3.1	2.8	2.4	4.1	2.7	2.8	3.7	3.9	3.3	3.0
400 percent or more	*	*	*	*2.0	*2.6	*2.6	*2.5	*2.6	*2.1	2.8	3.0
Geographic Region [4]											
Northeast	1.8	1.7	2.1	2.2	1.9	2.4	2.3	2.1	2.0	1.9	2.1
Midwest	2.2	2.4	2.4	2.5	2.5	2.5	2.6	2.6	2.6	2.4	2.5
South	2.5	2.7	2.5	2.8	2.9	3.0	3.2	3.0	2.9	3.0	2.9
West	2.0	2.4	2.7	2.4	2.1	2.2	2.2	2.3	2.4	2.4	2.4
Location of Residence [4]											
Within MSA[10]	2.1	2.3	2.4	2.4	2.4	2.5	2.6	2.4	2.4	2.4	2.4
Outside MSA[10]	2.5	2.5	2.5	2.8	2.9	2.9	3.0	3.3	3.4	3.2	3.3

NA = Not available.   * = Figure does not meet standards of reliability or precision. Data preceded by an asterisk have a relative standard error (RSE) of 20 percent to 30 percent. Data not shown have an RSE of greater than 30 percent.   1 Heart disease is based on self-reported responses to questions about whether respondents had ever been told by a doctor or other health professional that they had coronary heart disease, angina (angina pectoris), a heart attack (myocardial infarction), or any other kind or heart disease or heart condition.   2 Cancer is based on self-reported responses to a question about whether respondents had ever been told by a doctor or other health professional that they had cancer or a malignancy of any kind. Excludes squamous cell and basal cell carcinomas.   3 Stroke is based on self-reported responses to a question about whether respondents had ever been told by a doctor or other health professional that they had a stroke.   4 Estimates are age-adjusted to the year 2000 standard population using five age groups: 18 to 44 years, 45 to 54 years, 55 to 64 years, 65 to 74 years, and 75 years and over. Age-adjusted estimates in this table may differ from other age-adjusted estimates based on the same data and presented elsewhere if different age groups are used in the adjustment procedure.   5 Includes all other races not shown separately and unknown education level.   6 The race groups White, Black, American Indian or Alaska Native, Asian, Native Hawaiian or Other Pacific Islander, and two or more races, include persons of Hispanic and non-Hispanic origin. Persons of Hispanic origin may be of any race.   7 Estimates are for persons 25 years of age and over and are age-adjusted to the year 2000 standard population using five age groups: 25 to 44 years, 45 to 54 years, 55 to 64 years, 65 to 74 years, and 75 years and over.   8 GED is General Educational Development high school equivalency diploma.   9 Percent of poverty level is based on family income and family size and composition using U.S. Census Bureau poverty thresholds.   10 MSA = metropolitan statistical area.

Table 3-5A. Diabetes Prevalence and Glycemic Control Among Adults 20 Years of Age and Over, by Sex, Age, Race and Hispanic Origin, Selected Years 1988–1994 through 2009–2012

(Percent.)

Age, race, sex, and Hispanic origin	Physician-diagnosed and undiagnosed diabetes			Physician-diagnosed diabetes			Undiagnosed diabetes		
	1988–1994	2003–2006	2009–2012	1988–1994	2003–2006	2009–2012	1988–1994	2003–2006	2009–2012
20 Years and Over, Age-Adjusted									
All persons	8.8	10.6	11.7	5.2	7.7	8.4	3.6	3.0	3.3
Sex									
Male	9.6	11.1	13.2	5.5	7.0	9.0	4.1	4.1	4.2
Female	8.2	10.2	10.3	5.1	8.2	7.8	3.2	2.0	2.5
Hispanic Origin									
Not Hispanic or Latino									
White only	7.7	8.9	9.1	4.8	6.2	6.6	2.9	2.7	2.5
Black or African American only	16.3	16.7	17.9	9.1	13.0	13.3	7.2	3.8	4.7
Mexican	15.6	17.1	20.5	10.7	12.9	13.9	5.0	4.2	6.6
Percent of Poverty Level									
Below 100 percent	14.2	14.8	17.1	8.8	12.4	12.1	*5.4	*	5.0
100 percent or more	8.1	10.1	10.8	4.8	7.1	7.8	3.3	3.0	3.0
100 percent to 199 percent	9.7	13.9	14.8	5.2	9.5	11.4	4.4	4.4	3.4
200 percent or more	7.8	8.9	9.4	4.7	6.3	6.5	3.1	2.6	2.9
200 percent to 399 percent	7.8	10.5	11.5	4.3	7.5	8.4	3.6	*3.1	3.1
400 percent or more	7.8	7.0	7.7	5.3	5.2	*5.2	2.5	*	2.5
20 Years and Over, Crude									
All persons	8.3	10.9	12.3	4.9	7.9	8.9	3.4	3.0	3.5
Sex									
Male	8.6	11.0	13.5	4.9	6.9	9.1	3.7	4.0	4.4
Female	8.0	10.8	11.2	5.0	8.7	8.7	3.1	2.1	2.6
Hispanic Origin									
Not Hispanic or Latino									
White only	7.6	9.6	10.5	4.7	6.7	7.6	2.9	3.0	2.8
Black or African American only	13.3	15.8	17.1	7.2	12.3	12.5	6.1	3.5	4.6
Mexican	10.4	12.6	15.8	6.3	8.8	10.1	4.1	*3.8	5.7
Percent of Poverty Level									
Below 100 percent	11.6	12.7	14.3	7.2	10.6	9.8	4.4	*	4.5
100 percent or more	7.6	10.5	11.8	4.5	7.3	8.6	3.1	3.1	3.3
100 percent to 199 percent	9.1	14.9	15.8	5.2	10.2	12.3	3.9	4.7	3.5
200 percent or more	7.1	9.1	10.4	4.3	6.5	7.3	2.8	2.7	3.2
200 percent to 399 percent	6.8	11.0	12.3	3.7	7.7	9.0	3.1	*3.2	3.3
400 percent or more	7.6	7.4	8.9	5.2	5.3	*5.8	*2.5	*2.2	*3.1
Age									
20 to 44 years	*2.1	3.9	3.7	*	2.8	2.1	1.1	*1.1	1.6
45 to 64 years	14.0	13.7	16.2	7.9	10.1	11.4	6.0	3.5	4.8
65 years and over	19.4	24.9	26.8	12.7	17.5	21.2	6.7	ˉ ⁴	5.5

Table 3-5B. Diabetes Prevalence and Glycemic Control Among Adults 20 Years of Age and Over, by Sex, Age, Race and Hispanic Origin, Selected Years 1988–1994 through 2009–2012

(Percent.)

Characteristic	2003–2006	2007–2010	2009–2012	1999–2002
Poor glycemic control (A1c greater than 9 percent) among persons with physician-diagnosed diabetes				
20 Years and Over, Age-Adjusted				
All persons	17.4	20.3	18.3	21.3
Sex				
Male	22.5	21.6	20.8	26.2
Female	11.6	19.2	15.8	16.5
Hispanic Origin				
Not Hispanic or Latino				
White only	*18.1	*15.2	*11.2	*
Black or African American only	*15.5	31.8	30.4	28.8
Mexican	23.7	*25.5	*24.3	32.5
Percent of Poverty Level				
Below 100 percent	*17.8	23.2	22.9	23.6
100 percent or more	*18.1	20.0	17.2	21.2
100 percent to 199 percent	*	*22.0	*	*20.0
200 percent or more	*22.6	19.4	18.0	*22.0
200 percent to 399 percent	*22.9	*16.3	*20.2	*21.4
400 percent or more	*	*22.4	*	*
20 Years and Over, Crude				
All persons				
	14.5	13.9	12.5	13.8
Sex				
Male	17.5	14.9	14.0	14.8
Female	11.6	12.9	11.0	12.8
Hispanic Origin				
Not Hispanic or Latino	11.5	10.5	9.5	9.5
White only	20.0	21.0	19.0	19.6
Black or African American only	23.0	21.7	19.6	23.5
Mexican				
Percent of Poverty Level	16.3	20.3	18.5	19.8
Below 100 percent	13.9	12.8	11.1	11.9
100 percent or more	*10.6	*11.8	9.8	12.4
100 percent to 199 percent	15.5	13.3	11.8	11.7
200 percent or more	15.6	*11.2	12.4	12.3
200 percent to 399 percent	15.5	*15.6	*11.2	*11.1
400 percent or more				
Age				
20 to 44 years	*20.0	28.1	24.9	30.1
45 to 64 years	19.5	15.4	14.1	14.4
65 years and over	*6.3	6.2	6.8	8.0

Table 3-5C. End-Stage Renal Disease Patients, by Selected Characteristics, Selected Years, 2000–2012

(Number, rate per million population.)

Characteristic	Incidence				Prevalence			
	Number of new patients				Number of patients alive on December 31			
	2000	2010	2011	2012	2000	2010	2011	2012
Total	91,241	113,380	111,209	112,596	378,074	577,675	597,620	620,136
Age								
Under 20 years	1,148	1,167	1,172	1,113	6,039	7,015	7,066	7,020
20 to 44 years	12,687	13,050	12,734	12,836	86,043	96,067	96,936	98,142
45 to 64 years	31,736	43,456	43,294	44,120	154,117	259,855	268,220	275,940
65 to 74 years	23,148	27,100	26,318	27,409	75,480	119,941	127,391	136,859
75 years and over	22,522	28,607	27,691	27,118	56,395	94,797	98,007	102,175
Sex								
Male	48,769	64,553	63,600	64,524	206,248	327,379	339,676	353,372
Female	42,472	48,827	47,609	48,072	171,826	250,296	257,944	266,764
Race [1]								
White	59,472	75,214	73,229	74,667	231,829	353,938	364,579	377,797
Black or African American	26,204	31,828	31,530	31,148	123,654	185,683	192,745	199,632
American Indian or Alaska Native	*	1,233	1,234	1,260	*	7,571	7,840	8,080
Asian or Pacific Islander	3,460	5,105	5,216	5,521	16,064	30,483	32,456	34,627
Hispanic Origin [2]								
Hispanic	10,053	15,251	15,582	15,399	40,627	85,228	90,856	95,819
Not Hispanic[3]	81,188	98,129	95,627	97,197	337,447	492,447	506,764	524,317
Primary Diagnosis								
Diabetes	40,489	50,020	49,151	49,258	133,128	217,165	225,110	234,160
Hypertension	24,490	32,317	31,506	32,293	92,817	143,951	149,710	156,595
Glomerulonephritis	9,958	9,311	9,218	8,988	75,477	98,822	101,103	103,312
Cystic kidney	2,140	2,582	2,476	2,495	17,685	27,492	28,407	29,389
Other urologic	1,610	526	429	533	7,996	7,499	7,287	7,253
Other cause	8,486	13,662	13,633	12,157	33,250	54,967	57,266	58,717
Unknown cause	3,712	4,262	4,026	3,469	15,539	24,232	24,733	24,923
Missing disease	356	700	770	3,403	2,182	3,547	4,004	5,787

*Data are considered unreliable and are not shown.   1 The race groups White, Black, American Indian or Alaska Native, and Asian or Pacific Islander, include persons of Hispanic and non-Hispanic origin.   2 Persons of Hispanic origin may be of any race.   3 Not Hispanic includes unknown ethnicity.

Table 3-6. End-Stage Renal Disease Patients, by Selected Characteristics, Selected Years, 2000–2012

(Number, rate per million population.)

Characteristic	New patients per million population				Patients alive on December 31 per million population			
	2000	2010	2011	2012	2000	2010	2011	2012
Total	323.3	366.5	356.9	358.6	1,333.2	1,860.7	1,910.8	1,968.2
Age								
Under 20 years	14.2	14.0	14.1	13.4	74.7	84.5	85.4	85.2
20 to 44 years	121.8	125.6	121.7	121.7	825.8	921.5	923.2	927.4
45 to 64 years	508.3	531.4	522.8	532.4	2,428.5	3,157.8	3,238.2	3,329.3
65 to 74 years	1,259.1	1,239.8	1,170.4	1,142.7	4,105.7	5,409.7	5,482.5	5,532.9
75 years and over	1,349.7	1,536.3	1,466.1	1,415.3	3,357.6	5,054.8	5,151.9	5,294.9
Sex								
Male	352.2	424.4	414.9	417.6	1,482.0	2,144.2	2,207.4	2,278.2
Female	295.5	310.5	300.7	301.5	1,189.9	1,586.3	1,623.5	1,667.5
Race [1]								
White	257.9	306.0	296.5	300.8	1,001.9	1,436.7	1,472.4	1,518.1
Black or African American	713.4	754.2	738.4	720.9	3,342.9	4,374.5	4,487.7	4,593.7
American Indian or Alaska Native	*	288.3	284.5	286.4	*	1,758.1	1,795.0	1,824.2
Asian or Pacific Islander	290.9	298.3	296.4	305.2	1,320.9	1,756.7	1,819.1	1,888.6
Hispanic Origin [1,2]								
Hispanic	281.8	300.5	300.3	290.3	1,116.0	1,660.8	1,732.0	1,787.6
Not Hispanic[3]	329.3	379.4	368.2	372.5	1,365.2	1,900.2	1,946.8	2,005.2
Primary Diagnosis								
Diabetes	143.4	161.7	157.7	156.9	469.4	699.5	719.7	743.1
Hypertension	86.7	104.4	101.1	102.8	327.3	463.6	478.6	497.0
Glomerulonephritis	35.2	30.1	29.5	28.6	266.1	318.3	323.2	327.8
Cystic kidney	7.5	8.3	7.9	7.9	62.3	88.5	90.8	93.2
Other urologic	5.7	1.7	1.3	1.6	28.1	24.1	23.2	23.0
Other cause	30.0	44.1	43.7	38.7	117.2	177.0	183.1	186.3
Unknown cause	13.1	13.7	12.9	11.0	54.7	78.0	79.0	79.1
Missing disease	1.2	2.2	2.4	10.8	7.6	11.4	12.8	18.3

*Data are considered unreliable and are not shown.   1 The race groups White, Black, American Indian or Alaska Native, and Asian or Pacific Islander, include persons of Hispanic and non-Hispanic origin.   2 Persons of Hispanic origin may be of any race.   3 Not Hispanic includes unknown ethnicity.

Table 3-7. Severe Headache or Migraine, Low Back Pain, and Neck Pain Among Adults 18 Years of Age and Over, by Selected Characteristics, 1997, 2000, 2010, and 2013

(Percent of adults with pain in the last 3 months.)

Characteristic	Severe headache or migraine[1]				Low back pain[1]				Neck pain[1]			
	1997	2000	2010	2013	1997	2000	2010	2013	1997	2000	2010	2013
18 years and over, age-adjusted[2,3]	15.8	14.7	16.6	16.0	28.2	27.3	28.4	28.4	14.7	14.4	15.4	14.4
18 years and over, crude[3]	16.0	14.8	16.4	15.6	28.1	27.2	28.8	29.0	14.6	14.4	15.8	14.9
Age												
18 to 44 years	18.7	17.2	20.4	18.8	26.1	24.6	25.2	23.8	13.3	12.6	13.1	11.2
18 to 24 years	18.7	16.1	19.6	17.1	21.9	20.9	19.4	18.0	9.8	8.7	8.3	6.7
25 to 44 years	18.7	17.6	20.7	19.5	27.3	25.8	27.2	26.0	14.3	13.9	14.8	12.9
45 to 64 years	15.8	14.8	15.6	15.6	31.3	30.4	32.4	33.7	17.0	17.7	20.0	19.4
45 to 54 years	17.8	16.3	16.7	17.9	31.3	29.4	31.3	32.5	17.3	17.8	19.1	19.4
55 to 64 years	12.7	12.3	14.1	13.0	31.2	32.0	33.8	35.0	16.6	17.6	21.0	19.4
65 years and over	7.0	7.0	6.4	7.3	29.5	30.0	31.8	33.7	15.0	14.0	14.8	15.9
65 to 74 years	8.2	7.9	7.4	8.1	30.2	29.6	32.5	33.3	15.0	13.9	15.5	17.3
75 years and over	5.4	6.0	5.1	6.2	28.6	30.6	30.9	34.2	15.0	14.2	14.0	14.1
Sex [2]												
Male	9.9	8.9	11.0	10.1	26.5	25.5	26.3	26.4	12.6	12.1	13.1	12.2
Female	21.4	20.3	22.1	21.6	29.6	28.8	30.3	30.2	16.6	16.5	17.6	16.5
Sex and Age												
Male												
18 to 44 years	11.9	10.4	13.5	12.0	24.8	23.4	23.2	21.4	11.6	10.6	11.0	9.3
45 to 54 years	10.3	9.1	10.4	10.7	29.4	27.4	29.6	31.4	13.9	14.8	16.3	16.3
55 to 64 years	8.8	7.6	9.6	9.1	30.7	29.6	32.8	34.9	14.6	15.1	17.6	17.8
65 to 74 years	5.0	5.1	5.5	4.5	29.0	27.5	28.4	32.2	13.6	12.0	12.8	16.0
75 years and over	*2.4	4.5	4.0	4.1	22.5	26.3	27.4	29.7	12.6	12.4	13.0	9.7
Female												
18 to 44 years	25.4	23.9	27.3	25.5	27.3	25.7	27.1	26.1	14.9	14.6	15.2	13.1
45 to 54 years	24.9	23.2	22.9	24.8	33.1	31.3	33.0	33.6	20.6	20.7	21.8	22.3
55 to 64 years	16.3	16.7	18.2	16.5	31.7	34.2	34.7	35.1	18.4	19.8	24.1	20.9
65 to 74 years	10.7	10.1	9.1	11.1	31.1	31.2	36.1	34.3	16.1	15.5	17.8	18.4
75 years and over	7.4	6.9	5.8	7.6	32.4	33.2	33.2	37.3	16.5	15.2	14.6	17.1
Race [2,4]												
White only	15.9	15.0	16.7	16.0	28.7	28.0	29.1	29.0	15.1	15.0	16.0	14.8
Black or African American only	16.7	13.9	18.2	16.9	26.9	24.3	27.2	27.9	13.3	10.7	13.3	13.1
American Indian or Alaska Native only	18.9	21.1	18.8	18.9	33.3	31.4	33.6	31.2	16.2	19.6	16.9	17.3
Asian only	11.7	12.0	10.1	10.9	21.0	19.0	19.1	18.8	9.2	11.0	9.6	9.5
Native Hawaiian or Other Pacific Islander only	NA	*	*	*	NA	*	*	*	NA	*	*	*
2 or more races	NA	19.9	21.5	24.7	NA	41.8	35.6	33.0	NA	22.1	22.0	21.3
Hispanic Origin and Race [2,4]												
Hispanic or Latino	15.5	13.5	16.2	15.6	26.4	25.0	27.4	25.1	13.9	13.4	15.1	13.3
Mexican	14.6	12.3	15.7	15.5	25.2	21.5	26.5	23.3	12.9	11.6	14.7	12.9
Not Hispanic or Latino	15.9	15.0	16.8	16.2	28.4	27.7	28.7	29.0	14.9	14.7	15.5	14.8
White only	16.1	15.4	17.0	16.5	29.1	28.4	29.7	30.0	15.4	15.4	16.3	15.4
Black or African American only	16.8	13.8	18.4	16.7	26.9	24.2	27.1	27.8	13.3	10.6	13.3	13.0
Education [5,6]												
25 years and over												
No high school diploma or GED	19.2	17.9	18.2	18.7	33.6	32.4	34.5	34.5	16.5	15.9	18.9	17.6
High school diploma or GED	16.0	14.8	17.4	16.5	30.2	29.4	31.9	31.9	15.5	15.4	16.8	16.4
Some college or more	13.8	13.4	15.1	15.0	26.9	26.3	28.0	28.4	14.6	15.0	15.8	15.0
Percent of Poverty Level [2,7]												
Below 100 percent	23.3	19.9	22.7	24.9	35.4	32.4	34.9	37.6	18.6	16.5	20.2	21.6
100 percent to 199 percent	18.9	17.7	19.5	18.4	30.8	30.6	32.5	32.8	16.1	15.3	17.7	16.3
200 percent to 399 percent	15.5	15.4	16.6	15.5	27.9	27.4	28.5	27.7	14.8	14.7	15.2	14.2
400 percent or more	12.4	11.8	13.3	12.1	24.8	24.5	24.7	23.8	12.8	13.4	13.1	11.8
Hispanic Origin and Race and Percent of Poverty Level [2,4,7]												
Hispanic or Latino												
Below 100 percent	18.9	18.1	19.6	19.5	29.5	28.4	29.0	29.7	16.4	15.6	17.4	17.0
100 percent to 199 percent	15.7	12.9	15.1	14.9	26.8	24.8	27.2	26.5	12.9	13.3	15.7	12.8
200 percent to 399 percent	14.0	13.6	16.5	14.6	25.0	23.5	27.5	24.1	13.8	13.6	12.9	12.5
400 percent or more	13.0	9.6	14.0	13.7	21.6	24.1	25.6	20.0	12.1	11.6	15.3	11.6
Not Hispanic or Latino												
White only												
Below 100 percent	26.1	21.3	24.8	29.0	38.9	36.6	40.5	44.3	20.5	18.7	23.7	25.9
100 percent to 199 percent	20.4	20.3	22.0	19.9	33.3	34.6	35.9	36.7	18.0	17.6	19.9	18.9
200 percent to 399 percent	16.3	16.5	16.9	16.3	29.1	28.5	30.5	29.6	15.9	16.0	16.8	15.3
400 percent or more	12.5	12.3	13.8	12.7	25.4	25.2	25.2	25.3	13.1	14.0	13.6	12.4

Table 3-7. Severe Headache or Migraine, Low Back Pain, and Neck Pain Among Adults 18 Years of Age and Over, by Selected Characteristics, 1997, 2000, 2010, and 2013— continued

(Percent of adults with pain in the last 3 months.)

Characteristic	Severe headache or migraine[1]				Low back pain[1]				Neck pain[1]			
	1997	2000	2010	2013	1997	2000	2010	2013	1997	2000	2010	2013
Black or African American only												
Below 100 percent	22.7	21.1	24.0	25.4	34.5	27.5	32.5	36.2	17.9	13.7	18.6	19.8
100 percent to 199 percent	17.6	16.3	19.6	18.6	27.7	26.2	31.2	31.1	14.0	11.1	14.4	13.5
200 percent to 399 percent	14.0	11.4	17.6	13.9	24.3	23.8	23.7	24.1	10.2	9.8	11.7	11.1
400 percent or more	12.9	8.2	12.2	9.2	21.5	20.3	21.0	20.2	11.9	8.1	8.5	8.0
Disability Measure [2,8]												
Any basic actions difficulty or complex activity limitation	29.3	28.3	30.1	30.6	48.0	49.0	49.5	50.2	27.2	29.0	28.1	28.1
Any basic actions difficulty	30.0	29.3	30.9	31.4	49.3	50.0	51.1	52.1	27.9	29.9	29.0	29.6
Any complex activity limitation	34.6	32.7	36.0	34.9	55.1	54.3	54.5	55.6	33.1	33.9	34.3	33.5
No disability	11.0	10.4	11.7	11.1	19.4	18.7	19.0	19.2	9.1	9.1	9.7	8.7
Geographic Region [2]												
Northeast	14.5	12.7	15.4	13.7	27.1	26.0	28.0	26.9	14.0	13.5	14.9	13.2
Midwest	15.6	15.1	16.8	17.1	28.7	28.2	28.1	29.7	15.3	14.5	16.0	14.5
South	17.1	14.9	18.2	16.5	27.5	26.5	28.3	27.9	13.9	13.7	14.6	13.8
West	15.3	15.9	15.1	15.9	30.0	28.6	29.3	29.0	16.1	16.5	16.5	16.2
Location of Residence [2]												
Within MSA[9]	15.2	14.4	16.3	15.5	27.0	26.6	27.5	27.8	14.2	14.3	14.9	14.1
Outside MSA[9]	18.1	16.1	18.6	18.9	32.5	29.6	33.8	31.5	16.4	14.9	18.1	16.4

NA = Not available.   * = Figure does not meet standards of reliability or precision. Data preceded by an asterisk have a relative standard error (RSE) of 20 percent to 30 percent. Data not shown have an RSE of greater than 30 percent.   1 In three separate questions, respondents were asked, "During the past 3 months, did you have a severe headache or migraine? ...low back pain? ...neck pain?" Respondents were instructed to report pain that had lasted a whole day or more, and not to report fleeting or minor aches or pains. Persons may be represented in more than one column.   2 Estimates are age adjusted to the year 2000 standard population using five age groups: 18 to 44 years, 45 to 54 years, 55 to 64 years, 65 to 74 years, and 75 years and over. Age-adjusted estimates in this table may differ from other age-adjusted estimates based on the same data and presented elsewhere if different age groups are used in the adjustment procedure.   3 Includes all other races not shown separately, unknown education level, and unknown disability status.   4 The race groups White, Black, American Indian or Alaska Native, Asian, Native Hawaiian or Other Pacific Islander, and two or more races, include persons of Hispanic and non-Hispanic origin. Persons of Hispanic origin may be of any race.   5 Estimates are for persons 25 years of age and over and are age-adjusted to the year 2000 standard population using five age groups: 25 to 44 years, 45 to 54 years, 55 to 64 years, 65 to 74 years, and 75 years and over.   6 GED is General Educational Development high school equivalency diploma.   7 Percent of poverty level is based on family income and family size and composition using U.S. Census Bureau poverty thresholds.   8 Any basic actions difficulty or complex activity limitation is defined as having one or more of the following limitations or difficulties: movement difficulty, emotional difficulty, sensory (seeing or hearing) difficulty, cognitive difficulty, self-care (activities of daily living or instrumental activities of daily living) limitation, social limitation, or work limitation.   9 MSA = metropolitan statistical area.

Table 3-8A. Joint Pain Among Adults 18 Years of Age and Over, by Selected Characteristics, Selected Years, 2002–2010

(Percent.)

Characteristic	Any joint pain[1]		
	2002	2005	2010
18 years and over, age-adjusted[2,3]	29.5	30.7	32.1
18 years and over, crude[3]	29.5	31.1	33.3
Age			
18 to 44 years	19.3	19.1	20.6
18 to 24 years	14.2	14.0	15.2
25 to 44 years	21.0	20.9	22.6
45 to 64 years	37.5	39.9	42.9
45 to 54 years	34.3	35.8	39.3
55 to 64 years	42.3	45.7	47.3
65 years and over	47.2	50.9	49.6
65 to 74 years	46.0	49.3	49.5
75 years and over	48.7	52.6	49.8
Sex [2]			
Male	28.0	28.9	30.8
Female	30.7	32.2	33.2
Sex and Age			
Male			
18 to 44 years	20.1	19.3	21.6
45 to 54 years	31.1	33.4	37.3
55 to 64 years	37.3	40.7	42.5
65 to 74 years	41.7	45.1	42.9
75 years and over	43.9	47.0	46.6
Female			
18 to 44 years	18.4	18.9	19.7
45 to 54 years	37.3	38.2	41.3
55 to 64 years	46.8	50.4	51.8
65 to 74 years	49.6	52.9	55.2
75 years and over	51.6	56.2	51.9
Race [2,4]			
White only	29.8	31.3	32.6
Black or African American only	30.8	28.5	32.0
American Indian or Alaska Native only	36.7	34.8	38.1
Asian only	18.1	18.5	20.4
Native Hawaiian or Other Pacific Islander only	*	*	*
2 or more races	42.7	46.2	43.5
Hispanic Origin and Race [2,4]			
Hispanic or Latino	23.4	24.2	25.4
Mexican	24.6	23.8	25.0
Not Hispanic or Latino	30.4	31.7	33.3
White only	30.8	32.8	34.3
Black or African American only	30.8	28.5	32.1
Education [5,6]			
25 years and over			
No high school diploma or GED	33.0	33.3	33.8
High school diploma or GED	32.9	33.1	36.8
Some college or more	31.1	33.2	34.0
Percent of Poverty Level [2,7]			
Below 100 percent	31.7	33.7	35.6
100 percent to 199 percent	31.7	31.9	34.0
200 percent to 399 percent	30.1	31.0	32.2
400 percent or more	27.6	29.3	30.5
Hispanic Origin and Race and Percent of Poverty Level [2,4,7]			
Hispanic or Latino			
Below 100 percent	26.8	24.5	25.3
100 percent to 199 percent	24.5	24.1	25.4
200 percent to 399 percent	21.6	23.6	24.8
400 percent or more	21.9	24.7	27.4
Not Hispanic or Latino			
White only			
Below 100 percent	34.2	39.3	40.1
100 percent to 199 percent	34.9	36.2	38.7
200 percent to 399 percent	32.0	33.6	34.8
400 percent or more	28.2	30.1	31.8
Black or African American only			
Below 100 percent	31.6	33.0	37.6
100 percent to 199 percent	34.0	28.6	33.0
200 percent to 399 percent	29.1	27.2	30.8
400 percent or more	29.8	25.8	26.8
Disability Measure [2,8]			
Any basic actions difficulty or complex activity limitation	52.5	54.8	54.6

Table 3-8A. Joint Pain Among Adults 18 Years of Age and Over, by Selected Characteristics, Selected Years, 2002–2010— continued

(Percent.)

Characteristic	Any joint pain[1]		
	2002	2005	2010
Any basic actions difficulty	54.0	56.7	56.2
Any complex activity limitation	56.4	57.8	56.5
No disability	19.6	20.3	21.5
Geographic Region [2]			
Northeast	27.5	28.6	28.9
Midwest	32.1	34.8	35.7
South	29.3	29.8	32.4
West	28.4	29.2	30.6
Location of Residence [2]			
Within MSA[9]	28.3	29.2	31.1
Outside MSA[9]	33.9	36.3	37.4

Table 3-8B. Joint Pain Among Adults 18 Years of Age and Over, by Selected Characteristics, Selected Years, 2002–2010

(Percent.)

Characteristic	Knee pain[1]			Shoulder pain[1]		
	2002	2005	2010	2002	2005	2010
18 years and over, age-adjusted[2,3]	16.5	18.2	19.6	8.6	9.2	9.0
18 years and over, crude[3]	16.5	18.5	20.3	8.7	9.3	9.4
Age						
18 to 44 years	10.5	11.6	12.6	4.9	4.9	5.2
18 to 24 years	8.3	8.8	9.8	3.4	2.4	3.5
25 to 44 years	11.2	12.6	13.6	5.4	5.8	5.8
45 to 64 years	20.4	23.2	26.1	12.3	12.9	13.2
45 to 54 years	18.4	20.6	23.5	10.5	11.5	12.0
55 to 64 years	23.4	26.9	29.3	15.1	14.9	14.8
65 years and over	28.6	30.2	30.5	14.1	16.0	13.6
65 to 74 years	27.6	29.7	30.2	14.0	15.7	13.5
75 years and over	29.7	30.8	30.9	14.1	16.2	13.7
Sex [2]						
Male	15.2	16.8	18.7	8.4	9.3	9.3
Female	17.6	19.4	20.3	8.8	9.0	8.6
Sex and Age						
Male						
18 to 44 years	10.7	12.0	12.9	5.5	5.4	6.1
45 to 54 years	16.2	18.9	22.3	9.5	11.4	12.2
55 to 64 years	20.1	23.1	27.4	13.7	14.7	15.3
65 to 74 years	24.1	25.1	25.3	13.3	15.7	11.8
75 years and over	25.7	25.7	28.7	11.4	15.1	13.1
Female						
18 to 44 years	10.2	11.2	12.2	4.2	4.5	4.3
45 to 54 years	20.5	22.3	24.8	11.4	11.5	11.8
55 to 64 years	26.4	30.5	31.0	16.3	15.1	14.3
65 to 74 years	30.5	33.6	34.4	14.7	15.7	15.0
75 years and over	32.1	34.0	32.4	15.7	16.9	14.1
Race [2,4]						
White only	16.3	18.5	19.7	8.8	9.5	9.1
Black or African American only	20.2	18.2	21.0	8.3	7.6	8.9
American Indian or Alaska Native only	24.5	15.0	26.9	*11.3	*8.1	10.1
Asian only	8.5	10.2	12.8	3.9	5.3	6.9
Native Hawaiian or Other Pacific Islander only	*	*	*	*	*	*
2 or more races	28.1	28.6	27.1	15.4	18.9	13.9
Hispanic Origin and Race [2,4]						
Hispanic or Latino	13.6	14.9	15.5	7.6	8.2	7.4
Mexican	14.1	14.9	15.4	8.3	8.5	7.3
Not Hispanic or Latino	17.0	18.9	20.3	8.9	9.4	9.3
White only	16.9	19.4	20.7	9.1	9.8	9.5
Black or African American only	20.1	18.1	21.0	8.3	7.6	8.9
Education [5,6]						
25 years and over						
No high school diploma or GED	19.5	20.7	22.0	10.8	11.7	10.9
High school diploma or GED	18.6	19.7	22.7	10.2	10.5	10.9
Some college or more	16.9	19.2	20.1	8.8	9.7	9.1
Percent of Poverty Level [2,7]						
Below 100 percent	19.9	21.4	22.9	11.2	11.2	11.1
100 percent to 199 percent	19.0	19.8	21.9	10.4	10.5	10.9
200 percent to 399 percent	16.4	18.4	19.3	8.8	9.2	9.0
400 percent or more	14.9	16.6	18.1	7.3	8.1	7.7
Hispanic Origin and Race and Percent of Poverty Level [2,7]						
Hispanic or Latino						
Below 100 percent	16.1	15.7	15.9	11.5	10.5	7.6
100 percent to 199 percent	14.4	15.2	16.1	8.2	8.3	8.0
200 percent to 399 percent	11.7	13.1	14.5	5.7	8.2	6.8
400 percent or more	12.3	15.6	16.3	4.9	*6.4	7.4
Not Hispanic or Latino						
White only						
Below 100 percent	21.3	24.7	25.2	12.4	13.4	12.6
100 percent to 199 percent	20.3	22.8	24.8	11.6	12.0	12.2
200 percent to 399 percent	17.0	20.1	20.9	9.6	10.1	10.0
400 percent or more	15.1	17.0	18.8	7.6	8.4	8.0
Black or African American only						
Below 100 percent	20.8	22.5	25.1	9.1	9.0	11.9
100 percent to 199 percent	23.2	18.3	22.6	10.9	8.3	10.0
200 percent to 399 percent	19.1	16.6	19.8	7.4	7.2	7.8
400 percent or more	18.2	15.8	15.7	*8.0	*5.7	6.5
Disability Measure [2,8]						
Any basic actions difficulty or complex activity limitation	32.1	35.7	35.9	17.8	18.8	16.8
Any basic actions difficulty	33.4	37.3	37.3	18.3	19.5	17.2

Table 3-8B. Joint Pain Among Adults 18 Years of Age and Over, by Selected Characteristics, Selected Years, 2002–2010— continued

(Percent.)

Characteristic	Knee pain[1]			Shoulder pain[1]		
	2002	2005	2010	2002	2005	2010
Any complex activity limitation	35.2	38.2	37.5	22.0	23.5	20.6
No disability	9.4	10.4	11.6	4.6	4.8	4.9
Geographic Region [2]						
Northeast	15.8	16.7	17.9	7.9	8.1	8.3
Midwest	18.4	21.6	22.3	8.6	10.1	10.0
South	16.7	17.9	19.8	9.1	8.9	9.0
West	14.6	16.3	17.9	8.6	9.6	8.5
Location of Residence [2]						
Within MSA[9]	16.0	17.2	19.0	8.1	8.4	8.3
Outside MSA[9]	18.7	22.3	23.0	10.8	12.2	12.3

Table 3-8C. Joint Pain Among Adults 18 Years of Age and Over, by Selected Characteristics, Selected Years, 2002–2010

(Percent.)

Characteristic	Finger pain[1]			Hip pain[1]		
	2002	2005	2010	2002	2005	2010
18 years and over, age-adjusted[2,3]	7.5	7.4	7.1	6.6	7.1	7.0
18 years and over, crude[3]	7.5	7.6	7.5	6.6	7.2	7.3
Age						
18 to 44 years	3.4	2.8	3.1	3.2	3.2	3.2
18 to 24 years	2.0	*1.0	1.7	1.6	2.1	*1.5
25 to 44 years	3.9	3.5	3.6	3.8	3.6	3.8
45 to 64 years	11.0	11.2	10.5	9.1	9.7	10.0
45 to 54 years	9.1	9.2	8.4	7.8	7.6	9.0
55 to 64 years	13.9	14.0	13.2	11.0	12.6	11.3
65 years and over	13.9	15.2	14.2	12.9	14.6	13.5
65 to 74 years	14.4	14.9	15.3	12.6	13.7	13.3
75 years and over	13.3	15.4	12.8	13.3	15.7	13.7
Sex [2]						
Male	5.8	6.0	5.8	5.1	5.4	5.3
Female	8.9	8.7	8.2	8.0	8.6	8.6
Sex and Age						
Male						
18 to 44 years	3.0	2.6	3.0	2.5	2.4	2.0
45 to 54 years	6.6	7.5	7.3	5.6	5.7	6.8
55 to 64 years	10.5	10.4	9.9	8.0	9.5	8.7
65 to 74 years	11.2	11.4	10.9	10.5	10.8	10.3
75 years and over	10.0	12.1	9.5	10.1	12.7	12.9
Female						
18 to 44 years	3.8	3.0	3.1	3.9	4.0	4.5
45 to 54 years	11.5	10.9	9.4	9.9	9.5	11.1
55 to 64 years	17.0	17.4	16.2	13.7	15.4	13.7
65 to 74 years	17.1	17.9	19.0	14.2	16.2	15.8
75 years and over	15.3	17.5	15.1	15.2	17.5	14.3
Race [2,4]						
White only	7.6	7.8	7.4	6.9	7.4	7.2
Black or African American only	6.5	4.6	5.6	5.6	6.1	6.0
American Indian or Alaska Native only	*12.9	*13.0	*7.2	*10.4	*	*9.9
Asian only	*3.2	4.1	3.3	*2.3	*2.1	*2.4
Native Hawaiian or Other Pacific Islander only	*	*	*	*	*	*
2 or more races	12.8	10.5	12.2	10.0	13.7	11.7
Hispanic Origin and Race [2,4]						
Hispanic or Latino	6.8	6.0	6.0	3.8	4.1	4.3
Mexican	7.8	7.0	6.3	4.0	4.1	3.9
Not Hispanic or Latino	7.6	7.6	7.3	6.9	7.4	7.3
White only	7.8	8.2	7.7	7.3	7.8	7.7
Black or African American only	6.5	4.7	5.6	5.7	6.2	6.1
Education [5,6]						
25 years and over						
No high school diploma or GED	9.5	8.8	8.5	7.3	8.5	7.9
High school diploma or GED	8.3	8.8	9.1	7.3	7.5	9.0
Some college or more	8.2	8.1	7.4	7.5	7.8	7.3
Percent of Poverty Level [2,7]						
Below 100 percent	9.8	8.0	9.1	8.5	8.9	9.7
100 percent to 199 percent	8.9	8.2	8.3	7.5	8.1	8.5
200 percent to 399 percent	7.9	7.9	7.2	6.8	6.9	6.8
400 percent or more	6.2	6.6	6.0	5.8	6.3	5.7
Hispanic Origin and Race and Percent of Poverty Level [2,4,7]						
Hispanic or Latino						
Below 100 percent	8.6	6.4	6.4	5.9	4.4	5.6
100 percent to 199 percent	8.2	5.7	5.2	3.9	3.9	4.5
200 percent to 399 percent	6.2	6.5	6.8	3.2	4.2	3.1
400 percent or more	*5.3	*5.1	5.8	*1.8	*4.3	*5.2
Not Hispanic or Latino						
White only						
Below 100 percent	10.9	9.9	11.1	9.9	11.6	12.0
100 percent to 199 percent	9.9	9.6	9.8	9.1	9.8	10.6
200 percent to 399 percent	8.5	8.9	7.8	7.5	7.8	7.8
400 percent or more	6.5	7.0	6.3	6.2	6.8	6.0
Black or African American only						

Table 3-8C. Joint Pain Among Adults 18 Years of Age and Over, by Selected Characteristics, Selected Years, 2002–2010— continued

(Percent.)

Characteristic	Finger pain[1]			Hip pain[1]		
	2002	2005	2010	2002	2005	2010
Below 100 percent	7.9	5.7	7.8	8.1	7.7	9.0
100 percent to 199 percent	7.4	6.0	6.2	6.4	6.3	5.9
200 percent to 399 percent	6.0	3.9	4.3	4.7	6.0	5.2
400 percent or more	*4.8	*2.8	*4.2	*4.5	*5.5	4.7
Disability Measure [2,8]						
Any basic actions difficulty or complex activity limitation	14.5	14.2	12.8	13.8	14.6	14.2
Any basic actions difficulty	14.9	14.8	13.3	14.4	15.2	14.6
Any complex activity limitation	17.8	16.9	15.0	17.8	19.7	18.7
No disability	4.0	4.1	4.2	3.1	3.3	3.1
Geographic Region [2]						
Northeast	6.6	6.2	5.5	5.7	6.4	5.5
Midwest	7.5	8.5	7.9	6.9	7.9	8.5
South	7.6	7.3	7.4	7.0	7.1	7.2
West	8.0	7.5	7.1	6.4	6.6	6.3
Location of Residence [2]						
Within MSA[9]	7.2	7.0	7.0	6.2	6.5	6.5
Outside MSA[9]	8.4	9.1	7.9	8.0	9.3	9.4

* = Figure does not meet standards of reliability or precision. Data preceded by an asterisk have a relative standard error (RSE) of 20 percent to 30 percent. Data not shown have an RSE of greater than 30 percent.   1 Starting with 2002 data, respondents were asked, "During the past 30 days, have you had any symptoms of pain, aching, or stiffness in or around a joint?" Respondents were instructed not to include the back or neck. To facilitate their responses, respondents were shown a card illustrating the body joints. Respondents reporting more than one type of joint pain were included in each response category. This table shows the most commonly reported joints.   2 Estimates are age adjusted to the year 2000 standard population using five age groups: 18 to 44 years, 45 to 54 years, 55 to 64 years, 65 to 74 years, and 75 years and over. Age-adjusted estimates in this table may differ from other age-adjusted estimates based on the same data and presented elsewhere if different age groups are used in the adjustment procedure.   3 Includes all other races not shown separately, unknown education level, and unknown disability status.   4 The race groups White, Black, American Indian or Alaska Native, Asian, Native Hawaiian or Other Pacific Islander, and two or more races, include persons of Hispanic and non-Hispanic origin. Persons of Hispanic origin may be of any race.   5 Estimates are for persons 25 years of age and over and are age-adjusted to the year 2000 standard population using five age groups: 25 to 44 years, 45 to 54 years, 55 to 64 years, 65 to 74 years, and 75 years and over.   6 GED is General Educational Development high school equivalency diploma.   7 Percent of poverty level is based on family income and family size and composition using U.S. Census Bureau poverty thresholds.   8 Any basic actions difficulty or complex activity limitation is defined as having one or more of the following limitations or difficulties: movement difficulty, emotional difficulty, sensory (seeing or hearing) difficulty, cognitive difficulty, self-care (activities of daily living or instrumental activities of daily living) limitation, social limitation, or work limitation.   9 MSA = metropolitan statistical area.

Table 3-9. Basic Actions Difficulty and Complex Activity Limitation Among Adults 18 Years of Age and Over, by Selected Characteristics, Selected Years, 1997–2013

(Number, percent.)

Characteristic	18 years and over				18 to 64 years				65 years and over			
	1997	2005	2010[1]	2013[1]	1997	2005	2010[1]	2013[1]	1997	2005	2010[1]	2013[1]
Number in Millions												
At least one basic actions difficulty or complex activity limitation[2,3]	60.9	66.5	73.7	75.4	41.3	45.4	50.7	49.8	19.6	21.1	23.0	25.6
At least one basic actions difficulty[2]	56.7	62.4	69.2	70.9	38.1	42.1	47.2	46.3	18.6	20.3	22.0	24.6
At least one complex activity limitation[3]	29.0	31.3	35.0	37.5	18.1	19.9	22.9	23.9	11.0	11.5	12.1	13.6
Percent with At Least One Basic Actions Difficulty or Complex Activity Limitation[2,3]												
Total, age-adjusted[4,5]	32.5	31.0	31.9	31.4	X	X	X	X	X	X	X	X
Total, crude[4]	31.8	31.2	32.8	32.9	25.8	25.3	27.1	26.6	62.2	62.4	61.7	61.1
Percent with At Least One Basic Actions Difficulty[2]												
Total, age-adjusted[4,5]	30.1	29.1	29.9	29.5	X	X	X	X	X	X	X	X
Total, crude[4]	29.4	29.3	30.8	30.9	23.6	23.5	25.1	24.7	58.8	60.1	59.3	58.9
Sex												
Male	25.6	25.2	26.3	26.3	20.7	20.3	21.4	21.0	54.5	55.2	53.8	52.8
Female	32.9	33.1	35.1	35.2	26.4	26.6	28.8	28.3	61.9	63.7	63.6	63.7
Race[6]												
White only	29.6	29.7	31.2	31.4	23.5	23.5	25.1	24.7	58.5	60.0	59.2	58.4
Black or African American only	31.4	30.4	32.3	33.6	26.9	26.1	28.4	29.0	64.4	63.2	62.9	63.8
American Indian or Alaska Native only	43.8	25.6	41.6	35.7	41.9	25.2	38.5	30.4	66.0	*	74.0	74.3
Asian only	15.5	15.7	17.5	17.6	13.0	11.8	12.8	12.3	46.4	46.2	50.1	53.4
Native Hawaiian or Other Pacific Islander only	NA	*	*	*	NA	*	*	*	NA	*	*	*
Two or more races	NA	40.0	36.3	34.7	NA	34.9	33.9	30.8	NA	90.4	65.4	71.6
Hispanic Origin and Race[6]												
Hispanic or Latino	23.8	21.6	24.7	23.3	21.0	18.7	21.2	19.9	54.6	56.2	61.5	56.9
Not Hispanic or Latino	30.0	30.4	31.8	32.3	23.9	24.3	25.9	25.7	59.0	60.3	59.1	59.1
White only	30.3	31.1	32.4	33.0	23.8	24.5	26.0	25.9	58.7	60.3	59.0	58.7
Black or African American only	31.5	30.7	32.6	34.1	27.0	26.3	28.6	29.5	64.4	63.5	63.2	63.7
Percent of Poverty Level[7]												
Below 100 percent	41.9	40.2	40.6	43.7	36.2	34.9	36.3	38.9	74.1	73.1	72.7	75.0
100 percent to 199 percent	38.2	38.4	38.7	39.4	29.2	29.6	30.5	30.6	66.6	68.5	69.5	70.2
200 percent to 399 percent	28.4	29.7	31.1	30.2	22.0	22.8	24.1	22.7	56.1	59.0	58.9	59.5
400 percent or more	21.0	21.4	23.0	22.4	18.2	18.1	19.3	18.0	45.5	48.2	47.0	45.4
Location of Residence												
Within MSA[8]	27.7	27.5	29.2	29.3	22.3	22.1	23.6	23.3	56.6	58.3	59.2	58.3
Outside MSA[8]	35.6	36.3	39.3	40.0	28.6	29.5	33.8	33.2	65.8	65.5	59.9	61.3
Percent with At Least One Complex Activity Limitation[3]												
Total, age-adjusted[4,5]	15.6	14.5	14.9	15.2	X	X	X	X	X	X	X	X
Total, crude[4]	15.1	14.6	15.5	16.0	11.2	11.0	12.1	12.4	35.1	33.6	32.3	32.0
Sex												
Male	13.7	12.9	14.0	14.8	10.6	10.1	11.3	12.0	31.9	29.4	30.1	29.1
Female	16.5	16.1	16.8	17.0	11.9	11.8	12.9	12.9	37.4	36.7	34.0	34.3
Race[6]												
White only	15.0	14.4	15.2	16.0	10.9	10.7	11.7	12.2	34.3	33.1	31.7	31.4
Black or African American only	19.0	17.1	19.7	19.0	15.2	14.0	17.0	15.9	47.1	40.9	39.9	39.7
American Indian or Alaska Native only	23.7	14.2	15.4	22.2	22.1	13.0	14.5	19.4	*42.6	*	*	42.7
Asian only	5.7	6.6	7.7	7.4	4.9	4.7	5.0	4.7	*14.8	*20.8	26.7	26.0
Native Hawaiian or Other Pacific Islander only	NA	*	*	*	NA	*	*	*	NA	*	*	*
Two or more races	NA	26.2	19.6	19.7	NA	21.8	17.0	17.8	NA	69.7	53.6	37.9
Hispanic Origin and Race[6]												
Hispanic or Latino	11.9	9.8	10.4	10.5	9.8	7.6	7.9	8.3	33.9	35.0	37.6	32.9
Not Hispanic or Latino	15.5	15.3	16.3	16.9	11.4	11.5	12.9	13.3	35.1	33.5	31.9	31.9
White only	15.4	15.2	16.1	17.1	11.1	11.3	12.5	13.2	34.4	32.9	31.1	31.4
Black or African American only	18.8	17.3	20.0	19.4	15.0	14.1	17.3	16.3	46.8	40.9	40.0	39.7
Percent of Poverty Level[7]												
Below 100 percent	30.0	27.3	27.5	29.6	25.2	23.4	24.0	26.1	56.9	51.5	54.5	52.7
100 percent to 199 percent	23.3	22.7	23.7	23.9	16.7	17.2	18.4	17.9	43.9	41.3	43.7	45.1
200 percent to 399 percent	13.3	14.0	14.5	14.9	9.3	9.9	10.8	10.7	30.6	31.8	29.3	31.6
400 percent or more	7.3	7.3	7.7	7.8	5.8	5.5	5.8	6.0	20.2	21.5	19.8	17.2
Location of Residence												
Within MSA[8]	14.1	13.2	14.2	14.8	10.6	9.9	10.9	11.5	32.7	31.7	31.6	31.2
Outside MSA[8]	19.0	20.0	22.2	22.3	13.6	15.4	18.8	18.2	42.8	39.7	35.2	35.3

Characteristic	18 years and over				18 to 64 years				65 years and over			
	1997	2005	2010[1]	2013[1]	1997	2005	2010[1]	2013[1]	1997	2005	2010[1]	2013[1]

NA = Not available.   X = Not applicable.   * = Figure does not meet standards of reliability or precision. Data preceded by an asterisk have a relative standard error (RSE) of 20 percent to 30 percent. Data not shown have an RSE of greater than 30 percent.   1 Starting with 2007 data, the hearing question, a component of the basic actions difficulty measure, was revised. Consequently, data for basic actions difficulty prior to 2007 are not comparable with 2007 data and beyond.   2 A basic actions difficulty is defined as having one or more of the following difficulties: movement, emotional, sensory (seeing or hearing), or cognitive.   3 A complex activity limitation is defined as having one or more of the following limitations: self-care (activities of daily living or instrumental activities of daily living), social, or work.   4 Includes all other races not shown separately.   5 Estimates are for persons 25 years of age and over and are age-adjusted to the year 2000 standard population using five age groups: 25 to 44 years, 45 to 54 years, 55 to 64 years, 65 to 74 years, and 75 years and over.   6 The race groups, White, Black, American Indian or Alaska Native, Asian, Native Hawaiian or Other Pacific Islander, and 2 or more races, include persons of Hispanic and non-Hispanic origin. Persons of Hispanic origin may be of any race.   7 Percent of poverty level is based on family income and family size and composition using U.S. Census Bureau poverty thresholds.   8 MSA = metropolitan statistical area.

Table 3-10. Selected Vision and Hearing Limitations Among Adults 18 Years of Age and Over, by Selected Characteristics, Selected Years, 1997–2013

(Percent.)

Characteristic	Any trouble seeing, even with glasses or contacts[1]					A lot of trouble hearing or deaf[2]				
	1997	2000	2005	2010	2013	2007	2010	2011	2012	2013
Percent of Adults										
18 years and over, age-adjusted[3,4]	10.0	9.0	9.2	9.1	8.7	2.3	2.1	2.2	2.0	2.0
18 years and over, crude[4]	9.8	8.9	9.3	9.4	9.1	2.3	2.2	2.2	2.0	2.1
Age										
18 to 44 years	6.2	5.3	5.5	6.2	5.5	0.4	0.5	0.6	0.4	0.4
18 to 24 years	5.4	4.2	5.0	5.8	5.5	*	*	*	*	*
25 to 44 years	6.5	5.7	5.7	6.3	5.5	0.5	0.5	0.7	0.5	0.4
45 to 64 years	12.0	10.7	11.2	11.6	11.1	2.0	1.9	1.9	1.7	1.7
45 to 54 years	12.2	10.9	11.0	10.7	10.6	1.2	1.2	1.5	1.3	1.1
55 to 64 years	11.6	10.5	11.5	12.7	11.7	3.0	2.7	2.4	2.0	2.4
65 years and over	18.1	17.4	17.4	13.9	14.3	8.7	7.6	7.7	7.0	7.4
65 to 74 years	14.2	13.6	13.2	12.2	11.5	4.7	4.6	4.6	4.0	4.4
75 years and over	23.1	21.9	22.0	16.1	18.0	13.3	11.1	11.6	11.1	11.4
Sex [3]										
Male	8.8	7.9	7.9	7.9	7.5	3.1	2.8	2.7	2.6	2.5
Female	11.1	10.1	10.5	10.3	9.8	1.6	1.6	1.7	1.5	1.6
Sex and Age										
Male										
18 to 44 years	5.3	4.4	4.5	5.2	4.5	*0.5	*0.7	*0.6	*0.5	*0.4
45 to 54 years	10.1	8.8	8.8	9.1	9.4	1.5	*1.1	*1.8	1.6	*1.4
55 to 64 years	10.5	9.5	10.5	10.7	10.4	4.7	3.9	3.2	2.8	3.1
65 to 74 years	13.2	12.8	11.4	10.5	10.9	7.0	6.7	6.0	5.9	6.0
75 years and over	21.4	20.7	20.4	15.7	14.7	16.9	14.5	14.7	14.2	14.1
Female										
18 to 44 years	7.1	6.2	6.5	7.1	6.5	*0.3	*0.3	0.5	0.4	*0.4
45 to 54 years	14.2	12.8	13.2	12.3	11.8	*1.0	*1.3	1.1	*1.1	*0.9
55 to 64 years	12.6	11.5	12.4	14.6	12.9	*1.3	1.6	1.6	1.3	1.7
65 to 74 years	15.0	14.4	14.8	13.6	12.1	2.8	2.9	3.3	*2.2	3.1
75 years and over	24.2	22.7	23.0	16.4	20.3	11.1	8.9	9.5	9.0	9.5
Race [3,5]										
White only	9.7	8.8	9.1	8.8	8.7	2.4	2.3	2.3	2.1	2.2
Black or African American only	12.8	10.6	10.9	12.1	10.0	1.2	1.1	1.2	1.1	1.0
American Indian or Alaska Native only	19.2	16.6	*14.9	15.0	13.7	*3.8	*	*	*	*
Asian only	6.2	6.3	5.5	5.3	4.9	*	*1.0	*1.8	*1.2	*1.1
Native Hawaiian or Other Pacific Islander only	NA	*	*	*	*	*	*	*	*	*
Two or more races	NA	16.2	16.4	13.1	11.8	*4.9	*	*	*	*1.4
Hispanic Origin and Race [3,5]										
Hispanic or Latino	10.0	9.7	9.6	9.2	9.7	2.5	1.4	1.4	2.0	1.3
Mexican	10.2	8.3	9.9	9.0	10.9	2.5	*1.5	1.6	*2.0	1.5
Not Hispanic or Latino	10.0	9.1	9.2	9.2	8.6	2.3	2.2	2.3	2.0	2.1
White only	9.8	8.9	9.1	8.9	8.6	2.5	2.4	2.4	2.1	2.3
Black or African American only	12.8	10.6	10.9	12.2	10.1	1.2	1.1	1.2	1.1	1.0
Education [6,7]										
25 years of age and over										
No high school diploma or GED	15.0	12.2	13.5	14.1	12.8	4.1	3.2	3.1	2.5	3.0
High school diploma or GED	10.6	9.5	10.3	10.5	10.0	2.8	2.5	2.8	2.6	2.5
Some college or more	8.9	8.9	8.6	8.0	8.0	1.9	2.0	2.0	1.9	1.9
Percent of Poverty Level [3,8]										
Below 100 percent	17.0	12.9	15.3	14.8	15.6	3.4	2.7	2.7	2.7	2.5
100 percent to 199 percent	12.9	11.6	11.5	12.2	11.2	2.8	2.5	2.5	2.3	2.4
200 percent to 399 percent	9.1	8.8	8.9	9.0	7.6	2.4	2.1	2.4	1.9	2.1
400 percent or more	7.3	7.1	6.9	6.4	6.4	1.6	1.8	1.7	1.7	1.6
Hispanic Origin and Race, and Percent of Poverty Level [3,5,8]										
Hispanic or Latino										
Below 100 percent	12.8	11.0	13.6	10.8	13.1	*	*	*1.3	*1.8	*
100 percent to 199 percent	11.2	9.4	8.8	10.8	10.6	*2.1	*2.3	*1.8	*	*1.6
200 percent to 399 percent	8.1	9.2	8.2	8.9	7.4	*	*	*1.3	*2.0	*
400 percent or more	*8.1	10.5	8.0	5.3	9.0	*	*	*	*	*
Not Hispanic or Latino										
White only										
Below 100 percent	17.9	13.1	16.2	16.8	17.7	4.3	3.7	3.6	3.6	3.2
100 percent to 199 percent	13.1	12.0	12.7	12.6	11.8	3.3	3.0	2.8	2.7	2.9
200 percent to 399 percent	9.2	9.2	9.0	8.8	7.8	2.6	2.3	2.8	2.0	2.4

Table 3-10. Selected Vision and Hearing Limitations Among Adults 18 Years of Age and Over, by Selected Characteristics, Selected Years, 1997–2013 — continued

(Percent.)

Characteristic	Any trouble seeing, even with glasses or contacts[1]					A lot of trouble hearing or deaf[2]				
	1997	2000	2005	2010	2013	2007	2010	2011	2012	2013
400 percent or more	7.3	7.0	6.9	6.7	6.4	1.7	2.0	1.8	1.8	1.8
Black or African American only										
Below 100 percent	17.9	13.6	16.0	15.8	15.3	*	*1.5	*1.6	*2.1	*1.4
100 percent to 199 percent	16.0	12.9	11.3	14.9	11.4	*	*0.7	*1.5	*1.2	*1.1
200 percent to 399 percent	9.3	7.7	9.7	12.0	8.0	*	*	*1.0	*	*
400 percent or more	7.7	8.3	6.4	6.6	6.7	*	*	*	*	*
Geographic Region[3]										
Northeast	8.6	7.4	8.1	7.8	7.4	1.7	1.4	2.3	1.6	1.8
Midwest	9.5	9.6	9.7	9.1	9.0	2.3	2.3	1.9	2.0	2.3
South	11.4	9.2	9.8	10.6	8.9	2.5	2.6	2.4	2.2	2.1
West	9.7	9.9	8.6	8.0	9.1	2.4	1.9	2.1	1.9	1.8
Location of Residence[3]										
Within MSA[9]	9.5	8.5	8.6	8.6	8.4	2.1	1.9	2.0	1.9	1.8
Outside MSA[9]	12.0	11.1	11.7	11.6	10.6	3.3	3.0	3.0	2.4	2.9

NA = Not available.   * = Figure does not meet standards of reliability or precision. Data preceded by an asterisk have a relative standard error (RSE) of 20 percent to 30 percent.   1 Respondents were asked, "Do you have any trouble seeing, even when wearing glasses or contact lenses?" Respondents were also asked, "Are you blind or unable to see at all?" In this analysis, any trouble seeing and blind are combined into one category. In 2011, 0.4 percent of adults 18 years of age and over identified themselves as blind.   2 Starting in 2007, respondents were asked, "WITHOUT the use of hearing aids or other listening devices,is your hearing excellent, good, a little trouble hearing, moderate trouble, a lot of trouble, or are you deaf?"   3 Estimates are age adjusted to the year 2000 standard population using five age groups: 18 to 44 years, 45 to 54 years, 55 to 64 years, 65 to 74 years, and 75 years and over. Age-adjusted estimates in this table may differ from other age-adjusted estimates based on the same data and presented elsewhere if different age groups are used in the adjustment procedure.   4 Includes all other races not shown separately and unknown education level.   5 The race groups White, Black, American Indian or Alaska Native, Asian, Native Hawaiian or Other Pacific Islander, and two or more races, include persons of Hispanic and non-Hispanic origin. Persons of Hispanic origin may be of any race.   6 Estimates are for persons 25 years of age and over and are age-adjusted to the year 2000 standard population using five age groups: 25 to 44 years, 45 to 54 years, 55 to 64 years, 65 to 74 years, and 75 years and over.   7 GED is General Educational Development high school equivalency diploma.   8 Percent of poverty level is based on family income and family size and composition using U.S. Census Bureau poverty thresholds.   9 MSA = metropolitan statistical area.

Table 3-11. Respondent-Assessed Health Status, by Selected Characteristics, Selected Years, 1991–2013

(Percent.)

Characteristic	1991[1]	1995[1]	2000	2005	2010	2011	2012	2013
Percent of Persons with Fair or Poor Health [2]								
All ages, age-adjusted[3,4]	10.4	10.6	9.0	9.2	9.6	9.8	9.5	9.4
All ages, crude[4]	10.0	10.1	8.9	9.3	10.1	10.4	10.3	10.2
Age								
Under 18 years	2.6	2.6	1.7	1.8	2.0	2.0	2.1	1.7
Under 6 years	2.7	2.7	1.5	1.6	1.8	1.5	1.5	1.6
6 to 17 years	2.6	2.5	1.8	1.9	2.2	2.2	2.4	1.8
18 to 44 years	6.1	6.6	5.1	5.5	6.3	6.5	6.4	6.2
18 to 24 years	4.8	4.5	3.3	3.3	3.9	4.2	3.8	3.6
25 to 44 years	6.4	7.2	5.7	6.3	7.2	7.3	7.4	7.2
45 to 54 years	13.4	13.4	11.9	11.6	13.3	14.1	14.2	14.1
55 to 64 years	20.7	21.4	17.9	18.3	19.4	19.1	19.3	19.2
65 years and over	29.0	28.3	26.9	26.6	24.4	24.7	22.7	23.1
65 to 74 years	26.0	25.6	22.5	23.4	21.2	21.5	19.6	19.7
75 years and over	33.6	32.2	32.1	30.2	28.3	28.6	26.6	27.6
Sex [3]								
Male	10.0	10.1	8.8	8.8	9.2	9.4	9.2	9.0
Female	10.8	11.1	9.3	9.5	10.0	10.1	9.9	9.8
Race [3,5]								
White only	9.6	9.7	8.2	8.6	8.8	9.0	8.8	8.7
Black or African American only	16.8	17.2	14.6	14.3	14.9	15.0	14.9	14.3
American Indian or Alaska Native only	18.3	18.7	17.2	13.2	17.8	14.4	16.5	15.3
Asian only	7.8	9.3	7.4	6.8	8.1	8.7	7.9	7.7
Native Hawaiian or Other Pacific Islander only	NA	NA	*	*	*	*	*	*
Two or more races	NA	NA	16.2	14.5	15.6	14.2	13.0	13.9
Black or African American; White	NA	NA	*14.5	8.3	*16.7	16.7	16.3	*19.0
American Indian and Alaska Native; White	NA	NA	18.7	17.2	19.0	16.5	14.4	16.2
Hispanic Origin and Race [3,5]								
Hispanic or Latino	15.6	15.1	12.8	13.3	13.1	13.2	13.3	12.7
Mexican	17.0	16.7	12.8	14.3	13.7	14.0	13.6	13.3
Not Hispanic or Latino	10.0	10.1	8.7	8.7	9.2	9.4	9.1	9.0
White only	9.1	9.1	7.9	8.0	8.2	8.4	8.1	8.2
Black or African American only	16.8	17.3	14.6	14.4	14.9	15.0	15.0	14.2
Percent of Poverty Level [3,6]								
Below 100 percent	22.8	23.7	19.6	20.4	20.9	21.5	21.6	21.8
100 percent to 199 percent	14.7	15.5	14.1	14.4	15.2	15.0	14.9	14.4
200 percent to 399 percent	7.9	7.9	8.4	8.3	8.3	8.7	8.4	8.2
400 percent or more	4.9	4.7	4.5	4.7	4.3	4.3	3.9	4.0
Hispanic Origin and Race and Percent of Poverty Level [3,5,6]								
Hispanic or Latino								
Below 100 percent	23.6	22.7	18.7	20.2	19.2	21.0	20.9	20.3
100 percent to 199 percent	18.0	16.9	15.3	15.3	15.6	14.4	14.5	14.3
200 percent to 399 percent	10.3	10.1	10.3	10.3	10.3	10.8	10.0	10.3
400 percent or more	6.6	4.0	5.5	7.6	6.4	5.0	6.7	5.3
Not Hispanic or Latino								
White only								
Below 100 percent	21.9	22.8	18.8	20.1	20.9	21.2	21.1	22.2
100 percent to 199 percent	14.0	14.8	13.4	13.8	14.8	15.0	15.3	14.4
200 percent to 399 percent	7.5	7.3	7.9	7.9	7.7	8.1	7.7	7.7
400 percent or more	4.7	4.6	4.2	4.3	4.0	4.1	3.5	3.8
Black or African American only								
Below 100 percent	25.8	27.7	23.8	23.3	23.9	24.7	25.0	24.8
100 percent to 199 percent	17.0	19.3	18.2	17.6	18.3	18.5	16.9	17.5
200 percent to 399 percent	12.0	11.4	11.7	11.2	11.2	10.7	11.9	9.8
400 percent or more	5.9	6.5	7.3	7.1	6.8	6.9	6.6	5.0
Disability Measure Among Adults 18 Years and Over [3,7]								
Any basic actions difficulty or complex activity limitation	NA	NA	27.6	28.5	28.7	30.1	30.2	30.5
Any basic actions difficulty	NA	NA	27.7	29.1	28.9	30.6	30.6	30.7
Any complex activity limitation	NA	NA	45.6	46.3	46.0	48.3	46.6	47.8
No disability	NA	NA	3.8	3.6	3.5	3.6	3.6	3.8
Geographic Region [3]								

Table 3-11. Respondent-Assessed Health Status, by Selected Characteristics, Selected Years, 1991–2013— continued

(Percent.)

Characteristic	1991[1]	1995[1]	2000	2005	2010	2011	2012	2013
Northeast	8.3	9.1	7.6	7.5	7.9	8.4	8.0	8.2
Midwest	9.1	9.7	8.0	8.3	9.0	8.8	9.1	8.8
South	13.1	12.3	10.7	11.0	11.1	11.2	10.8	10.6
West	9.7	10.1	8.8	8.6	9.2	9.5	9.1	9.1
Location of Residence [3,8]								
Within MSA	9.9	10.1	8.5	8.7	9.2	9.4	9.0	9.1
Outside MSA	11.9	12.6	11.1	11.2	11.9	11.7	12.3	11.4

NA = Not available.   * = Figure does not meet standards of reliability or precision. Data preceded by an asterisk have a relative standard error (RSE) of 20 percent to 30 percent. Data not shown have an RSE of greater than 30 percent.   1 Data prior to 1997 are not strictly comparable with data for later years due to the 1997 questionnaire redesign.   2 See Appendix II, Health status, respondent-assessed, in Health, United States, 2014.   3 Estimates are age-adjusted to the year 2000 standard population using six age groups: under 18 years, 18 to 44 years, 45 to 54 years, 55 to 64 years, 65 to 74 years, and 75 years and over. The disability measure is age-adjusted using the five adult age groups. The disability measure is age-adjusted using the five adult age groups.   4 Includes all other races not shown separately and unknown disability status.   5 The race groups White, Black, American Indian or Alaska Native, Asian, Native Hawaiian or Other Pacific Islander, and two or more races, include persons of Hispanic and non-Hispanic origin. Persons of Hispanic origin may be of any race.   6 Percent of poverty level is based on family income and family size and composition using U.S. Census Bureau poverty thresholds.   7 Any basic actions difficulty or complex activity limitation is defined as having one or more of the following limitations or difficulties: movement difficulty, emotional difficulty, sensory (seeing or hearing) difficulty, cognitive difficulty, self-care (activities of daily living or instrumental activities of daily living) limitation, social limitation, or work limitation.   8 MSA = metropolitan statistical area.

Table 3-12. Serious Psychological Distress in the Past 30 Days Among Adults 18 Years of Age and Over, by Selected Characteristics, Annual Average, Selected Years, 1997–1998 through 2012–2013

(Percent of persons with serious psychological distress[1].)

Characteristic	1997–1998	2004–2005	2009–2010	2010–2011	2011–2012	2020–2013
18 years and over, age-adjusted[2,3]	3.2	3.0	3.2	3.3	3.1	3.4
18 years and over, crude[3]	3.2	3.0	3.3	3.4	3.2	3.4
Age	2.9	2.8	3.1	2.9	2.8	3.1
18 to 44 years	2.7	2.5	2.4	2.4	2.3	2.4
18 to 24 years	3.0	2.9	3.4	3.1	3.0	3.3
25 to 44 years	3.7	3.7	4.1	4.5	4.2	4.4
45 to 64 years	3.9	3.9	4.1	4.2	4.0	4.4
45 to 54 years	3.4	3.4	4.0	4.7	4.4	4.4
55 to 64 years						
	3.1	2.5	2.1	2.4	2.3	2.5
65 years and over	2.5	2.2	2.0	2.6	2.5	2.7
65 to 74 years	3.8	2.9	2.3	2.1	1.9	2.2
75 years and over						
Sex[2]	2.5	2.3	2.8	2.8	2.5	2.7
Male	3.8	3.7	3.7	3.7	3.7	4.0
Female						
Race[2,4]	3.1	2.9	3.2	3.2	3.1	3.3
White only	4.0	3.6	3.8	3.7	3.3	3.3
Black or African American only	7.8	*3.5	*5.2	5.6	6.5	4.1
American Indian or Alaska Native only	2.0	1.7	1.6	1.7	1.9	2.1
Asian only						
Native Hawaiian or Other Pacific Islander only	NA	*	*	*	*	*
Two or more races	NA	7.9	5.2	5.6	6.7	7.8
Hispanic Origin and Race[2,4]						
Hispanic or Latino	5.0	3.7	3.6	4.0	3.8	3.8
Mexican	5.2	3.6	2.8	3.6	3.4	3.6
Not Hispanic or Latino	3.0	3.0	3.2	3.2	3.1	3.3
White only	2.9	2.9	3.1	3.2	3.1	3.3
Black or African American only	3.9	3.6	3.8	3.7	3.3	3.2
Percent of Poverty Level[2,5]						
Below 100 percent	9.1	8.6	8.4	8.2	8.2	9.2
100 percent to 199 percent	5.0	5.0	4.8	5.0	4.9	5.3
200 percent to 399 percent	2.5	2.5	2.8	2.9	2.6	2.4
400 percent or more	1.3	1.1	1.2	1.2	1.1	1.3
Hispanic Origin and Race and Percent of Poverty Level[2,4,5]						
Hispanic or Latino						
Below 100 percent	8.6	6.6	6.4	7.5	7.4	7.0
100 percent to 199 percent	5.4	3.9	4.1	4.3	3.9	3.9
200 percent to 399 percent	3.4	2.6	2.6	3.1	2.3	2.6
400 percent or more	*	*1.9	*1.5	*1.4	*1.4	*1.7
Not Hispanic or Latino						
White only						
Below 100 percent	9.6	10.2	10.1	9.6	9.4	11.4
100 percent to 199 percent	5.2	5.6	5.5	5.6	5.8	6.7
200 percent to 399 percent	2.5	2.6	3.2	3.2	2.8	2.5
400 percent or more	1.3	1.1	1.1	1.1	1.0	1.3
Black or African American only						
Below 100 percent	8.7	7.6	8.3	7.7	7.3	7.8
100 percent to 199 percent	4.3	4.8	3.5	4.4	3.5	3.0
200 percent to 399 percent	2.2	2.1	2.5	1.9	2.0	2.2
400 percent or more	*	*	*1.6	*1.5	*1.0	*
Geographic Region[2]						
Northeast	2.7	2.5	3.1	3.0	2.7	2.9
Midwest	2.6	2.7	3.3	3.1	3.0	3.5
South	3.8	3.7	3.5	3.6	3.5	3.6
West	3.3	2.8	2.9	3.3	3.1	3.1
Location of Residence[2,6]						
Within MSA	3.0	2.8	3.1	3.1	3.0	3.2
Outside MSA	3.9	4.0	4.1	4.0	4.1	4.3

NA = Not available.   * = Figure does not meet standards of reliability or precision. Data preceded by an asterisk have a relative standard error (RSE) of 20 percent to 30 percent. Data not shown have an RSE of greater than 30 percent.   1 Serious psychological distress is measured by a six-question scale that asks respondents how often they experienced each of six symptoms of psychological distress in the past 30 days.   2 Estimates are age adjusted to the year 2000 standard population using five age groups: 18 to 44 years, 45 to 54 years, 55 to 64 years, 65 to 74 years, and 75 years and over.   3 Includes all other races not shown separately.   4 The race groups White, Black, American Indian or Alaska Native, Asian, Native Hawaiian or Other Pacific Islander, and two or more races, include persons of Hispanic and non-Hispanic origin. Persons of Hispanic origin may be of any race.   5 Percent of poverty level is based on family income and family size and composition using U.S. Census Bureau poverty thresholds.   6 MSA = metropolitan statistical area.

Table 3-13. Children Under 18 Years of Age Who Suffer from Asthma, by Selected Characteristics, Annual Average, Selected Years, 1997–1999 through 2011–2013

(Percent of children.)

Characteristic	Current asthma[1]					Asthma attack in the past 12 months[2]				
	1997–1999	2000–2002	2009–2011	2010–2012	2011–2013	1997–1999	2000–2002	2009–2011	2010–2012	2011–2013
Children Under 18 Years[3]	NA	NA	9.5	9.4	9.0	5.4	5.7	5.6	5.5	5.3
Age										
0 to 4 years	NA	NA	6.4	6.1	5.5	4.3	4.7	4.5	4.2	3.6
5 to 17 years	NA	NA	10.7	10.7	10.4	5.7	6.1	6.0	6.1	5.9
5 to 9 years	NA	NA	10.2	10.3	9.8	5.6	6.3	6.2	6.6	6.2
10 to 17 years	NA	NA	11.1	10.9	10.8	5.8	5.9	5.8	5.7	5.7
Sex										
Male	NA	NA	10.7	10.2	9.8	6.2	6.6	6.3	6.3	5.9
Female	NA	NA	8.3	8.5	8.2	4.5	4.7	4.8	4.8	4.7
Hispanic Origin and Race[4]										
Race[4]										
White only	NA	NA	8.1	8.1	7.8	5.0	5.2	4.8	4.9	4.7
Black or African American only	NA	NA	16.4	16.0	15.3	7.0	8.0	8.8	8.9	8.5
American Indian or Alaska Native only	NA	NA	*6.6	9.4	9.5	6.4	*8.7	*3.5	*5.5	*5.8
Asian only	NA	NA	7.7	6.8	5.6	4.3	4.7	5.2	4.4	3.2
Native Hawaiian or Other Pacific Islander only	NA	NA	*	*	*	NA	*	*	*	*
Two or more races	NA	NA	13.3	12.7	13.1	NA	7.3	8.0	7.1	7.1
Hispanic Origin										
Hispanic or Latino	NA	NA	8.5	8.8	8.6	4.8	4.2	4.7	4.9	4.6
Not Hispanic or Latino	NA	NA	9.8	9.6	9.2	5.5	6.0	5.8	5.7	5.5
White only	NA	NA	8.2	8.0	7.7	5.1	5.5	5.0	5.0	4.8
Black or African American only	NA	NA	16.4	16.1	15.2	7.0	7.9	8.8	9.0	8.5
Percent of Poverty Level[5]										
Below 100 percent	NA	NA	12.7	12.5	12.4	6.1	7.1	7.5	7.5	7.2
100 percent to 199 percent	NA	NA	9.9	9.9	9.2	5.3	5.4	5.9	6.0	5.2
200 percent to 399 percent	NA	NA	8.3	8.7	8.3	5.0	5.3	4.6	4.7	4.7
400 percent or more	NA	NA	7.8	7.0	6.7	5.2	5.5	4.7	4.4	4.3
Health Insurance Status at the Time of Interview[6]										
Insured	NA	NA	9.7	9.6	9.2	5.6	5.9	5.7	5.7	5.4
Private	NA	NA	8.2	8.1	7.7	5.0	5.3	4.9	4.8	4.6
Medicaid	NA	NA	12.0	11.9	11.4	7.7	7.7	6.9	7.0	6.4
Uninsured	NA	NA	6.8	6.7	6.9	3.9	4.3	3.6	4.0	4.3

NA = Not available.   * = Figure does not meet standards of reliability or precision. Data preceded by an asterisk have a relative standard error (RSE) of 20 percent to 30 percent. Data not shown have an RSE of greater than 30 percent.   1 Based on parent or knowledgeable adult responding to both questions, "Has a doctor or other health professional ever told you that your child had asthma?" and "Does your child still have asthma?"   2 Based on parent or knowledgeable adult responding to both questions, "Has a doctor or other health professional ever told you that your child had asthma?" and "During the past 12 months, did your child have an episode of asthma or an asthma attack?"   3 Includes all other races not shown separately, unknown poverty level, and unknown health insurance status.   4 The race groups White, Black, American Indian or Alaska Native, Asian, Native Hawaiian or Other Pacific Islander, and two or more races, include persons of Hispanic and non-Hispanic origin. Persons of Hispanic origin may be of any race.   5 Percent of poverty level is based on family income and family size and composition using U.S. Census Bureau poverty thresholds. Missing family income data were imputed for 1997 and beyond.   6 Health insurance categories are mutually exclusive. Persons who reported both Medicaid and private coverage are classified as having private coverage. Starting with 1997 data, state-sponsored health plan coverage is included as Medicaid coverage. Starting with 1999 data, coverage by the Children's Health Insurance Program (CHIP) is included as Medicaid coverage. In addition to private and Medicaid, the insured category also includes military, other government, and Medicare coverage. Persons not covered by private insurance, Medicaid, CHIP, state-sponsored or other government-sponsored health plans, Medicare, or military plans are considered to have no health insurance coverage. Persons with only Indian Health Service coverage are considered to have no health insurance coverage.

Table 3-14. Hypertension Among Persons 20 Years of Age and Over, by Selected Characteristics, Selected Years, 1988–1994 through 2009–2012

(Percent.)

Sex, age, race and Hispanic origin[1], and percent of poverty level	Hypertension[2,3]			Uncontrolled high blood pressure among persons with hypertension[4]		
	1988–1994	2001–2004	2009–2012	1988–1994	2001–2004	2005–2008
20 Years and Over, Age-Adjusted [5]						
Both Sexes [6]	25.5	30.9	30.0	77.2	66.0	55.1
Male	26.4	30.3	30.6	83.2	68.3	62.0
Female	24.4	31.0	29.3	68.5	57.6	44.7
Not Hispanic or Latino						
White only, male	25.6	29.3	29.6	82.6	67.8	58.7
White only, female	23.0	29.0	27.5	67.0	52.7	42.8
Black or African American only, male	37.5	41.5	42.5	84.0	70.8	68.9
Black or African American only, female	38.3	44.3	44.2	71.1	65.4	46.8
Mexican origin, male	26.9	26.1	27.3	87.9	76.4	76.4
Mexican origin, female	25.0	29.7	29.3	77.6	63.8	47.1
Percent of Poverty Level [7]						
Below 100 percent	31.7	35.5	33.4	75.0	66.1	56.3
100 percent to 199 percent	26.6	34.0	33.1	76.0	70.1	57.6
200 percent to 399 percent	24.7	31.4	30.6	76.2	67.8	51.5
400 percent or more	22.6	27.9	27.3	81.5	60.8	60.2
20 Years and Over, Crude						
Both Sexes [6]	24.1	30.8	32.2	73.9	63.0	47.4
Male	23.8	29.0	31.6	79.3	62.1	50.7
Female	24.4	32.5	32.8	68.8	63.7	44.2
Not Hispanic or Latino						
White only, male	24.3	29.9	33.1	78.0	59.4	47.2
White only, female	24.6	32.9	33.7	67.8	63.8	42.6
Black or African American only, male	31.1	36.7	39.9	83.3	68.7	60.5
Black or African American only, female	32.5	41.6	44.5	70.0	61.9	45.8
Mexican male	16.4	15.8	19.1	86.5	73.6	69.8
Mexican female	15.9	19.0	22.0	80.6	69.8	52.8
Percent of Poverty Level [7]						
Below 100 percent	25.7	28.3	27.3	74.0	67.3	54.8
100 percent to 199 percent	26.7	34.6	35.3	75.1	64.5	49.8
200 percent to 399 percent	22.4	31.5	33.4	73.4	63.4	45.7
400 percent or more	22.0	28.4	31.5	74.3	59.2	43.1
Male						
20 to 44 years	10.9	12.3	11.2	90.5	71.0	70.3
20 to 34 years	7.1	7.0	5.8	92.6	87.1	88.4
35 to 44 years	17.1	19.2	19.1	89.0	63.2	62.0
45 to 64 years	34.2	39.9	42.2	73.1	61.1	50.2
45 to 54 years	29.2	35.9	33.6	76.2	64.9	47.7
55 to 64 years	40.6	47.5	51.9	70.3	55.5	52.0
65 to 74 years	54.4	61.7	61.7	74.3	49.5	36.9
75 years and over	60.4	67.1	75.1	82.5	68.3	48.9
Female						
20 to 44 years	6.5	7.7	8.7	63.4	51.0	46.5
20 to 34 years	2.9	*2.7	3.9	82.2	*50.2	49.0
35 to 44 years	11.2	14.0	15.5	56.8	51.2	45.5
45 to 64 years	32.8	42.6	39.5	62.1	60.9	36.5
45 to 54 years	23.9	35.2	29.5	58.5	66.1	36.2
55 to 64 years	42.6	54.4	51.0	64.3	55.6	36.8
65 to 74 years	56.2	72.9	66.7	68.7	67.2	45.4
75 years and over	73.6	82.0	79.3	81.9	72.4	57.8

* = Figure does not meet standards of reliability or precision. Data preceded by an asterisk have a relative standard error (RSE) of 20 percent to 30 percent.   1 Persons of Mexican origin may be of any race.   2 Hypertension is defined as having measured high blood pressure and/or taking antihypertensive medication. High blood pressure is defined as having measured systolic pressure of at least 140 mmHg or diastolic pressure of at least 90 mmHg. Those with high blood pressure also may be taking prescribed medicine for high blood pressure. Those taking antihypertensive medication may not have measured high blood pressure but are still classified as having hypertension.   3 Respondents were asked, "Are you now taking prescribed medicine for your high blood pressure?"   4 Uncontrolled high blood pressure among persons with hypertension is defined as measured systolic pressure of at least 140 mmHg or diastolic pressure of at least 90 mmHg, among those with measured high blood pressure or reporting taking antihypertensive medication.   5 Age-adjusted to the 2000 standard population using five age groups: 20 to 34 years, 35 to 44 years, 45 to 54 years, 55 to 64 years, and 65 years and over.   6 Includes persons of all races and Hispanic origins, not just those shown separately.   7 Percent of poverty level is based on family income and family size. Persons with unknown percent of poverty level are excluded (8 percent in 2007-2010).

Table 3-15. Cholesterol Among Persons 20 Years of Age and Over, by Selected Characteristics, Selected Years, 1988–1994 through 2009–2012

(Percent, number.)

Characteristic[1]	1988–1994	2007–2010	2009–2012
PERCENT OF POPULATION WITH HYPERCHOLESTEROLEMIA[2]			
20 Years and Over, Age-Adjusted [3]			
Both Sexes [4]	22.8	27.4	27.8
Male	21.1	28.0	27.9
Female	24.0	26.7	27.5
Not Hispanic or Latino			
White only, male	21.1	28.1	28.1
White only, female	24.2	27.4	28.2
Black or African American only, male	18.6	25.4	25.6
Black or African American only, female	23.1	25.6	26.3
Mexican origin, male	19.9	28.6	27.2
Mexican origin, female	19.8	25.5	26.2
Percent of Poverty Level [5]			
Below 100 percent	23.0	26.5	28.7
100 percent to 199 percent	22.1	27.6	27.1
200 percent to 399 percent	23.1	28.9	28.1
400 percent or more	21.7	26.6	27.4
20 Years and Over, Crude			
Both Sexes [4]	21.5	28.7	29.5
Male	19.6	28.7	28.8
Female	23.2	28.7	30.1
Not Hispanic or Latino			
White only, male	20.0	30.4	30.9
White only, female	24.5	31.4	33.4
Black or African American only, male	16.0	24.1	24.4
Black or African American only, female	19.7	24.7	25.5
Mexican origin, male	16.2	23.7	21.9
Mexican origin, female	14.9	21.0	19.4
Percent of Poverty Level [5]			
Below 100 percent	19.4	22.3	24.1
100 percent to 199 percent	21.3	28.7	28.2
200 percent to 399 percent	21.3	30.6	30.5
400 percent or more	21.9	29.6	31.6
Male			
20 to 44 years	13.1	14.3	12.6
20 to 34 years	8.2	8.5	6.6
35 to 44 years	21.0	22.5	21.2
45 to 64 years	30.1	39.0	39.8
45 to 54 years	29.6	34.0	35.7
55 to 64 years	30.8	46.2	44.5
65 to 74 years	27.4	48.9	50.7
75 years and over	24.4	45.2	51.2
Female			
20 to 44 years	9.9	10.6	9.4
20 to 34 years	7.3	6.8	6.3
35 to 44 years	13.5	15.7	14.0
45 to 64 years	36.4	39.1	42.4
45 to 54 years	28.2	29.1	31.2
55 to 64 years	45.8	51.4	55.3
65 to 74 years	46.9	53.3	57.7
75 years and over	41.2	52.5	53.3
PERCENT OF POPULATION WITH HIGH CHOLESTEROL[6]			
20 Years and Over, Age-Adjusted [3]			
Both Sexes [4]	20.8	13.7	12.9
Male	19.0	12.6	11.7
Female	22.0	14.4	14.0
Not Hispanic or Latino			
White only, male	18.8	12.2	11.6
White only, female	22.2	15.3	14.7
Black or African American only, male	16.9	10.8	9.0
Black or African American only, female	21.4	11.5	10.8
Mexican origin, male	18.5	15.1	13.5
Mexican origin, female	18.7	13.6	12.8
Percent of Poverty Level [5]			
Below 100 percent	20.6	14.4	13.4
100 percent to 199 percent	20.6	15.0	13.2
200 percent to 399 percent	20.8	14.4	13.2

Table 3-15. Cholesterol Among Persons 20 Years of Age and Over, by Selected Characteristics, Selected Years, 1988–1994 through 2009–2012— continued

(Percent, number.)

Characteristic[1]	1988–1994	2007–2010	2009–2012
400 percent or more	19.5	12.3	12.3
20 Years and Over, Crude			
Both Sexes [4]	19.6	14.1	13.4
Male	17.7	12.9	11.8
Female	21.3	15.2	14.9
Not Hispanic or Latino			
White only, male	18.0	12.6	11.8
White only, female	22.5	16.7	16.5
Black or African American only, male	14.7	10.9	8.8
Black or African American only, female	18.2	11.3	10.6
Mexican origin, male	15.4	14.7	13.0
Mexican origin, female	14.3	12.3	10.9
Percent of Poverty Level [5]			
Below 100 percent	17.6	12.8	12.0
100 percent to 199 percent	19.8	14.6	12.9
200 percent to 399 percent	19.3	14.6	13.9
400 percent or more	19.9	13.7	13.6
Male			
20 to 44 years	12.5	11.1	10.0
20 to 34 years	8.2	7.6	6.0
35 to 44 years	19.4	16.2	15.8
45 to 64 years	27.2	17.7	16.2
45 to 54 years	26.6	18.7	18.0
55 to 64 years	28.0	16.3	14.1
65 to 74 years	21.9	7.5	8.1
75 years and over	20.4	6.8	*5.5
Female			
20 to 44 years	9.4	8.4	7.6
20 to 34 years	7.3	5.8	5.7
35 to 44 years	12.3	11.9	10.4
45 to 64 years	33.4	21.3	22.4
45 to 54 years	26.7	17.7	18.7
55 to 64 years	40.9	25.6	26.6
65 to 74 years	41.3	20.6	19.6
75 years and over	38.2	20.2	16.2
MEAN SERUM TOTAL CHOLESTEROL LEVEL, MG/DL			
20 Years and Over, Age-Adjusted [3]			
Both Sexes [4]	206	196	195
Male	204	194	192
Female	207	198	198
Not Hispanic or Latino			
White only, male	205	193	192
White only, female	208	199	199
Black or African American only, male	202	191	188
Black or African American only, female	207	192	192
Mexican origin, male	206	200	197
Mexican origin, female	206	196	194
Percent of Poverty Level [5]			
Below 100 percent	205	196	196
100 percent to 199 percent	205	198	194
200 percent to 399 percent	207	196	195
400 percent or more	205	195	196
20 Years and Over, Crude			
Both Sexes [4]	204	197	196
Male	202	194	193
Female	206	199	199
Not Hispanic or Latino			
White only, male	203	193	193
White only, female	208	201	202
Black or African American only, male	198	191	187
Black or African American only, female	201	191	191
Mexican origin, male	199	200	198
Mexican origin, female	198	195	193
Percent of Poverty Level [5]			
Below 100 percent	200	194	192
100 percent to 199 percent	202	197	193
200 percent to 399 percent	205	197	196
400 percent or more	206	198	199

Table 3-15. Cholesterol Among Persons 20 Years of Age and Over, by Selected Characteristics, Selected Years, 1988–1994 through 2009–2012— continued

(Percent, number.)

Characteristic[1]	1988–1994	2007–2010	2009–2012
Male			
20 to 44 years	194	194	191
20 to 34 years	186	186	182
35 to 44 years	206	205	204
45 to 64 years	216	202	200
45 to 54 years	216	204	203
55 to 64 years	216	199	198
65 to 74 years	212	182	184
75 years and over	205	176	173
Female			
20 to 44 years	189	187	187
20 to 34 years	184	181	180
35 to 44 years	195	195	196
45 to 64 years	225	211	212
45 to 54 years	217	208	209
55 to 64 years	235	214	216
65 to 74 years	233	207	206
75 years and over	229	203	201

1 Persons of Mexican origin may be of any race.   2 Hypercholesterolemia is defined as measured serum total cholesterol greater than or equal to 240 mg/dL or reporting taking cholesterol-lowering medications. Respondents were asked, "Are you now following this advice [from a doctor or health professional] to take prescribed medicine [to lower your cholesterol]?"   3 Age adjusted to the 2000 standard population using five age groups: 20 to 34 years, 35 to 44 years, 45 to 54 years, 55 to 64 years, and 65 years and over.   4 Includes persons of all races and Hispanic origins, not just those shown separately. 5 Percent of poverty level is based on family income and family size. Persons with unknown percent of poverty level are excluded (8 percent in 2007–2010).   6 High cholesterol is defined as serum total cholesterol greater than or equal to 240 mg/dL (6.20 mmol/L), regardless of whether the respondent reported taking cholesterol-lowering medications.

Table 3-16. Mean Energy and Macronutrient Intake Among Persons 20 Years of Age and Over, by Sex and Age, Selected Years, 1988–1994 through 2009–2012

(Percent, number.)

Characteristic	1988–1994	1999–2002	2003–2006	2007–2010	2009–2012
Percent kcal from carbohydrates					
Both sexes, age-adjusted[1]	49.8	50.7	48.9	49.5	49.5
Both sexes, crude	49.8	50.7	48.9	49.4	49.4
20-44 years	49.2	51.3	49.3	50.1	49.9
45-64 years	49.7	49.3	47.5	48.2	48.5
65-74 years	51.1	50.5	49.2	49.0	49.0
75 years and over	53.0	52.6	51.5	51.1	51.0
Male, age-adjusted[1]	48.5	49.5	47.8	48.0	48.1
Male, crude	48.4	49.4	47.7	47.9	48.0
20-44 years	48.1	50.2	48.4	48.7	48.5
45-64 years	48.3	48.0	46.3	46.4	47.2
65-74 years	49.4	49.4	47.6	47.5	47.0
75 years and over	50.9	51.0	50.3	50.4	50.3
Female, age-adjusted[1]	51.0	51.9	49.9	50.8	50.8
Female, crude	51.0	51.9	49.9	50.7	50.7
20-44 years	50.3	52.5	50.2	51.4	51.3
45-64 years	51.0	50.6	48.7	49.8	49.8
65-74 years	52.5	51.4	50.6	50.4	50.9
75 years and over	54.2	53.7	52.4	51.6	51.6
Percent kcal from protein					
Both sexes, age-adjusted[1]	15.5	15.3	15.6	15.8	15.7
Both sexes, crude	15.4	15.3	15.6	15.8	15.7
20-44 years	15.0	14.9	15.3	15.6	15.6
45-64 years	15.9	15.6	16.0	16.0	15.8
65-74 years	16.2	16.3	15.9	16.2	16.4
75 years and over	16.0	15.4	15.6	15.8	15.8
Male, age-adjusted[1]	15.5	15.4	15.6	16.0	16.0
Male, crude	15.4	15.4	15.6	16.0	16.0
20-44 years	15.0	15.0	15.4	15.8	15.8
45-64 years	15.9	15.7	15.8	16.3	16.0
65-74 years	15.9	16.3	16.0	16.3	16.6
75 years and over	16.3	15.7	15.8	15.9	16.0
Female, age-adjusted[1]	15.5	15.2	15.6	15.6	15.5
Female, crude	15.4	15.2	15.6	15.6	15.5
20-44 years	14.9	14.8	15.2	15.4	15.3
45-64 years	15.9	15.5	16.1	15.8	15.5
65-74 years	16.5	16.3	15.9	16.1	16.2
75 years and over	15.9	15.3	15.5	15.7	15.6
Percent kcal from total fat					
Both sexes, age-adjusted[1]	33.5	33.0	33.7	33.1	32.9
Both sexes, crude	33.5	33.0	33.7	33.2	33.0
20-44 years	34.0	32.4	33.1	32.3	32.3
45-64 years	33.4	33.9	34.6	34.1	33.5
65-74 years	32.3	33.4	34.3	34.1	33.7
75 years and over	32.0	32.8	33.1	33.3	33.3
Male, age-adjusted[1]	33.8	33.0	33.5	33.1	33.0
Male, crude	33.9	33.0	33.6	33.2	33.0
20-44 years	34.1	32.2	32.6	32.2	32.2
45-64 years	33.9	34.0	34.8	34.3	33.8
65-74 years	33.0	33.4	34.5	34.4	34.1
75 years and over	33.0	33.2	33.3	33.2	33.1
Female, age-adjusted[1]	33.2	33.1	33.8	33.1	32.8
Female, crude	33.2	33.1	33.9	33.2	32.9
20-44 years	33.9	32.6	33.6	32.4	32.4
45-64 years	32.9	33.9	34.4	33.9	33.2
65-74 years	31.6	33.3	34.1	33.9	33.3
75 years and over	31.5	32.6	32.9	33.4	33.5
Percent kcal from saturated fat					
Both sexes, age-adjusted[1]	11.2	10.7	11.2	10.8	10.6
Both sexes, crude	11.2	10.7	11.2	10.9	10.6
20-44 years	11.5	10.8	11.1	10.6	10.5
45-64 years	11.1	10.8	11.4	11.1	10.8
65-74 years	10.7	10.5	11.2	11.1	10.7
75 years and over	10.7	10.3	11.0	10.9	10.8

Table 3-16. Mean Energy and Macronutrient Intake Among Persons 20 Years of Age and Over, by Sex and Age, Selected Years, 1988–1994 through 2009–2012— continued

(Percent, number.)

Characteristic	1988–1994	1999–2002	2003–2006	2007–2010	2009–2012
Male, age-adjusted[1]	11.3	10.7	11.1	10.8	10.6
Male, crude	11.4	10.7	11.1	10.9	10.6
20-44 years	11.5	10.8	11.0	10.6	10.4
45-64 years	11.2	10.7	11.3	11.2	10.9
65-74 years	10.9	10.6	11.2	11.0	10.8
75 years and over	11.2	10.7	11.2	10.9	10.7
Female, age-adjusted[1]	11.1	10.7	11.2	10.9	10.6
Female, crude	11.1	10.7	11.3	10.9	10.6
20-44 years	11.4	10.8	11.2	10.7	10.5
45-64 years	10.9	10.9	11.5	11.0	10.6
65-74 years	10.4	10.4	11.3	11.2	10.7
75 years and over	10.5	10.1	10.8	11.0	10.9

1 Age adjusted to the 2000 standard population using four age groups: 20 to 44 years, 45 to 64 years, 65 to 74 years, and 75 years and over.

Table 3-17. Participation in Leisure-Time Aerobic and Muscle-Strengthening Activities That Meet the 2008 Federal Physical Activity Guidelines for Adults 18 Years of Age and Over, by Selected Characteristics, 2000 and 2013

(Percent.)

| Characteristic | 2008 Physical Activity Guidelines for Americans[1] | | | | | | | |
| | Met both aerobic activity and muscle-strengthening guidelines | | Met neither aerobic activity nor muscle-strengthening guideline | | Met aerobic activity guideline | | Met muscle-strengthening guideline | |
	2000	2013	2000	2013	2000	2013	2000	2013
18 years and over, age-adjusted[2,3]	15.0	21.0	54.7	46.5	42.2	50.1	18.0	24.4
18 years and over, crude[3]	15.1	20.4	54.6	47.2	42.4	49.4	18.1	23.9
Age								
18 to 44 years	18.9	25.7	49.1	40.3	47.7	56.9	22.1	28.5
18 to 24 years	23.8	30.3	44.5	35.5	52.2	61.5	27.2	33.3
25 to 44 years	17.3	24.0	50.6	42.0	46.3	55.1	20.5	26.8
45 to 64 years	12.8	17.8	57.6	50.2	39.7	46.4	15.5	21.3
45 to 54 years	14.5	20.1	55.4	48.4	42.1	48.4	17.0	23.3
55 to 64 years	10.1	15.3	61.0	52.1	36.1	44.1	13.1	19.0
65 years and over	6.8	11.7	67.0	59.4	30.1	35.8	9.8	16.7
65 to 74 years	8.4	14.7	60.3	54.0	36.8	41.8	11.3	19.2
75 years and over	4.9	7.6	75.0	66.8	22.1	27.6	8.0	13.4
Sex [2]								
Male	17.9	25.0	49.6	42.0	47.4	54.3	20.8	28.7
Female	12.3	17.2	59.4	50.7	37.6	46.2	15.4	20.2
Sex and Age								
Male								
18 to 44 years	23.0	31.7	43.0	34.7	53.6	61.8	26.3	35.2
45 to 54 years	16.0	22.3	52.7	46.3	45.2	50.4	18.0	25.5
55 to 64 years	11.3	17.6	58.7	49.6	38.9	46.7	13.8	21.1
65 to 74 years	9.4	15.9	55.3	49.7	41.8	46.5	12.2	20.0
75 years and over	7.1	7.8	66.7	60.6	30.7	33.2	10.1	14.3
Female								
18 to 44 years	15.0	19.8	55.0	45.7	42.0	52.0	17.9	22.0
45 to 54 years	13.1	18.0	57.9	50.5	39.1	46.4	16.1	21.2
55 to 64 years	9.0	13.2	63.1	54.4	33.5	41.7	12.4	17.1
65 to 74 years	7.7	13.6	64.3	57.7	32.6	37.7	10.5	18.5
75 years and over	3.6	7.5	80.0	71.0	16.8	23.7	6.7	12.7
Race [2,4]								
White only	15.7	21.7	53.1	45.2	44.1	51.5	18.5	25.0
Black or African American only	12.2	17.7	64.6	54.7	31.7	41.4	16.0	21.7
American Indian or Alaska Native only	*10.6	16.8	67.1	50.8	29.7	47.4	13.9	20.0
Asian only	14.1	18.3	55.0	47.6	41.7	49.5	17.2	21.0
Native Hawaiian or Other Pacific Islander only	*	*	*	*	*	*	*	*
Two or more races	19.0	22.4	52.8	44.4	43.9	51.6	22.2	26.7
Hispanic Origin and Race [2,4]								
Hispanic or Latino	9.2	16.6	66.5	53.8	30.8	42.9	11.9	19.8
Mexican	8.1	15.0	67.0	53.4	30.0	43.5	11.3	18.1
Not Hispanic or Latino	15.8	21.9	53.2	45.2	43.7	51.5	18.8	25.2
White only	16.5	22.9	51.4	43.1	45.7	53.6	19.3	26.2
Black or African American only	12.2	17.8	64.6	54.7	31.7	41.4	16.0	21.8
Education [5,6]								
No high school diploma or GED	4.3	8.0	74.0	66.6	23.9	30.7	6.6	10.9
High school diploma or GED	9.5	13.8	61.7	57.0	35.7	39.9	12.1	16.9
Some college or more	18.9	24.4	47.1	40.6	49.4	55.7	22.4	28.1
Percent of Poverty Level [2,7]								
Below 100 percent	9.3	12.6	68.0	59.5	29.3	37.2	12.3	15.9
100 percent to 199 percent	9.0	14.3	65.5	56.7	32.0	39.5	11.5	18.0
200 percent to 399 percent	13.2	19.2	56.8	48.0	39.9	48.8	16.5	22.4
400 percent or more	20.5	29.1	45.0	35.6	52.0	61.1	23.4	32.5
Hispanic Origin and Race and Percent of Poverty Level [2,7]								
Hispanic or Latino								
Below 100 percent	4.4	8.7	75.2	65.1	22.1	32.2	7.2	11.6
100 percent to 199 percent	5.0	12.2	72.2	60.1	25.8	36.4	7.1	15.6
200 percent to 399 percent	10.2	20.6	63.1	48.5	33.0	48.6	14.0	23.5
400 percent or more	19.6	27.6	52.8	39.5	45.1	56.8	21.7	31.2
Not Hispanic or Latino								
White only								
Below 100 percent	11.7	14.9	63.5	56.2	34.0	40.0	14.7	18.5
100 percent to 199 percent	10.3	15.7	62.6	53.8	34.8	42.7	12.9	19.0
200 percent to 399 percent	13.9	19.0	54.7	46.8	42.3	50.1	16.9	22.0
400 percent or more	21.0	30.0	43.7	33.9	53.4	62.7	23.8	33.3

Table 3-17. Participation in Leisure-Time Aerobic and Muscle-Strengthening Activities That Meet the 2008 Federal Physical Activity Guidelines for Adults 18 Years of Age and Over, by Selected Characteristics, 2000 and 2013— continued

(Percent.)

| Characteristic | 2008 Physical Activity Guidelines for Americans[1] | | | | | | | |
| | Met both aerobic activity and muscle-strengthening guidelines | | Met neither aerobic activity nor muscle-strengthening guideline | | Met aerobic activity guideline | | Met muscle-strengthening guideline | |
	2000	2013	2000	2013	2000	2013	2000	2013
Black or African American only								
Below 100 percent	9.5	11.6	72.1	63.5	25.4	33.4	12.1	14.8
100 percent to 199 percent	9.5	13.8	69.2	62.0	28.0	33.0	12.3	18.9
200 percent to 399 percent	11.8	17.1	64.3	52.7	31.4	42.9	16.2	21.6
400 percent or more	17.6	28.5	54.9	39.4	40.3	57.0	22.4	32.8
Disability Measure [2,8]								
Any basic actions difficulty or complex activity limitation	10.3	14.1	62.2	56.9	34.2	38.6	14.0	18.5
Any basic actions difficulty	10.3	13.8	62.1	57.3	34.0	38.3	14.2	18.2
Any complex activity limitation	7.2	10.8	71.2	65.1	24.9	29.5	11.3	16.2
No disability	17.0	24.2	50.6	40.2	46.6	56.7	19.8	27.4
Geographic Region [2]								
Northeast	17.0	22.2	51.8	47.1	45.3	49.2	20.0	26.0
Midwest	16.4	21.7	53.4	46.3	43.5	50.0	19.3	25.3
South	12.1	18.2	59.7	49.5	37.3	47.3	15.1	21.5
West	16.7	23.7	50.1	41.5	46.9	55.4	19.7	26.9
Location of residence [2,9]								
Within MSA	15.7	21.9	54.1	45.3	42.9	51.3	18.6	25.4
Outside MSA	12.3	15.7	56.9	53.5	39.9	43.4	15.5	18.7

* = Figure does not meet standards of reliability or precision. Data preceded by an asterisk have a relative standard error (RSE) of 20 percent to 30 percent. Data not shown have an RSE of greater than 30 percent.   1 Starting with Health, United States, 2010, measures of physical activity shown in this table changed to reflect the 2008 federal Physical Activity Guidelines for Americans (available from http://www.health.gov/PAGuidelines/).   2 Estimates are age adjusted to the year 2000 standard population using five age groups: 18 to 44 years, 45 to 54 years, 55 to 64 years, 65 to 74 years, and 75 years and over.   3 Includes all other races not shown separately, unknown education level, and unknown disability status.   4 The race groups White, Black, American Indian or Alaska Native, Asian, Native Hawaiian or Other Pacific Islander, and two or more races, include persons of Hispanic and non-Hispanic origin. Persons of Hispanic origin may be of any race.   5 Estimates are for persons 25 years of age and over and are age-adjusted to the year 2000 standard population using five age groups: 25–44 years, 45–54 years, 55–64 years, 65–74 years, and 75 years and over.   6 GED is General Educational Development high school equivalency diploma.   7 Percent of poverty level is based on family income and family size and composition using U.S. Census Bureau poverty thresholds.   8 Any basic actions difficulty or complex activity limitation is defined as having one or more of the following limitations or difficulties: movement difficulty, emotional difficulty, sensory (seeing or hearing) difficulty, cognitive difficulty, self-care (activities of daily living or instrumental activities of daily living) limitation, social limitation, or work limitation.   9 MSA = metropolitan statistical area.

Table 3-18A. Healthy Weight, Overweight, and Obesity Among Persons 20 Years of Age and Over, by Selected Characteristics, Selected Years, 1988–1994 through 2009–2012

(Percent.)

Sex, age, race and Hispanic origin[1], and percent of poverty level	Healthy weight (BMI from 18.5 to 24.9)[2]						
	1988–1994	1999–2002	2001–2004	2003–2006	2005–2008	2007–2010	2009–2012
20 Years and Over, Age-Adjusted [3]							
Both Sexes [4]	41.6	33.0	32.3	31.6	30.8	29.8	29.6
Male	37.9	30.2	28.3	26.6	26.1	25.7	26.2
Female	45.0	35.7	36.1	36.5	35.2	33.7	32.8
Not Hispanic or Latino							
White only, male	37.3	29.6	28.0	26.8	26.0	25.5	26.2
White only, female	48.7	39.5	39.8	39.6	37.8	36.9	36.0
Black or African American only, male	40.1	34.7	30.8	27.0	26.7	28.5	28.0
Black or African American only, female	29.2	21.6	18.9	19.2	20.4	17.9	16.4
Mexican origin, male	30.2	26.5	25.3	23.8	21.8	18.5	17.5
Mexican origin, female	29.7	27.5	26.5	25.1	24.1	21.3	20.9
Percent of Poverty Level [5]							
Below 100 percent	37.5	32.7	34.3	32.1	29.1	27.3	27.3
100 percent to 199 percent	39.3	30.5	31.9	31.3	28.3	27.6	26.5
200 percent to 399 percent	41.8	29.6	29.4	29.7	30.0	29.7	30.0
400 percent or more	45.5	36.5	35.1	33.7	33.5	32.1	32.0
20 Years and Over, Crude							
Both Sexes [4]	42.6	32.9	32.2	31.4	30.5	29.6	29.2
Male	39.4	30.4	28.4	26.6	26.1	25.8	26.2
Female	45.7	35.4	35.8	35.9	34.8	33.2	31.9
Not Hispanic or Latino							
White only, male	38.2	29.2	27.4	26.2	25.4	24.8	25.6
White only, female	48.8	38.7	38.8	38.2	36.9	35.7	34.2
Black or African American only, male	41.5	35.9	31.5	27.1	27.4	29.4	28.5
Black or African American only, female	31.2	21.8	19.3	19.2	20.3	17.6	16.1
Mexican origin, male	35.2	29.4	28.1	25.2	22.8	19.5	17.9
Mexican origin, female	32.4	29.5	28.0	25.8	24.7	22.3	22.2
Percent of Poverty Level [5]							
Below 100 percent	39.8	34.5	36.2	33.2	30.9	29.2	29.2
100 percent to 199 percent	41.5	31.5	32.6	31.7	28.8	28.0	26.8
200 percent to 399 percent	42.9	29.7	29.3	29.6	30.0	29.5	29.6
400 percent or more	44.6	35.3	33.5	32.1	31.8	30.5	30.3
Male							
20 to 34 years	51.1	40.3	38.3	35.9	38.0	37.5	37.5
35 to 44 years	33.4	29.0	26.5	24.1	20.9	19.8	21.0
45 to 54 years	33.6	24.0	21.2	20.8	21.7	21.8	20.0
55 to 64 years	28.6	23.8	22.2	19.3	18.5	19.4	21.9
65 to 74 years	30.1	22.8	23.1	21.2	20.2	21.6	22.4
75 years and over	40.9	32.0	32.1	33.1	28.1	25.4	28.2
Female							
20 to 34 years	57.9	42.5	44.2	45.1	40.5	41.1	40.8
35 to 44 years	47.1	37.1	38.3	37.6	36.2	34.4	35.2
45 to 54 years	37.2	33.1	31.0	31.1	32.1	30.7	27.3
55 to 64 years	31.5	27.6	29.2	29.5	29.9	26.7	23.8
65 to 74 years	37.0	26.4	27.0	28.5	28.8	23.9	23.5
75 years and over	43.0	36.9	34.6	35.4	36.3	35.4	35.3

Table 3-18B. Healthy Weight, Overweight, and Obesity Among Persons 20 Years of Age and Over, by Selected Characteristics, Selected Years, 1988–1994 through 2009–2012

(Percent.)

Sex, age, race and Hispanic origin[1], and percent of poverty level	Overweight (includes obesity; BMI greater than or equal to 25.0)[2]						
	1988–1994	1999–2002	2001–2004	2003–2006	2005–2008	2007–2010	2009–2012
20 Years and Over, Age-Adjusted [3]							
Both Sexes [4]	56.0	65.1	66.0	66.7	67.5	68.5	68.7
Male	60.9	68.8	70.5	72.1	72.9	73.3	72.9
Female	51.4	61.6	61.6	61.3	62.5	63.9	64.6
Not Hispanic or Latino							
White only, male	61.6	69.4	71.0	71.8	72.9	73.6	73.2
White only, female	47.5	57.2	57.6	57.9	59.6	60.3	60.9
Black or African American only, male	57.8	62.6	67.0	71.6	71.7	70.0	70.2
Black or African American only, female	68.2	77.2	79.6	79.8	78.0	80.0	81.8
Mexican origin, male	68.9	73.2	74.6	75.8	77.7	81.3	81.9
Mexican origin, female	68.9	71.2	73.0	73.9	74.8	78.0	78.3
Percent of Poverty Level [5]							
Below 100 percent	59.6	64.7	63.4	65.7	67.7	69.7	70.0
100 percent to 199 percent	58.0	67.3	66.2	66.5	69.6	70.5	71.7
200 percent to 399 percent	56.0	68.6	68.8	69.0	68.7	68.6	68.3
400 percent or more	52.4	62.2	63.7	64.7	65.3	66.9	66.8
20 Years and Over, Crude							
Both Sexes [4]	54.9	65.2	66.1	66.9	67.8	68.7	69.1
Male	59.4	68.6	70.4	72.1	72.8	73.2	72.9
Female	50.7	62.0	61.9	61.9	63.0	64.5	65.5
Not Hispanic or Latino							
White only, male	60.6	69.9	71.6	72.5	73.4	74.2	73.8
White only, female	47.4	58.2	58.7	59.4	60.7	61.7	62.9
Black or African American only, male	56.7	61.7	66.3	71.6	71.1	69.1	69.6
Black or African American only, female	66.0	76.9	79.1	79.7	78.1	80.2	82.1
Mexican origin, male	63.9	70.1	71.8	74.6	76.8	80.2	81.4
Mexican origin, female	65.9	69.3	71.4	73.0	73.9	77.1	76.9
Percent of Poverty Level [5]							
Below 100 percent	56.8	62.5	61.4	64.4	65.9	67.8	68.0
100 percent to 199 percent	55.7	66.2	65.3	66.0	69.1	70.1	71.4
200 percent to 399 percent	54.9	68.5	69.0	69.0	68.7	68.8	68.8
400 percent or more	53.3	63.7	65.5	66.5	67.2	68.5	68.6
Male							
20 to 34 years	47.5	57.4	59.0	61.6	60.5	61.1	60.9
35 to 44 years	65.5	70.5	72.9	75.2	78.8	80.2	78.9
45 to 54 years	66.1	75.7	78.5	78.5	76.8	76.8	79.3
55 to 64 years	70.5	75.4	77.3	79.7	80.5	79.8	77.4
65 to 74 years	68.5	76.2	76.1	78.0	79.1	77.5	76.9
75 years and over	56.5	67.4	66.8	65.8	70.8	73.2	70.4
Female							
20 to 34 years	37.0	52.9	51.6	50.9	55.6	55.4	55.2
35 to 44 years	49.6	60.6	60.1	60.7	62.1	63.9	62.4
45 to 54 years	60.3	65.1	67.4	67.3	65.8	66.2	70.5
55 to 64 years	66.3	72.2	69.9	69.6	69.4	72.2	75.1
65 to 74 years	60.3	70.9	71.5	70.5	69.6	74.2	73.8
75 years and over	52.3	59.9	63.7	62.6	61.3	63.2	62.4

Table 3-18C. Healthy Weight, Overweight, and Obesity Among Persons 20 Years of Age and Over, by Selected Characteristics, Selected Years, 1988–1994 through 2009–2012

(Percent.)

Sex, age, race and Hispanic origin[1], and percent of poverty level	Obesity (BMI greater than or equal to 30.0)[2]						
	1988–1994	1999–2002	2001–2004	2003–2006	2005–2008	2007–2010	2009–2012
20 Years and Over, Age-Adjusted [3]							
Both Sexes [4]	22.9	30.4	31.4	33.4	34.0	34.7	35.3
Male	20.2	27.5	29.5	32.4	32.7	33.9	34.6
Female	25.5	33.2	33.2	34.3	35.4	35.5	35.9
Not Hispanic or Latino							
White only, male	20.3	28.0	30.2	32.4	32.6	34.1	34.4
White only, female	22.9	30.7	30.7	31.6	33.1	32.5	32.3
Black or African American only, male	20.9	27.8	30.8	35.7	37.5	38.3	38.1
Black or African American only, female	38.3	48.6	51.1	53.4	51.0	54.0	57.5
Mexican origin, male	23.8	27.8	29.1	29.5	32.0	36.3	40.2
Mexican origin, female	35.2	38.0	39.4	41.8	43.3	44.6	46.3
Percent of Poverty Level [5]							
Below 100 percent	28.1	34.7	33.7	35.0	35.9	37.2	38.3
100 percent to 199 percent	26.1	34.1	33.6	35.9	38.0	37.3	40.1
200 percent to 399 percent	22.7	32.1	33.3	35.7	35.7	36.8	37.0
400 percent or more	18.7	25.5	27.3	28.9	29.4	31.3	30.2
20 Years and Over, Crude							
Both Sexes [4]	22.3	30.5	31.5	33.5	34.3	34.9	35.5
Male	19.5	27.5	29.5	32.4	32.8	33.9	34.6
Female	25.0	33.4	33.3	34.6	35.6	35.9	36.4
Not Hispanic or Latino							
White only, male	19.9	28.4	30.5	32.6	33.1	34.4	34.7
White only, female	22.7	31.3	31.2	32.2	33.3	33.2	33.5
Black or African American only, male	20.7	27.5	30.7	35.8	37.2	38.1	37.9
Black or African American only, female	36.7	48.7	51.1	53.2	51.0	54.2	57.6
Mexican origin, male	20.6	26.0	27.8	29.0	30.9	35.6	40.2
Mexican origin, female	33.3	37.0	38.5	41.2	42.9	44.2	45.2
Percent of Poverty Level [5]							
Below 100 percent	25.9	33.0	33.0	34.6	35.4	36.5	37.0
100 percent to 199 percent	24.3	32.8	32.6	35.0	37.0	36.8	40.0
200 percent to 399 percent	22.1	31.8	33.2	35.5	35.6	36.8	37.1
400 percent or more	19.3	27.2	28.6	30.7	31.7	32.4	31.7
Male							
20 to 34 years	14.1	21.7	23.2	26.2	25.4	27.1	28.9
35 to 44 years	21.5	28.5	33.8	37.0	35.9	37.2	38.1
45 to 54 years	23.2	30.6	31.8	34.6	35.9	36.6	38.1
55 to 64 years	27.2	35.5	36.0	39.3	40.4	37.3	38.1
65 to 74 years	24.1	31.9	32.1	33.0	36.2	41.5	36.4
75 years and over	13.2	18.0	19.9	24.0	25.6	26.6	27.4
Female							
20 to 34 years	18.5	28.3	28.6	28.4	31.4	30.4	30.0
35 to 44 years	25.5	32.1	33.3	36.1	36.7	37.1	36.0
45 to 54 years	32.4	36.9	38.0	40.0	39.1	36.9	38.3
55 to 64 years	33.7	42.1	39.0	41.0	42.3	43.4	42.9
65 to 74 years	26.9	39.3	37.9	36.4	35.6	40.3	44.2
75 years and over	19.2	23.6	23.2	24.2	25.9	28.7	29.8

NA = Not available.   * = Figure does not meet standards of reliability or precision. Data preceded by an asterisk have a relative standard error (RSE) of 20 percent to 30 percent. Data not shown have an RSE of greater than 30 percent.   1 Persons of Hispanic origin may be of any race.   2 Body mass index (BMI) equals weight in kilograms divided by height in meters squared.   3 Age adjusted to the year 2000 standard population using five age groups: 20 to 34 years, 35 to 44 years, 45 to 54 years, 55 to 64 years, and 65 years and over (65 to 74 years for estimates for 20 to 74 years).   4 Includes all other races and origins not shown separately.   5 Percent of poverty level is based on family income and family size. Persons with unknown percent of poverty level are excluded (8 percent in 2007–2010).

Table 3-19. Untreated Dental Caries, by Selected Characteristics, Selected Years, 1988–1994 through 2011–2012

(Percent.)

Sex, race and Hispanic origin[1], and percent of poverty level	Age 5–19 years		Age 20–44 years		Age 45-64 years		Age 65 years and over	
	1988–1994	2011–2012	1988–1994	2011–2012	1988–1994	2011–2012	1988–1994	2011–2012
Total [2]	24.3	17.5	29.5	27.4	25.4	25.8	27.1	18.9
Sex								
Male	23.6	18.9	32.8	29.0	28.5	31.7	31.2	20.8
Female	25.0	16.1	26.4	25.9	22.6	20.3	24.1	17.3
Race and Hispanic Origin								
Not Hispanic or Latino								
White only	19.4	14.5	24.8	22.1	21.7	22.1	24.6	15.5
Black or African American only	33.9	23.2	49.2	41.4	46.2	43.2	51.2	40.9
Mexican origin	37.9	24.2	40.0	38.0	41.4	44.1	46.3	48.3
Percent of Poverty Level [3]								
Below 100 percent	39.0	24.6	47.8	40.2	49.5	51.6	46.8	39.5
100 percent to 199 percent	29.6	21.6	43.7	38.0	42.5	41.0	37.6	33.1
200 percent to 399 percent	16.6	15.4	24.5	22.0	25.0	28.1	24.1	*12.2
400 percent or more	*10.4	*4.8	12.5	*11.3	13.0	11.7	15.6	*
Race and Hispanic Origin, and Percent of Poverty Level [3]								
Not Hispanic or Latino								
White only								
Below 100% of poverty level	33.8	21.7	42.9	*39.0	47.6	*51.6	38.5	46.1
100% or more of poverty level	17.3	12.3	22.7	17.8	19.7	19.8	23.9	14.1
Black or African American only								
Below 100% of poverty level	37.4	29.2	60.0	48.0	62.9	69.7	56.3	*44.5
100% or more of poverty level	31.2	18.0	44.8	37.8	41.2	35.2	47.8	39.1
Mexican origin								
Below 100% of poverty level	47.5	24.2	52.7	38.0	52.7	*45.7	62.8	*56.7
100% or more of poverty level	28.0	22.8	31.2	35.1	34.5	43.4	35.4	*45.0

NOTE: Root caries are not included. Persons without at least one primary or one permanent tooth or one root tip were classified as edentulous and were excluded from this analysis. The majority of edentulous persons are 65 years of age and over. Estimates of edentulism among persons 65 years of age and over are 46 percent in 1971–1974, 33 percent in 1988–1994, and 23 percent in 2005–2008. For estimates prior to 2005–2008, only dental caries in primary teeth was evaluated for children 2–5 years of age. Caries in both permanent and primary teeth was evaluated for children 6–11 years of age. For children 12–19 years of age and adults, only dental caries in permanent teeth was evaluated. Starting with 2005–2006 data, dental caries data were collected using a simplified examination process that used health technologists to screen for caries instead of using dentists to conduct a comprehensive caries exam. In addition, dental caries data were not collected on children younger than 5 years of age. Because of this change in the examination process and because 2005–2008 dental caries data are based on both primary and permanent teeth, regardless of age, data for 2005–2008 need to be interpreted with caution, especially when comparing with earlier data.   * = Figure does not meet standards of reliability or precision. Data preceded by an asterisk have a relative standard error (RSE) of 20 percent to 30 percent. Data not shown have an RSE of greater than 30 percent.   1 Persons of Mexican origin may be of any race.   2 Includes persons of all races and Hispanic origins, not just those shown separately, and those with unknown percent of poverty level.   3 Percent of poverty level is based on family income and family size. Persons with unknown percent of poverty level are excluded (6 percent in 2011–2012).

Table 3-20. Selected Health Conditions and Risk Factors, Selected Years, 1988–1994 through 2011–2012

(Percent.)

Health condition	1988–1994	1999–2000	2001–2002	2003–2004	2005–2006	2007–2008	2009–2010	2011–2012
Diabetes [1]								
Total, age-adjusted[2]	9.1	9.0	10.5	10.8	10.4	11.5	11.5	NA
Total, crude	8.4	8.5	10.1	10.8	10.7	11.9	12.0	NA
High Cholesterol [3]								
Total, age-adjusted[4]	22.8	25.5	24.6	27.9	27.4	27.6	27.2	28.2
Total, crude	21.5	24.5	24.2	27.9	28.1	28.8	28.6	30.4
High Serum Total Cholesterol [5]								
Total, age-adjusted[4]	20.8	18.3	16.5	16.9	15.6	14.2	13.2	12.7
Total, crude	19.6	17.7	16.4	17.0	15.9	14.6	13.6	13.1
Hypertension [6]								
Total, age-adjusted[4]	25.5	30.0	29.7	32.1	30.5	31.2	30.0	30.0
Total, crude	24.1	28.9	28.9	32.5	31.7	32.6	31.9	32.5
Uncontrolled High Blood Pressure Among Persons with Hypertension [7]								
Total, age-adjusted[4]	77.2	71.9	68.3	63.8	63.0	56.2	55.7	54.6
Total, crude	73.9	69.1	65.4	60.8	56.6	51.8	46.7	48.0
Overweight (Includes Obesity) [8]								
Total, age-adjusted[4]	56.0	64.5	65.6	66.4	66.9	68.1	68.8	68.6
Total, crude	54.9	64.1	65.6	66.5	67.3	68.3	69.2	69.0
Obesity [9]								
Total, age-adjusted[4]	22.9	30.5	30.5	32.3	34.4	33.7	35.7	34.9
Total, crude	22.3	30.3	30.6	32.3	34.7	33.9	35.9	35.1
Untreated Dental Caries [10]								
Total, age-adjusted[4]	27.7	24.3	21.3	30.0	24.4	21.7	NA	NA
Total, crude	28.2	25.0	21.6	30.3	24.5	21.8	NA	NA
Percent of Persons Under 20 Years of Age								
Obesity [11]								
2 to 5 years	7.2	10.3	10.6	14.0	11.0	10.1	12.1	8.4
6 to 11 years	11.3	15.1	16.3	18.8	15.1	19.6	18.0	17.7
12 to 19 years	10.5	14.8	16.7	17.4	17.8	18.1	18.4	20.5
Untreated Dental Caries [10]								
6 to 19 years	23.6	22.7	20.6	25.2	NA	16.9	14.3	NA

NA = Not available.   1 Includes physician-diagnosed and undiagnosed diabetes. Estimates were obtained using fasting weights. was obtained by self-report and excludes women who reported having diabetes only during pregnancy. Undiagnosed diabetes is defined as a fasting plasma glucose (FPG) of at least 126 mg/dL or a hemoglobin A1c of at least 6.5% and no reported physician diagnosis.   2 Age adjusted to the 2000 standard population using three age groups: 20 to 44 years, 45 to 64 years, and 65 years and over.   3 Hypercholesterolemia is defined as measured serum total cholesterol greater than or equal to 240 mg/dL or reporting taking cholesterol-lowering medication. Respondents were asked, "Are you now following this advice [from a doctor or health professional] to take prescribed medicine [to lower your cholesterol]?"   4 Age adjusted to the 2000 standard population using five age groups: 20 to 34 years, 35 to 44 years, 45 to 54 years, 55 to 64 years, and 65 years and over.   5 Highcholesterol is defined as greater than or equal to 240 mg/dL (6.20 mmol/L).   6 Hypertension is defined as having measured high blood pressure and/or taking antihypertensive medication. High blood pressure is defined as having measured systolic pressure of at least 140 mmHg or diastolic pressure of at least 90 mmHg. Those with high blood pressure also may be taking prescribed medicine for high blood pressure. For antihypertensive medication use, respondents were asked, "Are you now taking prescribed medicine for your high blood pressure?"   7 Uncontrolled high blood pressure among persons with hypertension is defined as measured systolic pressure of at least 140 mmHg or diastolic pressure of at least 90 mmHg, among those with measured high blood pressure or reporting taking antihypertensive medication.   8 Excludes pregnant women. Overweight is defined as body mass index (BMI) greater than or equal to 25.0.   9 Excludes pregnant women. Obesity is defined as body mass index (BMI) greater than or equal to 30.0.   10 Untreated dental caries refers to decay on the crown or enamel surface of a tooth (i.e., coronal caries) that has not been treated or filled. The presence of caries was evaluated in primary and permanent teeth for persons aged 5 and older. The third molars were not included. Persons without at least one natural tooth (primary or permanent) were excluded.   11 Obesity is defined as body mass index (BMI) at or above the sex- and age-specific 95th percentile BMI cutoff points from the 2000 CDC growth charts for the United States.

Figure 3-2. Human Immunodeficiency Virus (HIV) Diagnosis by Race and Hispanic Origin, 2012

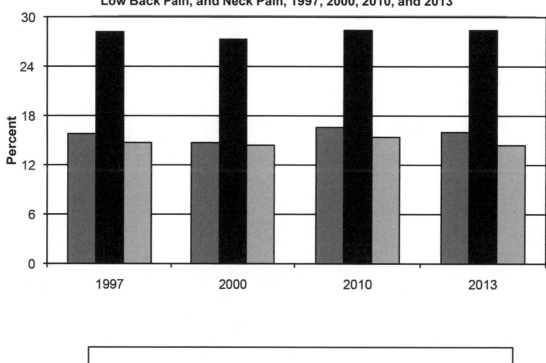

Native Hawaiian or Other Pacific Islander 0.2%

American Indian and Alaska Native 0.5%

Asian 2.0%

Multiple race 2.2%

Black or African American 47.0%

Hispanic or Latino (of any race) 20.5%

White 27.6%

Figure 3-3. Age-Adjusted Rates for Persons Age 18 Years and Over Suffering From Severe Headache or Migraine, Low Back Pain, and Neck Pain, 1997, 2000, 2010, and 2013

■ Severe headache or migraine   ■ Low back pain   ■ Neck pain

Figure 3-4. Age Adjusted Healthy Weight, Overweight, and Obesity Prevalence Among Persons 20–74 Years, Selected Years, 1960–1962 through 2009–2012

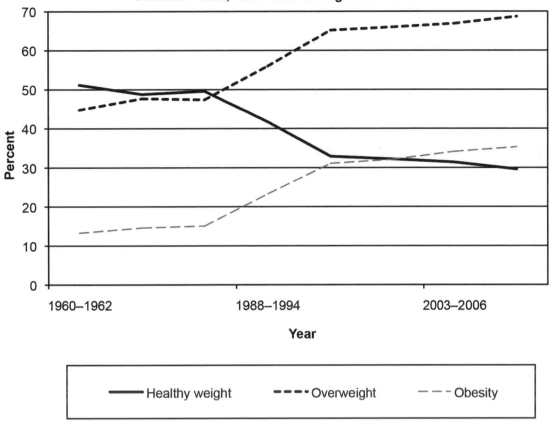

Figure 3-5. Obesity in Children and Adolescents Age 6 to 19 Years, Selected Years, 1971–1974 through 2009–2012

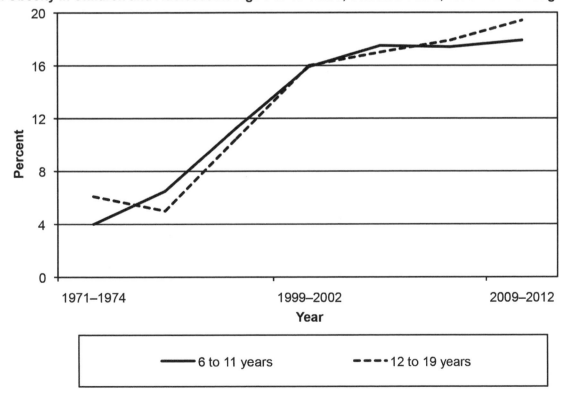

USE OF ADDICTIVE SUBSTANCES

Figure 3-6. Use of Selected Substances in the Past Month Among Persons 12 Years and Over, 2002, 2008, and 2013

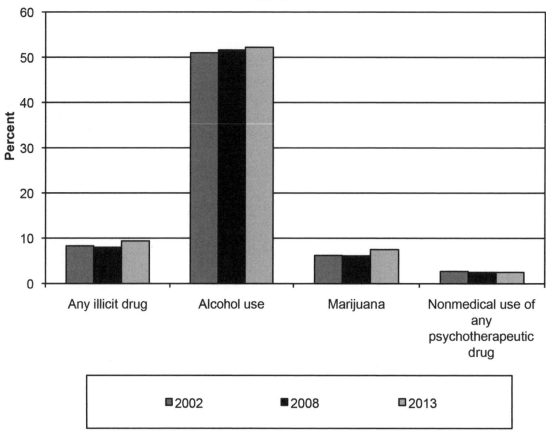

Figure 3-7. Current Cigarette Smoking Among Adults 18 Years and over, by Sex and Selected Race, Selected Years 1990–1992 to 2011–2013

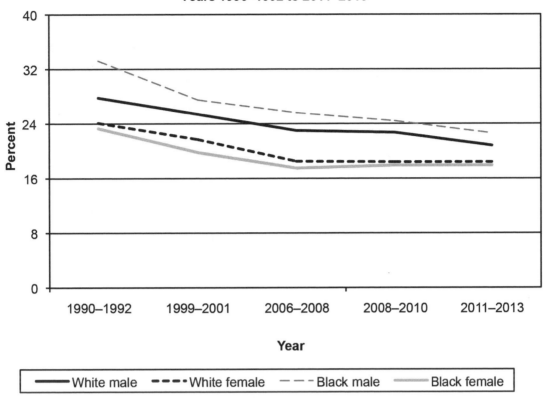

Table 3-21. Heavier Drinking and Drinking Five or More Drinks in a Day Among Adults 18 Years of Age and Over, by Selected Characteristics, Selected Years, 1997–2013

(Percent.)

Characteristic	Heavier drinker[1]				Five or more drinks in a day on at least 1 day in the past year[1]				Five or more drinks in a day on at least 12 days in the past year[1]			
	1997	2000	2010	2013	1997	2000	2010	2013	1997	2000	2010	2013
BOTH SEXES												
18 years and over, age-adjusted[2]	4.9	4.3	5.2	5.3	21.1	19.2	23.8	23.6	9.7	8.7	10.1	9.5
18 years and over, crude	5.0	4.3	5.2	5.3	21.5	19.3	23.2	22.6	9.8	8.7	9.9	9.2
Age												
All persons												
18 to 44 years	5.2	4.7	5.7	5.2	29.2	26.9	32.5	31.9	13.2	12.2	13.7	12.5
18 to 24 years	5.3	5.8	6.2	5.2	31.8	30.3	34.0	31.3	15.2	15.5	16.2	12.8
25 to 44 years	5.2	4.3	5.5	5.1	28.5	25.8	31.9	32.2	12.6	11.1	12.7	12.4
45 to 64 years	5.5	4.6	5.4	6.0	15.9	14.4	19.0	18.6	7.6	6.4	8.1	8.0
45 to 54 years	5.5	4.4	5.9	5.9	19.0	16.4	22.9	21.7	8.7	7.0	9.3	9.3
55 to 64 years	5.4	5.0	4.7	6.1	11.1	11.3	14.1	15.1	5.8	5.4	6.7	6.6
65 years and over	3.1	2.6	3.7	4.3	4.9	3.8	5.5	6.4	2.2	1.8	2.6	3.0
65 to 74 years	3.9	3.1	4.4	5.4	6.7	5.2	7.9	9.1	3.0	2.5	3.5	4.2
75 years and over	2.1	2.0	2.8	2.9	2.4	2.1	2.7	2.6	1.1	*0.9	*1.4	*1.4
Race [2,3]												
White only	5.2	4.5	5.6	5.7	22.9	20.8	26.3	26.0	10.3	9.2	11.1	10.5
Black or African American only	4.0	3.5	4.1	3.5	11.7	11.6	14.0	14.4	6.5	6.5	6.1	5.7
American Indian or Alaska Native only	*	*	*	*7.8	29.2	23.7	15.3	23.3	17.4	*12.1	*9.5	*12.4
Asian only	*1.9	*2.3	*1.3	*2.5	11.4	8.8	12.1	11.7	*4.8	3.6	4.3	4.2
Native Hawaiian or Other Pacific Islander only	NA	*	*	*	NA	*	*	*	NA	*	*	*
Two or more races	NA	*7.5	*5.9	*6.5	NA	28.0	25.7	26.3	NA	15.9	12.5	10.9
Hispanic Origin and Race [2,3]												
Hispanic or Latino	3.9	3.2	2.8	3.3	20.4	17.3	19.7	20.9	11.2	9.0	9.2	9.0
Mexican	4.4	3.8	3.1	3.8	21.2	19.9	21.4	21.8	12.6	10.8	10.1	10.0
Not Hispanic or Latino	5.1	4.5	5.6	5.6	21.3	19.7	24.7	24.2	9.5	8.8	10.3	9.6
White only	5.4	4.7	6.2	6.2	23.5	21.5	27.9	27.5	10.3	9.3	11.5	11.0
Black or African American only	3.9	3.4	4.2	3.5	11.6	11.5	13.9	14.3	6.5	6.5	6.1	5.5
Percent of Poverty Level [2,4]												
Below 100 percent	4.8	4.3	4.7	4.9	17.3	15.0	17.6	19.1	9.7	8.6	8.5	9.1
100 percent to 199 percent	4.9	4.2	4.9	4.5	18.4	15.7	20.9	20.3	9.8	8.0	9.8	8.4
200 percent to 399 percent	4.9	4.2	4.8	5.2	21.0	18.7	23.3	23.4	9.8	8.9	10.1	10.0
400 percent or more	5.1	4.4	6.0	5.9	24.3	22.1	28.1	26.7	9.7	8.9	10.9	9.9
Disability Measure [2,5]												
Any basic actions difficulty or complex activity limitation	5.7	5.2	5.5	4.9	20.2	18.8	21.9	20.7	10.2	9.3	9.5	8.6
Any basic actions difficulty	5.8	5.3	5.5	4.9	20.6	19.1	22.3	21.1	10.5	9.4	9.7	8.6
Any complex activity limitation	4.5	4.3	5.5	3.7	16.4	14.3	16.2	16.1	8.8	7.3	7.8	7.0
No disability	4.9	4.1	5.3	5.6	21.8	19.7	25.0	24.9	9.6	8.7	10.4	9.9
MALE												
18 years and over, age-adjusted[2]	6.1	5.1	5.7	5.7	30.7	28.3	32.4	32.1	15.8	14.4	15.6	15.1
18 years and over, crude	6.1	5.2	5.7	5.7	31.7	29.0	32.2	31.3	16.3	14.7	15.6	14.7
Age												
All persons												
18 to 44 years	6.5	5.6	6.1	5.5	40.6	37.8	42.5	41.4	21.1	19.6	20.6	19.1
18 to 24 years	6.0	6.3	6.0	5.4	40.6	38.0	39.9	37.7	22.9	22.9	21.5	17.9
25 to 44 years	6.6	5.3	6.2	5.6	40.6	37.7	43.5	42.8	20.6	18.5	20.2	19.6
45 to 64 years	6.6	5.5	5.8	6.3	25.3	23.5	27.3	27.0	12.7	11.3	13.2	13.0
45 to 54 years	6.6	5.7	5.9	6.4	29.4	26.3	32.0	30.3	14.5	12.3	14.5	14.3
55 to 64 years	6.6	5.4	5.7	6.3	18.9	19.0	21.4	23.5	10.0	9.8	11.6	11.5
65 years and over	3.7	3.1	4.0	5.2	9.3	7.4	9.8	11.4	4.7	3.7	4.7	6.0
65 to 74 years	4.8	3.9	4.4	6.3	12.2	9.5	13.5	15.2	6.1	4.9	6.3	7.6
75 years and over	*2.1	*2.0	*3.5	*3.4	5.1	4.4	4.6	5.4	*2.5	*2.0	*2.5	*3.4
Race [2,3]												
White only	6.3	5.1	6.1	6.0	32.8	29.9	35.3	34.9	16.7	14.9	17.1	16.5
Black or African American only	5.3	5.4	4.6	4.2	18.4	19.8	20.2	21.0	11.0	12.4	9.8	9.6
American Indian or Alaska Native only	*	*	*	*	45.7	29.2	*20.5	34.7	30.4	*14.0	*15.7	*19.4
Asian only	*2.3	*3.5	*1.4	*	17.8	14.1	17.2	17.0	*7.5	*5.9	6.8	6.5
Native Hawaiian or Other Pacific Islander only	NA	*	*	*	NA	*	*	*	NA	*	*	*
Two or more races	NA	*12.1	*8.4	*6.3	NA	39.2	37.6	34.8	NA	23.7	20.3	15.7
Hispanic Origin and Race [2,3]												
Hispanic or Latino	5.7	5.2	3.9	4.9	30.9	27.9	28.8	31.1	18.8	15.9	14.6	15.3
Mexican	6.9	6.6	4.4	5.4	34.2	32.2	32.2	33.4	21.9	19.1	16.3	17.3
Not Hispanic or Latino	6.1	5.2	6.0	5.8	30.7	28.6	33.3	32.3	15.5	14.3	15.9	15.0

Table 3-21. Heavier Drinking and Drinking Five or More Drinks in a Day Among Adults 18 Years of Age and Over, by Selected Characteristics, Selected Years, 1997–2013— continued

(Percent.)

Characteristic	Heavier drinker[1]				Five or more drinks in a day on at least 1 day in the past year[1]				Five or more drinks in a day on at least 12 days in the past year[1]			
	1997	2000	2010	2013	1997	2000	2010	2013	1997	2000	2010	2013
White only	6.4	5.2	6.5	6.3	33.3	30.6	36.9	36.1	16.6	15.0	17.6	16.8
Black or African American only	5.3	5.4	4.7	4.1	18.4	19.7	20.3	20.6	11.1	12.3	9.9	9.2
Percent of Poverty Level [2,4]												
Below 100 percent	6.8	6.4	6.5	6.8	26.9	24.8	26.0	27.3	16.5	15.7	14.1	15.5
100 percent to 199 percent	7.1	5.8	5.8	5.6	27.3	23.6	29.1	28.9	16.4	13.3	14.8	13.5
200 percent to 399 percent	6.6	5.3	5.8	6.1	30.4	27.4	31.8	31.0	16.0	14.7	16.4	15.6
400 percent or more	5.0	4.4	5.4	5.3	33.6	31.3	36.4	35.1	15.4	14.4	15.8	15.0
Disability Measure [2,5]												
Any basic actions difficulty or complex activity limitation	7.2	6.8	6.6	5.8	29.4	28.9	30.6	29.0	17.0	16.5	14.8	14.0
Any basic actions difficulty	7.5	6.8	6.7	5.8	30.4	29.8	31.8	30.2	17.7	16.8	15.5	14.6
Any complex activity limitation	5.4	5.8	6.6	4.3	23.1	20.5	21.1	21.3	14.2	11.9	11.3	10.7
No disability	5.8	4.8	5.4	5.7	31.5	28.5	33.5	33.3	15.6	14.1	15.9	15.4
FEMALE												
18 years and over, age-adjusted[2]	3.9	3.5	4.8	4.9	12.2	10.8	15.6	15.7	3.9	3.4	4.8	4.3
18 years and over, crude	3.9	3.5	4.8	4.9	12.1	10.6	14.9	14.6	3.9	3.3	4.6	4.1
Age												
All persons												
18 to 44 years	4.0	3.8	5.2	4.8	18.3	16.5	22.6	22.8	5.5	5.2	6.9	6.1
18 to 24 years	4.5	5.2	6.4	5.0	23.0	22.8	28.1	25.0	7.6	8.3	10.9	7.7
25 to 44 years	3.9	3.4	4.8	4.7	16.9	14.5	20.6	22.1	4.9	4.2	5.4	5.5
45 to 64 years	4.4	3.8	4.9	5.7	7.2	6.0	11.1	10.6	2.9	1.9	3.4	3.4
45 to 54 years	4.5	3.2	5.9	5.4	9.2	7.1	14.3	13.6	3.3	2.1	4.3	4.6
55 to 64 years	4.4	4.6	3.8	6.0	4.1	4.4	7.3	7.4	2.1	1.5	2.3	2.0
65 years and over	2.6	2.2	3.4	3.7	1.6	1.2	2.3	2.4	*0.4	*0.4	*	*0.7
65 to 74 years	3.1	2.5	4.5	4.6	2.3	1.7	*3.1	3.8	*	*	*	*1.2
75 years and over	2.0	1.9	2.3	2.5	*0.7	*	*1.4	*0.7	*	*	*	*
Race [2,3]												
White only	4.2	4.0	5.2	5.3	13.5	12.1	17.4	17.5	4.2	3.7	5.2	4.8
Black or African American only	2.9	2.0	3.8	3.0	6.5	5.2	9.0	9.2	2.9	1.9	3.1	2.6
American Indian or Alaska Native only	*	*	*	*4.0	18.1	*19.0	*11.7	*13.3	*	*	*	*
Asian only	*	*	*	*2.3	*5.2	*3.7	7.3	7.0	*	*	*	*2.2
Native Hawaiian or Other Pacific Islander only	NA	*	*	*	NA	*	*	*	NA	*	*	*
Two or more races	NA	*	*	*	NA	17.0	16.4	18.8	NA	*8.2	*6.3	*6.4
Hispanic Origin and Race [2,3]												
Hispanic or Latina	2.2	1.2	1.7	1.9	9.7	6.8	10.3	10.8	3.5	2.1	3.6	2.8
Mexican	*1.9	*1.1	*1.7	2.1	8.2	7.1	10.4	10.4	3.2	*2.2	3.7	2.7
Not Hispanic or Latina	4.1	3.8	5.3	5.4	12.6	11.5	16.6	16.7	4.0	3.6	5.0	4.6
White only	4.4	4.3	5.9	6.1	14.2	13.0	19.1	19.4	4.3	4.0	5.6	5.3
Black or African American only	2.9	2.0	3.8	3.1	6.2	5.2	8.9	9.2	2.9	1.9	3.0	2.6
Percent of Poverty Level [2,4]												
Below 100 percent	3.6	2.8	3.4	3.5	10.8	8.2	11.3	13.2	5.1	3.6	4.2	4.4
100 percent to 199 percent	3.1	2.9	4.1	3.6	10.5	9.0	13.5	13.3	4.0	3.5	5.1	4.1
200 percent to 399 percent	3.3	3.2	3.9	4.4	12.1	10.7	15.3	15.9	4.0	3.5	4.2	4.4
400 percent or more	5.2	4.5	6.7	6.6	14.2	12.6	19.2	17.8	3.4	3.3	5.6	4.6
Disability Measure [2,5]												
Any basic actions difficulty or complex activity limitation	4.5	4.1	4.7	4.3	13.1	11.3	15.2	14.5	5.0	4.1	5.4	4.5
Any basic actions difficulty	4.5	4.2	4.7	4.3	13.2	11.6	15.4	14.9	5.1	4.1	5.4	4.5
Any complex activity limitation	3.7	*3.2	4.6	3.2	10.8	9.1	12.3	11.5	4.2	*3.1	5.0	3.7
No disability	3.9	3.5	5.1	5.4	12.0	10.9	16.1	16.3	3.6	3.3	4.7	4.3

NA = Not available.   * = Figure does not meet standards of reliability or precision. Data preceded by an asterisk have a relative standard error (RSE) of 20 percent to 30 percent. Data not shown have an RSE of greater than 30 percent.   1 Heavier drinking is based on self–reported responses to questions about average alcohol consumption and is defined as more than 14 drinks per week for men and more than seven drinks per week for women on average. Respondents were also asked, "In the past year, on how many days did you have five or more drinks of any alcoholic beverage?"   2 Estimates are age adjusted to the year 2000 standard population using four age groups: 18 to 24 years, 25 to 44 years, 45 to 64 years, and 65 years and over. Age-adjusted estimates in this table may differ from other age–adjusted estimates based on the same data and presented elsewhere if different age groups are used in the adjustment procedure.   3 The race groups White, Black, American Indian or Alaska Native, Asian, Native Hawaiian or Other Pacific Islander, and two or more races, include persons of Hispanic and non–Hispanic origin. Persons of Hispanic origin may be of any race.   4 Percent of poverty level is based on family income and family size and composition using U.S. Census Bureau poverty thresholds. Missing family income data were imputed for 1997 and beyond.   5 Any basic actions difficulty or complex activity limitation is defined as having one or more of the following limitations or difficulties: movement difficulty, emotional difficulty, sensory (seeing or hearing) difficulty, cognitive difficulty, self–care (activities of daily living or instrumental activities of daily living) limitation, social limitation, or work limitation.

Table 3-22. Age-Adjusted Prevalence of Current Cigarette Smoking[1] Among Adults 25 Years of Age and Over, by Sex, Race, and Education Level, Selected Years, 1974–2013

(Percent.)

Sex, race, and education level	1974[2]	1985[2]	1990[2]	1995[2]	2000	2005	2010	2012	2013
25 YEARS AND OVER, AGE-ADJUSTED[3]									
All Persons [4]	36.9	30.0	25.4	24.5	22.6	20.3	19.2	18.3	17.8
No high school diploma or GED	43.7	40.8	36.7	35.6	31.6	28.2	26.9	26.3	25.8
High school diploma or GED	36.2	32.0	29.1	29.1	29.2	27.0	27.0	26.3	25.6
Some college, no bachelor's degree	35.9	29.5	23.4	22.6	21.7	21.8	21.3	19.6	19.5
Bachelor's degree or higher	27.2	18.5	13.9	13.6	10.9	9.1	8.3	7.8	7.7
All Males [4]	42.9	32.8	28.2	26.4	24.7	22.7	21.0	20.6	20.3
No high school diploma or GED	52.3	45.7	42.0	39.7	36.0	31.7	29.7	30.3	31.6
High school diploma or GED	42.4	35.5	33.1	32.7	32.1	29.9	29.3	29.6	28.8
Some college, no bachelor's degree	41.8	32.9	25.9	23.7	23.3	24.9	23.2	21.0	20.4
Bachelor's degree or higher	28.3	19.6	14.5	13.8	11.6	9.7	8.7	8.5	8.7
White Males [4,5]	41.9	31.7	27.6	25.9	24.7	22.4	21.0	20.5	20.1
No high school diploma or GED	51.5	45.0	41.8	38.7	38.2	31.6	29.4	29.6	30.2
High school diploma or GED	42.0	34.8	32.9	32.9	32.4	30.0	29.6	29.8	28.4
Some college, no bachelor's degree	41.6	32.2	25.4	23.3	23.5	24.5	23.4	20.3	20.3
Bachelor's degree or higher	27.8	19.1	14.4	13.4	11.3	9.3	8.8	8.9	8.8
Black or African American Males [4,5]	53.4	42.1	34.5	31.6	26.4	26.5	23.9	23.3	23.1
No high school diploma or GED	58.1	50.5	41.6	41.9	38.2	35.9	34.4	34.1	41.5
High school diploma or GED	*50.7	41.8	37.4	36.6	29.0	30.1	28.8	28.0	31.9
Some college, no bachelor's degree	*45.3	41.8	28.1	26.4	19.9	27.4	24.2	24.9	18.0
Bachelor's degree or higher	*41.4	*32.0	*20.8	*17.3	14.6	10.0	8.1	*7.3	7.7
All Females [4]	32.0	27.5	22.9	22.9	20.5	18.0	17.5	16.1	15.5
No high school diploma or GED	36.6	36.5	31.8	31.7	27.1	24.6	23.7	22.2	19.8
High school diploma or GED	32.2	29.5	26.1	26.4	26.6	24.1	24.9	22.6	22.0
Some college, no bachelor's degree	30.1	26.3	21.0	21.6	20.4	19.1	19.6	18.4	18.8
Bachelor's degree or higher	25.9	17.1	13.3	13.3	10.1	8.5	7.9	7.2	6.8
White Females [4,5]	31.7	27.3	23.3	23.1	21.0	18.6	18.3	16.9	16.2
No high school diploma or GED	36.8	36.7	33.4	32.4	28.4	24.6	24.0	22.4	19.0
High school diploma or GED	31.9	29.4	26.5	26.8	27.8	25.9	25.8	24.0	23.5
Some college, no bachelor's degree	30.4	26.7	21.2	22.2	21.1	19.5	21.0	19.0	19.8
Bachelor's degree or higher	25.5	16.5	13.4	13.5	10.2	9.1	8.7	7.7	7.3
Black or African American Females [4,5]	35.6	32.0	22.4	25.7	21.6	17.5	17.0	15.2	15.3
No high school diploma or GED	36.1	39.4	26.3	32.3	31.1	27.8	25.8	25.8	26.5
High school diploma or GED	40.9	32.1	24.1	27.8	25.4	18.2	22.9	17.0	17.0
Some college, no bachelor's degree	32.3	23.9	22.7	20.8	20.4	17.5	15.0	16.9	15.3
Bachelor's degree or higher	*36.3	26.6	17.0	17.3	10.8	*6.6	*6.6	7.1	7.3

* = Figure does not meet standards of reliability or precision. Data preceded by an asterisk have a relative standard error of 20 percent to 30 percent.   1 Starting with 1993 data, current cigarette smokers were defined as ever smoking 100 cigarettes in their lifetime and smoking now every day or some days.   2 Data prior to 1997 are not strictly comparable with data for later years due to the 1997 questionnaire redesign.   3 Estimates are age adjusted to the year 2000 standard population using four age groups: 25 to 34 years, 35 to 44 years, 45 to 64 years, and 65 years and over.   4 Includes unknown education level. Education categories shown are for 1997 and subsequent years. GED is General Educational Development high school equivalency diploma.   5 The race groups White and Black include persons of Hispanic and non-Hispanic origin.

Table 3-23. Current Cigarette Smoking[1] Among Adults, by Sex, Race, Hispanic Origin, Age, and Education Level, Average Annual, Selected Years 1990–1992 through 2011–2013

(Percent.)

Characteristic	Male					Female				
	1990–1992[2]	1999–2001	2006–2008	2008–2010	2011–2013	1990–1992[2]	1999–2001	2006–2008	2008–2010	2011–2013
18 Years and Over, Age-Adjusted [3]										
All persons[4]	27.9	25.0	22.8	22.4	20.8	23.7	21.1	18.0	18.0	16.1
Race [5]										
White only	27.4	25.1	22.9	22.6	20.9	24.3	22.2	18.9	18.8	17.0
Black or African American only	33.9	27.2	24.8	23.7	22.3	23.1	19.7	17.2	17.5	14.8
American Indian or Alaska Native only	34.2	30.3	31.5	25.1	25.6	36.7	34.7	22.2	21.0	19.1
Asian only	24.8	20.3	15.6	15.3	14.8	6.3	6.7	4.4	5.5	5.2
Native Hawaiian or Other Pacific Islander only	NA	*	*	*	*	NA	*	*	*	*
2 or more races	NA	34.4	25.1	27.7	27.1	NA	30.7	24.6	20.9	23.4
American Indian or Alaska Native; White	NA	38.7	34.6	34.6	35.1	NA	38.9	28.6	26.5	32.3
Hispanic Origin and Race [5]										
Hispanic or Latino	25.7	22.2	18.6	17.3	16.7	15.8	12.1	9.5	9.6	7.5
Mexican	26.2	21.9	18.7	17.5	16.4	14.8	10.6	8.8	8.4	6.9
Not Hispanic or Latino	28.1	25.5	23.7	23.4	21.7	24.4	22.3	19.4	19.5	17.6
White only	27.7	25.5	24.0	23.9	22.1	25.2	23.5	20.9	20.9	19.2
Black or African American only	33.9	27.2	25.1	24.0	22.5	23.2	19.7	17.2	17.7	14.9
18 Years and Over, Crude										
All persons[4]	28.4	25.5	23.1	22.7	20.9	23.6	21.0	17.9	17.8	15.9
Race [5]										
White only	27.8	25.4	23.0	22.7	20.8	24.1	21.7	18.5	18.4	16.6
Black or African American only	33.2	27.5	25.6	24.4	22.6	23.3	19.8	17.5	17.9	15.0
American Indian or Alaska Native only	35.5	31.8	30.7	25.6	26.2	37.3	36.9	23.0	21.6	19.5
Asian only	24.9	21.4	16.5	15.7	15.6	6.3	6.9	4.6	5.6	5.4
Native Hawaiian or Other Pacific Islander only	NA	*	*	*	*	NA	*	*	*	*
2 or more races	NA	35.9	27.0	29.2	27.8	NA	31.5	25.3	21.9	22.9
American Indian or Alaska Native; White	NA	41.1	33.5	33.9	33.5	NA	40.1	30.0	27.5	32.3
Hispanic Origin and Race [5]										
Hispanic or Latino	26.5	23.2	19.6	18.4	17.2	16.6	12.6	9.7	9.8	7.7
Mexican	27.1	22.8	19.4	18.6	16.6	15.0	11.0	8.8	8.5	7.0
Not Hispanic or Latino	28.5	25.8	23.7	23.4	21.5	24.2	21.9	19.1	19.0	17.2
White only	28.0	25.5	23.7	23.6	21.6	24.8	22.7	20.1	20.0	18.3
Black or African American only	33.3	27.5	26.0	24.7	22.7	23.3	19.8	17.6	18.0	15.2
Age and Hispanic Origin and Race [5]										
18 to 24 Years										
Hispanic or Latino	19.3	22.6	18.4	19.3	14.3	12.8	12.9	8.0	8.0	6.6
Not Hispanic or Latino										
White only	28.9	32.7	29.1	28.2	25.4	28.7	30.8	24.1	21.2	20.7
Black or African American only	17.7	21.9	23.6	18.4	14.8	10.8	13.0	13.5	14.9	9.9
25 to 34 Years										
Hispanic or Latino	29.9	23.2	20.4	20.1	20.4	19.2	12.5	9.5	9.6	8.7
Not Hispanic or Latino										
White only	32.7	30.8	31.6	30.8	29.6	30.9	27.4	26.7	26.5	23.6
Black or African American only	34.6	23.3	28.5	25.7	25.3	29.2	16.9	16.2	19.1	17.3
35 to 44 Years										
Hispanic or Latino	32.1	25.3	20.5	18.2	17.3	19.9	14.1	10.2	10.4	7.9
Not Hispanic or Latino										
White only	32.3	29.6	25.9	26.5	23.5	27.3	28.3	24.1	24.7	21.7
Black or African American only	44.1	32.0	20.9	23.2	25.0	31.3	27.5	19.4	19.0	15.4
45 to 64 Years										
Hispanic or Latino	26.6	24.7	21.4	19.2	17.4	17.1	13.5	12.5	12.2	9.0
Not Hispanic or Latino										
White only	28.4	25.1	23.5	24.1	22.4	26.1	22.1	20.7	21.0	20.5
Black or African American only	38.0	34.0	31.8	31.7	26.2	26.1	23.6	23.2	21.6	19.3
65 Years and Over										
Hispanic or Latino	16.1	12.6	9.4	8.2	12.4	6.6	5.9	4.7	5.5	3.8
Not Hispanic or Latino										
White only	14.2	10.0	10.5	9.8	9.5	12.3	9.8	8.6	9.5	7.8
Black or African American only	25.2	17.6	16.3	13.7	15.4	10.7	11.0	7.8	9.8	8.1
Percent of Poverty Level [2,6]										
Below 100 percent	40.5	36.5	32.1	32.5	34.2	30.7	29.1	28.1	28.6	25.1
100 percent to 199 percent	35.0	32.8	29.4	29.3	27.6	26.9	25.6	22.4	22.8	20.6
200 percent to 399 percent	26.5	27.3	24.8	24.3	21.8	22.6	22.3	18.5	18.5	16.5
400 percent or more	22.5	18.8	17.0	16.0	13.7	19.0	15.9	12.5	11.8	9.7

Table 3-23. Current Cigarette Smoking[1] Among Adults, by Sex, Race, Hispanic Origin, Age, and Education Level, Average Annual, Selected Years 1990–1992 through 2011–2013— continued

(Percent.)

Characteristic	Male					Female				
	1990–1992[2]	1999–2001	2006–2008	2008–2010	2011–2013	1990–1992[2]	1999–2001	2006–2008	2008–2010	2011–2013
Hispanic Origin and Race and Percent of Poverty Level [2,5,6]										
Hispanic or Latino										
Below 100 percent	29.2	25.3	20.8	20.2	19.8	16.3	14.4	11.9	11.4	9.9
100 percent to 199 percent	29.5	22.0	18.4	17.8	17.1	16.0	11.8	8.3	8.7	7.0
200 percent to 399 percent	23.7	23.6	19.7	16.6	16.7	15.9	12.0	8.6	10.2	7.3
400 percent or more	19.7	18.1	15.7	15.1	13.2	13.6	9.4	9.9	7.9	5.7
Not Hispanic or Latino										
White only										
Below 100 percent	44.2	40.7	38.6	40.6	43.4	37.8	38.3	38.0	39.4	36.9
100 percent to 199 percent	36.3	37.5	35.0	35.3	34.2	31.1	32.0	30.7	30.7	29.4
200 percent to 399 percent	26.4	28.5	27.0	27.4	23.6	23.7	24.8	22.1	21.9	19.8
400 percent or more	22.5	19.1	17.4	16.3	14.4	19.5	17.1	13.6	13.1	10.9
Black or African American only										
Below 100 percent	43.5	40.6	38.2	36.5	36.7	28.9	27.7	27.0	29.1	25.1
100 percent to 199 percent	36.0	33.9	30.9	30.4	26.7	20.3	21.3	18.6	19.6	15.0
200 percent to 399 percent	31.4	24.9	21.8	20.7	21.8	21.4	17.3	13.5	13.2	11.3
400 percent or more	24.3	17.9	18.4	15.6	10.9	19.2	12.6	10.3	8.2	7.5
Disability Measure [7]										
Any basic actions difficulty or complex activity limitation	NA	33.1	32.1	30.3	29.4	NA	28.1	26.8	26.8	25.2
Any basic actions difficulty	NA	33.2	32.5	30.5	30.1	NA	28.2	27.0	27.0	25.3
Any complex activity limitation	NA	37.6	34.2	33.2	31.5	NA	30.6	31.8	31.5	30.2
No disability	NA	22.8	20.1	19.8	17.9	NA	18.8	14.9	14.6	12.7
Education, Hispanic Origin, and Race [3,5]										
25 years and over, age-adjusted[9]										
No high school diploma or GED										
Hispanic or Latino	30.2	24.3	19.5	18.5	18.7	15.8	12.1	8.6	8.6	6.9
Not Hispanic or Latino										
White only	46.1	43.5	42.0	45.1	45.1	40.4	39.3	42.9	44.0	39.2
Black or African American only	45.4	40.0	35.9	37.2	37.1	31.3	29.4	28.7	29.9	28.3
High school diploma or GED										
Hispanic or Latino	29.6	24.1	21.7	20.3	21.2	18.4	12.5	10.7	11.4	9.3
Not Hispanic or Latino										
White only	32.9	31.8	32.7	34.4	31.7	28.4	29.2	28.8	30.3	29.6
Black or African American only	38.2	31.4	29.5	27.8	29.8	25.4	23.0	19.8	23.7	16.8
Some college or more										
Hispanic or Latino	20.4	17.1	15.8	12.9	12.2	14.3	11.1	10.3	9.9	7.5
Not Hispanic or Latino										
White only	19.3	17.6	16.2	15.9	14.9	18.1	16.7	14.7	15.5	14.1
Black or African American only	25.6	19.2	19.3	19.8	16.4	22.8	16.9	13.7	12.7	12.5

NA = Not available.   * = Figure does not meet standards of reliability or precision. Data preceded by an asterisk have a relative standard error (RSE) of 20 percent to 30 percent. Data not shown have an RSE of greater than 30 percent.   1 Starting with 1993 data, current cigarette smokers were defined as ever smoking 100 cigarettes in their lifetime and smoking now every day or some days.   2 Data prior to 1997 are not strictly comparable with data for later years due to the 1997 questionnaire redesign.   3 Estimates are age adjusted to the year 2000 standard population using five age groups: 18 to 24 years, 25 to 34 years, 35 to 44 years, 45 to 64 years, and 65 years and over. For age groups where smoking is 0 percent or 100 percent, the age-adjustment procedure was modified to substitute the percentage smoking from the previous 3-year period.   4 Includes all other races not shown separately, unknown education level, and unknown disability measure.   5 The race groups White, Black, American Indian or Alaska Native, Asian, Native Hawaiian or Other Pacific Islander, and two or more races include persons of Hispanic and non–Hispanic origin. Persons of Hispanic origin may be of any race.   6 Percent of poverty level is based on family income and family size and composition using U.S. Census Bureau poverty thresholds. Missing family income data were imputed for 1990 and beyond.   7 Any basic actions difficulty or complex activity limitation is defined as having one or more of the following limitations or difficulties: movement difficulty, emotional difficulty, sensory (seeing or hearing) difficulty, cognitive difficulty, self–care (activities of daily living or instrumental activities of daily living) limitation, social limitation, or work limitation.   8 Education categories shown are for 1997 and subsequent years. GED is General Educational Development high school equivalency diploma.   9 Estimates are age adjusted to the year 2000 standard using four age groups: 25 to 34 years, 35 to 44 years, 45 to 64 years, and 65 years and over.

Table 3-24. Current Cigarette Smoking[1] Among Adults 18 Years of Age and Over, by Sex, Race, and Age, Selected Years, 1965–2013

(Percent.)

Sex, race, and age	1965[2]	1985[2]	1995[2]	2005	2010	2011	2012	2013
18 Years and Over, Age-Adjusted[3]								
All persons	41.9	29.9	24.6	20.8	19.3	19.0	18.2	17.9
Male	51.2	32.2	26.5	23.4	21.2	21.2	20.6	20.5
Female	33.7	27.9	22.7	18.3	17.5	16.8	15.9	15.5
White male[4]	50.4	31.3	26.2	23.3	21.4	21.4	20.7	20.5
Black or African American male[4]	58.8	40.2	29.4	25.9	23.3	23.2	22.0	21.8
White female[4]	33.9	27.9	23.4	19.1	18.3	17.7	16.9	16.3
Black or African American female[4]	31.8	30.9	23.5	17.1	16.6	15.2	14.2	14.9
18 Years and Over, Crude								
All persons	42.4	30.1	24.7	20.9	19.3	19.0	18.1	17.8
Male	51.9	32.6	27.0	23.9	21.5	21.6	20.5	20.5
Female	33.9	27.9	22.6	18.1	17.3	16.5	15.8	15.3
White male[4]	51.1	31.7	26.6	23.6	21.4	21.6	20.3	20.3
Black or African American male[4]	60.4	39.9	28.5	26.5	24.3	23.8	22.0	21.9
White female[4]	34.0	27.7	23.1	18.7	17.9	17.2	16.6	15.9
Black or African American female[4]	33.7	31.0	23.5	17.3	17.0	15.3	14.7	15.1
All Males								
18 to 44 years	57.9	35.2	29.9	27.1	23.9	23.6	24.0	22.9
18 to 24 years	54.1	28.0	27.8	28.0	22.8	21.3	20.1	21.9
25 to 34 years	60.7	38.2	29.5	27.7	26.1	27.5	28.0	24.4
35 to 44 years	58.2	37.6	31.5	26.0	22.5	21.2	22.8	22.1
45 to 64 years	51.9	33.4	27.1	25.2	23.2	24.4	20.2	21.9
45 to 54 years	55.9	34.9	27.2	28.1	25.2	27.0	21.4	21.4
55 to 64 years	46.6	31.9	26.9	21.1	20.7	21.4	18.8	22.6
65 years and over	28.5	19.6	14.9	8.9	9.7	8.9	10.6	10.6
White Male [4]								
18 to 44 years	57.1	34.6	30.1	27.7	24.6	24.3	24.8	23.4
18 to 24 years	53.0	28.4	28.4	29.7	23.8	22.1	21.9	23.5
25 to 34 years	60.1	37.3	29.9	27.7	26.6	28.6	28.4	24.6
35 to 44 years	57.3	36.6	31.2	26.3	23.1	21.4	23.3	21.9
45 to 64 years	51.3	32.1	26.3	24.5	22.5	24.0	19.4	21.7
45 to 54 years	55.3	33.7	25.9	27.4	24.5	26.6	20.7	21.2
55 to 64 years	46.1	30.5	27.0	20.4	20.1	20.8	17.9	22.2
65 years and over	27.7	18.9	14.1	7.9	9.6	8.6	10.3	10.0
Black or African American Male [4]								
18 to 44 years	66.3	39.6	26.4	25.1	22.6	22.7	21.3	20.9
18 to 24 years	62.8	27.2	*	21.6	18.8	18.4	13.2	*13.2
25 to 34 years	68.4	45.6	25.1	29.8	25.7	25.0	24.9	24.8
35 to 44 years	67.3	45.0	36.3	23.3	22.6	24.3	24.7	24.0
45 to 64 years	57.9	46.1	33.9	32.4	31.8	28.9	24.6	25.7
45 to 54 years	62.4	47.7	36.9	33.9	33.2	29.2	23.3	25.7
55 to 64 years	51.8	44.4	29.1	29.8	29.6	28.4	26.4	25.6
65 years and over	36.4	27.7	28.5	16.8	10.0	13.7	17.4	15.5
All Females								
18 to 44 years	42.1	31.4	25.6	21.2	19.1	18.8	16.9	16.6
18 to 24 years	38.1	30.4	21.8	20.7	17.4	16.4	14.5	15.4
25 to 34 years	43.7	32.0	26.4	21.5	20.6	19.5	19.4	17.9
35 to 44 years	43.7	31.5	27.1	21.3	19.0	19.9	16.1	16.3
45 to 64 years	32.0	29.9	24.0	18.8	19.1	18.5	18.9	18.1
45 to 54 years	37.5	32.4	24.3	20.9	21.3	21.6	21.3	20.6
55 to 64 years	25.0	27.4	23.7	16.1	16.5	15.0	16.2	15.2
65 years and over	9.6	13.5	11.5	8.3	9.3	7.1	7.5	7.5
White Female [4]								
18 to 44 years	42.2	31.6	26.6	22.6	20.5	20.3	18.6	17.8
18 to 24 years	38.4	31.8	24.9	22.6	18.4	18.4	16.9	17.0
25 to 34 years	43.4	32.0	27.3	23.1	22.0	20.6	20.7	19.2
35 to 44 years	43.9	31.0	27.0	22.2	20.5	21.5	17.6	17.0
45 to 64 years	32.7	29.7	24.3	18.9	19.5	19.0	19.4	18.4
45 to 54 years	38.2	32.4	24.6	21.0	22.4	22.5	22.7	21.2
55 to 64 years	25.7	27.2	23.8	16.2	15.9	15.1	15.8	15.5
65 years and over	9.8	13.3	11.7	8.4	9.4	7.0	7.5	7.9

Table 3-24. Current Cigarette Smoking[1] Among Adults 18 Years of Age and Over, by Sex, Race, and Age, Selected Years, 1965–2013—continued

(Percent.)

Sex, race, and age	1965[2]	1985[2]	1995[2]	2005	2010	2011	2012	2013
Black or African American Female [4]								
18 to 44 years	42.9	33.5	24.0	16.9	17.1	15.0	12.3	15.1
18 to 24 years	37.1	23.7	*8.8	14.2	14.2	9.1	*7.4	11.8
25 to 34 years	47.8	36.2	26.7	16.9	19.3	17.5	17.3	16.4
35 to 44 years	42.8	40.2	31.9	19.0	17.2	17.4	11.2	16.4
45 to 64 years	25.7	33.4	27.5	21.0	19.8	18.3	20.4	18.8
45 to 54 years	32.3	36.4	28.3	22.2	20.4	20.1	20.1	22.2
55 to 64 years	16.5	29.8	26.3	19.1	18.9	16.0	20.8	14.8
65 years and over	7.1	14.5	13.3	10.0	9.4	9.1	9.1	6.5

* = Figure does not meet standards of reliability or precision. Data preceded by an asterisk have a relative standard error (RSE) of 20 percent to 30 percent. Data not shown have an RSE of greater than 30 percent.   1 Starting with 1993 data, current cigarette smokers were defined as ever smoking 100 cigarettes in their lifetime and smoking now every day or some days.   2 Data prior to 1997 are not strictly comparable with data for later years due to the 1997 questionnaire redesign.   3 Estimates are age adjusted to the year 2000 standard population using five age groups: 18 to 24 years, 25 to 34 years, 35 to 44 years, 45 to 64 years, and 65 years and over. For age groups where smoking is 0 percent or 100 percent, the age-adjustment procedure was modified to substitute the percentage smoking from the previous 3-year period.   4 The race groups White, Black, American Indian or Alaska Native, Asian, Native Hawaiian or Other Pacific Islander, and two or more races include persons of Hispanic and non–Hispanic origin. Persons of Hispanic origin may be of any race.

Table 3-25. Use of Selected Substances Among 12th Graders, 10th Graders, and 8th Graders, by Sex and Race, Selected Years, 1980–2013

(Percent.)

Substance, grade in school, sex, and race	1980	1990	2000	2005	2010	2011	2012	2013
Cigarettes								
All 12th graders	30.5	29.4	31.4	23.2	19.2	18.7	17.1	16.3
Male	26.8	29.1	32.8	24.8	21.9	21.5	19.3	18.4
Female	33.4	29.2	29.7	20.7	15.7	15.1	14.5	13.2
White	31.0	32.5	36.6	27.0	22.2	22.2	20.1	18.5
Black or African American	25.2	12.0	13.6	10.0	10.7	8.7	8.4	10.8
All 10th graders	NA	NA	23.9	14.9	13.6	11.8	10.8	9.1
Male	NA	NA	23.8	14.5	15.0	13.4	12.0	10.5
Female	NA	NA	23.6	15.1	12.1	10.0	9.6	7.5
White	NA	NA	27.3	17.0	14.8	13.7	12.2	10.4
Black or African American	NA	NA	11.3	7.7	7.0	7.2	6.2	4.2
All 8th graders	NA	NA	14.6	9.3	7.1	6.1	4.9	4.5
Male	NA	NA	14.3	8.7	7.4	6.2	4.6	4.0
Female	NA	NA	14.7	9.7	6.8	5.7	4.9	4.7
White	NA	NA	16.4	9.5	7.9	6.5	5.0	4.3
Black or African American	NA	NA	8.4	6.7	4.0	4.2	3.8	3.3
Marijuana								
All 12th graders	33.7	14.0	21.6	19.8	21.4	22.6	22.9	22.7
Male	37.8	16.1	24.7	23.6	25.2	26.4	26.5	26.4
Female	29.1	11.5	18.3	15.8	16.9	18.4	18.8	18.7
White	34.2	15.6	22.0	21.7	21.6	22.9	22.3	21.3
Black or African American	26.5	5.2	17.5	15.1	19.7	22.2	22.4	25.7
All 10th graders	NA	NA	19.7	15.2	16.7	17.6	17.0	18.0
Male	NA	NA	23.3	16.7	20.1	20.8	19.8	20.6
Female	NA	NA	16.2	13.4	13.3	14.5	14.4	15.3
White	NA	NA	20.1	15.7	15.9	16.9	16.6	16.5
Black or African American	NA	NA	17.0	13.5	15.9	20.0	17.6	20.7
All 8th graders	NA	NA	9.1	6.6	8.0	7.2	6.5	7.0
Male	NA	NA	10.2	7.6	9.2	8.5	7.0	6.7
Female	NA	NA	7.8	5.7	6.8	5.7	6.0	7.2
White	NA	NA	8.3	6.0	7.1	5.9	4.7	4.8
Black or African American	NA	NA	8.5	8.2	8.2	8.0	7.1	9.3
Cocaine								
All 12th graders	5.2	1.9	2.1	2.3	1.3	1.1	1.1	1.1
Male	6.0	2.3	2.7	2.6	1.9	1.5	1.5	1.4
Female	4.3	1.3	1.6	1.8	0.7	0.7	0.6	0.5
White	5.4	1.8	2.2	2.3	1.2	1.2	1.0	0.7
Black or African American	2.0	0.5	1.0	0.5	0.9	0.8	0.5	0.6
All 10th graders	NA	NA	1.8	1.5	0.9	0.7	0.8	0.8
Male	NA	NA	2.1	1.9	1.1	0.8	0.8	1.2
Female	NA	NA	1.4	1.2	0.5	0.5	0.7	0.5
White	NA	NA	1.7	1.5	0.7	0.5	0.5	0.6
Black or African American	NA	NA	0.4	0.8	0.6	0.6	1.2	0.9
All 8th graders	NA	NA	1.2	1.0	0.6	0.8	0.5	0.5
Male	NA	NA	1.3	0.9	0.6	0.7	0.5	0.4
Female	NA	NA	1.1	1.0	0.6	0.7	0.4	0.5
White	NA	NA	1.1	0.9	0.5	0.5	0.3	0.4
Black or African American	NA	NA	0.5	0.3	0.3	0.5	0.5	0.5
Inhalants								
All 12th graders	1.4	2.7	2.2	2.0	1.4	1.0	0.9	1.0
Male	1.8	3.5	2.9	2.4	2.1	1.1	0.9	1.2
Female	1.0	2.0	1.7	1.6	0.7	0.9	0.8	0.7
White	1.4	3.0	2.1	2.1	1.1	0.9	0.6	0.6
Black or African American	1.0	1.5	2.1	1.4	1.5	1.3	0.9	1.3
All 10th graders	NA	NA	2.6	2.2	2.0	1.7	1.4	1.3
Male	NA	NA	3.0	1.9	1.6	1.5	1.2	1.4
Female	NA	NA	2.2	2.5	2.4	2.0	1.6	1.3
White	NA	NA	2.8	2.2	1.7	1.4	1.1	1.0
Black or African American	NA	NA	1.5	1.4	1.8	1.6	1.2	1.9
All 8th graders	NA	NA	4.5	4.2	3.6	3.2	2.7	2.3
Male	NA	NA	4.1	3.1	2.8	2.5	1.9	1.6
Female	NA	NA	4.8	5.3	4.4	3.9	3.4	2.9
White	NA	NA	4.8	4.0	3.2	2.7	2.1	1.7
Black or African American	NA	NA	2.3	2.9	2.2	2.8	3.0	2.4

Table 3-25. Use of Selected Substances Among 12th Graders, 10th Graders, and 8th Graders, by Sex and Race, Selected Years, 1980–2013— continued

(Percent.)

Substance, grade in school, sex, and race	1980	1990	2000	2005	2010	2011	2012	2013
MDMA (Ecstasy)								
All 12th graders	NA	NA	3.6	1.0	1.4	2.3	0.9	1.5
Male	NA	NA	4.1	1.0	1.5	2.8	1.2	2.1
Female	NA	NA	3.1	1.0	1.2	1.8	0.6	0.9
White	NA	NA	3.9	1.0	0.9	2.1	0.9	1.5
Black or African American	NA	NA	1.9	0.9	1.1	1.1	0.4	0.7
All 10th graders	NA	NA	2.6	1.0	1.9	1.6	1.0	1.2
Male	NA	NA	2.5	1.0	2.3	1.7	1.1	1.5
Female	NA	NA	2.5	0.9	1.5	1.3	1.0	1.0
White	NA	NA	2.5	1.0	1.5	1.1	1.0	0.9
Black or African American	NA	NA	1.8	0.3	1.1	1.1	1.1	0.4
All 8th graders	NA	NA	1.4	0.6	1.1	0.6	0.5	0.5
Male	NA	NA	1.6	0.8	1.2	0.7	0.4	0.4
Female	NA	NA	1.2	0.4	1.1	0.5	0.6	0.5
White	NA	NA	1.4	0.6	1.0	0.4	0.4	0.3
Black or African American	NA	NA	0.8	0.9	0.5	0.2	0.5	0.6
Alcohol[1]								
All 12th graders	72.0	57.1	50.0	47.0	41.2	40.0	41.5	39.2
Male	77.4	61.3	54.0	50.7	44.2	42.1	43.8	41.8
Female	66.8	52.3	46.1	43.3	37.9	37.5	38.8	36.3
White	75.8	62.2	55.3	52.2	44.1	43.4	44.3	42.8
Black or African American	47.7	32.9	29.3	28.8	30.8	29.4	29.8	27.0
All 10th graders	NA	NA	41.0	33.2	28.9	27.2	27.6	25.7
Male	NA	NA	43.3	32.8	30.1	28.2	28.0	26.0
Female	NA	NA	38.6	33.6	27.7	26.0	27.1	25.3
White	NA	NA	44.3	36.7	29.2	28.9	29.2	26.9
Black or African American	NA	NA	24.7	20.8	21.3	20.3	20.1	17.7
All 8th graders	NA	NA	22.4	17.1	13.8	12.7	11.0	10.2
Male	NA	NA	22.5	16.2	13.2	12.1	10.3	9.3
Female	NA	NA	22.0	17.9	14.3	12.8	11.5	11.2
White	NA	NA	23.9	17.3	12.8	11.8	9.6	9.4
Black or African American	NA	NA	15.1	13.9	12.7	10.5	9.4	9.9
Binge Drinking[2]								
All 12th graders	41.2	32.2	30.0	27.1				
Male	52.1	39.1	36.7	32.6	28.0	25.5	27.2	26.1
Female	30.5	24.4	23.5	21.6	18.4	17.6	19.7	18.1
White	44.6	36.2	34.4	31.8	26.5	25.3	26.2	25.0
Black or African American	17.0	11.6	11.0	10.9	12.6	10.0	13.0	12.0
All 10th graders	NA	NA	24.1	19.0	16.3	14.7	15.6	13.7
Male	NA	NA	27.6	19.9	17.9	16.5	16.4	14.7
Female	NA	NA	20.6	17.9	14.6	12.7	14.8	12.5
White	NA	NA	26.6	21.5	16.0	16.1	16.5	14.7
Black or African American	NA	NA	10.6	8.4	11.5	7.3	9.3	7.9
All 8th graders	NA	NA	11.7	8.4	7.2	6.4	5.1	5.1
Male	NA	NA	11.7	8.2	6.5	6.1	4.6	4.5
Female	NA	NA	11.3	8.6	7.8	6.5	5.5	5.7
White	NA	NA	12.5	8.4	6.7	5.8	3.9	4.6
Black or African American	NA	NA	6.2	5.8	5.9	4.4	4.2	4.8

NA = Not available.   1 In 1993, the alcohol question was changed to indicate that a drink meant more than a few sips.   2 Five or more alcoholic drinks in a row at least once in the prior 2-week period.

AMBULATORY CARE

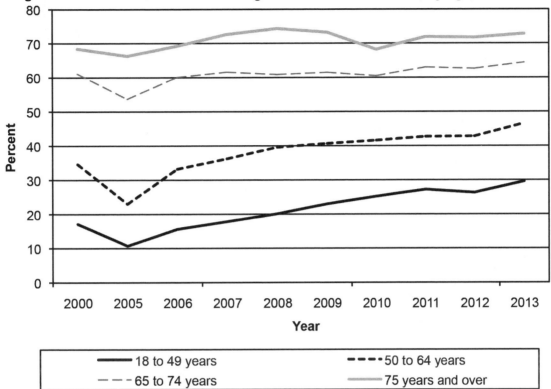

Figure 3-8. Influenza Vaccination Among Adults 18 Years and Over, By Age, 2000–2013

Figure 3-9. Percent of People with Reduced Access to Medical Care Due to Cost, Highest and Lowest Among States with the 25 Largest Populations, 2010–2011

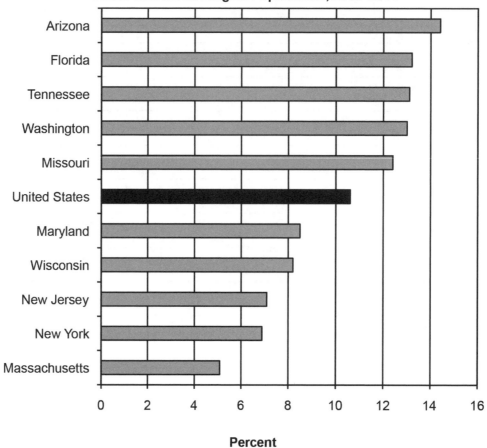

Percent

Table 3-26. No Usual Source of Health Care Among Children Under 18 Years of Age, by Selected Characteristics, Annual Average, Selected Years, 1993–1994 through 2012–2013

(Percent.)

Characteristic	Under 18 years			Under 6 years			6 to 17 years		
	1993–1994[1]	1999–2000	2012–2013	1993–1994[1]	1999–2000	2012–2013	1993–1994[1]	1999–2000	2012–2013
Percent of Children without a Usual Source of Health Care[2]									
All Children[3]	7.7	6.9	4.1	5.2	4.6	2.6	9.0	8.0	4.8
Sex									
Male	8.1	6.7	4.2	5.3	4.5	2.6	9.6	7.8	5.0
Female	7.3	7.1	3.9	5.0	4.7	2.6	8.5	8.2	4.6
Race[4]									
White only	7.0	6.3	4.1	4.7	4.4	2.7	8.3	7.2	4.7
Black or African American only	10.3	7.7	3.8	7.6	4.4	*1.6	11.9	9.1	4.9
American Indian or Alaska Native only	*9.3	*9.4	*5.0	*	*	*	*8.7	*9.4	*
Asian only	9.7	10.0	5.3	*3.4	*5.8	*3.8	13.5	12.2	6.1
Native Hawaiian or Other Pacific Islander only	NA	*	*	NA	*	*	NA	*	*
Two or more races	NA	*4.9	3.4	NA	*	*	NA	*7.2	4.2
Hispanic Origin and Race[4]									
Hispanic or Latino	14.3	14.2	6.5	9.3	9.0	4.1	17.7	17.2	7.9
Not Hispanic or Latino	6.7	5.5	3.3	4.4	3.6	2.1	7.8	6.3	3.9
White only	5.7	4.7	3.0	3.7	3.3	2.0	6.7	5.4	3.5
Black or African American only	10.2	7.6	3.9	7.7	4.5	*1.8	11.6	9.0	5.0
Percent of Poverty Level[5]									
Below 100 percent	13.9	13.1	6.1	9.4	7.6	4.2	16.8	16.2	7.2
100 percent to 199 percent	9.8	10.6	5.5	6.7	7.5	3.5	11.6	12.2	6.5
200 percent to 399 percent	3.7	4.8	3.5	1.9	3.2	1.8	4.5	5.6	4.2
400 percent or more	3.7	2.6	1.8	*1.6	1.5	*0.9	5.0	3.0	2.2
Hispanic Origin and Race and Percent of Poverty Level[4,5]									
Hispanic or Latino									
Below 100 percent	19.6	19.4	8.2	12.7	11.6	5.5	24.8	24.5	9.9
100 percent to 199 percent	15.3	17.1	6.6	9.9	11.3	*3.6	18.9	20.4	8.1
200 percent to 399 percent	5.2	8.3	5.2	*	*5.0	*3.1	6.7	10.1	6.4
400 percent or more	*	*3.8	*3.1	*	*	*	*	*5.0	*3.7
Not Hispanic or Latino									
White only									
Below 100 percent	10.2	10.7	5.3	6.5	*6.3	*4.2	12.7	13.1	5.9
100 percent to 199 percent	8.7	7.8	4.4	6.3	5.7	*3.5	10.1	8.8	4.8
200 percent to 399 percent	3.3	4.0	2.9	1.6	2.7	*1.4	4.0	4.6	3.5
400 percent or more	4.0	2.3	1.6	*1.7	*1.5	*	5.4	2.6	2.0
Black or African American only									
Below 100 percent	13.7	9.4	4.1	10.9	*4.7	*	15.5	11.8	5.1
100 percent to 199 percent	9.1	9.7	4.7	*6.0	*6.4	*	10.8	11.2	5.9
200 percent to 399 percent	5.0	5.0	*3.8	*	*	*	6.2	5.7	*5.1
400 percent or more	*	*3.5	*	*	*	*	*	*4.0	*
Health Insurance Status at the Time of Interview[6]									
Insured	5.0	3.9	2.5	3.3	2.6	1.7	5.9	4.5	2.9
Private	3.8	3.4	2.1	1.9	2.2	1.0	4.6	3.9	2.5
Medicaid	8.9	5.3	3.1	6.4	3.5	2.3	11.3	6.7	3.6
Uninsured	23.5	29.3	26.9	18.0	20.8	20.0	26.0	32.9	29.2
Health Insurance Status Prior to Interview[6]									
Insured continuously all 12 months	4.6	3.6	2.3	3.1	2.3	1.5	5.5	4.2	2.7
Uninsured for any period up to 12 months	15.3	15.0	12.7	10.9	12.5	10.1	18.1	16.4	14.1
Uninsured more than 12 months	27.6	35.8	33.7	21.4	26.8	23.5	30.0	39.1	36.3
Geographic Region									
Northeast									
Midwest	8.6	5.7	3.1	5.8	*2.7	2.7	10.7	7.5	3.3
South	21.7	19.8	16.9	18.0	*16.0	*	23.7	21.9	18.0
West	31.2	42.7	45.8	25.5	31.0	*29.6	33.4	47.1	50.1
Location of Residence									
Within MSA[7]	7.7	6.8	4.1	5.0	4.7	2.6	9.2	7.8	4.9
Outside MSA[7]	7.8	7.4	3.8	6.0	4.2	*2.5	8.7	8.7	4.4

NA = Not available.   * = Figure does not meet standards of reliability or precision. Data preceded by an asterisk have a relative standard error (RSE) of 20 percent to 30 percent. Data not shown have an RSE of greater than 30 percent.   1 Data prior to 1997 are not strictly comparable with data for later years due to the 1997 questionnaire redesign.   2 Persons who report the emergency department as their usual source of care are defined as having no usual source of care.   3 Includes all other races not shown separately and unknown health insurance status.   4 The race groups White, Black, American Indian or Alaska Native, Asian, Native Hawaiian or Other Pacific Islander, and two or more races include persons of Hispanic and non-Hispanic origin. Persons of Hispanic origin may be of any race.   5 Percent of poverty level is based on family income and family size and composition using U.S. Census Bureau poverty thresholds. Missing family income data were imputed starting in 1993.   6 Health insurance categories are mutually exclusive. Persons who reported both Medicaid and private coverage are classified as having private coverage. Medicaid includes other public assistance through 1996. Starting with 1997 data, state-sponsored health plan coverage is included as Medicaid coverage. Starting with 1999 data, coverage by the Children's Health Insurance Program (CHIP) is included with Medicaid coverage. Persons not covered by private insurance, Medicaid, CHIP, public assistance (through 1996), state-sponsored or other government-sponsored health plans (starting in 1997), Medicare, or military plans are considered to have no health insurance coverage. Persons with only Indian Health Service coverage are considered to have no health insurance coverage. Health insurance status was unknown for 8 to 9 percent of children in 1993-1996 and about 1 percent in 1997-2011.   7 MSA = metropolitan statistical area.

Table 3-27. No Usual Source of Health Care Among Adults 18 to 64 Years of Age, by Selected Characteristics, Annual Average, Selected Years, 1993–1994 through 2010–2011

(Percent.)

Characteristic	1993 to 1994[1]	1999 to 2000	2004 to 2005	2009 to 2010	2010 to 2011	2012 to 2013
PERCENT OF ADULTS WITHOUT A USUAL SOURCE OF HEALTH CARE [2]						
Total, 18 to 64 years [3]	18.9	17.8	18.0	20.3	19.6	19.7
Age						
18 to 44 years	21.7	21.6	22.8	26.0	25.2	25.4
18 to 24 years	26.6	27.2	29.9	29.8	28.1	28.7
19 to 25 years	28.0	29.0	31.3	33.1	30.9	30.8
25 to 44 years	20.3	19.9	20.3	24.7	24.1	24.2
45 to 64 years	12.8	10.9	10.6	12.3	11.8	12.0
45 to 54 years	14.1	12.0	11.9	14.7	14.0	14.0
55 to 64 years	11.1	9.2	8.8	9.3	9.0	9.6
Sex						
Male	23.9	24.1	23.3	25.9	24.6	24.5
Female	14.1	11.8	12.9	14.8	14.7	15.1
Race [3]						
White only	18.4	16.7	17.7	19.7	18.9	19.2
Black or African American only	20.0	19.2	19.3	22.4	22.5	21.4
American Indian or Alaska Native only	19.7	19.2	22.8	26.7	22.4	26.6
Asian only	24.8	22.1	18.8	20.8	20.8	19.9
Native Hawaiian or Other Pacific Islander only	NA	*	*	*	*	*
Two or more races	NA	21.0	18.1	27.5	24.4	23.5
American Indian or Alaska Native; White	NA	25.8	19.1	27.1	23.9	19.7
Hispanic Origin and Race [4]						
Hispanic or Latino	30.3	32.6	34.0	33.3	33.3	32.6
Mexican	32.4	36.5	37.8	35.7	35.2	34.5
Not Hispanic or Latino	17.7	15.8	15.4	17.9	17.0	17.1
White only	17.1	14.9	14.6	16.8	15.8	16.0
Black or African American only	19.7	19.2	19.0	22.2	22.1	21.3
Percent of Poverty Level [5]						
Below 100 percent	29.5	29.6	31.8	33.8	32.8	32.9
100 percent to 199 percent	25.4	27.1	27.1	30.5	30.4	29.4
200 percent to 399 percent	15.6	17.2	17.9	20.5	19.3	19.3
400 percent or more	13.4	11.6	10.3	10.8	9.7	10.1
Hispanic Origin and Race and Percent of Poverty Level [4,5]						
Hispanic or Latino						
Below 100 percent	40.0	44.4	44.5	45.5	44.3	43.5
100 percent to 199 percent	36.9	40.6	40.7	39.7	40.4	37.7
200 percent to 399 percent	20.7	26.9	30.1	29.1	28.9	28.8
400 percent or more	13.8	16.1	16.2	14.0	13.4	15.1
Not Hispanic or Latino						
White only						
Below 100 percent	28.2	24.2	26.8	28.8	27.5	28.9
100 percent to 199 percent	23.3	23.0	22.8	26.6	26.0	25.5
200 percent to 399 percent	14.8	15.3	15.6	18.6	17.2	16.8
400 percent or more	13.4	11.2	9.6	10.3	9.1	9.5
Black or African American only						
Below 100 percent	24.7	23.7	28.3	30.1	30.3	28.3
100 percent to 199 percent	22.3	24.4	22.1	28.5	29.6	27.3
200 percent to 399 percent	16.5	18.2	16.6	20.1	18.1	19.7
400 percent or more	11.7	12.0	11.3	10.5	10.6	9.7
Health Insurance Status at the Time of Interview [6]						
Insured	13.3	10.9	9.7	10.6	10.2	10.9
Private	13.1	11.1	9.5	10.6	10.1	10.6
Medicaid	16.3	9.9	12.1	12.5	12.3	13.2
Uninsured	43.1	49.2	52.5	55.6	54.2	54.2
Health Insurance Status Prior to Interview [6]						
Insured continuously all 12 months	12.7	10.3	8.9	9.8	9.3	10.0
Uninsured for any period up to 12 months	30.9	31.2	34.0	36.5	33.6	34.1
Uninsured more than 12 months	46.9	54.8	57.4	59.5	58.3	57.9
Percent of Poverty Level and Health Insurance Status Prior to Interview [5,6]						
Below 100 percent	16.7	11.6	12.7	13.0	13.4	14.3
Insured continuously all 12 months	33.6	31.9	39.4	37.8	36.6	38.7
Uninsured for any period up to 12 months	50.1	57.1	61.6	65.3	62.6	62.3
Uninsured more than 12 months						

Table 3-27. No Usual Source of Health Care Among Adults 18 to 64 Years of Age, by Selected Characteristics, Annual Average, Selected Years, 1993–1994 through 2010–2011— continued

(Percent.)

Characteristic	1993 to 1994[1]	1999 to 2000	2004 to 2005	2009 to 2010	2010 to 2011	2012 to 2013
100 percent to 199 percent	14.7	12.3	10.7	12.5	11.9	13.0
Insured continuously all 12 months	30.9	34.6	37.1	38.1	37.0	35.0
Uninsured for any period up to 12 months	47.6	54.9	56.0	58.5	58.2	56.8
Uninsured more than 12 months						
200 percent to 399 percent	11.7	10.6	9.5	10.6	10.0	10.4
Insured continuously all 12 months	29.2	29.0	31.9	37.6	33.7	34.2
Uninsured for any period up to 12 months	44.5	53.6	55.6	56.6	55.4	56.1
Uninsured more than 12 months						
400 percent or more	11.8	9.3	7.4	7.9	7.3	8.0
Insured continuously all 12 months	31.5	30.2	28.8	31.2	24.6	25.9
Uninsured for any period up to 12 months	36.5	51.8	56.5	53.8	52.5	52.7
Uninsured more than 12 months						
Disability Measure [7]						
Any basic actions difficulty or complex activity limitation	NA	14.1	15.0	16.8	16.2	16.1
Any basic actions difficulty	NA	14.1	15.2	16.7	16.2	15.9
Any complex activity limitation	NA	11.6	11.5	13.5	13.1	13.0
No disability	NA	18.8	18.8	21.5	20.7	20.9
Geographic Region						
Northeast	14.7	12.8	11.7	14.0	13.9	12.8
Midwest	16.2	17.0	15.4	17.5	16.7	18.0
South	21.8	19.7	21.0	23.5	22.3	22.3
West	21.1	20.1	21.2	22.9	22.4	22.6
Location of Residence						
Within MSA[8]	19.3	18.1	18.3	20.3	19.8	19.9
Outside MSA[8]	17.5	16.8	16.6	20.4	18.4	18.4

NA = Not available.   * = Figure does not meet standards of reliability or precision. Data not shown have an RSE of greater than 30 percent.   1Data prior to 1997 are not strictly comparable with data for later years due to the 1997 questionnaire redesign.   2Persons who report the emergency department as their usual source of care are defined as having no usual source of care.   3Includes all other races not shown separately, unknown health insurance status, and unknown disability status.   4The race groups White, Black, American Indian or Alaska Native, Asian, Native Hawaiian or Other Pacific Islander, and two or more races include persons of Hispanic and non-Hispanic origin. Persons of Hispanic origin may be of any race.   5Percent of poverty level is based on family income and family size and composition using U.S. Census Bureau poverty thresholds. Missing family income data were imputed starting in 1993.   6Health insurance categories are mutually exclusive. Persons who reported both Medicaid and private coverage are classified as having private coverage. Medicaid includes other public assistance through 1996. Starting with 1997 data, state-sponsored health plan coverage is included as Medicaid coverage. Starting with 1999 data, coverage by the Children's Health Insurance Program (CHIP) is included with Medicaid coverage. Persons not covered by private insurance, Medicaid, CHIP, public assistance (through 1996), state-sponsored or other government-sponsored health plans (starting in 1997), Medicare, or military plans are considered to have no health insurance coverage. Persons with only Indian Health Service coverage are considered to have no health insurance coverage. Health insurance status was unknown for 8 to 9 percent of children in 1993-1996 and about 1 percent in 1997-2011.   7Any basic actions difficulty or complex activity limitation is defined as having one or more of the following limitations or difficulties: movement difficulty, emotional difficulty, sensory (seeing or hearing) difficulty, cognitive difficulty, self-care (activities of daily living or instrumental activities of daily living) limitation, social limitation, or work limitation.   8MSA = metropolitan statistical area.

Table 3-28. Delay or Nonreceipt of Needed Medical Care, Nonreceipt of Needed Prescription Drugs, or Nonreceipt of Needed Dental Care During the Past 12 Months Due to Cost, by Selected Characteristics, Selected Years 1997–2013

(Percent.)

Characteristic	Delay or nonreceipt of needed medical care due to cost[1]				Delay or nonreceipt of needed prescription drugs due to cost[2]				Delay or nonreceipt of needed dental care due to cost[3]			
	1997	2005	2010	2013	1997	2005	2010	2013	1997	2005	2010	2013
TOTAL[4]	8.3	8.5	10.9	9.1	4.8	7.2	8.3	6.4	8.6	10.7	13.5	11.1
Age												
Under 19 years	4.5	4.3	4.5	3.2	2.1	3.0	2.8	2.2	6.0	7.3	6.6	5.3
Under 18 years	4.4	4.2	4.4	3.1	2.2	2.9	2.7	2.0	6.0	7.3	6.6	4.9
Under 6 years	3.3	3.3	3.7	2.2	1.6	2.5	2.5	1.7	3.9	3.7	3.9	2.7
6 to 17 years	4.9	4.7	4.8	3.5	2.4	3.1	2.8	2.2	6.8	8.4	7.5	5.7
18 to 64 years	10.7	11.0	14.7	12.4	6.3	9.4	11.2	8.8	10.6	13.0	17.3	14.3
18 to 44 years	11.0	11.3	14.5	11.9	6.9	9.8	11.2	8.2	11.7	14.1	17.9	14.2
18 to 24 years	10.2	11.3	13.5	10.1	6.7	9.6	9.7	7.2	11.6	13.7	17.4	11.4
25 to 34 years	11.4	11.8	15.3	13.0	6.9	10.2	12.0	9.3	12.3	15.1	18.3	16.0
35 to 44 years	11.0	10.8	14.4	12.1	7.1	9.6	11.3	8.0	11.2	13.3	17.8	14.3
19 to 25 years	11.1	12.5	14.8	11.2	7.7	10.3	10.9	7.6	13.1	14.8	18.9	11.8
45 to 64 years	10.1	10.6	14.9	13.2	5.1	8.7	11.3	9.6	8.4	11.5	16.5	14.5
45 to 54 years	10.6	10.8	15.0	13.4	5.6	9.2	11.5	10.3	9.4	12.1	17.8	15.1
55 to 64 years	9.3	10.4	14.6	13.0	4.2	8.0	11.0	8.8	7.0	10.7	14.9	13.8
65 years and over	4.6	4.6	5.0	4.2	2.8	5.1	4.7	3.4	3.5	5.2	6.9	6.4
65 to 74 years	5.0	5.4	6.3	4.9	3.4	6.4	6.3	4.1	4.2	6.2	9.0	7.5
75 years and over	4.1	3.7	3.4	3.2	2.0	3.6	2.8	2.4	2.6	4.0	4.3	4.9
18 TO 64 YEARS												
Sex												
Male	9.3	10.0	13.5	11.2	5.1	7.2	8.8	6.9	8.8	10.8	15.2	12.3
Female	12.0	12.1	15.7	13.6	7.4	11.4	13.5	10.6	12.4	15.2	19.4	16.2
Race[5]												
White only	10.8	11.1	14.5	12.3	5.9	9.1	10.8	8.5	10.6	12.8	17.1	14.2
Black or African American only	10.8	12.0	17.4	14.6	9.5	11.6	15.6	11.6	10.8	15.2	20.7	16.5
American Indian or Alaska Native only	14.5	13.2	*15.7	15.2	*10.1	*14.1	18.6	*11.3	18.8	19.2	23.1	13.5
Asian only	6.3	5.0	8.0	7.3	*2.8	*3.5	4.2	3.9	7.8	6.8	8.7	9.0
Native Hawaiian or Other Pacific Islander only	NA	*	*	*	NA	*	*	*	NA	*	*	*
Two or more races	NA	19.9	24.0	19.8	NA	22.9	16.6	14.8	NA	23.0	25.6	19.5
Hispanic Origin and Race[5]												
Hispanic or Latino	10.5	11.5	15.4	14.1	6.7	11.2	13.0	10.2	11.5	15.5	21.6	18.4
Mexican origin	9.7	11.4	15.6	14.0	6.5	12.0	13.5	10.7	11.3	16.3	22.0	19.8
Not Hispanic or Latino	10.7	11.0	14.5	12.1	6.3	9.0	10.9	8.5	10.5	12.6	16.6	13.5
White only	10.9	11.1	14.3	11.9	5.9	8.7	10.3	8.2	10.5	12.3	16.2	13.3
Black or African American only	10.8	12.0	17.5	14.5	9.5	11.4	15.6	11.7	10.8	15.3	20.8	16.3
Education[6]												
No high school diploma or GED	16.2	16.2	20.6	18.1	11.5	16.4	18.1	14.4	14.5	20.3	26.3	22.1
High school diploma or GED	11.1	11.7	16.1	14.8	7.0	10.5	13.8	10.9	11.4	14.6	20.1	17.0
Some college or more	9.2	9.8	13.4	11.2	4.3	7.1	9.2	7.4	8.8	10.4	14.4	12.7
Percent of Poverty Level[7]												
Below 100 percent	19.6	20.0	23.4	21.8	14.8	19.5	21.5	18.3	19.4	24.4	30.4	28.3
100 percent to 199 percent	17.9	18.9	24.0	20.3	11.6	16.3	18.4	14.4	18.3	21.0	29.2	23.5
200 percent to 399 percent	10.5	11.8	15.2	12.5	5.5	9.5	11.4	8.4	10.2	13.7	17.3	13.4
400 percent or more	4.6	5.0	6.8	5.1	1.7	3.3	3.9	2.8	4.5	5.9	7.0	5.2
Hispanic Origin and Race and Percent of Poverty Level[5,7]												
Hispanic or Latino												
Below 100 percent	14.6	14.8	19.0	18.9	10.6	17.3	18.9	16.8	16.1	23.5	30.5	27.2
100 percent to 199 percent	12.2	14.5	18.6	17.1	8.1	13.0	14.7	12.0	13.5	18.2	25.2	22.5
200 percent to 399 percent	8.0	9.6	13.9	12.0	4.4	9.1	11.5	6.8	9.2	12.5	18.1	14.4
400 percent or more	5.1	6.2	7.7	5.9	*	*4.2	4.6	*4.5	4.5	5.8	9.1	7.5
Not Hispanic or Latino												
White only												
Below 100 percent	24.3	23.6	26.1	24.1	17.3	20.5	24.6	20.4	23.4	25.1	31.8	31.2
100 percent to 199 percent	20.9	21.8	27.6	22.8	12.4	18.2	19.9	16.3	20.6	22.9	31.7	25.6
200 percent to 399 percent	11.4	13.1	16.0	13.2	5.4	10.0	11.3	8.7	10.6	14.4	18.0	13.6
400 percent or more	4.6	5.0	6.9	5.2	1.7	3.2	3.8	2.6	4.5	5.9	6.9	5.2
Black or African American only												
Below 100 percent	16.1	20.1	24.4	22.5	14.9	21.7	21.1	17.8	14.8	25.5	29.7	26.3
100 percent to 199 percent	14.3	16.2	22.9	18.7	13.9	14.3	21.3	15.0	16.4	19.0	28.2	20.4
200 percent to 399 percent	8.8	9.2	14.6	11.2	7.0	7.9	13.7	10.1	8.6	12.0	16.1	13.0
400 percent or more	4.6	5.5	8.1	6.1	*2.9	*4.1	5.6	*3.7	4.3	*7.0	9.1	*5.4

Table 3-28. Delay or Nonreceipt of Needed Medical Care, Nonreceipt of Needed Prescription Drugs, or Nonreceipt of Needed Dental Care During the Past 12 Months Due to Cost, by Selected Characteristics, Selected Years 1997–2013— continued

(Percent.)

Characteristic	Delay or nonreceipt of needed medical care due to cost[1]				Delay or nonreceipt of needed prescription drugs due to cost[2]				Delay or nonreceipt of needed dental care due to cost[3]			
	1997	2005	2010	2013	1997	2005	2010	2013	1997	2005	2010	2013
Health Insurance Status at the Time of Interview [8]												
Insured	6.8	6.8	9.1	7.4	3.7	6.0	7.3	5.8	7.2	8.7	11.8	9.8
Private	6.0	5.9	8.2	6.4	2.9	4.7	6.0	4.4	6.2	6.7	9.2	7.0
Medicaid	11.9	12.0	12.5	10.8	11.1	14.0	13.5	11.5	14.8	21.8	24.2	22.4
Uninsured	27.6	29.5	34.5	32.4	18.0	23.1	25.7	20.7	26.1	30.7	37.7	32.0
Health Insurance Status Prior to Interview [8]												
Insured continuously all 12 months	5.5	5.5	7.6	6.2	2.8	5.0	6.2	5.0	6.0	7.5	10.5	8.9
Uninsured for any period up to 12 months	28.7	31.7	35.1	31.8	17.7	23.5	25.1	20.5	25.2	30.3	33.6	28.3
Uninsured more than 12 months	30.6	31.1	35.9	33.8	18.9	24.5	26.2	20.9	28.0	32.1	39.4	33.1
Disability Measure [9]												
Any basic actions difficulty or complex activity limitation	23.3	24.8	28.9	26.3	14.8	20.0	22.6	20.2	19.8	23.8	28.8	26.6
Any basic actions difficulty	24.2	26.1	28.9	27.4	15.3	20.5	23.3	20.8	20.1	24.4	29.2	27.1
Any complex activity limitation	25.7	26.9	30.8	27.7	19.4	25.3	27.3	25.6	23.2	27.3	33.7	31.0
No disability	9.0	9.8	13.2	10.5	3.4	5.7	7.0	4.8	7.5	9.4	13.1	10.1
Geographic Region												
Northeast	8.8	8.7	10.2	9.0	4.9	7.2	7.7	6.4	8.9	10.6	12.9	10.4
Midwest	10.5	10.6	14.8	12.1	5.9	9.0	11.6	8.5	9.7	11.9	16.0	12.5
South	11.8	12.6	16.5	13.6	7.3	11.3	13.5	10.4	10.9	14.7	19.6	15.3
West	10.8	11.1	15.1	13.6	6.3	8.2	10.0	8.4	13.1	13.6	18.4	17.4
Location of Residence												
Within MSA[10]	10.2	10.6	14.2	12.1	5.9	8.8	10.8	8.5	10.0	12.7	17.0	14.0
Outside MSA[10]	12.5	12.8	17.4	14.6	7.9	11.8	13.6	10.8	12.9	14.6	19.1	15.9

NA = Not available.   * = Figure does not meet standards of reliability or precision. Data preceded by an asterisk have a relative standard error (RSE) of 20 percent to 30 percent. Data not shown have an RSE of greater than 30 percent.   1 Based on persons responding to the question, "During the past 12 months was there any time when person needed medical care but did not get it because person couldn't afford it?" and "During the past 12 months has medical care been delayed because of worry about the cost?"   2 Based on persons responding to the question, "During the past 12 months was there any time when person needed prescription medicine but didn't get it because person couldn't afford it?"   3 Based on persons responding to the question, "During the past 12 months was there any time when person needed dental care (including checkups) but didn't get it because person couldn't afford it?"   4 Includes all other races not shown separately, unknown health insurance status, unknown education level, and unknown disability status.   5 The race groups White, Black, American Indian or Alaska Native, Asian, Native Hawaiian or Other Pacific Islander, and two or more races include persons of Hispanic and non-Hispanic origin. Persons of Hispanic origin may be of any race.   6 Estimates are for persons 25 to 64 years of age. GED is General Educational Development high school equivalency diploma.   7 Percent of poverty level is based on family income and family size and composition using U.S. Census Bureau poverty thresholds. Missing family income data were imputed for 1997 and beyond.   8 For information on the health insurance categories, see Appendix II, Health insurance coverage, in Health: United States, 2014.   9 Any basic actions difficulty or complex activity limitation is defined as having one or more of the following limitations or difficulties: movement difficulty, emotional difficulty, sensory (seeing or hearing) difficulty, cognitive difficulty, self-care (activities of daily living or instrumental activities of daily living) limitation, social limitation, or work limitation.   10 MSA = metropolitan statistical area.

Table 3-29. Reduced Access to Medical Care During the Past 12 Months Due to Cost, 25 Largest States, Selected Annual Averages, 1997–1998 through 2010–2011

(Percent for the 25 states with the largest populations in 2010–2011.)

State	Did not get or delayed medical care due to cost[1]			Did not get prescription drugs due to cost[2]			Did not get dental care[3]		
	1997–1998	2000–2001	2010–2011	1997–1998	2000–2001	2010–2011	1997–1998	2000–2001	2010–2011
United States	7.9	7.5	10.6	4.5	5.3	8.0	8.1	8.4	13.2
Alabama	7.6	7.7	11.9	6.8	8.3	12.3	8.7	10.3	15.0
Arizona	8.0	7.4	14.4	4.1	4.6	11.1	9.4	8.4	20.6
California	6.8	6.6	10.4	3.9	4.7	7.2	8.3	8.1	15.0
Colorado	6.4	8.1	12.2	3.1	5.5	6.9	8.9	11.5	13.5
Florida	9.8	9.6	13.2	4.8	5.8	10.1	7.2	8.4	17.4
Georgia	8.0	7.7	12.1	4.2	4.0	9.7	5.8	5.3	13.8
Illinois	6.1	6.5	8.7	3.0	4.2	6.0	5.7	6.8	9.9
Indiana	9.0	8.6	12.0	5.1	6.8	11.9	7.2	6.9	12.2
Louisiana	9.8	11.1	11.4	8.7	9.8	12.0	11.3	16.4	18.0
Maryland	8.0	7.4	8.5	5.8	5.2	5.7	9.8	7.8	9.1
Massachusetts	5.1	4.3	5.1	*1.7	4.2	4.7	5.0	5.2	7.9
Michigan	7.2	7.0	11.4	3.8	5.1	9.8	7.5	7.9	15.9
Minnesota	8.1	7.0	10.3	3.6	3.9	6.0	8.7	8.3	10.7
Missouri	7.1	6.4	12.4	4.3	5.2	8.4	7.3	7.1	14.7
New Jersey	7.2	6.1	7.1	3.8	3.5	4.7	7.3	5.9	9.9
New York	6.4	5.8	6.9	2.8	3.8	5.4	5.6	7.5	7.8
North Carolina	7.8	7.9	11.3	4.0	5.8	7.9	8.2	7.9	12.4
Ohio	9.2	7.6	10.5	5.0	5.1	8.1	8.8	8.1	10.5
Pennsylvania	5.9	5.9	9.1	4.3	3.5	7.0	7.4	6.0	11.4
South Carolina	7.6	6.3	11.2	5.2	4.4	8.4	5.7	5.2	11.3
Tennessee	10.0	8.6	13.1	8.0	8.5	10.7	10.5	10.4	15.3
Texas	7.9	8.1	12.0	4.7	6.6	9.9	8.8	10.4	16.4
Virginia	6.2	7.2	9.3	4.1	5.2	6.9	8.3	7.4	9.6
Washington	8.6	9.2	13.0	4.8	6.8	8.3	11.6	11.9	17.6
Wisconsin	6.5	5.9	8.2	3.0	4.0	5.0	5.5	6.6	10.6

* = Figure does not meet standards of reliability or precision. Data preceded by an asterisk have a relative standard error (RSE) of 20 percent to 30 percent.   1Based on persons responding to the question, "During the past 12 months was there any time when person needed medical care but did not get it because person couldn't afford it?" and "During the past 12 months has medical care been delayed because of worry about the cost?"   2Based on persons responding to the question, "During the past 12 months was there any time when you needed prescription medicine but didn't get it because you couldn't afford it?"   3Based on persons responding to the question, "During the past 12 months was there any time when you needed dental care (including check ups) but didn't get it because you couldn't afford it?"

Table 3-30. No Health Care Visits[1] to an Office or Clinic Within the Past 12 Months Among Children Under 18 Years of Age, by Selected Characteristics, Selected Annual Averages, 1997–1998 through 2012–2013

(Percent.)

Characteristic	Under 18 years			Under 6 years			6 to 17 years		
	1997–1998	2005–2006	2012–2013	1997–1998	2005–2006	2012–2013	1997–1998	2005–2006	2012–2013
ALL CHILDREN [2]	12.8	11.7	8.8	5.7	6.1	5.0	16.3	14.4	10.7
Sex									
Male	12.9	12.0	8.8	4.9	6.2	4.9	16.8	14.7	10.7
Female	12.7	11.4	8.7	6.5	6.1	5.0	15.8	14.0	10.6
Race [3]									
White only	12.2	11.3	9.0	5.5	6.3	4.9	15.5	13.8	10.9
Black or African American only	14.3	11.7	8.1	6.5	4.6	5.3	18.1	15.1	9.5
American Indian or Alaska Native only	13.8	*15.7	*6.8	*	*	*	*17.6	*17.7	*8.7
Asian only	16.3	17.5	9.9	*5.6	10.5	*4.9	22.1	20.8	12.2
Native Hawaiian or Other Pacific Islander only	NA	*	*	NA	*	*	NA	*	*
Two or more races	NA	10.4	7.5	NA	*	*4.4	NA	14.8	9.3
Hispanic Origin and Race [3]									
Hispanic or Latino	19.3	17.4	11.7	9.7	9.6	6.4	25.3	21.9	14.6
Not Hispanic or Latino	11.6	10.3	7.9	4.8	5.1	4.4	14.9	12.6	9.5
White only	10.7	9.4	7.7	4.3	5.0	4.2	13.7	11.4	9.3
Black or African American only	14.5	11.7	8.1	6.5	*4.4	5.0	18.3	15.1	9.6
Percent of Poverty Level [4]									
Below 100 percent	17.6	14.2	10.7	8.1	7.7	7.3	23.6	18.2	12.8
100 percent to 199 percent	16.2	14.9	10.7	7.2	8.4	5.4	20.8	18.2	13.3
200 percent to 399 percent	11.7	11.1	8.7	4.9	6.1	4.2	14.8	13.4	10.7
400 percent or more	7.4	7.8	5.6	3.0	2.8	2.9	9.5	10.0	6.7
Hispanic Origin and Race and Percent of Poverty Level [3,4]									
Hispanic or Latino									
Below 100 percent	23.2	20.0	13.5	11.7	11.5	9.5	31.1	25.6	16.0
100 percent to 199 percent	20.9	19.1	12.8	9.7	10.1	5.0	28.1	24.4	16.8
200 percent to 399 percent	15.7	14.6	9.3	8.0	8.1	*3.5	19.7	17.9	12.6
400 percent or more	7.8	10.9	6.5	*	*	*	9.3	14.1	7.4
Not Hispanic or Latino									
White only									
Below 100 percent	14.0	9.4	9.5	*5.6	*5.6	*5.3	19.7	11.8	12.1
100 percent to 199 percent	14.1	13.2	9.7	6.0	8.5	*5.9	18.0	15.4	11.7
200 percent to 399 percent	10.9	9.7	8.3	4.3	5.8	4.3	13.9	11.4	10.0
400 percent or more	7.2	7.1	5.4	*2.8	*2.2	*2.4	9.1	9.2	6.7
Black or African American only									
Below 100 percent	15.8	12.1	8.5	7.6	*	*6.4	20.5	16.4	9.8
100 percent to 199 percent	16.4	13.1	8.2	*7.7	*	*	20.4	16.2	9.9
200 percent to 399 percent	13.3	11.7	9.2	*4.9	*	*	16.7	14.8	11.3
400 percent or more	8.3	*7.4	*4.0	*	*	*	10.7	*9.9	*
Health Insurance Status at the Time of Interview [5]									
Insured	10.4	9.5	7.5	4.5	4.9	4.5	13.4	11.9	9.0
Private	10.4	9.4	7.0	4.3	4.4	3.4	13.1	11.6	8.5
Medicaid	10.1	9.5	8.2	5.0	5.8	5.6	14.4	12.2	9.8
Uninsured	28.8	31.7	26.9	14.6	20.6	13.9	34.9	35.6	31.3
Health Insurance Status Prior to Interview [5]									
Insured continuously all 12 months	10.3	9.5	7.4	4.4	4.9	4.4	13.2	11.9	8.9
Uninsured for any period up to 12 months	15.9	15.8	12.4	7.7	9.3	*5.8	20.9	18.8	15.8
Uninsured more than 12 months	34.9	39.0	36.0	19.9	28.0	22.9	40.2	42.2	39.3
Percent of Poverty Level and Health Insurance Status Prior to Interview [4,5]									
Below 100 percent									
Insured continuously all 12 months	12.6	10.4	8.9	5.7	5.8	6.6	17.6	13.5	10.3
Uninsured for any period up to 12 months	19.9	17.5	11.4	*9.9	*	*	26.1	21.6	14.1
Uninsured more than 12 months	39.9	44.6	42.0	24.9	*32.3	*31.2	45.2	48.4	45.0
100 percent to 199 percent									
Insured continuously all 12 months	12.6	11.5	8.2	4.8	6.7	4.5	16.7	14.2	10.0
Uninsured for any period up to 12 months	15.6	17.7	15.5	*8.7	*10.8	*	20.2	20.4	19.5
Uninsured more than 12 months	33.7	39.2	37.7	21.3	26.0	*	37.9	42.9	40.9
200 percent to 399 percent									
Insured continuously all 12 months	10.5	9.8	7.8	4.5	5.2	3.9	13.2	12.0	9.6
Uninsured for any period up to 12 months	12.8	14.6	10.8	*	*	*	17.2	17.3	14.1
Uninsured more than 12 months	29.9	31.6	27.2	*11.8	*	*	36.5	33.2	30.7
400 percent or more									
Insured continuously all 12 months	7.0	7.4	5.3	2.9	2.5	2.7	8.8	9.5	6.4
Uninsured for any period up to 12 months	*10.8	*	*	*	*	*	*15.1	*	*
Uninsured more than 12 months	*28.8	*35.6	*30.3	*	*	*	*37.7	*38.3	*34.0

Table 3-30. No Health Care Visits[1] to an Office or Clinic Within the Past 12 Months Among Children Under 18 Years of Age, by Selected Characteristics, Selected Annual Averages, 1997–1998 through 2012–2013— continued

(Percent.)

Characteristic	Under 18 years			Under 6 years			6 to 17 years		
	1997–1998	2005–2006	2012–2013	1997–1998	2005–2006	2012–2013	1997–1998	2005–2006	2012–2013
Geographic Region									
Northeast	7.0	6.8	5.8	3.1	4.0	4.2	8.9	8.1	6.5
Midwest	12.2	9.8	8.3	5.9	5.2	3.1	15.3	12.0	10.9
South	14.3	12.4	9.2	5.6	6.2	5.9	18.5	15.5	10.8
West	16.3	16.5	10.7	7.9	8.8	5.7	20.7	20.3	13.1
Location of Residence									
Within MSA[6]	12.3	11.4	8.3	5.4	5.9	4.6	15.9	14.1	10.2
Outside MSA[6]	14.6	12.9	11.3	6.9	7.4	*7.0	17.9	15.4	13.4

NA = Not available.   * = Figure does not meet standards of reliability or precision. Data preceded by an asterisk have a relative standard error (RSE) of 20 percent to 30 percent. Data not shown have an RSE of greater than 30 percent.   1 Respondents were asked how many times a doctor or other health care professional was seen in the past 12 months at a doctor's office, clinic, or some other place. Excluded are visits to emergency rooms, hospitalizations, home visits, and telephone calls. Starting with 2000 data, dental visits were also excluded.   2 Includes all other races not shown separately and unknown health insurance status.   3 The race groups White, Black, American Indian or Alaska Native, Asian, Native Hawaiian or Other Pacific Islander, and two or more races include persons of Hispanic and non-Hispanic origin. Persons of Hispanic origin may be of any race.   4 Percent of poverty level is based on family income and family size and composition using U.S. Census Bureau poverty thresholds. Missing family income data were imputed starting in 1993.   5 Health insurance categories are mutually exclusive. Persons who reported both Medicaid and private coverage are classified as having private coverage. Medicaid includes other public assistance through 1996. Starting with 1997 data, state-sponsored health plan coverage is included as Medicaid coverage. Starting with 1999 data, coverage by the Children's Health Insurance Program (CHIP) is included with Medicaid coverage. Persons not covered by private insurance, Medicaid, CHIP, public assistance (through 1996), state-sponsored or other government-sponsored health plans (starting in 1997), Medicare, or military plans are considered to have no health insurance coverage. Persons with only Indian Health Service coverage are considered to have no health insurance coverage. Health insurance status was unknown for 8 to 9 percent of children in 1993-1996 and about 1 percent in 1997-2011.   6 MSA = metropolitan statistical area.

Table 3-31. Health Care Visits to Doctors' Offices, Emergency Departments, and Home Visits within the Past 12 Months, by Selected Characteristics, Selected Years, 1997–2013

(Percent distribution of health care visits to doctors' offices, emergency departments, and home visits during a 12-month period.)

Characteristic	None				1 to 3 visits				4 to 9 visits				10 or more visits			
	1997	2005	2010	2013	1997	2005	2010	2013	1997	2005	2010	2013	1997	2005	2010	2013
Total, age-adjusted[1,2]	16.5	15.5	15.6	16.1	46.2	45.9	45.4	47.6	23.6	25.1	25.8	24.0	13.7	13.6	13.2	12.3
Total, crude[1]	16.5	15.4	15.4	15.8	46.5	45.9	45.2	47.0	23.5	25.1	26.0	24.5	13.5	13.6	13.5	12.7
Age																
Under 18 years	11.8	10.2	8.1	8.2	54.1	56.0	55.6	59.7	25.2	26.5	28.2	25.1	8.9	7.4	8.2	7.1
Under 6 years	5.0	5.1	3.7	4.7	44.9	47.4	48.9	49.6	37.0	38.0	36.8	37.1	13.0	9.5	10.6	8.6
6 to 17 years	15.3	12.6	10.4	9.9	58.7	60.1	59.1	64.5	19.3	20.9	23.6	19.3	6.8	6.3	6.9	6.3
18 to 44 years	21.7	22.9	24.2	24.8	46.7	45.8	43.9	45.9	19.0	19.2	20.6	18.5	12.6	12.0	11.3	10.7
18 to 24 years	22.0	24.2	25.9	26.9	46.8	44.4	43.4	46.8	20.0	19.6	21.1	17.5	11.2	11.8	9.6	8.8
25 to 44 years	21.6	22.5	23.6	24.0	46.7	46.3	44.1	45.6	18.7	19.1	20.5	18.9	13.0	12.1	11.9	11.5
45 to 64 years	16.9	14.0	14.8	15.2	42.9	42.9	42.8	43.0	24.7	26.8	26.1	26.7	15.5	16.3	16.4	15.0
45 to 54 years	17.9	15.8	17.6	17.2	43.9	44.8	43.5	44.2	23.4	24.3	23.9	25.2	14.8	15.0	15.0	13.4
55 to 64 years	15.3	11.4	11.1	13.1	41.3	40.2	41.9	41.6	26.7	30.3	28.8	28.5	16.7	18.2	18.2	16.8
65 years and over	8.9	5.6	5.3	6.4	34.7	30.7	33.8	35.9	32.5	37.5	36.7	34.4	23.8	26.2	24.2	23.2
65 to 74 years	9.8	5.9	6.3	7.8	36.9	34.4	36.1	37.4	31.6	35.8	35.7	33.7	21.6	23.9	21.9	21.0
75 years and over	7.7	5.2	4.1	4.5	31.8	26.4	31.0	33.7	33.8	39.5	38.0	35.4	26.6	28.8	27.0	26.3
Sex[2]																
Male	21.3	20.4	20.4	21.0	47.1	46.7	46.4	47.7	20.6	22.2	22.7	21.2	11.0	10.7	10.5	10.1
Female	11.8	10.7	10.9	11.4	45.4	45.1	44.4	47.5	26.5	27.9	28.8	26.7	16.3	16.3	15.9	14.4
Race[2,3]																
White only	16.0	15.1	15.3	16.1	46.1	45.6	44.9	47.3	23.9	25.4	26.1	24.0	14.0	13.9	13.7	12.7
Black or African American only	16.8	15.9	15.7	15.2	46.1	47.4	47.2	47.6	23.2	23.8	24.7	25.7	13.9	12.9	12.4	11.5
American Indian or Alaska Native only	17.1	20.4	19.4	16.1	38.0	36.4	40.3	43.2	24.2	29.8	28.1	28.3	20.7	13.4	12.2	12.4
Asian only	22.8	21.5	20.4	18.4	49.1	49.3	49.9	53.1	19.7	20.8	22.1	21.3	8.3	8.4	7.6	7.2
Native Hawaiian and Other Pacific Islander only	NA	*	*	*	NA	*	*	*	NA	*	*	*	NA	*	*	*
Two or more races	NA	15.4	13.9	15.8	NA	37.3	42.3	42.6	NA	27.6	25.2	24.9	NA	19.7	18.6	16.8
Hispanic Origin and Race[2,3]																
Hispanic or Latino	24.9	23.9	23.5	24.0	42.3	42.1	43.2	45.8	20.3	22.2	22.6	20.5	12.5	11.8	10.7	9.7
Mexican	28.9	26.6	25.2	26.2	40.8	41.5	43.3	44.6	18.5	20.8	21.4	20.0	11.8	11.1	10.1	9.2
Not Hispanic or Latino	15.4	13.9	14.0	14.4	46.7	46.5	45.8	47.9	24.0	25.7	26.5	24.8	13.9	13.9	13.7	12.9
White only	14.7	13.0	13.2	13.9	46.6	46.4	45.3	47.6	24.4	26.2	27.1	25.0	14.3	14.5	14.4	13.5
Black or African American only	16.9	15.9	15.6	15.2	46.1	47.4	47.3	47.7	23.1	23.8	24.9	25.7	13.8	12.9	12.2	11.4
Percent of Poverty Level[2,4]																
Below 100 percent	20.6	20.7	20.4	20.1	37.8	37.3	37.5	39.8	22.7	24.7	25.1	23.5	18.9	17.3	17.0	16.6
100 percent to 199 percent	20.1	20.2	20.8	21.0	43.3	42.0	42.1	42.8	21.7	23.4	23.1	22.5	14.9	14.4	13.9	13.7
200 percent to 399 percent	16.4	15.9	16.2	16.7	47.2	47.3	46.3	48.9	23.6	24.0	25.4	23.0	12.8	12.8	12.1	11.3
400 percent or more	12.8	11.0	10.2	11.1	49.8	49.2	49.4	51.9	24.9	27.0	27.6	25.7	12.5	12.8	12.7	11.3
Hispanic Origin and Race, and Percent of Poverty Level[2,3,4]																
Hispanic or Latino																
Below 100 percent	32.3	27.9	28.7	26.4	33.3	37.2	36.5	38.6	19.2	20.2	22.5	13.2	15.1	14.6	12.3	13.2
100 percent to 199 percent	30.5	27.6	27.7	29.2	40.6	38.8	42.7	41.4	17.6	22.6	19.9	9.3	11.3	11.1	9.8	9.3
200 percent to 399 percent	24.2	22.7	21.6	19.6	45.5	44.9	45.0	45.9	19.9	23.1	23.1	10.3	10.3	9.2	10.3	10.3
400 percent or more	17.0	13.4	11.3	14.1	47.2	50.4	51.1	52.1	26.3	23.0	26.1	9.5	9.5	13.2	11.5	9.5
Not Hispanic or Latino																
White only																
Below 100 percent	18.0	16.4	15.0	15.6	36.9	36.1	37.0	38.8	25.3	28.0	27.4	19.2	19.8	19.5	20.6	19.2
100 percent to 199 percent	18.5	17.5	18.4	17.9	41.5	41.8	40.4	42.8	24.1	24.0	24.7	15.7	15.9	16.8	16.5	15.7
200 percent to 399 percent	15.3	13.8	14.7	14.4	44.6	47.3	46.0	47.7	26.1	24.7	26.3	13.7	13.9	14.2	13.0	13.7
400 percent or more	11.8	10.3	9.9	9.8	47.8	48.9	48.2	50.2	27.6	27.6	28.4	12.2	12.8	13.1	13.5	12.2
Black or African American only																
Below 100 percent	18.3	17.8	18.4	15.2	40.0	40.1	39.8	40.2	24.9	24.8	25.0	18.2	16.7	17.3	16.8	18.2
100 percent to 199 percent	20.8	16.1	17.6	17.2	44.2	47.0	45.7	45.5	20.7	24.3	24.3	13.0	14.3	12.6	12.5	13.0
200 percent to 399 percent	17.1	17.2	15.1	15.7	48.5	49.0	49.0	51.4	24.4	22.9	25.7	9.8	10.1	10.9	10.2	9.8
400 percent or more	11.3	12.1	10.0	10.4	52.2	52.0	58.2	54.7	24.8	24.7	22.5	11.6	11.7	11.2	9.3	11.6
Health Insurance Status at the Time of Interview[5,6]																
Under 65 years																
Insured	14.0	12.4	12.3	12.4	48.2	49.6	48.5	50.3	25.1	25.0	26.1	12.4	12.7	13.0	13.1	12.4
Private	14.3	12.8	12.4	12.7	49.9	51.5	51.0	53.1	24.8	24.5	25.5	9.9	11.0	11.2	11.1	9.9
Medicaid	10.4	9.9	10.9	10.6	32.4	37.8	38.2	40.0	27.6	26.8	28.0	23.0	29.6	25.5	23.0	23.0
Uninsured	36.8	37.5	37.2	37.1	41.9	42.0	42.2	43.5	14.1	14.7	15.2	5.5	7.2	5.8	5.4	5.5
Health Insurance Status Prior to Interview[5,6]																
Under 65 years																
Insured continuously all 12 months	13.9	12.3	12.1	12.2	48.5	49.8	48.6	50.5	25.1	25.0	26.2	12.3	12.6	12.9	13.0	12.3

Table 3-31. Health Care Visits to Doctors' Offices, Emergency Departments, and Home Visits within the Past 12 Months, by Selected Characteristics, Selected Years, 1997–2013— continued

(Percent distribution of health care visits to doctors' offices, emergency departments, and home visits during a 12-month period.)

Characteristic	None				1 to 3 visits				4 to 9 visits				10 or more visits			
	1997	2005	2010	2013	1997	2005	2010	2013	1997	2005	2010	2013	1997	2005	2010	2013
Uninsured for any period up to 12 months	20.4	18.9	18.5	19.0	44.1	44.9	47.8	47.3	21.5	22.5	22.0	12.2	13.9	13.7	11.6	12.2
Uninsured more than 12 months	43.1	43.5	43.8	43.0	39.5	40.0	39.7	41.7	12.3	12.3	12.6	4.1	5.1	4.2	3.9	4.1
Percent of Poverty Level and Health Insurance Status Prior to Interview (Under 65 Years) [4,5,6]																
Below 100 percent																
Insured continuously all 12 months	13.8	12.6	12.7	12.0	39.7	40.4	39.5	44.0	25.2	26.2	27.5	25.1	21.4	20.8	20.3	19.0
Uninsured for any period up to 12 months	19.7	18.9	16.9	19.2	37.6	37.4	43.0	40.8	21.9	23.7	25.0	22.4	20.9	20.0	15.1	17.6
Uninsured more than 12 months	41.2	46.0	45.0	44.8	39.9	35.2	38.1	37.1	12.2	14.4	13.6	13.8	6.6	4.3	3.3	4.2
100 percent to 199 percent																
Insured continuously all 12 months	16.0	14.8	14.8	14.9	46.4	45.7	44.4	45.3	21.9	24.3	24.8	24.2	15.8	15.2	16.0	15.6
Uninsured for any period up to 12 months	18.8	19.2	21.0	21.6	45.1	44.7	46.0	44.3	21.0	22.1	20.6	23.1	15.0	14.0	12.4	11.0
Uninsured more than 12 months	38.7	43.5	43.2	45.5	41.0	39.2	39.4	40.7	14.0	12.9	12.4	10.4	6.3	4.4	5.0	3.5
200 percent to 399 percent																
Insured continuously all 12 months	15.1	13.3	13.6	13.6	49.4	50.7	49.4	52.8	23.4	23.7	25.3	22.7	12.1	12.3	11.7	10.8
Uninsured for any period up to 12 months	17.9	19.9	18.8	19.5	49.3	45.7	49.7	50.9	20.0	22.3	19.7	20.3	12.8	12.2	11.8	9.4
Uninsured more than 12 months	37.0	42.0	43.8	45.0	43.8	44.0	40.7	42.4	12.6	10.3	13.3	8.3	6.6	3.7	*2.2	*4.4
400 percent or more																
Insured continuously all 12 months	12.4	10.6	9.7	10.9	52.2	52.1	51.8	54.2	23.9	25.9	26.8	25.0	11.5	11.4	11.6	9.9
Uninsured for any period up to 12 months	17.2	16.1	16.6	18.7	50.0	51.9	53.5	48.2	24.2	22.8	23.9	23.3	*8.5	9.2	*6.0	9.9
Uninsured more than 12 months	35.1	39.3	39.2	43.1	44.1	46.6	46.0	41.5	15.1	9.6	*8.8	*12.9	*5.7	*	*	*
Respondent-Assessed Health Status [2]																
Fair or poor	7.8	9.0	8.4	9.0	23.3	21.5	24.0	23.0	29.0	28.1	30.2	31.5	39.9	41.3	37.3	36.6
Good to excellent	17.2	16.1	16.3	16.8	48.4	48.2	47.5	50.0	23.3	24.8	25.5	23.6	11.1	10.8	10.7	9.6
Disability Measure Among Adults 18 Years of Age and Over [2,7]																
Any basic actions difficulty or complex activity limitation	11.1	9.6	11.5	11.9	32.0	29.7	30.9	28.7	27.9	29.6	29.3	30.6	29.1	31.1	28.3	28.8
Any basic actions difficulty	11.1	9.7	11.5	11.9	31.9	29.4	30.3	28.1	27.5	29.6	29.2	30.9	29.4	31.3	29.0	29.1
Any complex activity limitation	7.1	5.9	6.9	8.7	23.7	21.1	23.0	21.5	27.5	27.8	29.1	29.2	41.7	45.2	41.0	40.7
No disability	20.9	19.8	20.5	21.4	49.6	48.8	47.5	49.8	20.8	22.7	23.4	21.5	8.7	8.6	8.5	7.3
Geographic Region [2]																
Northeast	13.2	11.3	12.6	12.4	45.9	46.8	46.3	48.9	26.0	27.0	26.4	26.3	14.9	14.9	14.7	12.4
Midwest	15.9	13.8	13.4	14.9	47.7	47.2	46.8	48.8	22.8	25.2	26.4	23.2	13.6	13.9	13.3	13.1
South	17.2	16.0	16.1	16.7	46.1	45.7	44.2	46.2	23.3	25.1	26.6	24.8	13.5	13.3	13.2	12.3
West	19.1	20.0	19.1	19.1	44.8	44.2	45.2	47.6	22.8	23.3	23.5	21.8	13.3	12.5	12.2	11.6
Location of Residence [2]																
Within MSA[8]	16.2	15.5	15.6	15.9	46.4	46.2	45.8	48.1	23.7	24.9	25.6	23.9	13.7	13.3	13.0	12.2
Outside MSA[8]	17.3	15.3	15.9	17.6	45.4	44.5	42.7	44.5	23.3	25.6	27.0	24.8	13.9	14.6	14.4	13.1

* = Figure does not meet standards of reliability or precision. Data preceded by an asterisk have a relative standard error (RSE) of 20 percent to 30 percent. Data not shown have an RSE of greater than 30 percent.   Note: This table presents a summary measure of the number of visits to hospital emergency departments, home visits by a nurse or other health care professional, and visits to doctor offices/clinics during a 12-month period.   1 Includes all other races not shown separately, unknown health insurance status, and unknown disability status.   2 Estimates are age adjusted to the year 2000 standard population using six age groups: under 18 years, 18 to 44 years, 45 to 54 years, 55 to 64 years, 65 to 74 years, and 75 years and over.   3 The race groups White, Black, American Indian or Alaska Native, Asian, Native Hawaiian or Other Pacific Islander, and 2 or more races, include persons of Hispanic and non-Hispanic origin. Persons of Hispanic origin may be of any race.   4 Percent of poverty level is based on family income and family size and composition. Missing family income data were imputed for 1997 and beyond.   5 Estimates for persons under 65 years of age are age adjusted to the year 2000 standard population using four age groups: under 18 years, 18 to 44 years, 45 to 54 years, and 55 to64 years.   6 Health insurance categories are mutually exclusive. Persons who reported both Medicaid and private coverage are classified as having private coverage. Medicaid includes other public assistance through 1996. Starting with 1997 data, state-sponsored health plan coverage is included as Medicaid coverage. Starting with 1999 data, coverage by the Children's Health Insurance Program (CHIP) is included with Medicaid coverage. Persons not covered by private insurance, Medicaid, CHIP, public assistance (through 1996), state-sponsored or other government-sponsored health plans (starting in 1997), Medicare, or military plans are considered to have no health insurance coverage. Persons with only Indian Health Service coverage are considered to have no health insurance coverage. Health insurance status was unknown for 8 to 9 percent of children in 1993-1996 and about 1 percent in 1997-2011.   7 Any basic actions difficulty or complex activity limitation is defined as having one or more of the following limitations or difficulties: movement difficulty, emotional difficulty, sensory (seeing or hearing) difficulty, cognitive difficulty, self-care (activities of daily living or instrumental activities of daily living) limitation, social limitation, or work limitation.   8 MSA = metropolitan statistical area.

Table 3-32. Vaccination Coverage Among Children 19 to 35 Months of Age for Selected Diseases, by Race, Hispanic Origin, Poverty Level, and Location of Residence in Metropolitan Statistical Area, Selected Years, 1995–2013

(Percent.)

| Vaccination and year | Race and Hispanic origin[1] | | | | | | | Poverty level[2] | | | Location of residence | |
| | Not Hispanic or Latino | | | | | | Hispanic or Latino | Inside MSA[3] | | At or above poverty level | Central city | Outside MSA |
	White	Black or African American	American Indian or Alaska Native	Asian[4]	Native Hawaiian or Other Pacific Islander[5]	Two or more races			Below poverty level			
Combined Series (4:3:1:3*:3:1:4)[6]												
2009	45	40	*	39	*	41	46	41	46	45	45	42
2010	57	55	64	59	*	61	56	53	59	57	57	55
2011	69	64	66	71	*	71	70	64	72	70	68	67
2012	69	65	*	72	*	72	68	63	72	67	69	68
2013	72	65	70	73	*	72	69	64	74	69	73	69
DTP/DT/DTaP (4 Doses or More)[6]												
1995	80	74	71	84	*	NA	75	71	81	77	79	78
1996	83	79	85	85	*	NA	77	74	84	79	83	81
1997	84	77	80	80	*	NA	78	76	84	80	83	81
1998	87	77	83	89	*	NA	81	80	86	82	85	85
1999	86	79	80	87	*	NA	80	79	85	82	84	83
2000	84	76	75	85	*	NA	79	76	84	80	83	83
2001	84	76	77	84	*	NA	83	77	84	81	83	82
2002	84	76	*	88	*	78	79	75	84	79	84	80
2003	88	80	80	89	*	84	82	80	87	84	86	83
2004	88	80	77	90	*	86	84	81	87	84	87	85
2005	87	84	*	89	*	86	84	82	87	85	87	85
2006	87	81	83	86	*	84	85	81	87	84	86	85
2007	85	82	86	88	*	84	84	81	86	85	85	83
2008	85	80	82	92	*	88	85	80	87	85	85	82
2009	86	79	82	87	93	82	83	80	86	84	84	84
2010	85	84	82	88	*	83	84	81	86	84	85	84
2011	85	81	73	92	93	87	84	81	87	86	84	82
2012	84	80	88	88	*	86	81	79	85	82	83	81
2013	85	75	78	89	*	83	82	78	86	82	85	82
Polio (3 Doses or More)												
1995	89	84	86	90	*	NA	87	85	89	87	88	89
1996	92	90	90	90	*	NA	89	88	92	89	92	92
1997	92	89	90	89	*	NA	90	89	92	90	91	92
1998	92	88	85	93	*	NA	89	90	92	89	91	93
1999	90	87	88	90	*	NA	89	87	91	89	90	90
2000	91	87	90	93	*	NA	88	87	90	88	90	91
2001	90	85	88	90	*	NA	91	87	90	88	90	91
2002	91	87	*	92	95	87	90	88	91	89	91	90
2003	93	89	91	91	90	91	90	89	93	91	92	92
2004	92	90	87	93	*	92	91	90	92	91	92	92
2005	91	91	*	93	*	94	92	90	92	91	93	92
2006	93	90	91	92	96	92	93	92	93	93	93	93
2007	93	91	95	95	87	92	93	92	93	92	93	94
2008	94	92	91	97	*	94	94	92	94	94	94	93
2009	93	91	92	94	97	93	93	92	93	94	92	92
2010	93	94	95	93	95	90	94	92	94	93	94	93
2011	94	94	88	97	97	94	94	94	94	94	93	94
2012	93	93	95	92	*	93	93	92	93	93	93	93
2013	94	91	92	96	*	91	92	89	94	92	93	93
Measles, Mumps, Rubella												
1995	91	87	88	95	*	NA	88	86	91	90	90	89
1996	91	90	89	93	*	NA	88	87	92	90	91	91
1997	91	89	92	90	*	NA	88	86	92	90	91	91
1998	93	89	91	92	*	NA	91	90	93	92	92	93
1999	92	90	92	93	*	NA	90	90	92	91	92	90
2000	92	88	87	90	*	NA	90	89	91	90	91	91
2001	92	89	94	90	*	NA	92	89	92	91	92	91
2002	93	90	84	95	94	89	91	90	92	90	93	90
2003	93	92	92	96	*	94	93	92	93	93	93	92
2004	94	91	89	94	*	94	93	91	94	93	94	92
2005	91	92	90	92	90	94	91	89	92	92	92	90
2006	93	91	89	95	94	91	92	91	93	93	93	92
2007	92	92	96	94	88	95	93	91	93	92	93	92

Table 3-32. Vaccination Coverage Among Children 19 to 35 Months of Age for Selected Diseases, by Race, Hispanic Origin, Poverty Level, and Location of Residence in Metropolitan Statistical Area, Selected Years, 1995–2013— continued

(Percent.)

| Vaccination and year | Race and Hispanic origin[1] ||||||| Poverty level[2] || Location of residence |||
| | Not Hispanic or Latino ||||| | Hispanic or Latino | Inside MSA[3] || | | |
	White	Black or African American	American Indian or Alaska Native	Asian[4]	Native Hawaiian or Other Pacific Islander	Two or more races	Hispanic or Latino		Below poverty level	At or above poverty level	Central city	Outside MSA
2008	91	92	96	95	97	94	93	92	92	93	92	90
2009	91	88	95	91	97	89	89	89	91	91	89	89
2010	91	92	93	92	97	90	93	91	91	92	91	91
2011	91	91	95	94	99	91	92	91	92	92	91	92
2012	91	91	92	90	*	92	91	90	91	90	91	92
2013	92	91	96	97	90	92	92	91	93	92	92	91
Hib (full series)[7]												
2009	55	51	*	55	*	54	55	51	57	56	55	53
2010	68	65	77	70	*	70	65	61	70	67	68	63
2011	81	75	74	84	*	82	82	76	83	81	80	78
2012	82	78	85	86	*	83	80	76	84	81	82	80
2013	84	75	83	82	*	85	81	76	85	81	84	80
Hepatitis A (2 Doses or More)												
2008	NA	NA	NA	NA	NA	NA	NA	NA	NA	NA	NA	NA
2009	46	41	33	51	*	48	49	47	46	48	47	47
2010	46	49	*	51	*	50	57	51	49	52	49	45
2011	50	51	*	57	*	50	56	51	53	55	51	48
2012	53	52	*	58	*	49	54	49	55	55	53	48
2013	53	49	*	67	*	58	57	54	56	56	55	50
Hepatitis B (3 Doses or More)												
1995	68	66	52	80	*	NA	70	65	69	69	71	59
1996	82	82	79	85	*	NA	81	78	83	81	83	81
1997	85	82	83	88	*	NA	81	81	85	82	85	85
1998	88	84	82	89	*	NA	86	85	88	85	88	87
1999	89	87	*	88	*	NA	87	87	89	87	89	88
2000	91	89	91	91	*	NA	88	87	91	89	90	92
2001	90	85	86	90	*	NA	90	87	90	88	90	89
2002	91	88	*	94	94	84	90	88	90	89	91	90
2003	93	92	90	94	*	93	91	91	93	92	93	93
2004	93	91	91	93	*	94	92	91	93	92	93	93
2005	93	93	90	93	*	94	93	91	94	92	94	93
2006	94	92	95	92	97	92	94	93	94	93	94	93
2007	93	91	97	94	*	92	94	92	93	92	93	94
2008	93	92	92	98	*	95	94	91	94	93	94	93
2009	92	92	93	93	96	93	93	92	93	93	92	92
2010	91	92	97	92	97	90	93	92	92	91	92	93
2011	90	92	93	96	91	91	92	92	91	91	91	93
2012	89	90	94	93	*	92	89	89	90	90	90	91
2013	91	91	96	92	95	91	90	88	92	90	92	91
Varicella[8]												
1997	28	21	20	36	*	NA	22	17	29	26	29	17
1998	42	42	28	53	*	NA	47	41	44	45	45	34
1999	56	58	*	64	*	NA	61	55	58	59	61	47
2000	66	67	62	77	*	NA	70	64	69	69	70	60
2001	75	75	69	82	*	NA	80	74	77	78	78	68
2002	79	83	71	87	*	79	82	79	81	81	83	75
2003	84	85	81	91	*	86	86	84	85	86	86	80
2004	87	86	84	91	*	89	89	86	88	88	89	85
2005	86	91	82	92	*	90	89	87	88	88	88	86
2006	89	89	85	93	90	91	90	88	90	90	90	86
2007	89	90	95	94	89	92	91	89	90	90	90	89
2008	90	90	94	94	92	91	92	90	91	92	90	88
2009	89	88	89	90	98	91	91	89	90	91	89	89
2010	89	92	96	93	93	89	92	90	91	91	90	90
2011	90	91	90	94	99	92	92	90	91	91	91	90
2012	90	90	93	92	*	91	91	90	91	90	90	91
2013	90	92	95	96	89	91	92	90	92	91	92	90
PCV (4 doses or more)[9]												
2005	57	46	*	56	*	54	51	45	57	52	58	48
2006	71	61	63	65	*	71	67	62	71	69	71	62

Table 3-32. Vaccination Coverage Among Children 19 to 35 Months of Age for Selected Diseases, by Race, Hispanic Origin, Poverty Level, and Location of Residence in Metropolitan Statistical Area, Selected Years, 1995–2013— continued

(Percent.)

| Vaccination and year | Race and Hispanic origin[1] | | | | | | | Poverty level[2] | | | Location of residence | | |
| | Not Hispanic or Latino | | | | | | Hispanic or Latino | Inside MSA[3] | | | | | |
	White	Black or African American	American Indian or Alaska Native	Asian[4]	Native Hawaiian or Other Pacific Islander	Two or more races			Below poverty level	At or above poverty level	Central city	Remaining MSA	Outside MSA
2007	77	70	80	75	*	74	75	73	76	75	77	71
2008	81	76	71	82	*	85	79	74	83	81	81	75
2009	83	73	76	73	*	73	81	75	83	80	82	82
2010	84	80	85	79	*	83	84	79	86	83	84	83
2011	85	81	75	85	93	84	85	81	87	85	85	82
2012	84	77	*	81	*	84	82	77	85	80	84	81
2013	84	76	79	86	*	83	80	75	86	81	84	80
Rotavirus vaccine [10]												
2009	46	38	*	42	*	38	44	38	47	45	47	36
2010	60	53	*	63	*	58	61	52	63	59	62	52
2011	68	63	58	67	*	68	68	61	71	69	67	63
2012	71	60	*	70	*	69	70	63	73	69	71	63
2013	75	62	*	75	*	73	74	64	77	72	75	67

NOTE: Final estimates from the National Immunization Survey include an adjustment for children with missing immunization provider data. Poverty level is based on family income and family size using U.S. Census Bureau poverty thresholds. In 2011, 5.9 percent of all 19,144 children with provider-reported vaccination history data, 9.5 percent of Hispanic, 3.6 percent of non-Hispanic White, and 6.5% of non-Hispanic Black children were missing information about poverty level and were omitted from the estimates of vaccination coverage by poverty level.   NA = Not available.   * = Estimates are considered unreliable. For data prior to 2007, percents not shown if the unweighted sample size for the numerator was less than 30, or the confidence interval half-width divided by the estimate was greater than 50 percent, or the confidence interval half-width was greater than 10. Starting with 2007 data, percents not shown if the unweighted sample size for the denominator was less than 30, or the confidence interval half-width divided by the estimate was greater than 60 percent, or the confidence interval half-width was greater than 10.   1 Persons of Hispanic origin may be of any race.   2 Poverty level is based on family income and family size using U.S. Census Bureau poverty thresholds. In 2013, 2.9% of the 13,611 children with provider-reported vaccination history data, 0.9% of Hispanic, 1.3% of non-Hispanic white, and 0.4% of non-Hispanic black children, were missing information about poverty level and were omitted from the estimates of vaccination coverage by poverty level (unweighted percentages).   3 MSA = metropolitan statistical area.   4 Prior to data year 2002, the category Asian included Native Hawaiian and Other Pacific Islander.   5 The 4:3:1:3:3:1:4 combined series consists of 4 or more doses of diphtheria and tetanus toxoids and pertussis vaccine (DTP), diphtheria and tetanus toxoids (DT), or diphtheria and tetanus toxoids and acellular pertussis vaccine (DTaP);3 or more doses of any poliovirus vaccine; 1 or more doses of a measles-containing vaccine (MCV); 3 or more doses of Haemophilus influenzae type b vaccine (Hib); 3 or more doses of hepatitis B vaccine; 1 or more doses of varicella vaccine; and 4 or more doses of pneumococcal conjugate vaccine (PCV).   6 Diphtheria and tetanus toxoids and pertussis vaccine (DTP), diphtheria and tetanus toxoids (DT), and diphtheria and tetanus toxoids and acellular pertussis vaccine (DTaP).   7 Haemophilus influenzae type b vaccine (Hib) full series includes primary series plus the booster dose. Before January 2009, NIS did not distinguish between Hib vaccine product types; therefore, children who received 3 doses of a vaccine product that requires 4 doses were misclassified as fully vaccinated. In addition, there was a Hib vaccine shortage during December 2007-September 2009.   8 Recommended in 1996. Data collection for varicella began in July 1996.   9 PCV is pneumococcal conjugate vaccine. Recommended in 2000.   10 Rotavirus vaccine includes 2 or more or 3 or more doses, depending on the product type received.

Table 3-33. Vaccination Coverage Among Children 19 to 35 Months of Age, by State and Selected Urban Area, Selected Years 2002–2009

(Percent.)

State and selected urban area	2002	2005	2006	2007	2008	2009
Percent of Children 19 to 35 Months of Age with 4:3:1:3:3:1 Combined Series [1]						
United States	66	76	77	77	76	70
Alabama	73	82	79	78	75	73
Jefferson County (Birmingham)	74	85	NA	NA	NA	NA
Alaska	56	68	67	70	69	64
Arizona	59	75	71	75	76	70
Maricopa County (Phoenix)	62	76	68	NA	NA	NA
Arkansas	68	64	73	72	76	63
California	67	74	79	77	79	75
Alameda County	NA	71	NA	76	NA	NA
Fresno County	NA	NA	73	NA	NA	NA
Los Angeles County (Los Angeles)	72	78	79	78	76	78
Northern California	NA	NA	71	NA	69	NA
Santa Clara County (Santa Clara)	75	NA	78	NA	81	NA
Santa Bernadino County	NA	63	NA	70	NA	NA
San Diego County (San Diego)	71	NA	80	NA	NA	NA
Colorado	56	79	76	78	79	65
Denver	NA	79	NA	NA	NA	NA
Connecticut	73	82	82	87	70	47
Delaware	70	82	80	80	72	65
District of Columbia	68	72	79	82	78	75
Florida	66	78	79	80	80	75
Dade County (Miami)	60	NA	80	76	78	NA
Duval County (Jacksonville)	70	77	76	NA	NA	NA
Orange County	NA	NA	NA	NA	79	NA
Georgia	77	82	81	80	72	69
Fulton/DeKalb Counties (Atlanta)	75	72	75	NA	NA	NA
Hawaii	69	78	79	88	77	67
Idaho	53	68	68	66	60	52
Illinois	58	77	74	74	75	73
Chicago	58	70	77	71	78	72
Madison/St Clair County	NA	NA	NA	NA	75	NA
Indiana	59	70	76	74	76	66
Lake County	NA	NA	NA	NA	NA	65
Marion County (Indianapolis)	62	NA	77	71	NA	72
Iowa	58	76	79	76	75	66
Kansas	55	72	70	76	77	77
Eastern Kansas	NA	NA	74	NA	NA	NA
Kentucky	64	71	80	78	74	66
Louisiana	62	74	70	77	82	77
Orleans Parish (New Orleans)	53	NA	NA	NA	NA	NA
Maine	62	76	76	73	74	53
Maryland	71	79	78	91	80	80
Baltimore City	69	77	72	NA	75	63
Massachusetts	78	91	84	78	82	81
Boston	71	NA	82	NA	NA	NA
Michigan	72	81	78	79	75	71
Detroit	60	71	65	NA	NA	NA
Minnesota	62	78	78	81	75	58
Twin Cities	NA	NA	NA	NA	75	NA
Mississippi	64	79	73	77	76	73
Missouri	60	73	81	76	73	61
St. Louis County	NA	74	NA	NA	NA	NA
Montana	49	65	66	65	59	55
Nebraska	64	84	75	83	72	60
Nevada	65	63	60	63	68	59
Clark County	NA	59	NA	NA	NA	NA
New Hampshire	66	77	76	91	81	79
New Jersey	66	72	76	81	69	67
Newark	50	67	68	NA	NA	NA
New Mexico	59	75	72	76	77	68
New York	67	74	77	78	73	69
New York City	71	71	72	76	75	72
North Carolina	70	82	82	77	71	56
North Dakota	56	79	80	77	70	56
Ohio	64	78	75	78	82	74
Cuyahoga County (Cleveland)	65	77	77	NA	NA	NA
Franklin County (Columbus)	69	81	NA	NA	NA	NA
Oklahoma	60	72	78	79	72	70
Oregon	60	65	74	71	71	65
Pennsylvania	68	77	79	79	78	69
Allegheny County	NA	NA	74	NA	NA	NA
Philadelphia	68	77	80	82	80	74

Table 3-33. Vaccination Coverage Among Children 19 to 35 Months of Age, by State and Selected Urban Area, Selected Years 2002–2009— continued

(Percent.)

State and selected urban area	2002	2005	2006	2007	2008	2009
Rhode Island	81	80	81	76	78	51
South Carolina	74	76	81	80	78	67
South Dakota	62	80	74	77	77	75
Tennessee	67	80	77	79	81	74
Davidson County (Nashville)	67	81	NA	NA	NA	NA
Shelby County (Memphis)	61	74	73	NA	NA	NA
Texas	65	77	75	77	78	74
Bexar County (San Antonio)	72	71	75	80	76	71
Dallas County (Dallas)	68	73	73	72	74	74
El Paso County (El Paso)	61	69	69	77	75	71
Houston	56	77	70	73	72	70
Utah	61	68	78	74	77	70
Vermont	58	63	75	67	65	65
Virginia	65	82	77	76	73	70
Washington	52	66	71	69	74	70
Eastern Washington	NA	NA	72	NA	NA	NA
Eastern/Western Washington	NA	NA	NA	NA	76	67
King County (Seattle)	56	69	71	NA	NA	NA
Western Washington	NA	NA	NA	71	NA	NA
West Virginia	66	68	68	76	77	65
Wisconsin	68	77	81	77	80	59
Milwaukee County (Milwaukee)	60	74	78	NA	NA	NA
Wyoming	54	67	63	70	65	62

NA = Not available.   1 The 4:3:1:3:3:1 combined series consists of 4 or more doses of diphtheria and tetanus toxoids and pertussis vaccine (DTP), diphtheria and tetanus toxoids (DT), or diphtheria and tetanus toxoids and acellular pertussis vaccine (DTaP); 3 or more doses of any poliovirus vaccine; 1 or more doses of a measles-containing vaccine (MCV); 3 or more doses of Haemophilus influenzae type b vaccine (Hib) regardless of vaccine brand type; 3 or more doses of hepatitis B vaccine; and 1 or more doses of varicella vaccine. This series is the most complete series for which long-term state trend data are currently available.

Table 3-34A. Vaccination Coverage Among Adolescents 13 to 17 Years of Age for Selected Diseases, by Selected Characteristics, 2008–2013

(Percent.)

Vaccination coverage	2008	2009	2010	2011	2012	2013
Percent of Adolescents, 13 to 17 Years						
Measles, mumps, rubella (2 doses or more)	89.3	89.1	90.5	91.1	91.4	91.8
Hepatitis B (3 doses or more)	87.9	89.9	91.6	92.3	92.8	93.2
History of varicella or received varicella vaccine (2 doses or more)[1]	73.5	75.7	76.8	79.9	82.6	84.0
Tdap (1 dose or more)[2]	40.8	55.6	68.7	78.2	84.6	86.0
Meningococcal conjugate vaccine (MenACWY) (1 dose or more)[3]	41.8	53.6	62.7	70.5	74.0	77.8
Human papillomavirus (HPV) (3 doses or more among females)[4]	17.9	26.7	32.0	34.8	33.4	37.6
Human papillomavirus (HPV) (3 doses or more among males)[4]	X	X	X	1.3	6.8	13.9

Table 3-34B. Vaccination Coverage Among Adolescents 13 to 17 Years of Age for Selected Diseases, by Selected Characteristics, 2006–2013

(Percent.)

Vaccination coverage, 2013	Race and Hispanic origin[5]					Poverty level[6]		Location of residence		
	Not Hispanic or Latino				Hispanic or Latino	Below poverty level	At or above poverty level	Inside MSA[7]		Outside MSA[7]
	White	Black or African American	American Indian or Alaska Native	Asian				Central city	Remaining area	
Percent of Adolescents, 13 to 17 Years										
Measles, mumps, rubella (2 doses or more)	92.8	91.1	93.5	90.8	90.2	91.7	91.8	91.2	92.1	92.6
Hepatitis B (3 doses or more)	93.8	93.2	93.4	87.8	92.8	93.2	93.1	92.9	93.3	93.8
History of varicella or received varicella vaccine (2 doses or more)[1]	77.7	77.9	78.7	85.2	80.3	77.3	79.0	79.1	80.4	69.5
Tdap (1 dose or more)[2]	85.9	84.1	85.3	89.7	87.1	85.2	86.4	86.2	87.1	81.7
Meningococcal conjugate vaccine (MenACWY) (1 dose or more)[3]	75.6	77.0	71.7	83.8	83.4	78.4	77.5	80.5	79.7	63.1
Human papillomavirus (HPV) (3 doses or more among females)[4]	34.9	34.2	43.2	40.4	44.8	41.5	36.4	39.5	37.7	31.6
Human papillomavirus (HPV) (3 doses or more among males)[4]	11.1	15.7	*	9.1	20.3	16.7	13.0	16.9	13.0	8.0

X = Not applicable.   * = Estimates are not reliable and not shown if the unweighted sample size for the denominator is less than 30 or the confidence interval half-width divided by the estimate is greater than 0.588.   1 Varicella is chickenpox.   2 Tdap refers to tetanus toxoid-diphtheria vaccine (Td) or tetanus toxoid, reduced diphtheria toxoid, and acellular pertussis vaccine (Tdap) or tetanus-unknown type vaccine received since the age of 10 years.   3 Includes persons receiving MenACWY or meningococcal-unknown type vaccine.   4 For 2008, refers to HPV vaccine quadrivalent; for 2009 and beyond, refers to HPV vaccine quadrivalent or bivalent.   5 Persons of Hispanic origin may be of any race.   6 Poverty level is based on family income and family size using U.S. Census Bureau poverty thresholds. In 2011, less than 4 percent (unweighted) of adolescents with provider-reported vaccination data were missing information about poverty level and were not included in the estimates of vaccination coverage by poverty level.   7 MSA = metropolitan statistical area.

Table 3-35. Influenza Vaccination[1] Among Adults 18 Years of Age and Over, by Selected Characteristics, Selected Years, 1989–2013

(Percent.)

Characteristic	1989	1995	2000	2005	2010	2012	2013
18 years and over, age-adjusted[2,3]	9.6	23.7	28.7	21.6	35.1	36.6	39.7
18 years and over, crude[3]	9.1	23.0	28.4	21.4	35.8	37.7	41.0
Age							
18 to 49 years	3.4	13.1	17.1	10.7	25.2	26.3	29.6
50 years and over	19.9	41.9	47.9	38.1	50.5	52.4	55.4
50 to 64 years	10.6	27.0	34.6	23.0	41.6	42.8	46.6
65 years and over	30.4	58.2	64.4	59.7	63.9	66.5	67.9
65 to 74 years	28.0	54.9	61.1	53.7	60.5	62.6	64.4
75 years and over	34.2	63.0	68.4	66.3	68.2	71.7	72.8
50 YEARS AND OVER							
Sex							
Male	19.2	40.2	45.9	34.7	47.4	48.8	52.4
Female	20.6	43.4	49.5	40.9	53.2	55.6	58.1
Race [4]							
White only	20.9	43.6	49.8	39.7	51.5	53.7	57.0
Black or African American only	12.5	28.2	33.2	26.9	40.4	43.0	43.2
American Indian or Alaska Native only	26.2	*	43.6	*22.9	54.7	50.9	60.9
Asian only	*9.2	35.6	43.3	30.6	55.9	52.3	54.7
Native Hawaiian or Other Pacific Islander only	NA	NA	*	*	*	*	*
Two or more races	NA	NA	50.7	30.4	49.8	46.8	50.0
Hispanic Origin and Race [4]							
Hispanic or Latino	13.2	33.8	34.4	24.7	40.6	42.9	45.5
Mexican	13.0	35.4	33.0	26.1	41.3	42.7	48.0
Not Hispanic or Latino	20.3	42.4	48.8	39.1	51.5	53.4	56.4
White only	21.3	44.3	50.6	41.0	52.7	54.9	58.2
Black or African American only	12.4	28.5	33.2	26.9	40.0	43.2	43.3
Percent of Poverty Level [5]							
Below 100 percent	19.6	39.7	44.1	35.8	37.5	42.9	45.4
100 percent to 199 percent	24.0	43.2	50.7	41.2	47.6	49.4	52.7
200 percent to 399 percent	20.5	43.7	51.5	42.1	51.2	52.3	55.5
400 percent or more	17.5	39.3	44.3	33.9	54.3	56.0	59.0
Hispanic Origin and Race and Percent of Poverty Level [4,5]							
Hispanic or Latino							
Below 100 percent	12.7	29.7	35.8	22.3	36.3	39.0	42.8
100 percent to 199 percent	20.4	34.7	35.6	27.5	36.6	39.6	41.9
200 percent to 399 percent	12.7	34.2	33.7	22.3	41.8	43.6	46.0
400 percent or more	*9.8	39.1	32.2	26.6	47.7	50.2	51.0
Not Hispanic or Latino							
White only							
Below 100 percent	22.5	44.4	48.6	42.2	38.7	45.4	47.5
100 percent to 199 percent	26.1	46.7	54.8	46.1	51.1	53.0	57.0
200 percent to 399 percent	21.6	45.4	54.6	46.4	53.4	54.5	57.8
400 percent or more	18.1	40.8	46.0	35.1	54.9	57.1	60.6
Black or African American only							
Below 100 percent	14.6	31.8	35.5	28.9	32.4	39.4	38.5
100 percent to 199 percent	12.0	28.3	37.9	27.4	39.2	42.9	42.9
200 percent to 399 percent	14.1	29.0	31.0	25.7	42.6	43.7	45.3
400 percent or more	*8.8	*20.0	28.7	26.2	44.4	46.1	45.5
Disability Measure [6]							
Any basic actions difficulty or complex activity limitation	NA	NA	55.2	46.5	54.5	57.7	60.3
Any basic actions difficulty	NA	NA	55.3	46.7	54.8	57.8	60.7
Any complex activity limitation	NA	NA	57.1	50.3	55.3	60.0	60.3
No disability	NA	NA	41.3	29.7	47.0	47.8	51.3
Geographic Region							
Northeast	17.9	39.7	45.9	38.4	52.4	54.0	57.2
Midwest	20.0	43.2	49.3	39.9	51.8	53.9	56.0
South	20.2	41.4	46.8	37.3	49.3	51.8	54.3
West	21.8	43.8	50.1	36.8	49.5	50.7	55.3
Location of Residence							
Within MSA[7]	18.9	41.6	47.1	37.2	50.8	52.2	55.0
Outside MSA[7]	23.3	42.9	50.2	41.0	49.3	53.6	57.2

Characteristic	1989	1995	2000	2005	2010	2012	2013

NA = Not available.   * = Figure does not meet standards of reliability or precision.   1 Questions concerning use of influenza vaccination differed slightly on the National Health Interview Survey across the years for which data are shown.   2 Estimates are age adjusted to the year 2000 standard population using four age groups: 18 to 49 years, 50 to 64 years, 65 to 74 years, and 75 years and over.   3 Includes all other races not shown separately, unknown disability status, and unknown poverty level in 1989.   4 The race groups White, Black, American Indian or Alaska Native, Asian, Native Hawaiian or Other Pacific Islander, and two or more races, include persons of Hispanic and non-Hispanic origin. Persons of Hispanic origin may be of any race.   5 Percent of poverty level is based on family income and family size and composition using U.S. Census Bureau poverty thresholds. Poverty level was unknown for 11 percent of persons 18 years of age and over in 1989. Missing family income data were imputed for 1991 and beyond.   6 Any basic actions difficulty or complex activity limitation is defined as having one or more of the following limitations or difficulties: movement difficulty, emotional difficulty, sensory (seeing or hearing) difficulty, cognitive difficulty, self-care (activities of daily living or instrumental activities of daily living) limitation, social limitation, or work limitation.   7 MSA = metropolitan statistical area.

Table 3-36. Pneumococcal Vaccination[1] Among Adults 18 Years of Age and Over, by Selected Characteristics, Selected Years, 1989–2013

(Percent.)

Characteristic	1989	1995	2000	2005	2010	2012	2013
18 years and over, age-adjusted[2,3]	4.6	12.0	15.4	16.7	19.0	19.8	19.7
18 years and over, crude[3]	4.4	11.7	15.1	16.5	19.6	20.7	21.0
Age							
18 to 49 years	2.1	6.5	5.4	5.8	7.3	8.7	8.3
50 to 64 years	4.4	10.0	14.7	17.1	21.0	20.0	20.8
65 years and over	14.1	34.0	53.1	56.2	59.7	59.9	59.7
65 to 74 years	13.1	31.4	48.2	49.4	54.6	55.0	54.4
75 years and over	15.7	37.8	59.1	63.9	66.0	66.4	67.1
High-Risk Group [4]							
Total, 18 to 64 years	NA	NA	18.3	22.6	18.3	19.9	21.0
18 to 49 years	NA	NA	12.2	15.0	10.6	13.0	13.6
50 to 64 years	NA	NA	26.0	30.6	30.8	30.6	31.7
65 YEARS AND OVER							
Sex							
Male	13.9	34.6	52.1	53.4	57.6	55.8	57.1
Female	14.3	33.6	53.9	58.4	61.3	63.1	61.8
Race [5]							
White only	14.8	35.3	55.6	58.4	61.6	62.3	61.7
Black or African American only	6.4	21.9	30.6	40.2	45.5	46.0	48.4
American Indian or Alaska Native only	31.2	*	70.1	*	*48.5	*36.3	52.9
Asian only	*	*23.4	40.9	35.0	47.9	41.1	45.0
Native Hawaiian or Other Pacific Islander only	NA	NA	*	*	*	*	*
Two or more races	NA	NA	55.6	64.8	65.5	45.4	50.8
Hispanic Origin and Race [5]							
Hispanic or Latino	9.8	23.2	30.4	27.5	39.0	43.4	39.2
Mexican	12.9	*18.8	32.0	31.3	41.4	45.5	47.4
Not Hispanic or Latino	14.3	34.5	54.4	58.1	61.3	61.2	61.4
White only	15.0	35.9	56.8	60.6	63.5	64.0	63.6
Black or African American only	6.2	21.8	30.6	40.4	46.2	46.1	48.7
Percent of Poverty Level [6]							
Below 100 percent	11.2	28.7	40.6	46.7	42.6	39.5	50.5
100 percent to 199 percent	15.1	30.7	51.4	54.5	57.2	59.8	58.0
200 percent to 399 percent	15.1	36.1	55.8	60.8	62.2	63.6	61.7
400 percent or more	15.5	39.5	56.9	55.3	64.0	61.4	61.6
Hispanic Origin and Race and Percent of Poverty Level [5,6]							
Hispanic or Latino							
Below 100 percent	*	*14.1	23.8	20.9	30.2	30.9	35.3
100 percent to 199 percent	*11.0	*15.6	32.3	26.9	36.9	42.0	39.1
200 percent to 399 percent	*11.1	*34.4	37.6	35.2	45.8	54.5	36.1
400 percent or more	*	*55.1	*26.4	*25.2	43.0	46.4	49.1
Not Hispanic or Latino							
White only							
Below 100 percent	13.3	32.5	47.9	55.6	51.1	46.5	59.1
100 percent to 199 percent	16.0	33.5	56.1	60.5	61.3	66.1	63.3
200 percent to 399 percent	15.7	37.1	57.6	64.1	64.9	65.9	65.2
400 percent or more	15.9	39.3	59.5	57.4	66.0	63.5	63.2
Black or African American only							
Below 100 percent	*5.0	*22.6	28.8	42.3	34.9	36.1	48.9
100 percent to 199 percent	7.8	*20.9	28.1	36.6	46.4	44.5	46.9
200 percent to 399 percent	*5.9	*21.7	35.5	41.6	51.8	54.1	49.4
400 percent or more	*	*	*32.6	44.6	50.1	45.4	50.3
Any Basic Actions Difficulty or Complex Activity Limitation [7]							
Any basic actions difficulty or complex activity limitation	NA	NA	56.6	61.6	63.9	65.4	64.4
Any basic actions difficulty	NA	NA	56.8	61.6	64.2	66.0	64.9
Any complex activity limitation	NA	NA	58.0	63.3	65.2	65.7	66.1
No disability	NA	NA	48.0	47.8	53.3	53.2	53.1
Geographic Region							
Northeast	10.4	28.2	51.2	55.8	56.7	58.0	59.1
Midwest	13.7	31.0	52.6	58.5	61.2	63.8	62.3
South	14.9	35.9	51.3	57.4	60.9	59.5	59.3
West	17.9	41.1	59.7	51.4	58.9	58.2	58.3

Table 3-36. Pneumococcal Vaccination[1] Among Adults 18 Years of Age and Over, by Selected Characteristics, Selected Years, 1989–2013— continued

(Percent.)

Characteristic	1989	1995	2000	2005	2010	2012	2013
Location of Residence							
Within MSA[8]	13.1	33.8	52.4	55.1	58.8	59.3	59.0
Outside MSA[8]	17.1	34.8	55.4	59.8	63.3	62.4	62.8

NA = Not available.   * = Estimates are considered unreliable. Data preceded by an asterisk have a relative standard error (RSE) of 20 percent to 30 percent. Data not shown have an RSE of greater than 30 percent.   1 Respondents were asked, "Have you ever had a pneumonia shot? This shot is usually given only once or twice in a person's lifetime and is different from the flu shot. It is also called the pneumococcal vaccine."   2 Estimates are age adjusted to the year 2000 standard population using four age groups: 18 to 49 years, 50 to 64 years, 65 to 74 years, and 75 years and over.   3 Includes all other races not shown separately, unknown poverty level in 1989, and unknown disability status.   4 High-risk group membership is based on recommendations of the Advisory Committee on Immunization Practices (ACIP). The high-risk group includes persons who reported diabetes, cancer, heart, lung, liver, or kidney disease. Starting in 2009, this group also includes persons who reported asthma or cigarette smoking, to be consistent of the revised ACIP recommendation.   5 The race groups White, Black, American Indian or Alaska Native, Asian, Native Hawaiian or Other Pacific Islander, and two or more races, include persons of Hispanic and non-Hispanic origin. Persons of Hispanic origin may be of any race.   6 Percent of poverty level is based on family income and family size and composition using U.S. Census Bureau poverty thresholds. Poverty level was unknown for 11 percent of persons 18 years of age and over in 1989. Missing family income data were imputed for 1991 and beyond.   7 Any basic actions difficulty or complex activity limitation is defined as having one or more of the following limitations or difficulties: movement difficulty, emotional difficulty, sensory (seeing or hearing) difficulty, cognitive difficulty, self-care (activities of daily living or instrumental activities of daily living) limitation, social limitation, or work limitation.   8 MSA = metropolitan statistical area.

Table 3-37. Use of Mammography[1] Among Women 40 Years of Age and Over, by Selected Characteristics, Selected Years, 1987–2013

(Percent.)

Characteristic	1987	1990	1994	2000	2005	2010	2013
40 years and over, age-adjusted[2,3]	29.0	51.7	61.0	70.4	66.6	66.5	65.7
40 years and over, crude[2]	28.7	51.4	60.9	70.4	66.8	67.1	66.8
50 years and over, age-adjusted[2,3]	27.3	49.8	60.9	73.7	68.2	68.8	69.1
50 years and over, crude[2]	27.4	49.7	60.6	73.6	68.4	69.2	69.5
Age							
40 to 49 years	31.9	55.1	61.3	64.3	63.5	62.3	59.6
50 to 64 years	31.7	56.0	66.5	78.7	71.8	72.6	71.4
65 years and over	22.8	43.4	55.0	67.9	63.8	64.4	66.9
65 to 74 years	26.6	48.7	63.0	74.0	72.5	71.9	75.3
75 years and over	17.3	35.8	44.6	61.3	54.7	55.7	56.5
Race[4]							
40 years and over, crude							
White only	29.6	52.2	60.6	71.4	67.4	67.4	66.8
Black or African American only	24.0	46.4	64.3	67.8	64.9	67.9	67.1
American Indian or Alaska Native only	*	43.2	65.8	47.4	72.8	71.2	62.6
Asian only	*	46.0	55.8	53.5	54.6	62.4	66.6
Native Hawaiian or Other Pacific Islander only	NA	NA	NA	*	*	*	*
Two or more races	NA	NA	NA	69.2	63.7	51.4	65.4
Hispanic Origin and Race[4]							
40 years and over, crude							
Hispanic or Latina	18.3	45.2	51.9	61.2	58.8	64.2	61.4
Not Hispanic or Latina	29.4	51.8	61.5	71.1	67.5	67.4	67.5
White only	30.3	52.7	61.3	72.2	68.3	67.8	67.6
Black or African American only	23.8	46.0	64.4	67.9	65.2	67.4	67.2
Age, Hispanic Origin, and Race[4]							
40 to 49 years							
Hispanic or Latina	*15.3	45.1	47.5	54.1	54.2	59.8	56.4
Not Hispanic or Latina							
White only	34.3	57.0	62.0	67.2	65.5	62.6	60.3
Black or African American only	27.8	48.4	67.2	60.9	62.1	63.5	59.4
50 to 64 years							
Hispanic or Latina	23.0	47.5	60.1	66.5	61.5	68.6	65.6
Not Hispanic or Latina							
White only	33.6	58.1	67.5	80.6	73.5	73.5	72.1
Black or African American only	26.4	48.4	63.6	77.7	71.6	74.0	71.7
65 years and over							
Hispanic or Latina	*	41.1	48.0	68.3	63.8	65.2	63.2
Not Hispanic or Latina							
White only	24.0	43.8	54.9	68.3	64.7	65.0	67.3
Black or African American only	14.1	39.7	61.0	65.5	60.5	60.9	68.8
Age and Percent of Poverty Level[5]							
40 years and over, crude							
Below 100 percent	14.6	30.8	44.2	54.8	48.5	51.4	49.9
100 percent to 199 percent	20.9	39.1	48.6	58.1	55.3	53.8	56.7
200 percent to 399 percent	29.7	53.3	65.0	68.8	67.2	66.2	66.0
400 percent or more	42.9	68.7	74.1	81.5	76.6	78.1	77.2
40 to 49 years							
Below 100 percent	18.6	32.2	43.0	47.4	42.5	48.1	43.3
100 percent to 199 percent	18.4	39.0	47.6	43.6	49.8	46.2	52.0
200 percent to 399 percent	31.2	55.2	64.5	60.2	61.8	59.2	58.5
400 percent or more	44.1	68.9	69.9	75.8	73.6	73.6	69.0
50 to 64 years							
Below 100 percent	14.6	29.9	46.2	61.7	50.4	54.7	55.0
100 percent to 199 percent	24.2	39.8	49.0	68.3	58.8	57.3	57.2
200 percent to 399 percent	29.7	56.2	69.6	75.1	70.7	70.7	69.5
400 percent or more	44.7	71.6	78.0	86.9	80.6	82.8	80.9
65 years and over							
Below 100 percent	13.1	30.8	43.9	54.8	52.3	50.6	49.8
100 percent to 199 percent	19.9	38.6	48.8	60.3	56.1	55.5	59.3
200 percent to 399 percent	27.7	47.4	61.0	71.1	68.6	67.2	68.1
400 percent or more	34.7	61.2	73.0	81.9	72.6	74.5	79.0
Health Insurance Status at the Time of Interview[6]							
40 to 64 years							
Insured	NA	NA	68.3	76.0	72.5	74.1	72.1
Private	NA	NA	69.4	77.1	74.5	75.6	73.4
Medicaid	NA	NA	54.5	61.7	55.6	64.4	63.5
Uninsured	NA	NA	34.0	40.7	38.1	36.0	37.3
Health Insurance Status Prior to Interview[6]							
40 to 64 years							
Insured continuously all 12 months	NA	NA	68.6	76.8	73.1	74.7	72.7
Uninsured for any period up to 12 months	NA	NA	49.9	53.0	51.3	57.3	54.5
Uninsured more than 12 months	NA	NA	26.6	34.0	32.9	30.0	32.8
Age and Education[7]							
40 years and over, crude							

Table 3-37. Use of Mammography[1] Among Women 40 Years of Age and Over, by Selected Characteristics, Selected Years, 1987–2013—continued

(Percent.)

Characteristic	1987	1990	1994	2000	2005	2010	2013
No high school diploma or GED	17.8	36.4	48.2	57.7	52.8	53.0	53.6
High school diploma or GED	31.3	52.7	61.0	69.7	64.9	64.4	63.4
Some college or more	37.7	62.8	69.7	76.2	72.7	72.1	71.6
40 to 49 years							
No high school diploma or GED	15.1	38.5	50.4	46.8	51.2	44.9	46.9
High school diploma or GED	32.6	53.1	55.8	59.0	58.8	58.4	51.8
Some college or more	39.2	62.3	68.7	70.6	68.3	66.5	64.3
50 to 64 years							
No high school diploma or GED	21.2	41.0	51.6	66.5	56.9	56.7	58.2
High school diploma or GED	33.8	56.5	67.8	76.6	70.1	69.9	66.9
Some college or more	40.5	68.0	74.7	84.2	77.0	77.0	75.7
65 years and over							
No high school diploma or GED	16.5	33.0	45.6	57.4	50.7	54.1	53.4
High school diploma or GED	25.9	47.5	59.1	71.8	64.3	62.5	66.5
Some college or more	32.3	56.7	64.3	74.1	73.0	70.9	73.6
Disability Measure [8]							
40 years and over, crude							
Any basic actions difficulty or complex activity limitation	NA	NA	NA	67.8	63.5	63.3	63.5
Any basic actions difficulty	NA	NA	NA	67.9	63.5	63.3	63.8
Any complex activity limitation	NA	NA	NA	64.1	59.9	58.2	58.4
No disability	NA	NA	NA	72.6	69.8	70.8	69.8

NA = Not available.   * = Estimates are considered unreliable. Data preceded by an asterisk have a relative standard error (RSE) of 20 percent to 30 percent. Data not shown have an RSE of greater than 30 percent.   1 Questions concerning use of mammography differed slightly on the National Health Interview Survey across the years for which data are shown.   2 Includes all other races not shown separately, unknown poverty level in 1987, unknown health insurance status, unknown education level, and unknown disability status.   3 Estimates for women 40 years of age and over are age-adjusted to the year 2000 standard population using four age groups: 40 to 49 years, 50 to 64 years, 65 to 74 years, and 75 years and over. Estimates for women 50 years of age and over are age-adjusted using three age groups.   4 The race groups White, Black, American Indian or Alaska Native, Asian, Native Hawaiian or Other Pacific Islander, and two or more races, include persons of Hispanic and non-Hispanic origin. Persons of Hispanic origin may be of any race.   5 Percent of poverty level is based on family income and family size and composition using U.S. Census Bureau poverty thresholds. Poverty level was unknown for 11 percent of women 40 years of age and over in 1987. Missing family income data were imputed for 1997 and beyond.   6 Health insurance categories are mutually exclusive. Persons who reported both Medicaid and private coverage are classified as having private coverage. Medicaid includes other public assistance through 1996. Starting with 1997 data, state-sponsored health plan coverage is included as Medicaid coverage. Starting with 1999 data, coverage by the Children's Health Insurance Program (CHIP) is included with Medicaid coverage. Persons not covered by private insurance, Medicaid, CHIP, public assistance (through 1996), state-sponsored or other government-sponsored health plans (starting in 1997), Medicare, or military plans are considered to have no health insurance coverage. Persons with only Indian Health Service coverage are considered to have no health insurance coverage. Health insurance status was unknown for 8 to 9 percent of children in 1993-1996 and about 1 percent in 1997-2011.   7 Education categories shown are for 1998 and subsequent years. GED is General Educational Development high school equivalency diploma. In years prior to 1998, the following categories based on number of years in school completed were used: less than 12 years, 12 years, and 13 years or more.   8 Any basic actions difficulty or complex activity limitation is defined as having one or more of the following limitations or difficulties: movement difficulty, emotional difficulty, sensory (seeing or hearing) difficulty, cognitive difficulty, self-care (activities of daily living or instrumental activities of daily living) limitation, social limitation, or work limitation.

Table 3-38. Percent of Women 18 Years of Age and Over Who Have Had a Pap Smear[1] Within the Last Three Years, by Selected Characteristics, Selected Years, 1987–2013

(Percent.)

Characteristic	1987	1994	2000	2005	2010	2013
18 years and over, age-adjusted[2,3]	74.1	76.8	81.3	77.9	73.7	70.4
18 years and over, crude[2]	74.4	76.8	81.2	77.7	73.2	69.4
Age						
18 to 44 years	83.3	82.8	84.9	83.6	80.4	77.2
18 to 24 years	74.8	76.6	73.5	74.5	69.0	NA
25 to 44 years	86.3	84.6	88.5	86.8	84.6	83.2
45 to 64 years	70.5	77.4	84.6	80.6	76.9	73.9
45 to 54 years	75.7	81.9	86.3	83.4	79.9	78.6
55 to 64 years	65.2	71.0	82.0	76.8	73.2	68.6
65 years and over	50.8	57.3	64.5	54.9	47.1	42.7
65 to 74 years	57.9	64.9	71.6	66.3	58.0	54.5
75 years and over	40.4	47.3	56.7	42.7	34.6	27.9
Race [4]						
18 years and over, crude						
White only	74.1	76.2	81.3	77.7	72.8	68.7
Black or African American only	80.7	83.5	85.1	81.1	77.9	75.3
American Indian or Alaska Native only	85.4	73.5	76.8	75.2	73.4	70.1
Asian only	51.9	66.4	66.4	64.1	68.0	65.3
Native Hawaiian or Other Pacific Islander only	NA	NA	*	*	*	*
Two or more races	NA	NA	80.0	86.2	70.8	70.8
Hispanic Origin and Race [4]						
18 years and over, crude						
Hispanic or Latina	67.6	74.4	77.0	75.5	73.6	70.5
Not Hispanic or Latina	74.9	77.0	81.7	78.0	73.1	69.2
White only	74.7	76.5	81.8	78.1	72.8	68.4
Black or African American only	80.9	83.8	85.1	81.2	77.4	75.1
Age, Hispanic Origin, and Race [4]						
18 to 44 years						
Hispanic or Latina	73.9	80.6	78.1	76.5	75.9	72.3
Not Hispanic or Latina						
White only	84.5	82.9	86.6	85.8	82.1	79.0
Black or African American only	89.1	89.1	88.5	86.4	84.2	82.8
45 to 64 years						
Hispanic or Latina	57.7	70.1	77.8	78.4	75.4	74.4
Not Hispanic or Latina						
White only	71.2	77.5	85.9	81.4	77.2	73.6
Black or African American only	76.2	82.2	85.7	80.5	78.2	76.0
65 years and over						
Hispanic or Latina	41.7	43.8	66.8	60.0	54.2	49.4
Not Hispanic or Latina						
White only	51.8	58.2	64.2	54.1	46.5	41.4
Black or African American only	44.8	59.5	67.2	60.1	48.0	45.8
Age and Percent of Poverty Level [5]						
18 years and over, crude						
Below 100 percent	64.3	68.8	72.0	68.7	65.1	60.6
100 percent to 199 percent	68.2	68.8	73.4	69.0	64.3	59.8
200 percent to 399 percent	77.6	80.1	80.2	77.9	71.3	68.5
400 percent or more	83.6	85.4	89.1	85.7	83.1	79.4
18 to 44 years						
Below 100 percent	77.1	78.9	77.1	76.2	73.0	69.2
100 percent to 199 percent	80.4	78.2	79.4	78.1	75.7	72.6
200 percent to 399 percent	84.8	84.5	86.1	85.5	79.8	78.6
400 percent or more	88.9	88.7	89.8	88.7	88.9	84.5
45 to 64 years						
Below 100 percent	53.6	62.0	73.6	65.9	61.7	54.9
100 percent to 199 percent	60.4	66.2	76.1	69.6	63.2	61.2
200 percent to 399 percent	71.0	80.3	80.0	79.3	75.2	73.7
400 percent or more	79.1	84.0	91.5	87.4	85.7	82.8
65 years and over						
Below 100 percent	33.2	44.0	53.7	44.4	35.1	34.1
100 percent to 199 percent	50.4	51.5	61.0	49.5	40.7	33.0
200 percent to 399 percent	58.0	63.7	65.1	56.8	47.1	39.6
400 percent or more	65.2	76.2	75.4	64.6	57.7	58.1
Health Insurance Status at the Time of Interview [6]						
18 to 64 years, crude						
Insured	NA	83.8	87.8	85.6	82.8	80.0
Private	NA	83.6	88.0	86.5	84.2	81.3
Medicaid	NA	86.2	85.8	80.9	78.0	75.7
Uninsured	NA	68.6	70.4	67.7	61.9	57.6
Health Insurance Status Prior to Interview [6]						
18 to 64 years, crude						
Insured continuously all 12 months	NA	83.7	88.0	85.8	83.2	80.4
Uninsured for any period up to 12 months	NA	83.4	83.7	81.3	78.3	72.3

Table 3-38. Percent of Women 18 Years of Age and Over Who Have Had a Pap Smear[1] Within the Last Three Years, by Selected Characteristics, Selected Years, 1987–2013— continued

(Percent.)

Characteristic	1987	1994	2000	2005	2010	2013
Uninsured more than 12 months	NA	63.6	65.1	62.0	55.2	52.7
Age and Education [7]						
25 years and over, crude						
No high school diploma or GED	57.1	60.9	69.9	64.1	56.7	56.2
High school diploma or GED	76.4	76.0	79.8	73.8	66.8	62.0
Some college or more	84.0	85.2	88.0	84.6	80.7	77.1
25 to 44 years						
No high school diploma or GED	75.1	73.6	79.6	75.5	69.1	71.7
High school diploma or GED	85.6	82.4	86.2	83.1	79.0	79.5
Some college or more	90.1	89.1	91.4	90.5	89.0	86.1
45 to 64 years						
No high school diploma or GED	58.0	66.1	75.7	69.7	63.4	63.0
High school diploma or GED	72.3	75.9	81.8	79.0	72.4	67.0
Some college or more	80.1	84.7	89.1	84.1	81.5	78.7
65 years and over						
No high school diploma or GED	44.0	47.7	56.6	46.0	37.7	33.8
High school diploma or GED	55.4	61.2	66.9	52.5	42.6	38.8
Some college or more	59.4	66.5	69.8	63.8	54.9	49.7
Disability measure [8]						
18 years and over, crude						
Any basic actions difficulty or complex activity limitation	NA	NA	75.4	69.1	63.8	59.3
Any basic actions difficulty	NA	NA	75.1	69.1	63.6	59.2
Any complex activity limitation	NA	NA	71.0	62.2	58.5	52.8
No disability	NA	NA	84.1	82.6	78.9	75.2

NA = Not available.   * = Figure does not meet standards of reliability or precision. Data not shown have an RSE of greater than 30 percent.   1 Questions concerning use of Pap smears differed slightly on the National Health Interview Survey across the years for which data are shown.   2 Includes all other races not shown separately, unknown poverty level in 1987, unknown health insurance status, unknown education level, and unknown disability status.   3 Estimates are age adjusted to the year 2000 standard population using five age groups: 18 to 44 years, 45 to 54 years, 55 to 64 years, 65 to 74 years, and 75 years and over.   4 The race groups White, Black, American Indian or Alaska Native, Asian, Native Hawaiian or Other Pacific Islander, and two or more races, include persons of Hispanic and non-Hispanic origin. Persons of Hispanic origin may be of any race.   5 Percent of poverty level is based on family income and family size and composition. Missing family income data were imputed for 1993 and beyond.   6 Health insurance categories are mutually exclusive. Persons who reported both Medicaid and private coverage are classified as having private coverage. Medicaid includes other public assistance through 1996. Starting with 1997 data, state-sponsored health plan coverage is included as Medicaid coverage. Starting with 1999 data, coverage by the Children's Health Insurance Program (CHIP) is included with Medicaid coverage. Persons not covered by private insurance, Medicaid, CHIP, public assistance (through 1996), state-sponsored or other government-sponsored health plans (starting in 1997), Medicare, or military plans are considered to have no health insurance coverage. Persons with only Indian Health Service coverage are considered to have no health insurance coverage. Health insurance status was unknown for 8 to 9 percent of children in 1993-1996 and about 1 percent in 1997-2011.   7 Education categories shown are for 1998 and subsequent years. GED is General Educational Development high school equivalency diploma. In years prior to 1998, the following categories based on number of years in school completed were used: less than 12 years, 12 years, and 13 years or more.   8 Any basic actions difficulty or complex activity limitation is defined as having one or more of the following limitations or difficulties: movement difficulty, emotional difficulty, sensory (seeing or hearing) difficulty, cognitive difficulty, self-care (activities of daily living or instrumental activities of daily living) limitation, social limitation, or work limitation.

Table 3-39. Emergency Department Visits Within the Past 12 Months Among Children Under 18 Years of Age, by Selected Characteristics, Selected Years, 1997–2013

(Percent.)

Characteristic	Under 18 years			Under 6 years			6 to 17 years		
	1997	2005	2013	1997	2005	2013	1997	2005	2013
PERCENT OF CHILDREN WITH ONE OR MORE EMERGENCY DEPARTMENT VISITS[1]									
All children [2]	19.9	20.5	17.6	24.3	26.8	23.6	17.7	17.4	14.8
Sex									
Male	21.5	21.7	18.4	25.2	27.6	25.4	19.6	18.8	15.0
Female	18.3	19.2	16.9	23.3	25.9	21.7	15.7	15.9	14.5
Race [3]									
White only	19.4	19.8	17.1	22.6	25.3	22.5	17.8	17.1	14.6
Black or African American only	24.0	23.8	22.6	33.1	31.6	31.3	19.4	20.0	18.3
American Indian or Alaska Native only	*24.1	*32.1	18.8	*24.3	67.1	*22.2	*24.0	*	*16.3
Asian only	12.6	14.6	8.8	20.8	20.2	15.1	8.6	12.3	5.9
Native Hawaiian and Other Pacific Islander only	NA	*	*	NA	*	*	NA	*	*
Two or more races	NA	24.8	19.9	NA	38.3	25.0	NA	17.1	16.8
Hispanic Origin and Race [3]									
Hispanic or Latino	21.1	19.5	17.3	25.7	28.0	22.7	18.1	14.5	14.4
Not Hispanic or Latino	19.7	20.7	17.8	24.0	26.5	23.9	17.6	18.0	14.9
White only	19.2	19.9	17.2	22.2	24.5	22.8	17.7	17.9	14.7
Black or African American only	23.6	23.8	22.4	32.7	31.8	30.9	19.2	20.0	18.2
Percent of Poverty Level [4]									
Below 100 percent	25.1	27.3	24.1	29.5	33.5	30.8	22.2	23.5	20.2
100 percent to 199 percent	22.0	21.8	20.1	28.0	30.8	27.5	19.0	17.4	16.4
200 percent to 399 percent	18.0	18.9	15.5	21.4	25.9	21.1	16.4	15.7	13.0
400 percent or more	16.3	16.8	12.3	19.1	19.1	15.3	15.1	15.8	11.0
Hispanic Origin and Race and Percent of Poverty Level [3,4]									
Hispanic or Latino									
Below 100 percent	21.9	21.8	19.0	25.0	28.4	25.9	19.6	17.4	15.0
100 percent to 199 percent	20.8	17.8	17.6	28.8	26.1	21.4	15.6	13.1	15.6
200 percent to 399 percent	21.4	20.2	16.3	24.6	31.7	21.3	19.6	14.3	13.5
400 percent or more	17.7	15.3	12.1	*20.2	23.3	*16.7	16.4	*11.5	*10.0
Not Hispanic or Latino									
White only									
Below 100 percent	25.5	34.1	29.9	27.2	37.3	34.8	24.4	32.2	26.8
100 percent to 199 percent	22.3	22.8	22.6	25.8	30.7	32.9	20.7	19.1	17.1
200 percent to 399 percent	17.8	17.9	15.1	20.9	22.9	19.2	16.3	15.7	13.4
400 percent or more	16.5	16.8	12.2	19.0	18.7	14.8	15.4	16.0	11.1
Black or African American only									
Below 100 percent	29.3	27.1	26.9	39.5	34.8	36.0	23.0	22.6	21.6
100 percent to 199 percent	22.5	24.1	22.4	31.7	33.3	29.3	18.5	20.3	19.4
200 percent to 399 percent	18.5	22.6	17.9	23.9	33.3	29.8	16.3	17.8	13.1
400 percent or more	16.1	16.9	17.1	*18.8	*	*	15.2	17.4	16.0
Health Insurance Status at the Time of Interview [5]									
Insured	19.8	20.7	17.8	24.4	26.8	23.5	17.5	17.7	15.0
Private	17.5	17.4	13.2	20.9	21.7	17.2	15.9	15.5	11.5
Medicaid	28.2	28.5	24.0	33.0	35.5	29.9	24.1	23.6	20.4
Uninsured	20.2	18.4	15.1	23.0	26.6	23.3	18.9	15.4	12.1
Health Insurance Status Prior to Interview [5]									
Insured continuously all 12 months	19.6	20.5	17.7	24.1	26.7	23.5	17.3	17.3	14.8
Uninsured for any period up to 12 months	24.0	26.0	21.7	27.1	34.4	26.3	21.9	22.4	19.2
Uninsured more than 12 months	18.4	14.4	10.0	19.3	*15.7	*	18.1	14.0	9.1
Geographic Region									
Northeast	18.5	20.9	19.3	20.7	26.3	24.5	17.4	18.5	16.8
Midwest	19.5	21.8	18.5	26.0	30.1	26.0	16.4	17.8	15.1
South	21.8	21.7	18.2	25.6	27.1	24.7	19.9	18.8	15.0
West	18.5	16.7	14.8	23.5	22.9	19.1	15.9	13.8	12.7
Location of Residence									
Within MSA[6]	19.7	20.0	17.0	23.9	25.7	22.4	17.4	17.2	14.4
Outside MSA[6]	20.8	22.4	21.2	26.2	31.8	30.3	18.6	18.2	16.7
PERCENT OF CHILDREN WITH TWO OR MORE EMERGENCY DEPARTMENT VISITS									
All children [2]	7.1	6.8	5.8	9.6	9.8	8.0	5.8	5.4	4.8
Sex									
Male	7.3	7.2	5.8	9.9	10.7	8.6	6.0	5.4	4.5
Female	6.9	6.5	5.8	9.4	8.9	7.3	5.7	5.3	5.0
Race [3]									
White only	6.6	6.3	5.5	8.4	9.1	7.3	5.7	4.9	4.7
Black or African American only	9.6	9.2	8.3	14.9	12.7	12.6	6.9	7.5	6.1
American Indian or Alaska Native only	*	*	*	*	*	*	*	*	*
Asian only	*5.7	*4.6	*	*12.9	*	*	*	*3.9	*

Table 3-39. Emergency Department Visits Within the Past 12 Months Among Children Under 18 Years of Age, by Selected Characteristics, Selected Years, 1997–2013— continued

(Percent.)

Characteristic	Under 18 years			Under 6 years			6 to 17 years		
	1997	2005	2013	1997	2005	2013	1997	2005	2013
Native Hawaiian and Other Pacific Islander only	NA	*	*	NA	*	*	NA	*	*
Two or more races	NA	*8.6	7.1	NA	*13.2	*9.8	NA	*	*5.4
Hispanic Origin and Race [3]									
Hispanic or Latino	8.9	7.7	6.0	11.8	12.1	8.4	7.0	5.2	4.8
Not Hispanic or Latino	6.8	6.6	5.7	9.2	9.2	7.8	5.7	5.4	4.8
White only	6.2	5.9	5.4	7.8	8.2	7.0	5.5	4.9	4.7
Black or African American only	9.3	9.1	8.1	14.6	12.4	11.9	6.8	7.5	6.2
Percent of Poverty Level [4]									
Below 100 percent	11.1	11.2	9.2	14.5	15.9	12.4	8.9	8.4	7.4
100 percent to 199 percent	8.3	7.9	7.3	12.2	12.7	10.9	6.3	5.5	5.5
200 percent to 399 percent	6.2	5.7	4.8	7.4	7.6	5.9	5.6	4.8	4.3
400 percent or more	4.0	4.4	2.7	5.0	5.1	*3.0	3.6	4.0	2.6
Hispanic Origin and Race and Percent of Poverty Level [3,4]									
Hispanic or Latino									
Below 100 percent	10.4	10.0	6.8	13.9	13.8	10.0	8.0	7.4	5.0
100 percent to 199 percent	8.2	6.1	7.1	12.0	*8.7	9.5	5.7	*4.7	5.9
200 percent to 399 percent	8.5	7.7	*5.1	10.0	14.2	*6.2	*7.6	*4.4	*
400 percent or more	*5.0	*5.4	*	*	*	*	*	*	*
Not Hispanic or Latino									
White only									
Below 100 percent	10.7	13.5	11.8	12.2	18.6	14.0	9.8	10.4	10.4
100 percent to 199 percent	8.0	8.2	7.8	11.2	13.7	12.7	6.4	*5.5	*5.2
200 percent to 399 percent	6.0	5.1	4.3	6.7	6.1	*3.9	5.6	4.6	4.4
400 percent or more	3.7	3.7	3.1	4.6	4.1	*3.4	3.3	3.5	2.9
Black or African American only									
Below 100 percent	12.7	11.4	10.7	19.1	16.2	15.6	8.8	8.6	*7.9
100 percent to 199 percent	9.2	8.4	7.6	*13.5	*13.3	*9.8	*7.2	*6.5	*6.6
200 percent to 399 percent	5.8	*7.6	*7.1	*8.9	*	*	*4.5	*7.5	*4.9
400 percent or more	*	*7.2	*	*	*	*	*	*	*
Health Insurance Status at the Time of Interview [5]									
Insured	7.0	6.8	5.9	9.6	9.7	8.0	5.7	5.3	4.8
Private	5.2	5.0	3.4	6.8	6.2	4.5	4.5	4.4	2.9
Medicaid	13.1	11.1	9.4	16.2	15.8	11.9	10.4	7.7	7.9
Uninsured	7.7	7.0	5.2	9.8	11.5	*7.7	6.8	5.4	*4.3
Health Insurance Status Prior to Interview [5]									
Insured continuously all 12 months	6.9	6.7	5.9	9.4	9.7	8.0	5.7	5.2	4.8
Uninsured for any period up to 12 months	8.5	8.9	6.0	11.5	13.6	*8.9	6.6	6.9	4.4
Uninsured more than 12 months	6.8	5.5	*4.5	*8.6	*	*	6.2	5.3	*
Geographic Region									
Northeast	6.2	6.2	6.3	7.6	8.9	8.7	5.4	5.0	5.1
Midwest	6.6	6.9	6.9	10.4	9.6	11.1	4.8	5.5	4.9
South	8.0	7.9	6.3	10.1	10.8	8.1	6.9	6.3	5.3
West	7.1	5.5	3.8	10.0	9.1	4.3	5.6	3.9	3.5
Location of Residence									
Within MSA[6]	7.2	6.7	5.6	9.6	9.5	7.4	5.9	5.2	4.7
Outside MSA[6]	6.8	7.5	7.1	9.7	11.2	11.2	5.6	5.9	5.0

NA = Not available. * = Figure does not meet standards of reliability or precision. Data preceded by an asterisk have a relative standard error (RSE) of 20 percent to 30 percent. Data not shown have an RSE of greater than 30 percent. 1 See Appendix II of Health, United States, 2014, for more information. 2 Includes all other races not shown separately and unknown health insurance status. 3 The race groups, White, Black, American Indian or Alaska Native, Asian, Native Hawaiian or Other Pacific Islander, and 2 or more races, include persons of Hispanic and non-Hispanic origin. Persons of Hispanic origin may be of any race. 4 Percent of poverty level is based on family income and family size and composition using U.S. Census Bureau poverty thresholds. Missing family data were imputed for 1997 and beyond. 5 Health insurance categories are mutually exclusive. Persons who reported both Medicaid and private coverage are classified as having private coverage. Medicaid includes other public assistance through 1996. Starting with 1997 data, state-sponsored health plan coverage is included as Medicaid coverage. Starting with 1999 data, coverage by the Children's Health Insurance Program (CHIP) is included with Medicaid coverage. Persons not covered by private insurance, Medicaid, CHIP, public assistance (through 1996), state-sponsored or other government-sponsored health plans (starting in 1997), Medicare, or military plans are considered to have no health insurance coverage. Persons with only Indian Health Service coverage are considered to have no health insurance coverage. Health insurance status was unknown for 8 to 9 percent of children in 1993-1996 and about 1 percent in 1997-2011. 6 MSA = metropolitan statistical area.

Table 3-40. Emergency Department Visits Within the Past 12 Months Among Adults 18 Years of Age and Over, by Selected Characteristics, Selected Years, 1997–2013

(Percent.)

Characteristic	One or more emergency department visits					Two or more emergency department visits				
	1997	2000	2005	2010	2013	1997	2000	2005	2010	2013
18 years and over, age-adjusted[1,2]	19.6	20.2	20.5	21.4	18.8	6.7	6.9	7.1	7.8	6.9
18 years and over, crude[1]	19.6	20.1	20.4	21.3	18.7	6.7	6.8	7.0	7.7	6.8
Age										
18 to 44 years	20.7	20.5	20.8	22.0	18.5	6.8	7.0	7.1	8.4	6.9
18 to 24 years	26.3	25.7	25.3	25.4	20.8	9.1	8.8	8.9	9.6	8.1
25 to 44 years	19.0	18.8	19.2	20.7	17.7	6.2	6.4	6.5	8.0	6.5
45 to 64 years	16.2	17.6	18.2	19.2	17.6	5.6	5.6	6.4	6.7	6.5
45 to 54 years	15.7	17.9	17.6	18.6	17.2	5.5	5.8	6.1	6.6	6.8
55 to 64 years	16.9	17.0	19.0	19.8	18.1	5.7	5.3	6.8	6.8	6.3
65 years and over	22.0	23.7	23.7	23.7	21.3	8.1	8.6	8.2	7.7	7.0
65 to 74 years	20.3	21.6	20.8	20.7	18.4	7.1	7.4	7.4	6.4	6.0
75 years and over	24.3	26.2	27.1	27.4	25.3	9.3	10.0	9.1	9.4	8.4
Sex [2]										
Male	19.1	18.7	18.6	18.5	16.5	5.9	5.7	5.9	6.0	5.4
Female	20.2	21.6	22.3	24.3	21.0	7.5	7.9	8.2	9.6	8.3
Race [2,3]										
White only	19.0	19.4	19.8	20.7	18.1	6.2	6.4	6.5	7.2	6.3
Black or African American only	25.9	26.5	26.3	28.6	25.4	11.1	10.8	11.9	12.6	11.1
American Indian or Alaska Native only	24.8	30.3	31.0	22.6	26.7	13.1	*12.6	*11.1	*11.8	*9.0
Asian only	11.6	13.6	15.4	13.3	10.1	*2.9	*3.8	*3.8	3.3	3.3
Native Hawaiian and Other Pacific Islander only	NA	*	*	*	*	NA	*	*	*	*
Two or more races	NA	32.5	25.7	29.7	27.2	NA	11.3	12.8	11.1	13.1
American Indian or Alaska Native; White	NA	33.9	29.3	31.1	30.4	NA	*9.4	*15.3	*15.2	16.7
Hispanic Origin and Race [2,3]										
Hispanic or Latino	19.2	18.3	20.1	19.8	17.4	7.4	7.0	7.1	6.9	6.1
Mexican	17.8	17.4	17.2	18.1	16.0	6.4	7.1	5.8	6.1	5.4
Not Hispanic or Latino	19.7	20.6	20.7	21.9	19.1	6.7	6.9	7.1	8.1	7.1
White only	19.1	19.8	20.1	21.1	18.5	6.2	6.4	6.4	7.4	6.5
Black or African American only	25.9	26.5	26.2	29.0	25.5	11.0	10.8	11.9	12.7	11.2
Percent of Poverty Level [2,4]										
Below 100 percent	28.1	29.0	29.8	30.6	30.0	12.8	13.3	13.7	14.9	15.0
100 percent to 199 percent	23.8	23.9	23.2	25.6	22.9	9.3	9.6	9.6	10.5	9.8
200 percent to 399 percent	18.3	19.8	20.2	20.4	17.7	5.9	6.3	6.5	6.8	5.8
400 percent or more	15.9	16.8	16.9	17.0	13.4	3.9	4.5	4.5	4.7	3.3
Hispanic Origin and Race and Percent of Poverty Level [2,3,4]										
Hispanic or Latino										
Below 100 percent	22.1	22.4	24.0	23.6	22.7	9.8	9.7	9.2	11.5	9.3
100 percent to 199 percent	19.2	18.1	18.7	19.9	17.4	8.1	6.7	7.1	6.3	6.8
200 percent to 399 percent	18.5	17.3	18.9	18.1	15.3	6.0	7.4	5.9	5.2	4.7
400 percent or more	14.6	16.4	20.9	18.8	15.0	*3.8	*4.3	*6.9	*5.5	*3.7
Not Hispanic or Latino										
White only										
Below 100 percent	29.5	30.1	30.8	33.3	32.0	13.0	13.9	13.7	15.5	16.3
100 percent to 199 percent	24.3	25.5	24.3	26.8	25.0	9.1	10.4	9.8	11.2	10.7
200 percent to 399 percent	18.1	20.1	20.7	20.3	18.1	5.8	6.3	6.4	6.5	6.0
400 percent or more	15.8	16.3	16.2	16.9	13.4	3.8	4.1	4.0	4.9	3.2
Black or African American only										
Below 100 percent	34.6	35.4	35.4	36.9	36.8	17.5	17.4	18.3	20.2	20.5
100 percent to 199 percent	29.2	28.5	28.9	33.5	28.1	12.8	12.2	14.2	15.9	12.8
200 percent to 399 percent	20.8	23.2	21.5	25.7	21.0	8.1	8.0	8.7	10.2	7.1
400 percent or more	18.2	22.6	22.6	18.8	16.4	5.9	8.8	*9.2	*4.0	4.7
Health Insurance Status at the Time of Interview [5,6]										
18 to 64 years										
Insured	18.8	19.5	20.0	20.8	18.1	6.1	6.4	6.6	7.5	6.5
Private	16.9	17.6	17.3	17.4	14.1	4.7	5.1	4.8	5.2	3.9
Medicaid	37.6	42.2	40.1	40.2	38.0	19.7	21.0	20.1	21.1	19.0
Uninsured	20.0	19.3	19.5	21.3	18.5	7.5	6.9	8.0	8.9	8.1
Health Insurance Status Prior to Interview [5,6]										
18 to 64 years										
Insured continuously all 12 months	18.3	19.0	19.4	20.2	17.4	5.8	6.1	6.3	7.1	6.1
Uninsured for any period up to 12 months	25.5	28.2	28.0	26.0	26.6	9.4	10.3	12.4	12.5	11.3
Uninsured more than 12 months	18.9	17.3	18.0	20.6	17.1	7.1	6.4	7.0	8.1	7.6

Table 3-40. Emergency Department Visits Within the Past 12 Months Among Adults 18 Years of Age and Over, by Selected Characteristics, Selected Years, 1997–2013— continued

(Percent.)

Characteristic	One or more emergency department visits					Two or more emergency department visits				
	1997	2000	2005	2010	2013	1997	2000	2005	2010	2013
Percent of Poverty Level and Health Insurance Status Prior to Interview [4,5,6]										
18 to 64 years										
Below 100 percent										
Insured continuously all 12 months	30.2	31.6	33.6	35.2	33.3	14.7	15.4	15.3	18.3	16.5
Uninsured for any period up to 12 months	34.1	43.7	39.1	34.2	37.5	16.1	18.1	21.5	16.5	20.4
Uninsured more than 12 months	20.8	20.5	20.5	23.4	21.7	8.1	9.1	8.5	11.7	11.4
100 percent to 199 percent										
Insured continuously all 12 months	24.5	25.5	23.7	26.1	23.6	8.9	10.2	9.8	10.8	10.3
Uninsured for any period up to 12 months	28.7	27.7	28.4	29.7	28.5	12.3	11.7	12.7	15.6	11.5
Uninsured more than 12 months	19.0	17.4	18.5	21.2	17.2	8.3	6.4	7.7	7.8	7.9
200 to 399 percent										
Insured continuously all 12 months	17.5	19.5	19.7	19.6	16.6	5.3	6.3	6.4	6.0	5.5
Uninsured for any period up to 12 months	21.6	24.6	26.8	25.4	23.7	6.6	7.3	10.6	12.2	9.1
Uninsured more than 12 months	16.8	15.6	14.7	17.6	14.5	5.9	4.5	4.5	5.7	4.5
400 percent or more										
Insured continuously all 12 months	14.9	15.5	15.6	15.9	12.6	3.7	3.7	3.6	4.5	3.1
Uninsured for any period up to 12 months	18.0	20.1	20.2	12.5	14.2	*3.1	6.4	7.2	*	*
Uninsured more than 12 months	19.1	15.8	17.9	19.4	*8.4	*	*5.2	*7.4	*	*
Disability Measure [2,7]										
Any basic actions difficulty or complex activity limitation	30.8	32.0	34.4	34.9	32.4	13.5	14.6	15.6	16.8	16.4
Any basic actions difficulty	30.5	32.4	34.9	35.0	32.7	13.5	14.9	15.8	17.2	16.8
Any complex activity limitation	39.7	41.5	42.3	43.8	41.0	19.9	21.2	22.4	24.5	23.1
No disability	14.5	15.3	14.9	16.1	13.4	3.7	3.9	3.9	4.4	3.4
Geographic Region [2]										
Northeast	19.5	20.0	21.6	22.6	19.9	6.9	6.2	7.2	8.4	6.6
Midwest	19.3	20.1	21.6	22.3	20.0	6.2	6.9	7.2	8.2	7.6
South	20.9	21.2	20.7	22.1	19.2	7.3	7.6	7.6	8.0	7.4
West	17.7	18.6	17.8	18.9	16.3	6.0	6.3	6.0	6.7	5.4
Location of Residence [2]										
Within MSA[8]	19.1	19.6	20.1	20.8	18.3	6.4	6.6	6.8	7.5	6.6
Outside MSA[8]	21.5	22.5	22.3	25.5	22.2	7.8	7.8	8.1	9.8	8.8

NA = Not available.   * = Figure does not meet standards of reliability or precision. Data preceded by an asterisk have a relative standard error (RSE) of 20 percent to 30 percent. Data not shown have an RSE of greater than 30 percent.   1 Includes all other races not shown separately, unknown health insurance status, and unknown disability status.   2 Estimates are for persons 18 years of age and over and are age adjusted to the year 2000 standard population using five age groups: 18 to 44 years, 45 to 54 years, 55 to 64 years, 65 to 74 years, and 75 years and over.   3 The race groups White, black, American Indian or Alaska Native, Asian, Native Hawaiian or Other Pacific Islander, and two or more races include persons of Hispanic and non-Hispanic origin. Persons of Hispanic origin may be of any race.   4 Percent of poverty level is based on family income and family size and composition using U.S. Census Bureau poverty thresholds. Missing family income data were imputed for 1997 and beyond.   5 Estimates for persons 18 to 64 years of age are age adjusted to the year 2000 standard population using three age groups: 18 to 44 years, 45 to 54 years, and 55 to 64 years.   6 Health insurance categories are mutually exclusive. Persons who reported both Medicaid and private coverage are classified as having private coverage. Medicaid includes other public assistance through 1996. Starting with 1997 data, state-sponsored health plan coverage is included as Medicaid coverage. Starting with 1999 data, coverage by the Children's Health Insurance Program (CHIP) is included with Medicaid coverage. Persons not covered by private insurance, Medicaid, CHIP, public assistance (through 1996), state-sponsored or other government-sponsored health plans (starting in 1997), Medicare, or military plans are considered to have no health insurance coverage. Persons with only Indian Health Service coverage are considered to have no health insurance coverage. Health insurance status was unknown for 8 to 9 percent of children in 1993-1996 and about 1 percent in 1997-2011.   7 Any basic actions difficulty or complex activity limitation is defined as having one or more of the following limitations or difficulties: movement difficulty, emotional difficulty, sensory (seeing or hearing) difficulty, cognitive difficulty, self-care (activities of daily living or instrumental activities of daily living) limitation, social limitation, or work limitation.   8 MSA = metropolitan statistical area.

Table 3-41. Initial Injury-Related Visits to Hospital Emergency Departments, by Sex, Age, and Intent and Mechanism of Injury, Selected Annual Averages, 2005–2006 through 2010–2011

(Numbers in thousands; rate per 10,000 population.)

Sex, age, and intent and mechanism of injury[1]	Initial injury-related visits in thousands					Initial injury-related visits per 10,000 persons				
	2005–2006	2007–2008	2008–2009	2009–2010	2010–2011	2005–2006	2007–2008	2008–2009	2009–2010	2010–2011
Both Sexes										
All ages, age-adjusted[2,3]	31,706	28,699	31,328	32,204	33,007	1,076.4	960.9	1,040.8	1,063.2	1,084.0
All ages, crude[2]	31,706	28,699	31,328	32,204	33,007	1,068.6	951.3	1,029.4	1,049.7	1,067.9
Unintentional injuries[4]	25,658	23,670	25,725	26,523	27,275	864.7	784.6	845.3	864.5	882.4
Falls	8,100	8,144	8,900	9,393	9,932	273.0	270.0	292.4	306.2	321.3
Struck by or against objects or persons	2,935	2,746	2,916	3,055	3,166	98.9	91.0	95.8	99.6	102.4
Motor vehicle traffic	3,714	3,387	3,508	3,622	3,557	125.2	112.3	115.3	118.1	115.1
Cut or pierce	2,145	1,944	2,008	1,829	1,922	72.3	64.4	66.0	59.6	62.2
Intentional injuries	1,977	1,888	2,313	2,418	2,446	66.6	62.6	76.0	78.8	79.1
Male										
All ages, age-adjusted[2,3]	16,966	15,332	16,640	17,124	17,483	1,166.1	1,039.7	1,118.0	1,143.0	1,164.5
All ages, crude[2]	16,966	15,332	16,640	17,124	17,483	1,164.2	1,033.8	1,111.8	1,133.8	1,150.5
Unintentional injuries[4]	13,736	12,611	13,590	14,083	14,451	942.5	850.3	908.0	932.4	951.0
Falls	3,685	3,581	3,944	4,285	4,689	252.9	241.4	263.5	283.7	308.6
Struck by or against objects or persons	1,833	1,771	1,863	1,931	2,008	125.8	119.4	124.4	127.8	132.2
Motor vehicle traffic	1,733	1,693	1,734	1,762	1,710	118.9	114.2	115.8	116.7	112.5
Cut or pierce	1,392	1,270	1,263	1,183	1,236	95.5	85.7	84.4	78.3	81.4
Intentional injuries	1,135	1,020	1,266	1,348	1,396	77.8	68.8	84.6	89.3	91.8
Under 18 years[2]	5,072	4,602	5,132	5,403	5,309	1,346.6	1,216.8	1,351.1	1,416.3	1,397.8
Unintentional injuries[4]	4,391	3,995	4,509	4,817	4,724	1,165.8	1,056.3	1,187.1	1,262.9	1,243.9
Falls	1,362	1,305	1,512	1,647	1,737	361.5	345.0	398.1	431.8	457.4
Struck by or against objects or persons	816	850	909	1,022	997	216.6	224.6	239.2	267.9	262.6
Motor vehicle traffic	357	265	305	309	301	94.8	70.0	80.3	81.0	79.1
Cut or pierce	291	264	284	248	238	77.3	69.8	74.8	64.9	62.7
Intentional injuries	190	198	194	173	167	50.4	52.2	51.1	45.3	44.1
18 to 24 years[2]	2,552	2,305	2,562	2,516	2,511	1,729.5	1,547.4	1,695.5	1,630.1	1,612.1
Unintentional injuries[4]	1,985	1,788	1,947	1,878	1,890	1,345.4	1,200.6	1,288.6	1,216.7	1,213.7
Falls	318	309	366	375	390	215.2	207.7	242.4	243.0	250.4
Struck by or against objects or persons	290	280	283	216	259	196.9	188.0	187.4	140.2	166.6
Motor vehicle traffic	386	366	373	406	357	261.6	245.8	247.0	263.2	229.3
Cut or pierce	265	190	215	187	192	179.5	127.8	142.6	121.4	123.5
Intentional injuries	273	308	381	389	403	185.2	206.9	252.2	252.2	258.7
25 to 44 years[2]	5,199	4,471	4,611	4,719	4,850	1,243.6	1,072.7	1,109.5	1,140.9	1,184.3
Unintentional injuries[4]	4,001	3,531	3,540	3,577	3,690	957.1	847.0	851.8	864.8	901.1
Falls	763	677	703	739	815	182.4	162.5	169.2	178.7	199.1
Struck by or against objects or persons	472	384	401	400	452	112.9	92.1	96.4	96.8	110.4
Motor vehicle traffic	629	638	578	585	591	150.5	153.0	139.1	141.5	144.3
Cut or pierce	480	426	401	380	423	114.8	102.2	96.5	91.9	103.2
Intentional injuries	436	350	495	586	589	104.4	83.9	119.2	141.6	143.8
45 to 64 years[2]	2,842	2,707	2,996	3,071	3,270	790.0	718.3	780.7	788.7	822.7
Unintentional injuries[4]	2,275	2,223	2,437	2,531	2,741	632.5	590.0	635.1	649.9	689.6
Falls	599	651	669	775	909	166.6	172.8	174.2	199.0	228.6
Struck by or against objects or persons	208	205	216	208	204	57.9	54.3	56.4	53.3	51.4
Motor vehicle traffic	262	331	375	334	334	72.9	87.9	97.7	85.9	84.0
Cut or pierce	285	309	306	297	294	79.2	81.9	79.7	76.2	73.9
Intentional injuries	205	145	168	180	219	57.1	38.4	43.9	46.2	55.2
65 years and over[2]	1,301	1,247	1,340	1,415	1,544	837.5	768.6	805.1	824.7	871.6
Unintentional injuries[4]	1,082	1,073	1,157	1,280	1,406	696.8	661.7	695.2	746.1	793.5
Falls	644	638	694	749	838	414.5	393.2	416.7	436.3	473.0
Struck by or against objects or persons	46	*52	*54	84	95	29.8	*32.3	*32.2	49.1	53.6
Motor vehicle traffic	98	93	103	127	128	63.4	57.4	61.7	74.1	72.1
Cut or pierce	70	81	*57	71	90	45.3	50.0	*34.0	41.1	50.6
Intentional injuries	*	*	*	*	*	*	*	*	*	*
Female										
All ages, age-adjusted[2,3]	14,740	13,367	14,688	15,080	15,524	980.5	874.2	955.6	976.8	997.2
All ages, crude[2]	14,740	13,367	14,688	15,080	15,524	976.3	871.6	949.7	968.2	988.0
Unintentional injuries[4]	11,922	11,060	12,134	12,439	12,824	789.7	721.1	784.6	798.6	816.1
Falls	4,415	4,564	4,956	5,109	5,243	292.4	297.6	320.4	328.0	333.6
Struck by or against objects or persons	1,102	976	1,053	1,124	1,158	73.0	63.6	68.1	72.2	73.7
Motor vehicle traffic	1,981	1,695	1,774	1,860	1,847	131.2	110.5	114.7	119.4	117.6
Cut or pierce	753	673	745	646	685	49.9	43.9	48.2	41.5	43.6
Intentional injuries	843	867	1,048	1,070	1,050	55.8	56.5	67.7	68.7	66.8
Under 18 years[2]	3,625	3,062	3,508	3,645	3,673	1,008.7	848.2	967.5	1,001.6	1,013.2
Unintentional injuries[4]	3,058	2,690	3,008	3,115	3,120	851.1	745.3	829.5	855.9	860.7

Table 3-41. Initial Injury-Related Visits to Hospital Emergency Departments, by Sex, Age, and Intent and Mechanism of Injury, Selected Annual Averages, 2005–2006 through 2010–2011— continued

(Numbers in thousands; rate per 10,000 population.)

Sex, age, and intent and mechanism of injury[1]	Initial injury-related visits in thousands					Initial injury-related visits per 10,000 persons				
	2005–2006	2007–2008	2008–2009	2009–2010	2010–2011	2005–2006	2007–2008	2008–2009	2009–2010	2010–2011
Falls	1,039	1,014	1,096	1,144	1,138	289.1	280.9	302.3	314.3	314.0
Struck by or against objects or persons	419	391	439	454	425	116.7	108.3	121.1	124.7	117.2
Motor vehicle traffic	367	282	249	285	302	102.1	78.2	68.6	78.3	83.4
Cut or pierce	160	145	154	139	158	44.4	40.1	42.4	38.2	43.7
Intentional injuries	188	163	222	207	196	52.3	45.1	61.4	56.8	54.1
18 to 24 years[2]	1,882	1,698	1,736	1,854	1,936	1,329.3	1,186.5	1,194.5	1,259.9	1,297.1
Unintentional injuries[4]	1,431	1,318	1,325	1,437	1,530	1,010.5	921.0	911.7	976.4	1,025.0
Falls	290	301	307	299	305	205.0	210.5	210.9	203.5	204.5
Struck by or against objects or persons	146	106	110	135	171	103.4	74.0	75.4	91.6	114.7
Motor vehicle traffic	397	378	360	426	460	280.6	264.5	247.5	289.8	308.1
Cut or pierce	116	89	77	*81	*94	82.2	61.9	53.2	*55.1	*63.3
Intentional injuries	176	209	232	262	251	124.2	145.8	159.7	177.9	168.4
25 to 44 years[2]	4,173	3,733	4,087	4,152	4,233	1,004.2	905.4	996.6	1,016.6	1,034.6
Unintentional injuries[4]	3,266	2,865	3,179	3,244	3,308	785.8	694.7	775.1	794.2	808.5
Falls	873	900	1,004	986	941	210.1	218.2	244.7	241.4	229.9
Struck by or against objects or persons	309	216	198	250	284	74.3	52.4	48.3	61.2	69.4
Motor vehicle traffic	719	572	621	612	616	173.1	138.8	151.3	149.9	150.5
Cut or pierce	269	214	270	230	219	64.7	51.8	65.9	56.4	53.6
Intentional injuries	313	345	396	396	408	75.4	83.6	96.5	96.9	99.8
45 to 64 years[2]	2,904	2,681	3,061	3,106	3,101	767.8	677.5	760.0	759.3	741.9
Unintentional injuries[4]	2,278	2,209	2,539	2,536	2,519	602.2	558.3	630.4	619.9	602.7
Falls	865	886	1,012	1,067	1,075	228.7	223.9	251.2	260.8	257.1
Struck by or against objects or persons	160	171	216	205	197	42.2	43.2	53.5	50.0	47.2
Motor vehicle traffic	359	345	399	403	345	94.8	87.3	99.0	98.4	82.6
Cut or pierce	158	163	190	159	157	41.7	41.1	47.2	38.8	37.6
Intentional injuries	149	130	161	184	182	39.4	32.9	39.9	45.0	43.5
65 years and over[2]	2,155	2,193	2,294	2,322	2,582	1,002.9	989.9	1,016.3	1,014.2	1,110.7
Unintentional injuries[4]	1,889	1,978	2,083	2,108	2,348	879.1	892.5	922.8	920.4	1,009.8
Falls	1,347	1,463	1,538	1,612	1,784	626.9	660.1	681.2	704.1	767.2
Struck by or against objects or persons	69	91	91	81	81	31.9	41.2	40.4	35.5	34.7
Motor vehicle traffic	139	116	146	134	124	64.5	52.5	64.7	58.3	53.5
Cut or pierce	*50	*64	*54	*37	*56	*23.3	*28.8	*23.9	*16.3	*24.2
Intentional injuries	*	*	*	*	*	*	*	*	*	*

NOTE: An emergency department visit was considered injury related if the first-listed diagnosis was injury related (ICD-9-CM 800-909.2, 909.4, 909.9-994.9, 995.50-995.59, and 995.80-995.85) or the first-listed external cause code (E code) was injury related (ICD-9-CM E800-E869, E880-E929, and E950-E999). * = Figure does not meet standards of reliability or precision. Data preceded by an asterisk have a relative standard error (RSE) of 20 percent to 30 percent. Data not shown have an RSE greater than 30 percent. 1 Intent and mechanism of injury are based on the first-listed external cause of injury code (E code). Intentional injuries include suicide attempts and assaults. 2 Includes all injury-related visits not shown separately in table, including those with undetermined intent (1 percent in 2010 to 2011) and insufficient or no information to code cause of injury (9 percent in 2010 to 2011). 3 Rates are age adjusted to the year 2000 standard population using six age groups: under 18 years, 18 to 24 years, 25 to 44 years, 45 to 64 years, 65 to 74 years, and 75 years and over. 4 Includes unintentional injury-related visits with mechanism of injury not shown in table.

Table 3-42. Visits to Physician Offices, Hospital Outpatient Departments, and Hospital Emergency Departments, by Age, Sex, and Race, Selected Years, 1995–2011

(Number; rate.)

Age, sex, and race	All places[1]			Physician offices			Hospital outpatient departments			Hospital emergency departments		
	1995	2000	2011	1995	2000	2011	1995	2000	2011	1995	2000	2011
Number of Visits in the thousands												
Age												
Total	860,859	1,014,848	NA	697,082	823,542	NA	67,232	83,289	125,721	96,545	108,017	136,296
Under 18 years	194,644	212,165	NA	150,351	163,459	NA	17,636	21,076	27,651	26,657	27,630	29,451
18 to 44 years	285,184	315,774	NA	219,065	243,011	NA	24,299	26,947	37,557	41,820	45,816	56,646
45 to 64 years	188,320	255,894	NA	159,531	216,783	NA	14,811	20,772	37,980	13,978	18,339	29,828
45 to 54 years	104,891	142,233	NA	88,266	119,474	NA	8,029	11,558	19,310	8,595	11,201	17,595
55 to 64 years	83,429	113,661	NA	71,264	97,309	NA	6,782	9,214	18,670	5,383	7,138	12,232
65 years and over	192,712	231,014	NA	168,135	200,289	NA	10,486	14,494	22,534	14,090	16,232	20,372
65 to 74 years	102,605	116,505	NA	90,544	102,447	NA	6,004	7,515	12,529	6,057	6,543	8,208
75 years and over	90,106	114,510	NA	77,591	97,842	NA	4,482	6,979	10,005	8,033	9,690	12,163
Total, age-adjusted[2]	334	374	NA	271	304	NA	26	31	40	37	40	45
Total, crude	329	370	NA	266	300	NA	26	30	41	37	39	44
Under 18 years	275	293	NA	213	226	NA	25	29	37	38	38	40
18 to 44 years	264	291	NA	203	224	NA	22	25	34	39	42	51
45 to 64 years	364	422	NA	309	358	NA	29	34	46	27	30	36
45 to 54 years	339	385	NA	286	323	NA	26	31	44	28	30	40
55 to 64 years	401	481	NA	343	412	NA	33	39	49	26	30	32
65 years and over	612	706	NA	534	612	NA	33	44	56	45	50	51
65 to 74 years	560	656	NA	494	577	NA	33	42	56	33	37	37
75 years and over	683	766	NA	588	654	NA	34	47	56	61	65	68
Sex and Age												
Male, age-adjusted[2]	290	325	NA	232	261	NA	21	26	32	37	38	42
Male, crude	277	314	NA	220	251	NA	21	25	33	36	38	41
Under 18 years	273	302	NA	209	231	NA	25	29	37	40	41	41
18 to 44 years	190	203	NA	139	148	NA	14	17	20	37	38	43
45 to 54 years	275	316	NA	229	260	NA	20	26	34	26	30	38
55 to 64 years	351	428	NA	300	367	NA	26	32	45	25	30	34
65 to 74 years	508	614	NA	445	539	NA	29	38	52	34	36	37
75 years and over	711	771	NA	616	670	NA	34	42	49	61	59	62
Female, age-adjusted[2]	377	420	NA	309	345	NA	31	35	48	37	41	48
Female, crude	378	424	NA	310	348	NA	31	35	49	37	41	48
Under 18 years	277	285	NA	217	221	NA	25	29	38	35	35	39
18 to 44 years	336	377	NA	265	298	NA	31	33	47	40	46	59
45 to 54 years	400	451	NA	339	384	NA	32	36	53	29	31	41
55 to 64 years	446	529	NA	382	453	NA	38	45	54	26	31	31
65 to 74 years	603	692	NA	534	609	NA	36	46	60	32	37	37
75 years and over	666	763	NA	571	645	NA	34	49	61	61	69	72
Race and Age [3]												
White, age-adjusted[2]	339	380	NA	282	315	NA	23	28	37	34	37	42
White, crude	338	381	NA	281	316	NA	23	28	38	34	37	41
Under 18 years	295	306	NA	237	243	NA	23	27	37	35	36	37
18 to 44 years	267	301	NA	211	239	NA	20	23	31	36	39	47
45 to 54 years	334	386	NA	286	330	NA	23	28	37	25	28	35
55 to 64 years	397	480	NA	345	416	NA	28	36	44	24	28	30
65 to 74 years	557	641	NA	496	568	NA	29	38	49	32	35	34
75 years and over	689	764	NA	598	658	NA	31	44	52	60	63	65
Black or African American, age-adjusted[2]	309	353	NA	204	239	NA	48	51	51	58	62	85
Black or African American, crude	281	324	NA	178	214	NA	45	48	50	58	62	83
Under 18 years	193	264	NA	100	167	NA	39	40	48	53	57	72
18 to 44 years	260	257	NA	158	149	NA	38	40	37	64	68	96
45 to 54 years	387	383	NA	281	269	NA	55	61	54	51	53	83
55 to 64 years	414	495	NA	294	373	NA	73	70	73	47	52	60
65 to 74 years	553	656	NA	429	512	NA	*77	85	*85	47	59	73
75 years and over	534	745	NA	395	568	NA	66	85	*74	73	92	118

NA = Not available.   * = Estimates are considered unreliable. Data preceded by an asterisk have a relative standard error (RSE) of 20 percent to 30 percent. Data not shown have an RSE greater than 30 percent.   1 All places includes visits to physician offices and hospital outpatient and emergency departments.   2 Estimates are age adjusted to the year 2000 standard population using six age groups: under 18 years, 18 to 44 years, 45 to 54 years, 55 to 64 years, 65 to 74 years, and 75 years and over.   3 Estimates by racial group should be used with caution because information on race was collected from medical records. In 2010, race data were missing and imputed for 23 percent of visits to physician offices, 14 percent of visits to hospital outpatient departments, and 11 percent of visits to hospital emergency departments.

Table 3-43A. Visits to Primary Care Generalist and Specialist Physicians, by Selected Characteristics and Type of Physician, Selected Years, 1980–2010

(Percent.)

Age, sex, and race	Type of primary care generalist physician[1]								
	All primary care generalists			General and family practice			Internal medicine		
	1980	1990	2000	1980	1990	2000	1980	1990	2000
Age									
Total	66.2	63.6	58.9	33.5	29.9	24.1	12.1	13.8	15.3
Under 18 years	77.8	79.5	79.7	26.1	26.5	19.9	2.0	2.9	*
18 to 44 years	65.3	65.2	62.1	34.3	31.9	28.2	8.6	11.8	12.7
45 to 64 years	60.2	55.5	51.2	36.3	32.1	26.4	19.5	18.6	20.1
45 to 54 years	60.2	55.6	52.3	37.4	32.0	27.8	17.1	17.1	18.7
55 to 64 years	60.2	55.5	49.9	35.4	32.1	24.7	21.8	20.0	21.7
65 years and over	61.6	52.6	46.5	37.5	28.1	20.2	22.7	23.3	24.5
65 to 74 years	61.2	52.7	46.6	37.4	28.1	19.7	22.1	23.0	24.5
75 years and over	62.3	52.4	46.4	37.6	28.0	20.8	23.5	23.7	24.5
Sex and Age									
Male									
Under 18 years	77.3	78.1	77.7	25.6	24.1	18.3	2.0	3.0	*
18 to 44 years	50.8	51.8	51.5	38.0	35.9	34.2	11.5	15.0	14.4
45 to 64 years	55.6	50.6	49.4	34.4	31.0	28.7	20.5	19.2	19.8
65 years and over	58.2	51.2	43.1	35.6	27.7	19.3	22.3	23.3	23.8
Female									
Under 18 years	78.5	81.1	82.0	26.6	29.1	21.7	2.0	2.8	*
18 to 44 years	72.1	71.3	67.2	32.5	30.0	25.3	7.3	10.3	11.9
45 to 64 years	63.4	58.8	52.5	37.7	32.8	24.9	18.9	18.2	20.2
65 years and over	63.9	53.5	48.9	38.7	28.3	20.9	22.9	23.3	25.0
Race and Age [2]									
White									
Under 18 years	77.6	79.2	78.5	26.4	27.1	21.2	2.0	2.3	*
18 to 44 years	64.8	64.4	61.4	34.5	31.9	29.2	8.6	10.6	11.0
45 to 64 years	59.6	54.2	49.3	36.0	31.5	27.3	19.2	17.6	17.1
65 years and over	61.4	51.9	45.1	36.6	27.5	20.3	23.3	23.1	23.0
Black or African American									
Under 18 years	79.9	85.5	87.3	23.7	20.2	*	*2.2	9.8	*
18 to 44 years	68.5	68.3	65.0	31.7	31.9	22.0	9.0	18.1	20.9
45 to 64 years	66.1	61.6	61.7	38.6	31.2	23.3	22.6	26.9	35.9
65 years and over	64.6	58.6	52.8	49.0	28.9	*18.5	14.2	28.7	33.4

Table 3-43B. Visits to Primary Care Generalist and Specialist Physicians, by Selected Characteristics and Type of Physician, Selected Years, 1980–2010

(Percent.)

Age, sex, and race	Type of primary care generalist physician[1]						Specialty care physicians		
	Obstetrics and gynecology			Pediatrics					
	1980	1990	2000	1980	1990	2000	1980	1990	2000
Age									
Total	9.6	8.7	7.8	10.9	11.2	11.7	33.8	36.4	41.1
Under 18 years	1.3	1.2	*1.1	48.5	48.9	57.3	22.2	20.5	20.3
18 to 44 years	21.7	20.8	20.4	0.7	0.7	*0.9	34.7	34.8	37.9
45 to 64 years	4.2	4.6	4.5	*	*	*	39.8	44.5	48.8
45 to 54 years	5.6	6.3	5.6	*	*	*	39.8	44.4	47.7
55 to 64 years	2.9	3.1	3.3	*	*	*	39.8	44.5	50.1
65 years and over	1.4	1.1	1.5	*	*	*	38.4	47.4	53.5
65 to 74 years	1.7	1.6	2.0	*	*	*	38.8	47.3	53.4
75 years and over	1.0	*0.6	*1.0	*	*	*	37.7	47.6	53.6
Sex and Age									
Male									
Under 18 years	X	X	X	49.4	50.7	58.0	22.7	21.9	22.3
18 to 44 years	X	X	X	1.0	0.7	*1.7	49.2	48.2	48.5
45 to 64 years	X	X	X	*	*	*	44.4	49.4	50.6
65 years and over	X	X	X	*	*	*	41.8	48.8	56.9
Female									
Under 18 years	2.5	2.3	2.1	47.4	46.9	56.5	21.5	18.9	18.0
18 to 44 years	31.7	30.4	29.6	0.6	0.7	*	27.9	28.7	32.8
45 to 64 years	6.7	7.7	7.3	*	*	*	36.6	41.2	47.5
65 years and over	2.1	1.8	2.6	*	*	*	36.1	46.5	51.1
Race and Age[2]									
White									
Under 18 years	1.1	1.0	*1.2	48.2	48.8	54.7	22.4	20.8	21.5
18 to 44 years	21.0	21.1	20.4	0.7	0.7	*0.8	35.2	35.6	38.6
45 to 64 years	4.1	4.8	4.7	*	*	*	40.4	45.8	50.7
65 years and over	1.4	1.2	1.5	*	*	*	38.6	48.1	54.9
Black or African American									
Under 18 years	2.8	*3.4	*	51.2	52.1	75.0	20.1	14.5	*12.7
18 to 44 years	27.1	17.9	20.7	*	*	*	31.5	31.7	35.0
45 to 64 years	4.8	3.5	*2.4	*	*	*	33.9	38.4	38.3
65 years and over	*	*	*	*	*	*	35.4	41.4	47.2

NOTE: This table presents data on visits to physician offices and excludes visits to other sites, such as hospital outpatient and emergency departments.   X = Not applicable.   * = Figure does not meet standards of reliability or precision. Data preceded by an asterisk have a relative standard error (RSE) of 20 percent to 30 percent. Data not shown have a RSE greater than 30 percent.   1 Type of physician is based on physician's self-designated primary area of practice. Primary care generalist physicians are defined as practitioners in the fields of general and family practice, general internal medicine, general obstetrics and gynecology, and general pediatrics and exclude primary care specialists. Primary care generalists in general and family practice exclude primary care specialties, such as sports medicine and geriatrics. Primary care internal medicine physicians exclude internal medicine specialists, such as allergists, cardiologists, and endocrinologists. Primary care obstetrics and gynecology physicians exclude obstetrics and gynecology specialties, such as gynecological oncology, maternal and fetal medicine, obstetrics and gynecology critical care medicine, and reproductive endocrinology. Primary care pediatricians exclude pediatric specialists, such as adolescent medicine specialists, neonatologists, pediatric allergists, and pediatric cardiologists.   2 Estimates by racial group should be used with caution because information on race was collected from medical records. In 2010, race data were missing and imputed for 23 percent of visits.

Table 3-44. Dental Visits in the Past Year, by Selected Characteristics, Selected Years, 1997–2013

(Percent.)

Characteristic	2 years and over			2 to 17 years			18 to 64 years			65 years and over[1]		
	1997	2000	2013	1997	2000	2013	1997	2000	2013	1997	2000	2013
Total with Dental Visit [2,3]	65.1	66.2	66.2	72.7	74.1	83.0	64.1	65.1	61.7	54.8	56.6	60.6
Sex												
Male	62.9	63.5	63.4	72.3	73.7	82.6	60.4	60.7	57.1	55.4	56.1	60.5
Female	67.1	68.8	68.9	73.0	74.6	83.5	67.7	69.4	66.2	54.4	56.9	60.8
Race [3]												
White only	66.4	67.9	67.1	74.0	75.8	83.6	65.7	67.2	62.9	56.8	58.4	62.5
Black or African American only	58.9	59.5	61.0	68.8	70.0	80.8	57.0	57.1	55.9	35.4	38.2	42.6
American Indian or Alaska Native only	55.1	58.6	60.1	66.8	71.3	81.9	49.9	55.0	52.7	*	*	50.9
Asian only	62.5	67.1	67.0	69.9	72.8	80.9	60.3	65.6	63.7	53.9	60.6	63.0
Native Hawaiian and Other Pacific Islander only	NA	*	*	NA	*	*	NA	*	*	NA	*	*
Two or more races	NA	65.1	67.4	NA	71.4	82.6	NA	60.5	55.8	NA	57.4	49.2
Black or African American; White	NA	63.5	72.9	NA	65.7	84.5	NA	60.7	54.2	NA	*	*
American Indian or Alaska Native; White	NA	61.7	58.7	NA	63.4	75.3	NA	61.6	53.7	NA	*57.8	47.6
Hispanic Origin and Race [4]												
Hispanic or Latino	54.0	52.3	59.4	61.0	60.6	80.7	50.8	48.6	50.2	47.8	44.5	47.7
Not Hispanic or Latino	66.4	68.2	67.6	74.7	76.8	83.8	65.7	67.5	64.1	55.2	57.2	61.7
White only	68.0	69.9	69.1	76.4	78.9	85.0	67.5	69.4	66.0	57.2	59.1	63.9
Black or African American only	58.8	59.4	60.6	68.8	70.0	80.5	56.9	57.2	55.7	35.3	38.0	42.4
Percent of Poverty Level [5]												
Below 100 percent	50.5	50.4	52.8	62.0	62.4	78.5	46.9	46.8	42.5	31.5	33.3	33.0
100 percent to 199 percent	50.8	52.2	52.7	62.5	66.1	78.3	48.3	48.4	45.4	40.8	43.0	40.1
200 percent to 399 percent	66.2	65.6	65.5	76.1	75.5	84.6	63.4	62.2	60.3	60.7	62.8	61.2
400 percent or more	78.9	79.5	80.6	85.7	85.9	89.2	77.7	78.5	78.1	74.7	73.8	82.9
Hispanic Origin and Race and Percent of Poverty Level [4,5]												
Hispanic or Latino												
Below 100 percent	45.7	43.4	54.4	55.9	54.2	79.9	39.2	36.8	36.5	33.6	31.3	36.2
100 percent to 199 percent	47.2	45.5	53.8	53.8	56.9	80.2	43.5	39.2	41.2	47.9	42.9	34.0
200 percent to 399 percent	61.2	57.2	60.7	70.5	65.6	80.6	57.5	53.7	54.3	57.0	54.8	60.5
400 percent or more	73.0	70.0	76.6	82.4	78.4	85.6	70.8	68.7	75.0	64.9	53.4	66.8
Not Hispanic or Latino												
White only												
Below 100 percent	51.7	53.6	49.8	64.4	65.0	74.7	50.6	53.3	44.6	32.0	37.2	32.2
100 percent to 199 percent	52.4	53.8	52.2	66.1	69.7	77.8	50.4	51.7	48.1	42.2	43.4	41.2
200 percent to 399 percent	67.5	67.6	66.9	77.1	78.3	86.2	65.0	64.4	62.0	61.9	63.9	62.6
400 percent or more	79.7	80.8	81.7	86.8	87.5	90.6	78.5	79.7	79.0	75.5	76.1	84.8
Black or African American only												
Below 100 percent	52.8	51.8	55.4	66.1	67.1	81.7	46.2	44.4	43.2	27.7	21.7	30.0
100 percent to 199 percent	48.7	52.4	51.4	61.2	67.3	75.9	46.3	48.0	44.7	26.9	35.2	32.3
200 percent to 399 percent	63.3	62.3	64.2	75.0	74.0	83.3	60.7	58.4	60.7	41.5	48.4	46.6
400 percent or more	74.6	72.8	74.0	81.8	74.2	81.1	73.4	73.3	73.6	66.1	60.5	65.0
Disability Measure [6]												
Any basic actions difficulty or complex activity limitation	X	X	X	X	X	X	55.1	57.3	52.9	49.0	50.7	53.6
Any basic actions difficulty	X	X	X	X	X	X	54.7	57.0	53.1	48.7	50.7	53.6
Any complex activity limitation	X	X	X	X	X	X	51.0	52.5	49.1	44.6	44.4	45.9
No disability	X	X	X	X	X	X	67.4	67.7	64.9	64.2	65.7	71.7
Geographic Region												
Northeast	69.6	72.3	71.2	77.5	81.1	86.9	69.6	72.1	68.5	55.5	58.1	62.2
Midwest	68.4	69.9	68.1	76.4	77.2	85.5	67.4	69.2	63.9	57.6	58.6	60.6
South	60.2	61.0	62.5	68.0	69.5	80.6	59.4	59.8	57.4	49.0	50.8	57.0
West	65.0	65.3	66.7	71.5	72.0	82.1	62.9	63.0	61.6	61.9	63.1	65.7
Location of Residence												
Within MSA[7]	66.7	67.5	67.4	73.6	74.3	83.3	65.7	66.5	63.0	57.6	58.9	62.6
Outside MSA[7]	59.1	61.2	59.6	69.3	73.3	81.3	58.0	59.7	53.9	46.1	49.3	52.9

NA = Not available.   X = Not applicable.   * = Estimates do not meet the standards of reliability and precision.   1 Based on the 1997-2013 National Health Interview Surveys, about 21 to 30 percent of persons 65 years and over were edentulous (having lost all their natural teeth). In 1997-2013, about 69 to 73 percent of older dentate persons, compared with 17 to 23 percent of older edentate persons, had a dental visit in the past year.   2 Respondents were asked, "About how long has it been since you last saw or talked to a dentist?"   3 Includes all other races not shown separately and unknown disability status.   4 The race groups White, Black, American Indian or Alaska Native, Asian, Native Hawaiian or Other Pacific Islander, and two or more races include persons of Hispanic and non-Hispanic origin. Persons of Hispanic origin may be of any race.   5 Percent of poverty level is based on family income and family size and composition using U.S. Census Bureau poverty thresholds. Missing family income data were imputed for 1997 and beyond.   6 Any basic actions difficulty or complex activity limitation is defined as having one or more of the following limitations or difficulties: movement difficulty, emotional difficulty, sensory (seeing or hearing) difficulty, cognitive difficulty, self-care (activities of daily living or instrumental activities of daily living) limitation, social limitation, or work limitation.   7 MSA = metropolitan statistical area.

Table 3-45. Prescription Drug Use in the Past 30 Days, by Sex, Age, and Race, Selected Years, 1988–1994 through 2009–2012

(Percent.)

Sex and age	All persons[1]			White only[2]			Black or African American only[2]		
	1988–1994	2001–2004	2009–2012	1988–1994	2001–2004	2009–2012	1988–1994	2001–2004	2009–2012
PERCENT OF POPULATION WITH AT LEAST ONE PRESCRIPTION DRUG IN PAST 30 DAYS									
Both Sexes, Age-Adjusted [3]	39.1	46.7	47.3	41.1	50.6	52.4	36.9	40.5	43.7
Male	32.7	41.6	42.7	34.2	45.0	47.2	31.1	36.2	37.5
Female	45.0	51.5	51.8	47.6	56.0	57.6	41.4	43.8	48.8
Both Sexes, Crude	37.8	46.5	48.7	41.4	52.6	56.5	31.2	36.5	42.0
Male	30.6	40.5	43.4	33.5	46.0	50.7	25.5	31.6	35.1
Female	44.6	52.2	53.9	48.9	59.0	62.1	36.2	40.7	48.0
Under 18 years	20.5	23.9	23.5	22.9	27.3	26.7	14.8	18.0	22.8
18 to 44 years	31.3	37.7	38.1	34.3	43.5	46.7	27.8	29.4	30.7
45 to 64 years	54.8	66.2	67.2	55.5	68.6	70.9	57.5	63.4	64.6
65 years and over	73.6	87.3	89.8	74.0	88.3	90.3	74.5	80.8	90.3
Male									
Under 18 years	20.4	25.3	23.1	22.3	29.4	24.8	15.5	18.8	23.6
18 to 44 years	21.5	29.2	29.6	23.5	33.4	37.3	21.1	22.6	20.2
45 to 64 years	47.2	58.7	63.1	48.1	60.8	67.3	48.2	58.0	55.6
65 years and over	67.2	83.6	87.7	67.4	84.8	88.7	64.4	75.9	88.0
Female									
Under 18 years	20.6	22.4	23.8	23.6	25.1	28.7	14.2	17.1	21.9
18 to 44 years	40.7	45.9	46.4	44.7	53.5	56.3	33.4	35.0	39.3
45 to 64 years	62.0	73.4	71.1	62.6	76.3	74.2	64.4	67.7	72.2
65 years and over	78.3	90.1	91.4	78.8	91.0	91.7	81.3	84.0	91.8
PERCENT OF POPULATION WITH THREE OR MORE PRESCRIPTION DRUGS IN PAST 30 DAYS									
Both Sexes, Age-Adjusted [3]	11.8	20.2	20.6	12.4	21.8	22.0	12.6	17.7	21.9
Male	9.4	17.3	19.1	9.9	18.7	20.2	10.2	15.1	19.2
Female	13.9	22.8	22.0	14.6	24.8	23.8	14.3	19.7	24.0
Both Sexes, Crude	11.0	19.9	21.8	12.5	23.6	25.9	9.2	14.7	20.2
Male	8.3	16.4	19.4	9.5	19.5	23.1	7.0	11.9	16.9
Female	13.6	23.4	24.1	15.4	27.6	28.5	11.1	17.1	23.1
Under 18 years	2.4	4.0	3.6	3.2	5.0	3.3	1.5	2.8	5.2
18 to 44 years	5.7	10.2	9.6	6.3	12.2	12.2	5.4	8.1	8.8
45 to 64 years	20.0	34.2	34.7	20.9	35.6	36.9	21.9	33.7	38.2
65 years and over	35.3	59.8	64.8	35.0	62.0	64.5	41.2	50.1	67.9
Male									
Under 18 years	2.6	4.1	4.1	3.3	4.9	3.2	1.7	3.4	6.4
18 to 44 years	3.6	8.0	7.5	4.1	9.8	9.4	4.2	6.1	6.6
45 to 64 years	15.1	28.3	31.4	15.8	29.1	34.0	18.7	28.2	31.1
65 years and over	31.3	54.2	64.6	30.9	56.4	64.5	31.7	44.0	64.0
Female									
Under 18 years	2.3	3.9	3.1	3.0	5.2	3.4	*1.2	2.1	3.9
18 to 44 years	7.6	12.3	11.8	8.5	14.7	15.1	6.4	9.7	10.7
45 to 64 years	24.7	39.9	37.8	25.8	41.9	39.6	24.3	38.1	44.3
65 years and over	38.2	64.0	64.9	38.0	66.2	64.5	47.7	54.2	70.5
PERCENT OF POPULATION WITH FIVE OR MORE PRESCRIPTION DRUGS IN PAST 30 DAYS									
Both Sexes, Age-Adjusted [3]	4.0	9.2	10.1	4.2	9.8	10.6	3.8	8.7	10.9
Male	2.9	7.9	9.3	3.1	8.4	9.6	2.9	7.6	9.5
Female	4.9	10.4	10.8	5.1	11.1	11.5	4.5	9.5	12.0
Both Sexes, Crude	3.6	9.0	10.7	4.2	10.8	12.8	2.6	7.1	9.8
Male	2.5	7.3	9.3	2.9	8.8	11.1	1.8	5.9	8.1
Female	4.7	10.7	12.0	5.4	12.8	14.4	3.3	8.2	11.3
Under 18 years	*	0.8	0.8	*	*0.9	0.8	*	*0.7	*1.2
18 to 44 years	1.2	3.3	3.3	1.4	3.8	4.3	1.0	4.1	*2.9
45 to 64 years	7.4	15.7	16.3	7.8	16.3	17.1	7.1	16.8	19.2
65 years and over	13.8	33.3	39.1	13.9	35.4	38.8	14.3	25.4	41.4
Male									
Under 18 years	*	*0.8	0.9	*	*	*0.9	*	*	*1.8
18 to 44 years	*0.8	2.6	2.8	*	2.9	*3.4	*	*3.2	*
45 to 64 years	4.8	12.5	14.2	5.0	13.2	14.7	5.9	15.0	16.9
65 years and over	11.3	30.6	37.9	11.6	31.9	37.5	9.9	22.3	37.1
Female									
Under 18 years	*	*0.7	*0.6	*	*0.9	*	*	*	*
18 to 44 years	1.7	3.9	3.9	1.8	4.6	5.1	1.2	4.7	*3.9

Table 3-45. Prescription Drug Use in the Past 30 Days, by Sex, Age, and Race, Selected Years, 1988–1994 through 2009–2012—continued

(Percent.)

Sex and age	All persons[1]			White only[2]			Black or African American only[2]		
	1988–1994	2001–2004	2009–2012	1988–1994	2001–2004	2009–2012	1988–1994	2001–2004	2009–2012
45 to 64 years	9.7	18.8	18.3	10.3	19.4	19.5	8.0	18.2	21.1
65 years and over	15.6	35.4	40.0	15.7	38.0	39.8	17.4	27.5	44.3

* = Figure does not meet standards of reliability or precision. Data preceded by an asterisk have a relative standard error (RSE) of 20 to 30 percent. Data not shown have an RSE of greater than 30 percent.   1 Includes persons of all races and Hispanic origins, not just those shown separately.   2 Starting with 1999 data, race-specific estimates are tabulated according to the 1997 Revisions to the Standards for the Classification of Federal Data on Race and Ethnicity and are not strictly comparable with estimates for earlier years. The two non-Hispanic race categories shown in the table conform to the 1997 Standards. Starting with 1999 data, race-specific estimates are for persons who reported only one racial group. Prior to data year 1999, estimates were tabulated according to the 1977 Standards. Estimates for single-race categories prior to 1999 included persons who reported one race or, if they reported more than one race, identified one race as best representing their race.   3 Age adjusted to the 2000 standard population using four age groups: under 18 years, 18 to 44 years, 45 to 64 years, and 65 years and over.

Table 3-46. Selected Prescription Drug Classes Used in the Past 30 Days, by Sex and Age, Selected Years, 1988–1994 through 2009–2012

(Percent.)

Age group and Multum Lexicon Plus therapeutic class[1] (common indications for use)	Total			Male			Female		
	1988–1994	1999–2002	2009–2012	1988–1994	1999–2002	2009–2012	1988–1994	1999–2002	2009–2012
All Ages									
Antihyperlipidemic agents (high cholesterol)	1.7	6.5	13.1	1.5	7.1	13.9	1.8	5.8	12.3
Analgesics (pain relief)	7.2	9.4	8.8	5.4	7.3	7.5	9.0	11.3	10.0
Antidepressants (depression and related disorders)	1.8	6.4	9.0	1.2	4.4	6.0	2.3	8.3	11.8
Proton pump inhibitors (gastrointestinal reflux, ulcers)[2]	2.8	5.3	8.2	2.4	4.7	7.3	3.0	5.9	9.1
Beta-adrenergic blocking agents (high blood pressure, heart disease)	3.1	4.4	7.7	2.7	4.1	7.3	3.5	4.6	8.1
ACE inhibitors (high blood pressure, heart disease)	2.4	4.6	6.8	2.4	4.7	7.6	2.4	4.5	6.1
Antidiabetic agents (diabetes)	2.6	3.7	5.9	2.5	3.7	6.2	2.6	3.8	5.6
Diuretics (high blood pressure, heart disease, kidney disease)[3]	3.4	4.1	5.6	2.3	3.1	4.5	4.4	5.1	6.6
Thyroid hormones (hypothyroidism)	2.3	3.9	5.0	0.8	1.5	2.3	3.7	6.2	7.5
Bronchodilators (asthma, breathing)	2.6	3.5	5.0	2.5	3.1	4.6	2.7	3.8	5.3
Sex hormones (contraceptives, menopause, hot flashes)[4]	X	X	X	X	X	X	9.8	15.2	8.6
Anxiolytics, sedatives, and hypnotics (anxiety, insomnia, and related disorders)	2.8	3.3	4.6	1.9	2.6	3.8	3.6	4.0	5.4
Antihypertensive combinations (high blood pressure)	2.4	2.9	4.3	1.4	1.9	3.7	3.3	3.8	4.8
Anticonvulsants (epilepsy, seizure, and related disorders)	1.4	2.4	4.1	1.2	2.1	3.5	1.6	2.7	4.6
Calcium channel blocking agents (high blood pressure, heart disease)	3.6	4.2	4.0	3.4	3.5	3.9	3.8	4.8	4.1
Under 18 Years									
Bronchodilators (asthma, breathing)	3.0	4.0	5.1	3.3	4.4	5.7	2.7	3.6	4.4
CNS stimulants (attention deficit disorder, hyperactivity)	*0.8	2.9	3.5	*1.2	4.4	5.0	*	1.4	1.9
Penicillins (bacterial infections)	6.1	5.1	3.3	5.9	5.2	2.7	6.4	5.0	3.8
Leukotriene modifiers (asthma, allergies)	X	0.7	2.0	X	*0.9	2.3	X	*	1.7
Antihistamines (allergies)	2.0	4.4	1.7	2.1	4.9	1.9	1.9	3.9	1.6
Respiratory inhalant products (asthma, chronic obstructive pulmonary disease, and related disorders)	*0.7	1.5	2.0	*	1.7	2.4	*	1.3	1.5
Adrenal cortical steroids (anti-inflammatory)	*0.5	0.8	1.4	*	*0.7	1.5	*0.5	0.9	*1.2
Nasal preparations (nose symptoms)	*	1.1	1.6	*	*1.3	1.9	*	1.0	*1.3
Antidepressants (depression and related disorders)	*	1.8	*1.2	*	2.2	*	*	*1.5	*
Upper respiratory combinations (cough and cold, congestion)	2.3	2.3	*0.8	2.6	*2.4	*0.9	2.0	*2.2	*
Analgesics (pain relief)	1.2	1.4	1.2	*1.2	1.3	*1.2	1.4	1.6	*1.1
Dermatological agents (skin symptoms)	0.7	1.1	1.4	*	1.1	*1.2	*1.0	*1.1	1.7
18 to 44 Years									
Analgesics (pain relief)	7.2	8.0	7.6	5.1	6.0	5.8	9.1	9.9	9.5
Antidepressants (depression and related disorders)	1.6	6.0	8.4	*1.0	3.6	5.9	2.3	8.5	10.8
Sex hormones (contraceptives, menopause, hot flashes)[4]	X	X	X	X	X	X	11.5	13.5	14.0
Proton pump inhibitors (gastrointestinal reflux, ulcers)[2]	2.0	3.0	4.8	1.6	3.0	5.1	2.4	3.0	4.4
Anxiolytics, sedatives, and hypnotics (generalized anxiety and related disorders)	1.4	2.1	4.0	*1.0	*1.7	3.2	1.9	2.5	4.7
Anticonvulsants (epilepsy, seizure, and related disorders)	0.8	1.6	3.2	*0.6	1.6	2.9	1.0	*1.5	3.6
Bronchodilators (asthma, breathing)	1.4	2.2	3.5	*1.1	1.6	2.7	*1.8	2.8	4.2
Antihyperlipidemic agents (high cholesterol)	*0.4	1.3	2.3	*	2.0	*2.8	*	*	1.8
Antihistamines (allergies)	2.5	3.9	1.9	1.8	3.6	*1.5	3.2	4.2	2.2
Thyroid hormones (hypothyroidism)	1.3	1.6	1.9	*	*	*0.8	2.1	2.8	3.1
ACE inhibitors (high blood pressure, heart disease)	0.7	1.4	1.8	*0.9	1.5	2.1	*0.6	*1.2	1.6
Antidiabetic agents (diabetes)	*1.0	1.5	2.1	*	*1.5	2.0	*1.0	*1.6	2.1
Muscle relaxants (muscle spasm and related disorders)	1.0	1.3	1.7	*1.3	*1.1	*1.5	*0.7	*1.4	1.9
Beta-adrenergic blocking agents (high blood pressure, heart disease)	1.1	*1.2	1.7	*0.9	*1.3	1.3	1.3	*	2.1
Nasal preparations (nose symptoms)	*0.6	1.5	1.5	*	*1.2	*1.1	*0.7	1.7	1.8
45 to 64 Years									
Antihyperlipidemic agents (high cholesterol)	4.3	13.8	23.8	4.4	17.2	26.3	4.2	10.7	21.4
Proton pump inhibitors (gastrointestinal reflux, ulcers)[2]	5.2	9.9	13.2	5.3	8.4	11.7	5.2	11.3	14.6
Antidepressants (depression and related disorders)	3.5	10.5	14.3	*2.3	7.0	9.6	4.6	13.8	18.6
Sex hormones (contraceptives, menopause, hot flashes)[4]	X	X	X	X	X	X	19.9	30.3	9.3
Analgesics (pain relief)	11.9	16.0	14.2	9.2	13.5	13.2	14.3	18.3	15.2
Beta-adrenergic blocking agents (high blood pressure, heart disease)	6.6	8.7	11.5	7.0	7.8	11.6	6.2	9.5	11.4
ACE inhibitors (high blood pressure, heart disease)	5.2	8.8	11.8	5.7	9.8	13.1	4.6	7.9	10.6
Antidiabetic agents (diabetes)	5.5	7.0	10.0	5.9	7.8	11.0	5.1	6.3	9.1
Thyroid hormones (hypothyroidism)	4.7	6.6	8.5	*1.2	*2.7	3.6	8.1	10.1	13.0
Antihypertensive combinations (high blood pressure)	5.3	5.6	8.0	3.3	*3.7	8.1	7.1	7.3	7.9
Anxiolytics, sedatives, and hypnotics (generalized anxiety and related disorders)	6.0	6.2	7.4	4.3	4.9	6.8	7.5	7.4	7.9
Diuretics (high blood pressure, heart disease, kidney disease)[3]	6.1	6.6	8.8	4.8	4.8	7.6	7.3	8.3	9.8
Anticonvulsants (epilepsy, seizure, and related disorders)	2.7	4.3	6.3	*2.5	3.5	5.5	2.9	5.1	7.0
Bronchodilators (asthma, breathing)	3.4	3.8	5.8	2.9	3.1	4.8	3.8	4.5	6.7
Calcium channel blocking agents (high blood pressure, heart disease)	7.0	6.7	5.4	8.2	5.9	5.9	5.9	7.5	5.0

Table 3-46. Selected Prescription Drug Classes Used in the Past 30 Days, by Sex and Age, Selected Years, 1988–1994 through 2009–2012— continued

(Percent.)

Age group and Multum Lexicon Plus therapeutic class[1] (common indications for use)	Total			Male			Female		
	1988–1994	1999–2002	2009–2012	1988–1994	1999–2002	2009–2012	1988–1994	1999–2002	2009–2012
65 Years and Over									
Antihyperlipidemic agents (high cholesterol)	5.9	23.4	46.8	5.3	24.3	51.9	6.4	22.7	42.8
Beta-adrenergic blocking agents (high blood pressure, heart disease)	11.8	15.9	31.2	10.4	17.5	32.6	12.8	14.8	30.0
Anticonvulsants (epilepsy, seizure, and related disorders)	16.2	19.2	21.6	12.2	17.1	19.4	19.1	20.7	23.3
ACE inhibitors (high blood pressure, heart disease)	9.5	16.9	23.3	9.8	18.0	28.8	9.3	16.1	19.0
Proton pump inhibitors (gastrointestinal reflux, ulcers)[2]	7.5	14.6	21.6	7.2	14.1	18.9	7.7	15.0	23.8
Antidiabetic agents (diabetes)	9.0	12.4	19.0	9.0	12.9	22.0	9.0	12.0	16.7
Anticoagulants or antiplatelet agents (blood clot prevention)[5]	6.1	9.1	16.3	6.8	11.5	20.3	5.6	7.4	13.0
Analgesics (pain relief)	13.8	18.4	15.8	11.4	15.0	14.5	15.6	20.9	16.9
Calcium channel blocking agents (high blood pressure, heart disease)	16.1	19.1	17.3	14.5	17.4	16.6	17.3	20.4	17.8
Thyroid hormones (hypothyroidism)	7.0	14.3	15.6	3.3	6.7	9.2	9.7	19.8	20.8
Antihypertensive combinations (high blood pressure)	9.6	9.8	13.1	6.0	7.4	9.2	12.2	11.6	16.3
Antidepressants (depression and related disorders)	3.0	9.3	15.0	*2.3	7.2	10.3	3.5	10.8	18.7
Angiotensin II inhibitors (high blood pressure, heart disease)	X	4.8	12.0	X	4.1	11.6	X	5.3	12.3
Antiarrhythmic agents (heart rhythm irregularities)	23.1	16.6	9.3	21.6	17.9	9.1	24.3	15.6	9.5
65 to 74 Years									
Antihyperlipidemic agents (high cholesterol)	7.3	26.2	45.8	6.2	26.6	49.4	8.1	25.9	42.6
Beta-adrenergic blocking agents (high blood pressure, heart disease)	11.3	14.8	26.2	10.6	16.0	29.4	11.9	13.9	23.3
ACE inhibitors (high blood pressure, heart disease)	9.6	17.2	21.9	10.6	18.1	28.5	8.9	16.4	16.0
Proton pump inhibitors (gastrointestinal reflux, ulcers)[2]	7.0	14.7	19.4	6.3	13.4	16.8	7.5	15.8	21.7
Antidiabetic agents (diabetes)	8.8	12.9	19.5	8.0	13.8	21.4	9.4	12.0	17.9
Diuretics (high blood pressure, heart disease, kidney disease)[3]	14.2	15.9	18.7	10.8	14.6	16.1	17.0	16.9	21.0
Analgesics (pain relief)	13.0	18.5	15.8	10.5	14.9	14.7	15.0	21.4	16.9
Antihypertensive combinations (high blood pressure)	8.1	8.0	13.1	4.8	*6.7	9.4	10.8	9.0	16.3
Anticoagulants or antiplatelet agents (blood clot prevention)[5]	5.4	6.7	11.3	6.3	9.8	16.0	4.6	*4.2	7.2
Antidepressants (depression and related disorders)	2.8	9.3	15.2	*2.3	5.8	10.8	3.1	12.1	19.1
Calcium channel blocking agents (high blood pressure, heart disease)	15.0	16.1	13.6	14.0	15.3	14.9	15.8	16.8	12.5
Thyroid hormones (hypothyroidism)	6.4	13.0	14.7	*3.4	*5.0	*8.5	8.9	19.7	20.2
Angiotensin II inhibitors (high blood pressure, heart disease)	X	4.2	11.2	X	*3.5	9.7	X	4.9	12.5
Antiarrhythmic agents (heart rhythm irregularities)	20.2	13.0	6.7	19.0	15.5	7.4	21.1	10.8	6.1
75 Years and Over									
Antihyperlipidemic agents (high cholesterol)	3.8	19.9	48.2	*3.5	21.1	55.7	4.0	19.2	43.1
Beta-adrenergic blocking agents (high blood pressure, heart disease)	12.5	17.3	37.9	9.8	19.6	37.6	14.1	15.8	38.1
Diuretics (high blood pressure, heart disease, kidney disease)[3]	19.2	23.2	25.4	14.7	20.5	24.5	21.9	24.9	26.1
ACE inhibitors (high blood pressure, heart disease)	9.3	16.4	25.3	8.5	17.7	29.2	9.8	15.6	22.6
Anticoagulants or antiplatelet agents (blood clot prevention)[5]	7.2	12.0	22.8	7.8	13.9	27.0	6.9	10.9	20.0
Proton pump inhibitors (gastrointestinal reflux, ulcers)[2]	8.3	14.6	24.6	9.0	15.3	22.1	7.9	14.2	26.4
Calcium channel blocking agents (high blood pressure, heart disease)	17.8	22.8	22.2	15.3	20.5	19.3	19.2	24.2	24.1
Thyroid hormones (hypothyroidism)	7.9	15.8	16.9	3.0	9.2	10.3	10.9	20.0	21.4
Analgesics (pain relief)	15.1	18.4	15.8	13.0	15.1	14.2	16.3	20.4	16.9
Antidiabetic agents (diabetes)	9.3	11.8	18.3	10.7	11.5	22.9	8.5	12.0	15.2
Antihypertensive combinations (high blood pressure)	11.9	12.0	13.2	8.3	*8.2	8.9	14.0	14.4	16.2
Antiarrhythmic agents (heart rhythm irregularities)	27.7	21.0	12.9	26.3	21.3	11.8	28.6	20.7	13.7
Angiotensin II inhibitors (high blood pressure, heart disease)	X	5.4	13.2	X	*4.9	14.6	X	5.8	12.2
Antidepressants (depression and related disorders)	3.4	9.3	14.7	*2.3	9.2	9.6	4.0	9.4	18.3

X = Not applicable.   * = Figure does not meet standards of reliability or precision. Data preceded by an asterisk have a relative standard error (RSE) of 20 to 30 percent. Data not shown have an RSE of greater than 30 percent.   1 The drug therapeutic class is based on the December 2012 Lexicon Plus, a proprietary database of Cerner Multum, Inc. Lexicon Plus is a comprehensive database of all prescription and some nonprescription drug products available in the U.S. drug market. Data on prescription drug use are collected by the National Health and Nutrition Examination Survey. Respondents were asked if they had taken a prescription drug in the past 30 days. Those who answered "yes" were asked to show the interviewer the medication containers for all prescriptions. If no container was available, the respondent was asked to verbally report the name of the medication. Each drug's complete name was recorded and classified. Data presented are based on the second level classification of prescription drugs. Up to four classes are assigned to each drug. Drugs classified into more than one class were counted in each class. Some drug classes were not available in 1988-1994 and are coded as not applicable.   2 The drugs classes proton pump inhibitors (272) and H2 antagonists (94) have been combined because of their similar indications for use.   3 This category includes carbonic anhydrase inhibitors which are primarily used to treat glaucoma.   4 Although sex hormones may be used by males, most are used by females. Therefore, data for sex hormones are only presented for females.   5 The drugs classes anticoagulants (82) and antiplatelet agents (83) have been combined because of their similar indications for use.

Table 3-47. Dietary Supplement Use Among Persons 20 Years of Age and Over, by Selected Characteristics, Selected Years, 1988–1994 Through 2005–2008

(Percent.)

Sex, age, race and Hispanic origin[1], and percent of poverty level	Any supplement use in past 30 days[2]			Any vitamin D supplement use in past 30 days[3]			Any folic acid supplement use in past 30 days[4]		
	1988–1994	2001–2004	2005–2008	1988–1994	2001–2004	2005–2008	1988–1994	2001–2004	2005–2008
20 YEARS AND OVER, AGE-ADJUSTED [5]									
Sex									
Both sexes[6]	42.1	53.1	50.9	28.4	38.8	38.0	30.3	38.6	37.5
Male	35.7	47.0	44.4	24.3	33.3	32.2	26.2	34.7	32.9
Female	47.8	58.7	56.9	32.2	43.8	43.4	34.2	42.3	42.0
Race									
Not Hispanic or Latino									
White only, male	37.5	51.4	48.7	26.1	36.8	35.8	28.2	38.4	36.6
White only, female	50.9	64.5	61.3	35.4	49.9	47.7	37.7	48.5	46.1
Black or African American only, male	29.5	32.3	31.0	18.5	20.3	22.6	18.2	22.1	23.0
Black or African American only, female	38.2	38.3	43.0	22.7	25.2	30.5	23.7	25.2	30.3
Mexican male	28.9	31.9	30.0	17.1	20.9	19.6	18.6	21.1	19.2
Mexican female	36.8	43.8	41.5	21.9	30.8	28.1	23.3	28.0	26.5
Percent of Poverty Level [7]									
Below 199 percent	30.0	37.1	33.5	16.8	24.2	23.2	18.3	23.4	21.7
100 percent to 199 percent	36.0	45.9	43.9	23.3	30.1	30.3	24.1	29.3	30.4
200 percent to 399 percent	44.0	52.5	52.5	30.2	39.8	39.4	32.5	39.1	38.8
400 percent or more	51.0	63.9	60.8	35.8	48.8	47.7	38.5	49.3	47.3
20 YEARS AND OVER, CRUDE									
Sex									
Both sexes[6]	41.8	52.7	51.3	28.4	38.6	38.3	30.3	38.4	37.8
Male	35.3	46.2	44.2	24.2	32.8	32.1	26.0	34.1	32.8
Female	47.7	58.8	57.8	32.2	43.9	44.1	34.3	42.4	42.5
Race									
Not Hispanic or Latino									
White only, male	37.4	51.5	49.7	26.0	37.0	36.4	28.1	38.6	37.3
White only, female	51.1	65.5	63.3	35.4	50.5	49.1	37.7	48.9	47.2
Black or African American only, male	28.9	31.0	30.3	18.8	19.4	22.6	18.5	21.0	22.7
Black or African American only, female	37.0	37.6	42.4	22.9	24.7	30.4	23.9	24.8	30.1
Mexican male	25.6	26.6	24.1	15.5	17.3	16.0	17.1	17.3	15.7
Mexican female	34.9	39.1	37.6	21.9	27.1	26.5	23.1	25.8	25.8
Percent of Poverty Level [6]									
Below 199 percent	29.4	34.9	31.9	17.1	23.2	22.4	18.4	22.5	21.2
100 percent to 199 percent	36.8	46.7	45.2	24.0	30.6	31.3	24.9	29.9	31.1
200 percent to 399 percent	43.6	52.2	53.1	30.4	39.6	39.9	32.7	38.9	39.1
400 percent or more	50.8	63.7	61.0	36.0	48.6	47.6	38.7	49.1	47.3
Male									
20 to 34 years	31.0	34.7	31.2	21.9	24.2	22.9	23.5	24.9	23.0
35 to 44 years	36.8	43.2	38.4	26.3	31.1	29.2	28.5	32.5	29.6
45 to 54 years	32.8	47.9	47.0	23.6	35.3	32.4	25.3	36.1	33.9
55 to 64 years	42.9	55.9	56.6	28.1	41.5	42.1	30.2	43.2	43.0
65 to 74 years	39.4	64.4	60.0	24.4	43.8	43.7	26.3	46.6	44.3
75 years and over	40.9	64.0	64.0	23.0	41.7	44.7	24.1	44.4	45.1
Female									
20 to 34 years	43.6	47.9	44.4	33.1	36.3	35.6	35.5	37.1	35.6
35 to 44 years	46.5	52.0	49.7	32.2	38.7	37.9	34.8	37.9	38.2
45 to 54 years	47.8	62.7	60.3	32.3	45.6	44.9	33.7	44.5	43.2
55 to 64 years	52.3	72.6	70.2	33.4	55.7	53.8	35.8	51.3	52.0
65 to 74 years	52.9	69.3	75.5	30.0	51.6	57.7	31.2	46.8	52.1
75 years and over	54.0	72.2	71.1	29.8	53.1	50.6	30.7	48.6	44.8

1 Persons of Mexican origin may be of any race.   2 Respondents were asked "Have you used or taken any vitamins, minerals, herbals, or other dietary supplements in the past 30 days? Include prescription and non-prescription supplements." To facilitate their response, respondents were shown a card with some examples of different types of dietary supplements. The question wording differs slightly on the earlier, 1988-1994, survey.   3 Includes supplements with vitamin D, cholecalciferol, calciferol, ergocalciferol, or calcitriol as an ingredient.   4 Includes supplements with folic acid as an ingredient.   5 Age adjusted to the 2000 standard population using five age groups: 20 to 34 years, 35 to 44 years, 45 to 54 years, 55 to 64 years, and 65 years and over.   6 Includes persons of all races and Hispanic origins, not just those shown separately.   7 Percent of poverty level is based on family income and family size. Persons with unknown percent of poverty level are excluded (5 percent in 2005-2008).

INPATIENT CARE

Figure 3-10. Percent of Persons with a Hospital Stay in the Past Year, by Age, 2013

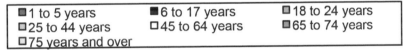

Figure 3-11. Average Length of Stay in Non-Federal, Short-Stay Hospitals, by Sex, Selected Years 1990–2009

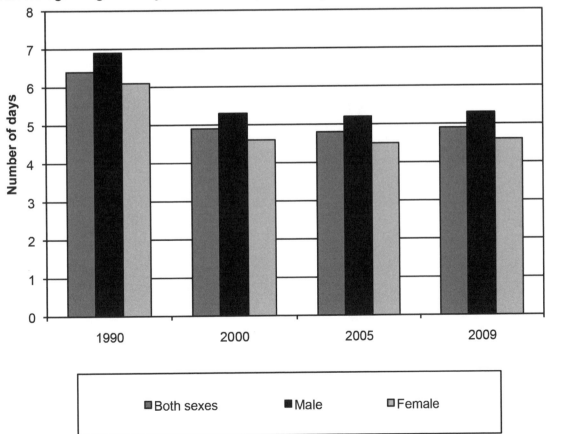

Table 3-48. Persons with Hospital Stays in the Past Year, by Selected Characteristics, Selected Years, 1997–2013

(Percent.)

Characteristic	One or more hospital stays[1]					Two or more hospital stays[1]				
	1997	2000	2005	2010	2013	1997	2000	2005	2010	2013
1 year and over, age-adjusted[2,3]	7.8	7.6	7.4	7.0	6.7	1.8	1.8	1.7	1.8	1.7
1 year and over, crude[2]	7.7	7.5	7.4	7.2	6.9	1.7	1.8	1.8	1.9	1.8
Age										
1 to 17 years	2.8	2.5	2.5	2.4	2.1	0.5	0.4	0.4	0.5	0.4
1 to 5 years	3.9	3.8	3.7	3.4	3.4	0.7	0.7	0.8	0.6	0.6
6 to 17 years	2.3	1.9	2.0	1.9	1.6	0.4	0.3	0.3	0.5	0.3
18 to 44 years	7.4	7.0	6.7	6.3	6.1	1.2	1.1	1.1	1.3	1.1
18 to 24 years	7.9	7.0	6.3	5.7	5.3	1.3	1.1	1.0	1.1	1.0
25 to 44 years	7.3	7.0	6.9	6.6	6.4	1.2	1.2	1.2	1.3	1.2
45 to 64 years	8.2	8.4	8.2	8.3	7.8	2.2	2.2	2.2	2.5	2.2
45 to 54 years	6.9	7.3	7.1	7.3	6.2	1.7	1.8	1.8	2.1	1.8
55 to 64 years	10.2	10.0	9.8	9.5	9.7	2.9	2.8	2.9	2.9	2.6
65 years and over	18.0	18.2	17.8	16.1	15.3	5.4	5.8	5.4	4.9	4.7
65 to 74 years	16.1	16.1	14.5	13.6	12.6	4.8	4.9	4.5	3.8	3.4
75 years and over	20.4	20.7	21.4	19.0	19.0	6.2	6.8	6.4	6.2	6.5
75 to 84 years	19.8	20.1	19.9	18.3	17.6	6.1	6.2	6.1	6.1	6.0
85 years and over	22.8	23.4	26.6	20.8	22.4	6.2	9.0	7.4	6.6	7.9
1 to 64 Years										
Total, 1 to 64 years[2,4]	6.3	6.1	5.9	5.7	5.3	1.3	1.2	1.2	1.3	1.2
Sex										
Male, crude	4.4	4.2	4.5	4.2	4.1	0.9	1.0	1.1	1.1	1.0
1 to 17 years	2.9	2.4	2.8	2.4	2.1	0.6	0.4	0.5	0.5	0.4
18 to 44 years	3.6	3.1	3.2	2.9	2.9	0.6	0.6	0.7	0.7	0.7
45 to 64 years	6.0	7.0	6.6	6.4	5.9	1.4	1.8	1.9	1.9	1.7
65 years and over	11.1	10.2	10.3	9.3	9.8	3.0	3.0	3.4	2.8	2.4
Female, crude	8.0	7.9	7.5	7.6	7.0	1.6	1.5	1.4	1.7	1.5
1 to 17 years	2.6	2.5	2.2	2.3	2.1	0.5	0.4	0.4	0.5	0.4
18 to 44 years	11.2	10.8	10.2	9.8	9.2	1.8	1.7	1.6	1.9	1.6
45 to 64 years	7.6	7.6	7.6	8.3	6.5	2.0	1.9	1.7	2.3	2.0
65 years and over	9.4	9.8	9.3	9.7	9.6	2.9	2.7	2.4	2.9	2.7
Race[4,5]										
White only	6.2	5.9	5.9	5.6	5.2	1.2	1.1	1.1	1.3	1.1
Black or African American only	7.6	7.4	6.6	6.7	6.2	1.9	1.9	1.8	1.9	1.8
American Indian or Alaska Native only	7.6	7.0	6.9	*7.6	8.9	*	*	*2.5	*2.4	*2.6
Asian only	3.9	3.9	3.9	3.6	3.6	*0.5	*0.6	*0.5	*0.4	0.6
Native Hawaiian and Other Pacific Islander only	NA	*	*	*	*	NA	*	*	*	*
Two or more races	NA	8.8	6.0	7.7	7.6	NA	*1.6	*1.9	*2.4	*1.7
Hispanic Origin and Race[4,5]										
Hispanic or Latino	6.8	5.5	5.4	5.2	4.8	1.3	0.9	1.2	1.1	1.1
Not Hispanic or Latino	6.2	6.1	6.0	5.8	5.4	1.3	1.3	1.2	1.4	1.2
White only	6.1	6.0	6.0	5.7	5.4	1.2	1.2	1.1	1.3	1.1
Black or African American only	7.5	7.4	6.6	6.7	6.2	1.9	1.9	1.7	1.9	1.8
Percent of Poverty Level[4,6]										
Below 100 percent	10.3	9.1	8.8	8.3	8.6	2.8	2.6	2.5	2.7	2.7
100 percent to 199 percent	7.3	7.3	7.4	7.0	6.0	1.7	1.9	1.9	1.9	1.6
200 percent to 399 percent	6.0	6.0	5.4	5.2	4.8	1.2	1.1	1.1	1.1	1.1
400 percent or more	4.7	5.0	4.8	4.5	4.2	0.7	0.8	0.8	0.8	0.6
Hispanic Origin and Race and Percent of Poverty Level[4,5,6]										
Hispanic or Latino										
Below 100 percent	9.1	7.4	7.6	7.3	6.4	2.0	1.6	2.0	2.0	2.0
100 percent to 199 percent	5.9	5.4	5.9	4.8	4.4	1.0	0.8	1.4	1.1	1.0
200 percent to 399 percent	5.9	4.6	4.4	4.3	4.3	1.1	0.7	0.8	0.7	0.8
400 percent or more	5.5	4.7	3.8	4.4	4.2	*1.1	*0.6	*0.6	*0.8	*0.6
Not Hispanic or Latino										
White only										
Below 100 percent	10.7	9.6	9.3	8.8	9.5	3.2	2.7	2.5	2.9	2.7
100 percent to 199 percent	7.7	7.8	8.2	7.8	6.9	1.8	2.2	2.0	2.2	1.9
200 percent to 399 percent	6.1	6.1	5.8	5.5	5.1	1.2	1.1	1.1	1.2	1.1
400 percent or more	4.7	5.0	4.9	4.6	4.2	0.7	0.8	0.7	0.8	0.6
Black or African American only										
Below 100 percent	11.4	10.8	9.4	9.4	9.4	3.3	3.4	3.1	3.1	3.6
100 percent to 199 percent	8.0	8.5	7.7	7.7	6.5	2.1	2.3	2.0	2.3	1.6
200 percent to 399 percent	6.2	6.1	5.2	5.3	4.5	1.5	1.3	1.3	1.4	1.2
400 percent or more	4.7	5.8	5.1	4.5	4.7	*0.9	*1.3	*1.2	*1.0	*1.0

Table 3-48. Persons with Hospital Stays in the Past Year, by Selected Characteristics, Selected Years, 1997–2013— continued

(Percent.)

Characteristic	One or more hospital stays[1]					Two or more hospital stays[1]				
	1997	2000	2005	2010	2013	1997	2000	2005	2010	2013
Health Insurance Status at the Time of Interview [4,7]										
Insured	6.6	6.4	6.3	6.2	5.7	1.3	1.3	1.3	1.4	1.2
Private	5.6	5.5	5.2	5.0	4.5	1.0	1.0	0.9	0.9	0.8
Medicaid	16.1	15.9	14.6	12.7	11.5	4.9	4.7	4.1	4.5	3.8
Uninsured	4.8	4.5	4.4	4.0	4.0	1.0	0.9	0.9	0.9	1.0
Health Insurance Status Prior to Interview [4,7]										
Insured continuously all 12 months	6.5	6.3	6.1	6.0	5.5	1.3	1.2	1.2	1.4	1.2
Uninsured for any period up to 12 months	8.5	8.4	9.0	7.9	7.5	1.8	1.9	2.4	1.9	1.9
Uninsured more than 12 months	3.8	3.5	3.2	3.0	3.3	0.8	0.8	0.6	0.8	0.9
Disability Measure Among Adults 18 to 64 Years [4,8]										
Any basic actions difficulty or complex activity limitation	14.1	15.1	15.2	14.3	14.2	4.1	4.4	4.9	5.2	4.6
Any basic actions difficulty	13.9	15.1	15.1	14.2	14.2	4.1	4.4	4.9	5.1	4.8
Any complex activity limitation	21.5	22.6	23.2	21.2	20.5	7.7	8.8	8.6	8.6	8.2
No disability	5.8	5.6	5.4	5.4	4.8	0.6	0.7	0.6	0.8	0.6
Geographic Region [4]										
Northeast	6.0	5.5	5.8	5.2	5.3	1.2	1.0	1.1	1.2	1.2
Midwest	6.5	6.3	6.3	6.3	5.6	1.5	1.3	1.3	1.5	1.3
South	6.8	6.6	6.3	6.0	5.7	1.4	1.5	1.4	1.5	1.3
West	5.4	5.2	4.8	4.9	4.5	0.8	0.9	0.8	1.1	0.8
Location of Residence [4]										
Within MSA[9]	6.1	5.8	5.7	5.5	5.2	1.2	1.1	1.2	1.3	1.1
Outside MSA[9]	7.0	6.9	6.8	6.9	6.3	1.6	1.5	1.4	1.6	1.7
65 Years and Over										
Total, 65 years and over[2,10]	18.1	18.3	17.8	16.2	15.7	5.4	5.8	5.4	4.9	4.9
65 to 74 years	16.1	16.1	14.5	13.6	12.6	4.8	4.9	4.5	3.8	3.4
75 years and over	20.4	20.7	21.4	19.0	19.0	6.2	6.8	6.4	6.2	6.5
Sex [10]										
Male	19.0	19.5	18.6	16.2	16.1	5.8	5.8	6.0	5.4	4.8
Female	17.5	17.4	17.3	16.2	15.4	5.1	5.7	4.9	4.6	5.0
Hispanic Origin and Race [5,10]										
Hispanic or Latino	17.3	16.6	17.7	13.9	15.1	6.2	6.4	5.7	5.0	4.9
Not Hispanic or Latino	18.2	18.4	17.9	16.4	15.7	5.4	5.8	5.4	4.9	4.9
White only	18.3	18.4	17.9	16.5	15.8	5.4	5.7	5.4	4.9	4.9
Black or African American only	18.9	19.8	19.0	16.9	18.2	5.5	7.5	6.3	5.5	5.8
Percent of Poverty Level [6,10]										
Below 100 percent	20.9	20.9	22.1	18.8	18.3	6.4	7.5	7.9	5.1	6.8
100 percent to 199 percent	19.6	19.2	19.2	17.2	18.3	6.5	6.6	5.9	5.2	6.0
200 percent to 399 percent	17.3	18.1	17.2	16.0	15.4	4.9	5.8	4.8	5.5	4.5
400 percent or more	16.6	16.0	16.1	15.0	13.4	4.7	4.2	5.1	4.1	3.9
Disability Measure [8,10]										
Any basic actions difficulty or complex activity limitation	22.6	24.7	24.1	20.2	20.2	7.2	8.6	8.3	6.4	7.1
Any basic actions difficulty	22.7	24.7	24.2	20.4	20.4	7.2	8.7	8.5	6.6	7.2
Any complex activity limitation	29.0	31.5	29.3	25.4	26.6	10.8	12.2	11.1	9.2	10.8
No disability	7.8	9.7	8.3	10.6	8.8	1.1	1.9	*1.6	*1.6	*1.6
Geographic Region [10]										
Northeast	17.2	16.6	16.1	16.5	15.2	5.1	4.5	4.5	6.1	5.1
Midwest	18.2	19.5	18.9	16.4	16.2	5.6	7.2	5.8	4.7	4.6
South	19.4	19.5	19.7	16.4	16.4	6.1	6.3	6.3	4.7	5.3
West	16.5	16.4	15.0	15.3	14.5	4.4	4.4	4.3	4.5	4.3
Location of Residence [10]										
Within MSA[9]	17.8	17.8	17.4	15.9	15.6	5.2	5.4	5.2	4.8	4.9
Outside MSA[9]	19.1	19.6	19.2	17.3	16.0	6.3	6.9	6.2	5.6	5.0

NA = Not available.   * = Figure does not meet standards of reliability or precision. Data preceded by an asterisk have a relative standard error (RSE) of 20 to 30 percent. Data not shown have an RSE of greater than 30 percent.   1 These estimates exclude hospitalizations for institutionalized persons and those who died while hospitalized.   2 Includes all other races not shown separately, unknown health insurance status, and unknown disability status.   3 Estimates are for persons 1 year of age and over and are age adjusted to the year 2000 standard population using six age groups: 1 to 17 years, 18 to 44 years, 45 to 54 years, 55 to 64 years, 65 to 74 years, and 75 years and over.   4 Estimates are for persons 1 to 64 years of age and are age adjusted to the year 2000 standard population using four age groups: 1 to 17 years, 18 to 44 years, 45 to 54 years, and 55 to 64 years. The disability measure is age adjusted using the three adult age groups.   5 The race groups White, Black, American Indian or Alaska Native, Asian, Native Hawaiian or Other Pacific Islander, and two or more races include persons of Hispanic and non-Hispanic origin. Persons of Hispanic origin may be of any race.   6 Percent of poverty level is based on family income and family size and composition using U.S. Census Bureau poverty thresholds. Missing family data were imputed for 1997 and beyond.   7 Health insurance categories are mutually exclusive. Persons who reported both Medicaid and private coverage are classified as having private coverage. Medicaid includes other public assistance through 1996. Starting with 1997 data, state-sponsored health plan coverage is included as Medicaid coverage. Starting with 1999 data, coverage by the Children's Health Insurance Program (CHIP) is included with Medicaid coverage. Persons not covered by private insurance, Medicaid, CHIP, public assistance (through 1996), state-sponsored or other government-sponsored health plans (starting in 1997), Medicare, or military plans are considered to have no health insurance coverage. Persons with only Indian Health Service coverage are considered to have no health insurance coverage. Health insurance status was unknown for 8 to 9 percent of children in 1993-1996 and about 1 percent in 1997-2011.   8 Any basic actions difficulty or complex activity limitation is defined as having one or more of the following limitations or difficulties: movement difficulty, emotional difficulty, sensory (seeing or hearing) difficulty, cognitive difficulty, self–care (activities of daily living or instrumental activities of daily living) limitation, social limitation, or work limitation.   9 MSA = metropolitan statistical area.   10 Estimates are for persons 65 years of age and over and are age adjusted to the standard population using two age groups: 65 to 74 years and 75 years and over.

Table 3-49. Discharges, Days of Care, and Average Length of Stay in Nonfederal Short-Stay Hospitals, by Selected Characteristics, Selected Years, 1980 through 2009–2010

(Rate per 10,000 population, number.)

Characteristic	1980[1]	1985[1]	1990	1995	2000	2005	2009–2010[2]
DISCHARGES PER 10,000 POPULATION							
Total, age-adjusted[3]	1,744.5	1,522.3	1,252.4	1,180.2	1,132.8	1,162.4	1,125.1
Total, crude	1,676.8	1,484.1	1,222.7	1,157.4	1,128.3	1,174.4	1,160.3
Age							
Under 18 years	756.5	614.0	463.5	423.7	402.6	411.0	336.2
Under 1 year	2,317.6	2,137.9	1,915.3	1,977.6	2,027.6	1,949.3	1,542.6
1 to 4 years	864.6	650.2	466.9	457.1	458.0	429.7	340.8
5 to 17 years	609.3	477.4	334.1	290.2	268.6	286.5	239.5
18 to 44 years	1,578.8	1,301.2	1,026.6	914.3	849.4	898.0	867.3
18 to 24 years	1,570.3	1,297.8	1,065.3	928.9	854.1	862.4	789.0
25 to 44 years	1,582.8	1,302.5	1,013.8	909.9	847.9	910.3	896.0
25 to 34 years	1,682.9	1,416.9	1,140.3	1,015.0	942.5	1,007.8	981.9
35 to 44 years	1,438.3	1,153.1	868.8	808.0	764.8	821.5	809.3
45 to 64 years	1,947.6	1,707.8	1,354.5	1,185.4	1,114.2	1,147.0	1,200.5
45 to 54 years	1,750.2	1,470.7	1,123.9	984.7	920.8	964.3	999.3
55 to 64 years	2,153.6	1,948.0	1,632.6	1,483.4	1,415.0	1,402.4	1,453.1
65 years and over	3,836.9	3,698.0	3,341.2	3,477.4	3,533.6	3,595.6	3,436.1
65 to 74 years	3,158.4	2,972.6	2,616.3	2,600.0	2,546.0	2,628.9	2,487.1
75 years and over	4,893.0	4,756.1	4,340.3	4,590.7	4,619.6	4,588.4	4,493.8
75 to 84 years	4,638.6	4,464.2	3,957.0	4,155.7	4,124.4	4,131.7	3,982.8
85 years and over	5,764.6	5,728.9	5,606.3	5,925.1	6,050.9	5,758.1	5,667.7
Sex[3]							
Male	1,543.9	1,382.5	1,130.0	1,048.5	990.8	1,013.0	975.3
Female	1,951.9	1,675.6	1,389.5	1,317.3	1,277.3	1,319.6	1,283.5
Sex and Age							
Male, all ages	1,390.4	1,240.2	1,002.2	941.7	910.6	959.0	957.4
Under 18 years	762.6	626.4	463.1	431.3	408.6	412.2	343.1
18 to 44 years	950.9	776.9	579.2	507.2	450.0	471.1	434.0
45 to 64 years	1,953.1	1,775.6	1,402.7	1,212.0	1,127.4	1,148.8	1,209.8
65 to 74 years	3,474.1	3,255.2	2,877.6	2,762.2	2,649.1	2,742.6	2,598.5
75 to 84 years	5,093.5	5,031.8	4,417.3	4,361.1	4,294.1	4,388.1	4,137.3
85 years and over	6,372.3	6,406.9	6,420.9	6,387.9	6,166.6	5,984.1	6,193.4
Female, all ages	1,944.0	1,712.2	1,431.7	1,362.9	1,336.6	1,382.2	1,357.1
Under 18 years	750.2	601.0	464.1	415.7	396.2	409.8	329.0
18 to 44 years	2,180.2	1,808.3	1,468.0	1,318.0	1,248.1	1,330.9	1,310.2
45 to 64 years	1,942.5	1,645.9	1,309.7	1,160.5	1,101.7	1,145.3	1,191.6
65 to 74 years	2,916.6	2,754.8	2,411.2	2,469.4	2,461.0	2,533.1	2,391.0
75 to 84 years	4,370.4	4,130.4	3,678.9	4,024.1	4,013.5	3,957.7	3,871.9
85 years and over	5,500.3	5,458.0	5,289.6	5,743.7	6,003.3	5,654.4	5,415.6
Geographic Region[3]							
Northeast	1,622.9	1,428.7	1,332.2	1,335.3	1,274.8	1,245.9	1,299.6
Midwest	1,925.2	1,584.7	1,287.5	1,132.8	1,109.2	1,174.9	1,146.8
South	1,814.1	1,569.4	1,325.0	1,252.4	1,209.2	1,202.5	1,136.1
West	1,519.7	1,469.6	1,006.6	967.4	894.0	1,005.9	932.7
DAYS OF CARE PER 10,000 POPULATION							
Total, age-adjusted[3]	13,027.0	10,017.9	8,189.3	6,386.2	5,576.8	5,541.7	5,369.2
Total, crude	12,166.8	9,576.6	7,840.5	6,201.7	5,546.5	5,620.9	5,598.7
Age							
Under 18 years	3,415.1	2,812.3	2,263.1	1,846.7	1,789.7	1,918.3	1,479.5
Under 1 year	13,213.9	14,141.2	11,484.7	10,834.5	11,524.0	12,131.6	9,170.4
1 to 4 years	3,333.5	2,280.4	1,700.1	1,525.6	1,482.2	1,355.3	1,111.0
5 to 17 years	2,698.5	2,049.8	1,633.2	1,240.3	1,172.1	1,300.9	990.5
18 to 44 years	8,323.6	6,294.7	4,676.7	3,517.2	3,093.8	3,305.0	3,147.4
18 to 24 years	7,174.6	5,287.2	4,015.9	2,987.4	2,679.5	2,819.9	2,687.1
25 to 44 years	8,861.4	6,685.2	4,895.5	3,676.4	3,225.5	3,472.8	3,316.3
25 to 34 years	8,497.5	6,688.9	4,939.7	3,536.1	3,161.7	3,434.3	3,342.6
35 to 44 years	9,386.6	6,680.4	4,844.8	3,812.3	3,281.5	3,507.9	3,289.7
45 to 64 years	15,969.5	12,015.9	9,139.3	6,574.5	5,515.4	5,717.3	6,058.0
45 to 54 years	13,167.2	9,692.8	6,996.6	5,162.0	4,374.2	4,711.2	4,719.7
55 to 64 years	18,895.4	14,369.5	11,722.6	8,671.6	7,290.8	7,124.0	7,739.0
65 years and over	40,983.5	32,279.7	28,956.1	23,736.5	21,118.9	19,882.8	19,225.8
65 to 74 years	31,470.3	24,373.3	20,878.2	16,847.0	14,389.7	13,985.3	13,504.6
75 years and over	55,788.2	43,812.7	40,090.8	32,478.1	28,518.6	25,939.4	25,602.5
75 to 84 years	51,836.2	40,521.6	35,995.1	28,947.5	25,397.8	23,155.3	22,884.1
85 years and over	69,332.0	54,782.4	53,616.9	43,305.9	37,537.8	33,071.5	31,848.6
Sex[3]							
Male	12,475.8	9,792.1	8,057.8	6,239.0	5,358.8	5,301.3	5,158.3
Female	13,662.9	10,340.4	8,404.5	6,548.8	5,809.7	5,828.7	5,630.6
Sex and Age							
Male, all ages	10,674.1	8,518.8	6,943.0	5,507.5	4,860.8	4,979.7	5,043.5
Under 18 years	3,473.1	2,942.7	2,335.7	1,998.0	1,955.7	2,006.2	1,555.6

Table 3-49. Discharges, Days of Care, and Average Length of Stay in Nonfederal Short-Stay Hospitals, by Selected Characteristics, Selected Years, 1980 through 2009–2010— continued

(Rate per 10,000 population, number.)

Characteristic	1980[1]	1985[1]	1990	1995	2000	2005	2009–2010[2]
18 to 44 years	6,102.4	4,746.6	3,517.4	2,729.7	2,175.0	2,282.7	2,036.6
45 to 64 years	15,894.9	12,290.1	9,434.2	6,822.7	5,704.4	5,773.5	6,327.1
65 to 74 years	33,697.6	26,220.5	22,515.5	17,697.4	14,897.4	14,502.6	14,462.9
75 to 84 years	54,723.3	44,087.4	38,257.8	29,642.6	26,616.7	25,106.9	24,184.6
85 years and over	77,013.1	58,609.5	60,347.3	45,263.6	37,765.3	35,179.0	35,211.1
Female, all ages	13,560.1	10,566.3	8,691.1	6,863.4	6,202.7	6,239.5	6,137.1
Under 18 years	3,354.5	2,675.5	2,186.8	1,687.9	1,615.1	1,826.1	1,399.7
18 to 44 years	10,450.7	7,792.0	5,820.3	4,297.9	4,010.8	4,341.8	4,283.0
45 to 64 years	16,037.1	11,765.5	8,865.1	6,341.7	5,336.4	5,663.9	5,801.9
65 to 74 years	29,764.7	22,949.2	19,592.7	16,162.0	13,971.3	13,549.0	12,678.4
75 to 84 years	50,133.3	38,424.7	34,628.3	28,502.5	24,601.0	21,830.1	21,949.6
85 years and over	65,990.5	53,253.6	51,000.5	42,538.6	37,444.4	32,103.5	30,236.0
Geographic Region [3]							
Northeast	14,024.4	11,143.1	10,266.8	8,389.7	7,185.9	6,636.5	7,072.6
Midwest	14,871.9	10,803.6	8,306.5	5,908.8	5,005.3	4,954.3	4,932.7
South	12,713.5	9,642.6	8,204.1	6,659.9	5,925.1	5,830.4	5,514.2
West	9,635.2	8,300.7	5,755.1	4,510.6	4,082.0	4,690.3	4,084.4
AVERAGE LENGTH OF STAY IN DAYS							
Total, age-adjusted[3]	7.5	6.6	6.5	5.4	4.9	4.8	4.8
Total, crude	7.3	6.5	6.4	5.4	4.9	4.8	4.8
Age							
Under 18 years	4.5	4.6	4.9	4.4	4.4	4.7	4.4
Under 1 year	5.7	6.6	6.0	5.5	5.7	6.2	5.9
1 to 4 years	3.9	3.5	3.6	3.3	3.2	3.2	3.3
5 to 17 years	4.4	4.3	4.9	4.3	4.4	4.5	4.1
18 to 44 years	5.3	4.8	4.6	3.8	3.6	3.7	3.6
18 to 24 years	4.6	4.1	3.8	3.2	3.1	3.3	3.4
25 to 44 years	5.6	5.1	4.8	4.0	3.8	3.8	3.7
25 to 34 years	5.0	4.7	4.3	3.5	3.4	3.4	3.4
35 to 44 years	6.5	5.8	5.6	4.7	4.3	4.3	4.1
45 to 64 years	8.2	7.0	6.7	5.5	5.0	5.0	5.0
45 to 54 years	7.5	6.6	6.2	5.2	4.8	4.9	4.7
55 to 64 years	8.8	7.4	7.2	5.8	5.2	5.1	5.3
65 years and over	10.7	8.7	8.7	6.8	6.0	5.5	5.6
65 to 74 years	10.0	8.2	8.0	6.5	5.7	5.3	5.4
75 years and over	11.4	9.2	9.2	7.1	6.2	5.7	5.7
75 to 84 years	11.2	9.1	9.1	7.0	6.2	5.6	5.7
85 years and over	12.0	9.6	9.6	7.3	6.2	5.7	5.6
Sex [3]							
Male	8.1	7.1	7.1	6.0	5.4	5.2	5.3
Female	7.0	6.2	6.0	5.0	4.5	4.4	4.4
Sex and Age							
Male, all ages	7.7	6.9	6.9	5.8	5.3	5.2	5.3
Under 18 years	4.6	4.7	5.0	4.6	4.8	4.9	4.5
18 to 44 years	6.4	6.1	6.1	5.4	4.8	4.8	4.7
45 to 64 years	8.1	6.9	6.7	5.6	5.1	5.0	5.2
65 to 74 years	9.7	8.1	7.8	6.4	5.6	5.3	5.6
75 to 84 years	10.7	8.8	8.7	6.8	6.2	5.7	5.8
85 years and over	12.1	9.1	9.4	7.1	6.1	5.9	5.7
Female, all ages	7.0	6.2	6.1	5.0	4.6	4.5	4.5
Under 18 years	4.5	4.5	4.7	4.1	4.1	4.5	4.3
18 to 44 years	4.8	4.3	4.0	3.3	3.2	3.3	3.3
45 to 64 years	8.3	7.1	6.8	5.5	4.8	4.9	4.9
65 to 74 years	10.2	8.3	8.1	6.5	5.7	5.3	5.3
75 to 84 years	11.5	9.3	9.4	7.1	6.1	5.5	5.7
85 years and over	12.0	9.8	9.6	7.4	6.2	5.7	5.6
Geographic Region [3]							
Northeast	8.6	7.8	7.7	6.3	5.6	5.3	5.4
Midwest	7.7	6.8	6.5	5.2	4.5	4.2	4.3
South	7.0	6.1	6.2	5.3	4.9	4.8	4.9
West	6.3	5.6	5.7	4.7	4.6	4.7	4.4

1 Comparisons of data from 1980–1985 with data from subsequent years should be made with caution because estimates of change may reflect improvements in the survey design rather than true changes in hospital use.   2 Starting with 2008 data, the sample of nonfederal short–stay hospitals was cut in half. This smaller sample size has increased standard errors. Therefore, caution should be exercised in interpreting trends in these data.   3 Estimates are age adjusted to the year 2000 standard population using six age groups: under 18 years, 18 to 44 years, 45 to 54 years, 55 to 64 years, 65 to 74 years, and 75 years and over.

Table 3-50. Discharges in Nonfederal Short-Stay Hospitals, by Sex, Age, and Selected First-Listed Diagnosis, Selected Years, 1990 through 2009–2010

(Numbers in thousands.)

Age and first-listed diagnosis	Both sexes			Male			Female		
	1990	1995	2009–2010[1]	1990	1995	2009–2010[1]	1990	1995	2009–2010[1]
ALL AGES [2]	30,788	30,722	35,599	12,280	12,198	14,461	18,508	18,525	21,139
Under 18 Years [2]	3,072	3,002	*2,506	1,572	1,565	*1,309	1,500	1,437	*1,197
Dehydration	63	106	*64	32	59	*35	31	47	*29
Acute bronchitis and bronchiolitis	114	170	*119	67	109	*73	47	61	*46
Pneumonia	221	250	*167	126	143	*84	95	107	*83
Asthma	182	227	*140	111	137	*88	71	90	*52
Appendicitis	83	69	*72	50	41	*45	34	28	*26
Injury	329	286	*173	210	171	*104	119	115	*69
Fracture	117	102	*76	76	66	*48	42	36	*28
Complications of care and adverse effects	41	46	*39	22	25	*21	19	*21	*18
18 to 44 Years [2]	11,138	9,996	9,746	3,120	2,761	2,465	8,018	7,235	7,280
HIV/AIDS	*20	88	24	*15	66	17	*	22	*7
Cancer, all	181	150	114	64	47	40	116	102	74
Childbirth	X	X	X	X	X	X	3,815	3,574	3,851
Uterine fibroids	X	X	X	X	X	X	110	115	84
Diabetes	105	102	159	61	52	79	44	50	81
Alcohol and drug	284	363	215	199	255	147	84	107	69
Schizophrenia, mood disorders, delusional disorders, nonorganic psychoses	384	551	541	184	262	271	200	289	271
Schizophrenia	145	*181	140	88	*118	84	57	63	56
Mood disorders	211	324	368	83	121	166	128	203	202
Heart disease	236	265	228	163	157	140	73	108	88
Ischemic heart disease	129	130	68	95	90	47	34	39	21
Pneumonia	136	149	107	69	74	51	67	75	56
Asthma	106	119	85	27	30	26	79	89	59
Intervertebral disc disorders	222	157	96	138	94	49	84	62	47
Injury	935	688	503	641	465	316	294	223	187
Fracture	302	250	203	217	176	142	85	74	61
Poisoning and toxic effects	124	118	125	54	59	55	70	59	70
Complications of care and adverse effects	135	146	187	63	64	74	72	82	113
45 to 64 Years [2]	6,244	6,168	9,585	3,115	3,053	4,710	3,129	3,115	4,874
HIV/AIDS	*3	20	16	*3	15	12	*	*5	*4
Cancer, all	545	461	497	236	193	244	309	268	253
Colorectal cancer	59	29	60	33	17	30	26	13	29
Lung/bronchus/tracheal cancer	101	76	62	60	37	28	41	39	34
Breast cancer[3]	X	X	X	X	X	X	69	61	47
Prostate cancer	X	X	X	19	32	*53	X	X	X
Uterine fibroids	X	X	X	X	X	X	70	74	95
Diabetes	134	172	255	65	86	128	70	86	127
Alcohol and drug	100	128	194	77	100	142	23	28	52
Schizophrenia, mood disorders, delusional disorders, nonorganic psychoses	152	194	379	56	75	169	95	118	210
Schizophrenia	47	*67	115	19	*	61	28	36	54
Mood disorders	91	112	242	32	37	97	58	74	146
Heart disease	1,100	1,152	1,162	704	749	730	397	403	432
Ischemic heart disease	739	762	544	502	537	371	237	225	173
Heart attack	233	256	210	165	188	147	68	68	63
Arrhythmias	131	131	197	79	75	121	53	56	76
Heart failure	122	143	254	68	75	145	54	68	109
Hypertension	75	82	143	38	37	69	37	45	74
Stroke	162	182	288	91	96	160	72	86	127
Pneumonia	154	163	261	76	75	135	79	88	126
Chronic obstructive pulmonary disease	73	154	231	39	72	94	34	82	137
Asthma	86	87	125	26	21	34	59	66	92
Osteoarthritis	87	110	491	36	47	211	51	64	280
Intervertebral disc disorders	145	115	162	82	65	82	63	51	79
Injury	334	296	450	178	165	242	157	131	208
Fracture	149	147	233	74	74	122	75	72	111
Poisoning and toxic effects	29	30	95	10	13	43	19	17	52
Internal organ injury	36	38	56	23	27	35	14	11	*21
Complications of care and adverse effects	148	186	398	79	92	199	69	94	199
65 to 74 Years [2]	4,689	4,832	5,251	2,268	2,290	2,540	2,421	2,542	2,711
Septicemia	49	65	150	27	27	76	21	38	74
Cancer, all	436	416	311	222	203	171	214	212	140
Colorectal cancer	48	46	35	24	22	20	24	24	15
Lung/bronchus/tracheal cancer	77	73	58	50	44	33	26	29	25
Breast cancer[3]	X	X	X	X	X	X	42	35	19
Prostate cancer	X	X	X	40	41	29	X	X	X
Diabetes	93	93	96	34	44	45	59	49	51

Table 3-50. Discharges in Nonfederal Short-Stay Hospitals, by Sex, Age, and Selected First-Listed Diagnosis, Selected Years, 1990 through 2009–2010— continued

(Numbers in thousands.)

Age and first-listed diagnosis	Both sexes			Male			Female		
	1990	1995	2009–2010[1]	1990	1995	2009–2010[1]	1990	1995	2009–2010[1]
Schizophrenia, mood disorders, delusional disorders, nonorganic psychoses	59	80	*62	20	20	*21	39	60	*41
Dementia and Alzheimer's disease	10	18	*18	4	11	*	*6	7	*9
Heart disease	1,000	1,115	860	547	618	498	453	497	363
Ischemic heart disease	576	614	359	331	365	229	245	250	131
Heart attack	185	210	131	110	129	81	75	82	50
Arrhythmias	124	153	180	67	74	97	57	79	82
Heart failure	188	233	198	93	126	110	95	107	88
Hypertension	39	42	61	13	14	*24	26	28	38
Stroke	222	250	231	108	141	124	114	109	107
Pneumonia	176	214	177	90	105	85	86	109	92
Chronic obstructive pulmonary disease	81	191	208	41	83	91	40	107	117
Gallstones	79	78	47	30	31	23	49	46	24
Kidney disease	18	31	121	9	16	70	9	15	51
Urinary tract infection	54	50	80	17	20	25	37	30	56
Hyperplasia of the prostate	X	X	X	113	62	21	X	X	X
Osteoarthritis	122	154	339	44	53	133	78	101	206
Injury	193	176	203	71	67	75	122	109	128
Fracture	120	109	126	36	36	37	85	72	88
Hip fracture	48	44	39	12	15	12	36	29	27
Complications of care and adverse effects	125	144	203	68	66	102	57	78	101
75 to 84 Years [2]	3,949	4,590	5,257	1,660	1,880	2,283	2,289	2,710	2,973
Septicemia	54	87	183	24	38	84	30	50	99
Cancer, all	300	281	227	158	131	109	142	150	119
Colorectal cancer	50	46	39	20	22	17	29	24	22
Lung/bronchus/tracheal cancer	36	32	44	22	17	22	*15	15	22
Breast cancer[3]	X	X	X	X	X	X	24	24	13
Prostate cancer	X	X	X	37	18	*6	X	X	X
Diabetes	44	73	88	17	30	37	27	43	51
Schizophrenia, mood disorders, delusional disorders, nonorganic psychoses	39	44	*	*10	10	*	28	35	*24
Dementia and Alzheimer's disease	20	46	58	9	19	26	11	26	33
Heart disease	865	1,057	976	377	471	466	488	585	510
Ischemic heart disease	382	479	328	177	228	173	205	251	156
Heart attack	156	188	149	83	91	70	73	97	78
Arrhythmias	133	175	223	58	83	92	76	92	131
Heart failure	261	290	291	108	116	137	153	174	154
Hypertension	23	31	50	*	*11	*17	19	20	33
Stroke	258	297	260	104	129	116	154	169	144
Pneumonia	224	282	237	112	142	107	112	140	130
Chronic obstructive pulmonary disease	55	143	173	34	63	83	22	80	91
Gallstones	48	55	52	20	22	22	28	33	30
Kidney disease	24	28	145	10	17	68	*14	12	77
Urinary tract infection	86	99	162	25	35	48	61	64	114
Hyperplasia of the prostate	X	X	X	69	41	21	X	X	X
Osteoarthritis	69	115	213	25	34	84	44	80	129
Injury	259	270	313	58	77	104	201	193	208
Fracture	195	208	219	35	53	62	161	154	158
Hip fracture	115	122	92	20	29	25	95	93	66
Complications of care and adverse effects	81	108	162	38	40	83	43	68	79
85 Years and Over [2]	1,694	2,134	3,256	543	648	1,153	1,151	1,486	2,102
Septicemia	41	57	150	12	17	60	29	40	90
Cancer, all	77	77	83	31	32	39	45	45	44
Colorectal cancer	14	17	10	*5	*	*4	9	11	*6
Lung/bronchus/tracheal cancer	*6	*4	*14	*	*2	*	*	*	*6
Breast cancer[3]	X	X	X	X	X	X	*9	8	*5
Prostate cancer	X	X	X	*7	*	*4	X	X	X
Diabetes	16	22	34	*5	*	13	11	15	*21
Schizophrenia, mood disorders, delusional disorders, nonorganic psychoses	*8	16	*	*	*	*	*8	*7	*12	*
Dementia and Alzheimer's disease	15	28	44	*2	*6	18	13	22	26
Heart disease	335	446	606	112	135	228	223	311	378
Ischemic heart disease	128	144	142	49	48	60	79	96	82
Heart attack	60	73	92	23	28	37	37	44	56
Arrhythmias	51	72	122	16	20	40	35	51	82
Heart failure	126	181	259	39	52	98	87	129	161
Hypertension	*5	8	28	*	*	*9	*4	*6	19
Stroke	129	156	163	35	42	52	95	114	111
Pneumonia	151	194	204	64	73	80	88	121	124

Table 3-50. Discharges in Nonfederal Short-Stay Hospitals, by Sex, Age, and Selected First-Listed Diagnosis, Selected Years, 1990 through 2009–2010— continued

(Numbers in thousands.)

Age and first-listed diagnosis	Both sexes			Male			Female		
	1990	1995	2009–2010[1]	1990	1995	2009–2010[1]	1990	1995	2009–2010[1]
Chronic obstructive pulmonary disease	13	39	83	*6	18	32	*7	21	50
Gallstones	18	21	23	*6	*7	*8	13	15	15
Kidney disease	14	16	96	8	*8	43	*6	*9	53
Urinary tract infection	65	74	185	20	*18	40	45	56	144
Hyperplasia of the prostate	X	X	X	13	9	*6	X	X	X
Osteoarthritis	13	20	40	*	*6	*10	8	14	30
Injury	164	216	302	37	47	80	127	169	222
Fracture	133	172	228	28	32	51	104	140	177
Hip fracture	82	108	122	19	19	29	63	88	93
Complications of care and adverse effects	29	29	73	11	*10	30	18	19	43

X = Not applicable.   * = Figure does not meet standards of reliability or precision. Data preceded by an asterisk have a relative standard error (RSE) of 20 to 30 percent. Data not shown have an RSE of greater than 30 percent.   1 Starting with 2008 data, the sample of nonfederal short-stay hospitals was cut in half. This smaller sample size has increased standard errors. Therefore, caution should be exercised in interpreting trends in these data.   2 Includes discharges with first-listed diagnoses not shown in table.   3 Shown for women only.

Table 3-51. Discharge Rate in Nonfederal Short-Stay Hospitals, by Sex, Age, and Selected First-Listed Diagnosis, Selected Years 1990 through 2009–2010

(Number per 10,000 population.)

Age and first-listed diagnosis	Both sexes			Male			Female		
	1990	2000	2009–2010[†]	1990	2000	2009–2010[†]	1990	2000	2009–2010[†]
All Ages, Age-Adjusted [2,3]	1,252.4	1,132.8	1,125.1	1,130.0	990.8	975.3	1,389.5	1,277.3	1,283.5
All Ages, Crude [3]	1,222.7	1,128.3	1,160.3	1,002.2	910.6	957.4	1,431.7	1,336.6	1,357.1
Under 18 Years [3]	463.5	402.6	*336.2	463.1	408.6	*343.1	464.1	396.2	*329.0
Dehydration	9.5	15.7	*8.6	9.4	17.2	*9.1	9.7	14.2	*8.0
Acute bronchitis and bronchiolitis	17.2	27.8	*16.0	19.6	31.4	*19.1	14.6	24.1	*12.7
Pneumonia	33.3	25.2	*22.4	37.0	25.7	*22.0	29.5	24.6	*22.7
Asthma	27.5	29.6	*18.7	32.7	34.8	*23.1	22.0	24.0	*14.2
Appendicitis	12.6	11.9	*9.6	14.6	13.0	*11.9	10.5	10.8	*7.2
Injury	49.7	33.6	*23.2	62.0	42.0	*27.2	36.8	24.8	*19.1
Fracture	17.7	13.8	*10.2	22.3	18.3	*12.6	12.9	9.0	*7.8
Complications of care and adverse effects	6.2	*7.3	*5.2	6.5	*7.9	*5.5	5.9	*6.6	*4.9
18 to 44 Years [3]	1,026.6	849.4	867.3	579.2	450.0	434.0	1,468.0	1,248.1	1,310.2
HIV/AIDS	*1.8	4.3	2.2	*2.8	5.8	3.1	*	2.8	*1.2
Cancer, all	16.6	10.5	10.1	11.9	7.3	7.0	21.3	13.7	13.3
Childbirth	X	X	X	X	X	X	698.6	645.2	693.1
Uterine fibroids	X	X	X	X	X	X	20.2	21.7	15.2
Diabetes	9.7	11.5	14.2	11.3	13.0	13.9	8.1	9.9	14.5
Alcohol and drug	26.2	29.7	19.2	37.0	39.1	25.8	15.5	*20.2	12.4
Schizophrenia, mood disorders, delusional disorders, nonorganic psychoses	35.4	*53.6	48.2	34.1	*53.2	47.6	36.7	*53.9	48.7
Schizophrenia	13.4	*14.4	12.4	16.4	*18.6	14.8	10.5	*10.1	10.0
Mood disorders	19.4	*35.9	32.8	15.4	*31.0	29.3	23.4	*40.9	36.3
Heart disease	21.7	21.8	20.3	30.2	26.6	24.6	13.4	17.0	15.8
Ischemic heart disease	11.9	9.9	6.0	17.7	14.2	8.3	6.3	5.6	3.7
Pneumonia	12.5	10.9	9.5	12.8	10.0	8.9	12.2	11.9	10.1
Asthma	9.8	9.0	7.6	5.1	5.4	4.6	14.4	12.6	10.7
Intervertebral disc disorders	20.5	12.5	8.5	25.6	14.5	8.6	15.4	10.4	8.4
Injury	86.2	45.8	44.8	119.0	62.3	55.7	53.8	29.4	33.6
Fracture	27.8	17.8	18.1	40.2	25.4	25.0	15.5	10.2	11.0
Poisoning and toxic effects	11.4	8.5	11.2	10.0	6.7	9.7	12.7	10.3	12.6
Complications of care and adverse effects	12.5	12.2	16.6	11.7	11.2	13.1	13.3	13.1	20.3
45 to 64 Years [3]	1,354.5	1,114.2	1,200.5	1,402.7	1,127.4	1,209.8	1,309.7	1,101.7	1,191.6
HIV/AIDS	*0.6	*3.2	2.0	*1.2	*4.9	3.0	*	*	*1.1
Cancer, all	118.3	62.9	62.2	106.3	62.1	62.6	129.5	63.6	61.8
Colorectal cancer	12.7	7.9	7.5	14.8	8.9	7.8	10.8	6.9	7.2
Lung/bronchus/tracheal cancer	21.8	6.9	7.8	26.8	8.6	7.2	17.2	5.2	8.3
Breast cancer[4]	X	X	X	X	X	X	29.0	14.2	11.5
Prostate cancer	X	X	X	8.5	9.6	*13.5	X	X	X
Uterine fibroids	X	X	X	X	X	X	29.3	35.6	23.3
Diabetes	29.1	33.1	32.0	29.1	37.4	32.9	29.2	29.0	31.1
Alcohol and drug	21.7	23.3	24.2	34.6	33.5	36.4	9.6	13.7	12.7
Schizophrenia, mood disorders, delusional disorders, nonorganic psychoses	32.9	42.7	47.5	25.4	*39.6	43.5	39.8	45.6	51.3
Schizophrenia	10.1	12.8	14.4	8.4	*14.4	15.7	11.7	11.3	13.2
Mood disorders	19.6	*26.9	30.4	14.5	*21.6	24.9	24.4	*32.0	35.6
Heart disease	238.7	203.6	145.6	316.8	264.0	187.5	166.1	146.4	105.6
Ischemic heart disease	160.3	126.4	68.2	226.1	177.3	95.4	99.2	78.2	42.3
Heart attack	50.6	38.8	26.4	74.4	58.7	37.8	28.4	19.9	15.4
Arrhythmias	28.5	25.1	24.7	35.5	31.8	31.1	22.1	18.7	18.6
Heart failure	26.4	31.4	31.8	30.7	33.5	37.3	22.4	29.3	26.6
Hypertension	16.3	19.0	17.9	16.9	17.6	17.6	15.6	20.3	18.2
Stroke	35.2	36.7	36.0	40.8	38.3	41.2	30.1	35.2	31.1
Pneumonia	33.5	35.3	32.6	34.0	34.2	34.7	33.0	36.4	30.7
Chronic obstructive pulmonary disease	15.8	30.8	28.9	17.4	30.8	24.1	14.3	30.8	33.5
Asthma	18.6	13.4	15.7	11.8	6.2	8.7	24.9	20.2	22.4
Osteoarthritis	18.9	24.0	61.5	16.3	20.8	54.1	21.2	27.0	68.4
Intervertebral disc disorders	31.5	21.2	20.3	36.8	22.5	21.2	26.5	20.0	19.4
Injury	72.5	47.9	56.4	79.9	51.2	62.2	65.6	44.7	50.8
Fracture	32.4	26.2	29.2	33.4	25.3	31.3	31.5	27.0	27.2
Poisoning and toxic effects	6.3	6.3	11.9	4.5	5.5	11.0	8.0	7.1	12.7
Internal organ injury	7.9	4.5	7.1	10.2	5.9	9.1	5.7	3.2	*5.1
Complications of care and adverse effects	32.0	34.5	49.8	35.6	36.3	51.0	28.7	32.7	48.7
65 to 74 Years [3]	2,616.3	2,546.0	2,487.1	2,877.6	2,649.1	2,598.5	2,411.2	2,461.0	2,391.0
Septicemia	27.2	35.6	71.3	34.9	40.1	77.9	21.2	32.0	65.5
Cancer, all	243.1	159.0	147.5	281.4	176.4	175.3	213.0	144.7	123.6
Colorectal cancer	27.0	22.8	16.6	30.6	29.9	20.1	24.1	16.9	13.5
Lung/bronchus/tracheal cancer	42.9	26.1	27.3	63.9	28.2	33.6	26.4	24.5	21.9
Breast cancer[4]	X	X	X	X	X	X	42.3	31.2	16.7
Prostate cancer	X	X	X	50.6	37.1	30.1	X	X	X
Diabetes	51.8	46.4	45.4	43.6	46.8	45.7	58.3	46.2	45.2

Table 3-51. Discharge Rate in Nonfederal Short-Stay Hospitals, by Sex, Age, and Selected First-Listed Diagnosis, Selected Years 1990 through 2009–2010— continued

(Number per 10,000 population.)

Age and first-listed diagnosis	Both sexes			Male			Female		
	1990	2000	2009–2010[1]	1990	2000	2009–2010[1]	1990	2000	2009–2010[1]
Schizophrenia, mood disorders, delusional disorders, nonorganic psychoses	32.7	37.1	*29.2	25.3	*34.2	*21.6	38.6	39.6	*35.7
Dementia and Alzheimer's disease	5.6	*11.2	*8.3	4.9	*16.2	*	*6.1	*7.0	*7.6
Heart disease	558.1	604.8	407.4	694.2	706.4	509.0	451.3	521.0	319.8
Ischemic heart disease	321.3	307.0	170.2	419.9	396.5	233.9	243.9	233.2	115.2
Heart attack	103.3	100.3	62.0	139.8	124.7	82.8	74.6	80.2	44.1
Arrhythmias	69.1	102.6	85.1	84.7	108.3	99.4	56.9	97.9	72.7
Heart failure	105.2	131.6	93.9	118.0	136.4	112.3	95.1	127.6	78.0
Hypertension	21.8	21.5	29.1	16.2	16.5	*24.3	26.2	25.5	33.2
Stroke	123.9	127.1	109.5	137.5	131.8	126.6	113.1	123.2	94.7
Pneumonia	98.1	121.3	83.8	113.6	127.7	86.8	85.9	116.1	81.2
Chronic obstructive pulmonary disease	45.3	102.3	98.5	52.6	102.6	92.8	39.6	102.0	103.4
Gallstones	44.2	33.4	22.2	38.2	30.2	23.6	48.9	36.0	21.1
Kidney disease	9.9	19.1	57.1	11.0	21.0	71.3	9.0	17.5	44.9
Urinary tract infection	30.2	25.5	38.0	21.7	19.7	25.4	36.9	30.3	49.0
Hyperplasia of the prostate	X	X	X	143.5	53.6	21.6	X	X	X
Osteoarthritis	68.0	101.4	160.7	55.2	103.1	136.4	78.0	100.1	181.7
Injury	107.7	101.5	96.4	90.7	83.8	77.1	121.1	116.2	112.9
Fracture	67.2	63.3	59.5	45.2	46.8	38.0	84.4	76.9	77.9
Hip fracture	26.7	26.4	18.3	15.3	*20.0	12.2	35.7	31.7	23.6
Complications of care and adverse effects	69.7	80.0	96.3	85.7	95.7	104.5	57.2	67.1	89.3
75 to 84 Years [3]	3,957.0	4,124.4	3,982.8	4,417.3	4,294.1	4,137.3	3,678.9	4,013.5	3,871.9
Septicemia	53.9	68.3	138.7	63.8	78.1	151.6	47.9	61.9	129.3
Cancer, all	300.3	194.0	172.3	420.8	211.0	197.3	227.6	182.9	154.3
Colorectal cancer	49.8	33.0	29.8	54.0	37.5	30.8	47.3	30.1	29.1
Lung/bronchus/tracheal cancer	36.5	27.0	33.5	57.2	32.2	40.5	*24.0	23.6	28.5
Breast cancer[4]	X	X	X	X	X	X	38.7	30.8	16.5
Prostate cancer	X	X	X	99.2	27.4	*11.1	X	X	X
Diabetes	44.3	63.4	66.9	44.8	68.1	67.5	44.0	60.3	66.5
Schizophrenia, mood disorders, delusional disorders, nonorganic psychoses	38.8	41.4	*	*27.3	*30.6	*	45.7	48.5	*31.3
Dementia and Alzheimer's disease	20.0	36.5	44.0	22.8	36.8	46.2	18.3	36.3	42.3
Heart disease	866.6	954.8	739.5	1,003.8	1,062.5	844.7	783.7	884.3	663.8
Ischemic heart disease	382.4	416.7	248.7	470.5	528.5	312.9	329.1	343.6	202.7
Heart attack	155.9	166.9	112.8	220.9	212.8	127.7	116.7	136.9	102.2
Arrhythmias	133.4	176.8	168.7	153.3	174.4	165.9	121.4	178.3	170.7
Heart failure	261.4	263.1	220.7	286.2	271.1	248.3	246.4	257.9	200.9
Hypertension	22.6	39.7	38.0	*	*28.4	*31.7	30.7	47.1	42.5
Stroke	259.0	255.5	196.9	277.7	278.4	210.6	247.7	240.6	187.1
Pneumonia	224.6	263.5	179.3	297.8	310.8	193.3	180.4	232.6	169.3
Chronic obstructive pulmonary disease	55.4	146.2	131.4	89.4	179.6	149.9	34.8	124.3	118.0
Gallstones	47.6	39.6	39.1	51.9	41.4	39.0	45.0	38.5	39.1
Kidney disease	24.5	37.6	110.2	27.6	48.7	123.9	*22.6	30.4	100.3
Urinary tract infection	86.0	85.6	123.0	66.6	72.5	87.6	97.8	94.2	148.5
Hyperplasia of the prostate	X	X	X	183.3	67.2	38.5	X	X	X
Osteoarthritis	68.6	100.6	161.4	65.2	76.5	152.6	70.7	116.4	167.8
Injury	259.1	229.1	237.0	153.4	171.7	189.0	323.0	266.6	271.5
Fracture	195.8	170.2	166.2	92.6	116.4	111.8	258.1	205.4	205.3
Hip fracture	115.2	99.0	69.4	53.7	68.6	45.6	152.4	118.8	86.5
Complications of care and adverse effects	81.5	101.4	123.1	101.4	136.0	150.8	69.4	78.8	103.2
85 Years and Over [3]	5,606.3	6,050.9	5,667.7	6,420.9	6,166.6	6,193.4	5,289.6	6,003.3	5,415.6
Septicemia	135.6	153.9	261.4	139.0	207.3	320.8	134.3	131.9	232.8
Cancer, all	254.0	194.5	144.0	370.6	250.5	209.0	208.7	171.5	112.8
Colorectal cancer	47.6	49.7	17.0	*59.1	*58.8	*20.7	43.2	45.9	*15.2
Lung/bronchus/tracheal cancer	*19.1	12.1	*25.0	*	*20.9	*	*	*8.5	*15.2
Breast cancer[4]	X	X	X	X	X	X	*41.7	*20.5	*12.0
Prostate cancer	X	X	X	*87.8	*49.3	*20.0	X	X	X
Diabetes	53.0	65.6	58.7	*53.5	*54.2	69.4	52.8	70.3	*53.6
Schizophrenia, mood disorders, delusional disorders, nonorganic psychoses	*27.9	*37.3	*	*	*	*40.6	*30.7	*43.0	*
Dementia and Alzheimer's disease	49.7	107.0	77.2	*28.9	94.3	96.2	57.7	112.2	68.0
Heart disease	1,107.0	1,298.2	1,054.7	1,320.3	1,407.4	1,224.2	1,024.1	1,253.4	973.4
Ischemic heart disease	423.0	427.2	246.9	581.6	534.4	323.5	361.3	383.2	210.2
Heart attack	199.8	251.1	161.0	274.2	296.0	197.1	170.9	232.7	143.6
Arrhythmias	167.2	232.4	212.3	189.6	247.1	213.2	158.5	226.4	211.9
Heart failure	416.7	480.4	451.7	460.5	455.7	528.8	399.7	490.5	414.7
Hypertension	*17.9	41.1	49.1	*	*18.3	*47.6	*19.3	50.4	49.8
Stroke	427.2	373.8	284.1	408.2	396.7	278.5	434.6	364.3	286.8
Pneumonia	501.0	514.9	355.3	753.7	607.8	429.2	402.8	476.8	319.9

Table 3-51. Discharge Rate in Nonfederal Short-Stay Hospitals, by Sex, Age, and Selected First-Listed Diagnosis, Selected Years 1990 through 2009–2010— continued

(Number per 10,000 population.)

Age and first-listed diagnosis	Both sexes			Male			Female		
	1990	2000	2009–2010[1]	1990	2000	2009–2010[1]	1990	2000	2009–2010[1]
Chronic obstructive pulmonary disease	44.1	130.9	144.0	*72.9	150.4	173.4	*32.9	123.0	129.8
Gallstones	60.7	39.2	39.7	*68.2	*29.7	*40.6	57.8	*43.1	39.3
Kidney disease	47.1	49.5	167.4	92.4	*68.1	230.5	*29.4	*41.9	137.1
Urinary tract infection	216.5	191.5	321.9	239.3	153.1	217.0	207.6	207.2	372.1
Hyperplasia of the prostate	X	X	X	158.6	*69.9	*31.8	X	X	X
Osteoarthritis	44.5	56.0	70.2	*	*	*54.9	35.8	57.3	77.6
Injury	542.0	545.5	525.3	435.4	355.6	428.4	583.4	623.5	571.7
Fracture	439.0	450.9	396.6	335.7	252.4	275.7	479.2	532.4	454.6
Hip fracture	272.3	275.1	211.6	224.4	146.5	155.4	291.0	327.9	238.6
Complications of care and adverse effects	96.6	79.1	127.1	132.3	90.5	160.0	82.7	74.4	111.4

X = Not applicable.   * = Figure does not meet standards of reliability or precision. Data preceded by an asterisk have a relative standard error (RSE) of 20 to 30 percent. Data not shown have an RSE of greater than 30 percent.   1 Starting with 2008 data, the sample of nonfederal short-stay hospitals was cut in half. This smaller sample size has increased standard errors. Therefore, caution should be exercised in interpreting trends in these data.   2 Estimates are age adjusted to the year 2000 standard population using six age groups: under 18 years, 18 to 44 years, 45 to 54 years, 55 to 64 years, 65 to 74 years, and 75 years and over.   3 Includes discharges with first-listed diagnoses not shown in table.   4 Shown for women only.

Table 3-52. Discharges with at Least One Procedure in Nonfederal Short-Stay Hospitals, by Sex, Age, and Selected Procedures, Selected Years, 1990 through 2009–2010

(Percent; rate per 10,000 population.)

Age and procedure (any listed)	Both sexes			Male			Female		
	1990	2000	2009-2010[1]	1990	2000	2009-2010[1]	1990	2000	2009-2010[1]
18 Years and Over									
Hospital discharges with at least one procedure, crude (percent)[2]	67.4	62.1	63.2	65.2	59.2	59.9	68.7	63.9	65.3
Hospital discharges with at least one procedure, age-adjusted[2,3]	1,020.1	859.9		882.2	701.4		1,176.4	1,026.2	
Hospital discharges with at least one procedure, crude[2]	1,006.4	856.8	900.0	788.1	648.4	697.8	1,205.9	1,049.8	1,091.3
Operations on vessels of heart	28.3	41.2	33.1	41.9	56.9	46.7	15.8	26.7	20.2
Coronary angioplasty or arthrectomy	14.0	26.2	23.2	20.5	34.9	31.7	8.0	18.1	15.1
Coronary artery stent insertion	X	21.7	20.5	X	28.7	28.0	X	15.3	13.5
Drug-eluting stent insertion	X	X	15.0	X	X	20.4	X	X	9.9
Coronary artery bypass graft (CABG)	14.1	15.0	9.9	21.2	21.8	15.0	7.7	8.7	5.1
Cardiac catheterization	52.1	57.8	43.1	68.3	72.1	53.0	37.4	44.6	33.7
Pacemaker	8.6	8.5	8.7	10.1	8.5	9.0	7.1	8.5	8.4
Carotid (neck arteries) endarterectomy	3.6	5.9	4.1	4.1	6.6	4.7	3.1	5.3	3.5
Endoscopy of small intestine	40.8	42.5	44.6	38.6	39.1	40.7	42.8	45.6	48.3
Endoscopy of large intestine	27.9	25.0	20.6	22.5	20.2	18.0	32.8	29.4	23.1
Gall bladder removal	27.9	19.6	18.2	16.5	13.3	13.1	38.2	25.5	23.0
Laparoscopic gall bladder removal	X	14.8	14.8	X	9.2	9.6	X	20.1	19.7
Treatment of intra-abdominal scar tissue	17.0	14.4	14.7	6.5	5.7	7.8	26.6	22.4	21.3
Reduction of fracture	27.6	24.9	23.2	27.3	22.0	20.0	27.8	27.7	26.3
Excision of intervertebral disc and spinal fusion	18.7	18.2	21.8	22.3	20.0	21.4	15.4	16.4	22.1
Total hip replacement	6.4	7.3	13.9	5.4	6.8	13.6	7.3	7.7	14.1
Partial hip replacement	4.8	5.0	13.1	2.0	2.3	10.9	7.3	7.6	15.1
Total knee replacement	6.7	13.8	28.8	4.9	11.0	21.6	8.4	16.4	35.6
CT scan	68.4	29.2	*17.0	68.6	27.4	15.7	68.2	30.9	*18.2
Arteriography and angiocardiography with contrast	59.7	63.0	53.8	75.6	76.2	63.4	45.2	50.7	44.8
Diagnostic ultrasound	72.3	36.9	34.9	62.1	33.1	33.9	81.7	40.4	35.9
Magnetic resonance imaging	9.5	9.2	9.8	9.4	8.2	9.0	9.6	10.2	*10.6
Mechanical ventilation	17.6	23.0	32.4	18.8	23.9	34.0	16.4	22.1	30.9
18 to 44 Years									
Hospital discharges with at least one procedure, crude (percent)[2]	73.0	71.7	72.4	62.6	55.9	53.7	77.0	77.4	78.7
Hospital discharges with at least one procedure[2]	749.3	609.1	627.6	362.8	251.6	233.3	1,130.6	965.9	1,030.6
Operations on vessels of heart	3.0	3.9	2.8	4.9	5.5	4.1	*1.2	2.3	*1.5
Coronary angioplasty or arthrectomy	1.9	3.0	*2.3	3.0	4.3	3.4	*0.8	1.6	*1.2
Coronary artery stent insertion	X	2.5	*2.0	X	3.6	*2.9	X	1.4	*1.1
Drug-eluting stent insertion	X	X	*1.5	X	X	*2.1	X	X	*
Coronary artery bypass graft (CABG)	1.0	0.9	*0.5	*1.8	1.1	*0.8	*	*0.7	*
Cardiac catheterization	9.0	8.5	6.3	12.5	11.0	8.3	5.5	5.9	4.3
Endoscopy of small intestine	13.1	10.3	14.7	13.2	10.4	11.4	13.0	10.2	18.0
Endoscopy of large intestine.	6.9	5.5	6.2	5.6	4.7	5.3	8.1	6.3	7.0
Gall bladder removal	18.7	11.9	12.8	6.2	4.3	5.1	31.0	19.4	20.7
Laparoscopic gall bladder removal	X	9.9	11.0	X	3.0	3.7	X	16.8	18.4
Treatment of intra-abdominal scar tissue	14.1	10.8	10.5	2.0	1.5	*2.5	26.0	20.1	18.6
Hysterectomy	X	X	X	X	X	X	63.3	55.7	38.0
Abdominal hysterectomy	X	X	X	X	X	X	47.1	34.6	21.3
Vaginal hysterectomy	X	X	X	X	X	X	15.8	19.1	*12.3
Forceps, vacuum, and breech delivery	X	X	X	X	X	X	77.5	59.9	*43.9
Episiotomy	X	X	X	X	X	X	293.3	160.8	53.6
Other procedures inducing or assisting delivery	X	X	X	X	X	X	387.9	384.2	422.6
Medical induction of labor	X	X	X	X	X	X	41.1	77.7	125.9
Cesarean section	X	X	X	X	X	X	167.1	149.5	233.5
Reduction of fracture	19.1	13.7	11.6	27.9	19.0	15.3	10.4	8.4	7.9
Excision of intervertebral disc and spinal fusion	17.0	14.1	10.7	21.5	16.2	10.3	12.6	12.1	11.0
CT scan	27.5	10.6	*6.6	32.3	11.0	*6.1	22.7	10.3	*7.1
Arteriography and angiocardiography with contrast	12.5	10.3	9.1	17.4	12.9	9.9	7.6	7.7	8.2
Diagnostic ultrasound	34.2	11.6	10.0	19.3	8.3	7.2	48.9	14.9	12.8
Magnetic resonance imaging	4.9	3.8	*4.1	4.9	3.6	*2.9	4.9	*4.0	*5.4
Mechanical ventilation	4.6	7.0	9.9	5.4	8.2	11.2	3.8	5.8	8.6

Table 3-52. Discharges with at Least One Procedure in Nonfederal Short-Stay Hospitals, by Sex, Age, and Selected Procedures, Selected Years, 1990 through 2009–2010— continued

(Percent; rate per 10,000 population.)

Age and procedure (any listed)	Both sexes			Male			Female		
	1990	2000	2009-2010†	1990	2000	2009-2010†	1990	2000	2009-2010†
45 to 64 Years									
Hospital discharges with at least one procedure, crude (percent)²	68.2	62.3	63.0	68.9	63.4	63.3	67.6	61.3	62.8
Hospital discharges with at least one procedure²	924.2	694.6	756.7	965.9	714.4	766.2	885.4	675.9	747.7
Operations on vessels of heart	53.0	57.7	40.0	83.2	88.5	59.5	24.8	28.4	21.4
Coronary angioplasty or arthrecto-my	29.4	37.5	28.9	45.3	55.9	42.7	14.5	20.0	15.8
Coronary artery stent insertion	X	31.1	25.4	X	46.5	37.5	X	16.5	13.8
Drug-eluting stent insertion	X	X	18.7	X	X	27.5	X	X	10.2
Coronary artery bypass graft (CABG)	23.4	20.3	11.1	37.5	32.5	16.9	10.3	8.6	*5.5
Cardiac catheterization	98.2	83.0	54.4	136.8	113.9	72.3	62.3	53.7	37.2
Pacemaker	7.8	4.0	3.2	10.9	5.2	4.2	*4.9	2.8	*2.3
Carotid (neck arteries) endarterec-tomy	4.0	5.2	3.1	5.2	5.2	3.6	3.0	*5.2	*2.7
Endoscopy of small intestine	45.0	36.4	43.2	46.3	40.7	42.2	43.8	32.3	44.2
Endoscopy of large intestine	28.5	19.3	18.0	25.4	18.1	15.9	31.4	20.4	20.0
Gall bladder removal	36.4	20.6	18.0	22.3	16.3	13.8	49.5	24.6	21.9
Laparoscopic gall bladder removal	X	15.3	14.6	X	12.1	10.6	X	18.5	18.5
Treatment of intra-abdominal scar tissue	17.1	15.0	13.8	9.5	7.0	8.2	24.2	22.6	19.1
Removal of prostate	X	X	X	35.8	15.6	16.9	X	X	X
Transurethral prostatectomy	X	X	X	30.4	7.0	3.3	X	X	X
Hysterectomy	X	X	X	X	X	X	76.4	78.2	54.1
Abdominal hysterectomy	X	X	X	X	X	X	58.4	53.2	32.1
Vaginal hysterectomy	X	X	X	X	X	X	17.6	21.6	15.4
Reduction of fracture	20.3	18.5	18.2	19.5	17.6	18.1	21.0	19.3	18.3
Excision of intervertebral disc and spinal fusion	26.1	25.7	30.8	29.4	27.1	31.3	23.1	24.4	30.2
Total hip replacement	6.2	8.1	18.0	5.7	9.1	19.0	6.5	7.2	17.1
Partial hip replacement	*	*1.3	*13.8	*	*0.8	*13.7	*	*1.7	*13.8
Total knee replacement	6.7	12.7	37.1	5.8	8.7	27.8	*7.4	16.4	46.0
Mastectomy	X	X	X	X	X	X	21.2	10.6	9.3
CT scan	65.4	25.2	*17.1	69.9	25.9	17.4	61.2	24.5	*16.9
Arteriography and angiocardiogra-phy with contrast	105.4	85.3	64.3	138.5	111.4	83.3	74.6	60.7	46.3
Diagnostic ultrasound	69.5	34.3	31.8	73.8	38.0	36.3	65.5	30.9	27.5
Magnetic resonance imaging	10.9	8.9	9.2	10.7	9.4	9.2	11.0	8.4	9.2
Mechanical ventilation	17.6	21.2	32.9	18.6	22.9	34.4	16.7	19.6	31.5
65 to 74 Years									
Hospital discharges with at least one procedure, crude (percent)²	66.5	61.3	63.2	69.3	63.9	64.6	63.8	58.9	62.0
Hospital discharges with at least one procedure²	1,739.4	1,559.8	1,573.0	1,994.1	1,692.3	1,678.0	1,539.4	1,450.6	1,482.5
Operations on vessels of heart	97.0	139.8	104.2	148.9	195.3	152.6	56.3	94.1	62.4
Coronary angioplasty or arthrecto-my	44.1	86.3	69.4	64.9	116.0	96.6	27.8	61.9	45.9
Coronary artery stent insertion	X	71.7	61.1	X	94.9	83.3	X	52.5	42.0
Drug-eluting stent insertion	X	X	46.1	X	X	62.5	X	X	32.1
Coronary artery bypass graft (CABG)	52.1	53.9	34.7	83.1	79.7	55.9	27.7	32.6	16.5
Cardiac catheterization	164.0	174.2	120.4	213.8	222.7	153.7	124.9	134.2	91.7
Pacemaker	24.6	22.5	18.6	32.1	22.8	18.1	18.7	22.3	19.0
Carotid (neck arteries) endarterec-tomy	14.6	24.1	15.6	18.0	29.5	21.8	11.9	19.6	*10.3
Endoscopy of small intestine	92.8	106.6	93.2	91.5	102.4	99.0	93.7	110.0	88.2
Endoscopy of large intestine	70.3	64.8	44.3	62.5	59.7	41.6	76.5	69.0	46.7
Gall bladder removal	45.0	42.1	30.0	42.0	37.9	31.9	47.4	45.5	28.3
Laparoscopic gall bladder removal	X	29.5	22.0	X	24.4	21.2	X	33.7	22.6
Treatment of intra-abdominal scar tissue	23.1	21.4	29.0	17.1	14.5	24.3	27.7	27.1	33.0
Removal of prostate	X	X	X	201.1	83.7	50.8	X	X	X
Transurethral prostatectomy	X	X	X	180.9	59.4	24.1	X	X	X
Hysterectomy	X	X	X	X	X	X	37.4	35.9	30.2
Abdominal hysterectomy	X	X	X	X	X	X	20.8	20.5	15.0
Vaginal hysterectomy	X	X	X	X	X	X	16.5	14.7	*14.1
Reduction of fracture	36.2	36.4	32.9	24.3	26.2	18.4	45.5	44.8	45.5
Excision of intervertebral disc and spinal fusion	16.3	21.1	42.1	14.2	22.5	39.2	18.0	20.0	*44.5
Total hip replacement	24.0	25.4	39.3	23.0	26.4	37.1	24.9	24.5	41.2
Partial hip replacement	8.9	7.6	*25.3	*4.0	*	*19.1	*12.7	10.5	*30.7
Total knee replacement	33.2	65.4	108.3	26.4	64.5	84.0	38.6	66.0	129.3
Mastectomy	X	X	X	X	X	X	30.7	22.7	*12.9

Table 3-52. Discharges with at Least One Procedure in Nonfederal Short-Stay Hospitals, by Sex, Age, and Selected Procedures, Selected Years, 1990 through 2009–2010— continued

(Percent; rate per 10,000 population.)

Age and procedure (any listed)	Both sexes			Male			Female		
	1990	2000	2009-2010¹	1990	2000	2009-2010¹	1990	2000	2009-2010¹
CT scan	153.7	64.3	*29.4	163.4	65.7	*31.1	146.1	63.1	*27.9
Arteriography and angiocardiography with contrast	184.5	186.2	146.5	239.0	231.9	186.7	141.7	148.5	111.9
Diagnostic ultrasound	155.2	92.7	79.8	165.2	94.1	85.6	147.4	91.6	74.8
Magnetic resonance imaging	20.6	17.2	*18.3	19.2	*14.6	18.9	21.7	*19.3	*17.8
Mechanical ventilation	48.6	60.0	79.9	58.7	70.3	90.7	40.6	51.6	70.7
75 to 84 Years									
Hospital discharges with at least one procedure, crude (percent)²	59.0	53.6	56.4	61.7	56.3	59.0	57.0	51.8	54.5
Hospital discharges with at least one procedure²	2,332.9	2,212.3	2,247.8	2,723.9	2,416.5	2,441.4	2,096.7	2,078.8	2,108.7
Operations on vessels of heart	69.1	143.2	126.0	107.6	202.5	189.8	45.8	104.5	80.2
Coronary angioplasty or arthrectomy	22.4	84.7	82.7	33.7	109.3	116.8	15.7	68.7	58.2
Coronary artery stent insertion	X	69.8	75.3	X	86.5	107.5	X	58.8	52.2
Drug-eluting stent insertion	X	X	54.7	X	X	77.5	X	X	38.2
Coronary artery bypass graft (CABG)	47.0	57.7	42.7	74.7	90.5	*72.3	30.3	36.2	*21.5
Cardiac catheterization	116.6	190.2	149.3	166.0	236.9	179.9	86.8	159.6	127.4
Pacemaker	50.8	58.1	60.0	70.6	72.2	84.9	38.8	48.9	42.1
Carotid (neck arteries) endarterectomy	19.8	32.8	23.7	24.2	45.5	29.6	*17.1	24.5	19.5
Endoscopy of small intestine	171.4	189.7	166.0	188.9	193.8	164.2	160.8	187.0	167.3
Endoscopy of large intestine	131.1	123.7	87.9	126.1	113.8	83.9	134.1	130.1	90.7
Gall bladder removal	51.8	43.4	43.6	64.4	46.7	50.5	44.2	41.3	38.7
Laparoscopic gall bladder removal	X	28.9	35.9	X	29.6	39.2	X	28.5	33.6
Treatment of intra-abdominal scar tissue	34.0	28.6	30.2	28.2	26.3	28.7	37.5	30.2	31.3
Removal of prostate	X	X	X	273.5	98.0	41.2	X	X	X
Transurethral prostatectomy	X	X	X	257.5	89.0	36.6	X	X	X
Hysterectomy	X	X	X	X	X	X	28.5	25.5	18.5
Abdominal hysterectomy	X	X	X	X	X	X	18.8	16.2	*11.1
Vaginal hysterectomy	X	X	X	X	X	X	*9.4	8.1	*5.6
Reduction of fracture	86.2	80.1	68.1	43.4	57.2	46.0	112.1	95.0	84.0
Excision of intervertebral disc and spinal fusion	12.0	17.4	36.5	*13.2	*20.4	*39.9	11.3	15.3	34.0
Total hip replacement	30.7	26.3	49.4	*26.9	*21.3	47.2	33.1	29.6	51.1
Partial hip replacement	43.6	36.6	37.9	*14.3	20.0	*29.9	61.2	47.5	43.7
Total knee replacement	28.4	59.3	86.2	*19.5	48.7	80.4	33.9	66.3	90.4
Mastectomy	X	X	X	X	X	X	29.2	22.0	*11.3
CT scan	279.7	119.2	*55.2	307.2	127.9	*51.0	263.0	113.5	*58.3
Arteriography and angiocardiography with contrast	141.0	219.2	187.8	192.3	287.9	223.3	109.9	174.3	162.2
Diagnostic ultrasound	273.5	134.1	122.0	315.7	142.8	137.7	248.0	128.4	110.8
Magnetic resonance imaging	30.5	*37.3	*37.6	43.0	*33.6	*44.0	*23.0	*39.8	*33.0
Mechanical ventilation	79.8	91.1	102.0	110.3	106.5	119.5	61.3	80.9	89.5
85 Years and Over									
Hospital discharges with at least one procedure, crude (percent)²	49.3	44.6	46.8	52.4	45.4	50.5	47.8	44.3	44.7
Hospital discharges with at least one procedure²	2,762.1	2,700.5	2,650.6	3,367.3	2,797.9	3,125.0	2,526.8	2,660.6	2,423.0
Operations on vessels of heart	*14.0	51.1	55.5	*	83.0	98.6	*	38.0	34.8
Coronary angioplasty or arthrectomy	*	36.3	44.6	*	*52.9	74.6	*	29.5	*30.2
Coronary artery stent insertion	X	31.6	40.0	X	*48.9	66.6	X	*24.4	*27.2
Drug-eluting stent insertion	X	X	22.7	X	X	*36.9	X	X	*15.8
Coronary artery bypass graft (CABG)	*	*15.1	*10.1	*	*30.1	*22.5	*	*9.0	*4.2
Cardiac catheterization	*23.7	87.7	78.5	*	122.8	111.7	*19.0	73.2	62.6
Pacemaker	79.5	82.9	89.3	120.4	104.3	100.6	63.5	74.2	84.0
Carotid (neck arteries) endarterectomy	*	*12.0	*	*	*	*7.1	*	*4.8	*
Endoscopy of small intestine	228.8	262.4	192.2	288.7	245.1	228.5	205.5	269.5	174.7
Endoscopy of large intestine	180.8	158.1	98.1	188.0	133.3	128.9	178.0	168.3	83.4
Gall bladder removal	46.4	40.9	23.0	*68.4	*42.9	*30.2	37.8	*40.1	*19.5
Laparoscopic gall bladder removal	X	*30.4	15.4	X	*	*	X	*30.5	*14.0
Treatment of intra-abdominal scar tissue	29.6	24.3	23.0	*	*16.4	*13.9	33.7	*27.5	*27.4
Removal of prostate	X	X	X	257.2	*113.0	42.7	X	X	X
Transurethral prostatectomy	X	X	X	247.1	*110.0	41.8	X	X	X
Hysterectomy	X	X	X	X	X	X	*	*	*
Abdominal hysterectomy	X	X	X	X	X	X	*	*	*
Vaginal hysterectomy	X	X	X	X	X	X	*	*	*

Table 3-52. Discharges with at Least One Procedure in Nonfederal Short-Stay Hospitals, by Sex, Age, and Selected Procedures, Selected Years, 1990 through 2009–2010— continued

(Percent; rate per 10,000 population.)

Age and procedure (any listed)	Both sexes			Male			Female		
	1990	2000	2009-2010[1]	1990	2000	2009-2010[1]	1990	2000	2009-2010[1]
Reduction of fracture	196.2	200.5	180.3	150.6	93.8	132.8	213.9	244.3	203.0
Excision of intervertebral disc and spinal fusion	*	*2.3	*6.2	*	*	*	*	*	*
Total hip replacement	*27.8	*20.7	*25.5	*	*	*	*23.2	*26.3	*21.6
Partial hip replacement	67.4	82.2	77.1	*52.9	*44.1	66.2	73.1	97.9	82.3
Total knee replacement	*12.4	*22.9	34.0	*	*	*31.3	*	*16.2	35.3
Mastectomy	X	X	X	X	X	X	*28.9	*15.7	*
CT scan	378.4	158.7	*84.9	401.2	141.4	*84.8	369.5	165.9	*85.0
Arteriography and angiocardiography with contrast	50.6	120.8	135.6	*87.6	164.4	161.9	36.2	102.8	123.0
Diagnostic ultrasound	327.7	208.5	200.6	394.5	181.4	216.3	301.7	219.6	193.1
Magnetic resonance imaging	*18.5	*40.4	*35.7	*	*	*35.9	*16.2	*	*
Mechanical ventilation	91.5	106.0	130.3	97.9	116.5	172.2	89.1	101.7	110.2

X = Not applicable.   * = Figure does not meet standards of reliability or precision. Data preceded by an asterisk have a relative standard error (RSE) of 20 to 30 percent. Data not shown have an RSE of greater than 30 percent.   1 Starting with 2008 data, the sample of nonfederal short-stay hospitals was cut in half. This smaller sample size has increased standard errors. Therefore, caution should be exercised in interpreting trends in these data.   2 Includes discharges for procedures not shown separately.   3 Estimates are age-adjusted to the year 2000 standard population using five age groups: 18 to 44 years, 45 to 54 years, 55 to 64 years, 65 to 74 years, and 75 years and over.

HEALTH PERSONNEL

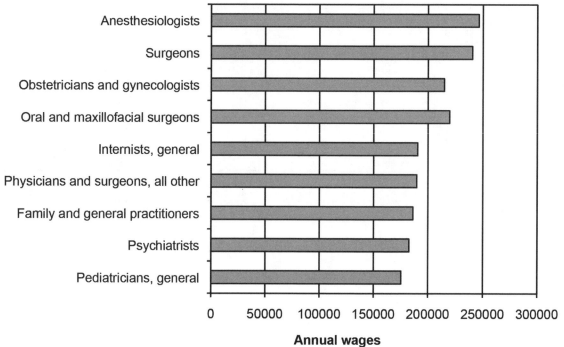

Figure 3-12. Annual Wages for Selected Specialties in Medicine, 2014

Table 3-53. Health Care Employment and Wages, by Selected Occupations, Selected Years, 2001–2013

(Number; dollars.)

Occupation title	Employment[1]					Mean hourly wage (dollars)[2]				
	2001	2005	2009	2012	2013	2001	2005	2009	2012	2013
Health Care Practitioners and Technical Occupations										
Audiologists	11,040	10,030	12,590	12,060	11,550	$23.89	$27.72	$32.14	$35.04	$35.75
Cardiovascular technologists and technicians	40,990	43,560	48,070	50,530	51,010	17.55	19.99	23.91	25.51	25.95
Dental hygienists	149,880	161,140	173,900	190,290	192,330	27.30	29.15	32.63	33.99	34.39
Diagnostic medical sonographers	32,990	43,590	51,630	57,700	58,250	23.08	26.65	30.60	31.90	32.29
Dietetic technicians	28,940	23,780	24,510	24,660	26,420	11.23	12.20	13.72	13.79	13.74
Dietitians and nutritionists	43,200	48,850	53,220	58,240	59,530	19.74	22.09	25.59	27.00	27.07
Emergency medical technicians and paramedics	170,690	196,880	217,920	232,860	237,660	12.24	13.68	15.88	16.53	16.77
Licensed practical and licensed vocational nurses	683,790	710,020	728,670	718,800	705,200	15.14	17.41	19.66	20.39	20.63
Magnetic resonance imaging technologists	NA	NA	NA	29,560	32,000	NA	NA	NA	31.45	31.71
Medical and clinical laboratory technicians	146,920	142,330	152,420	157,920	157,080	14.52	15.95	18.20	18.91	19.35
Medical and clininical laboratory technologists	145,400	155,250	166,860	160,700	162,630	20.70	23.37	26.74	28.19	28.59
Medical records and health information technicians	142,170	160,450	170,580	182,370	180,760	12.20	13.81	16.29	17.68	18.13
Nuclear medicine technologists	17,360	18,280	21,670	20,480	20,020	24.65	29.10	32.91	34.06	34.60
Nurse anesthetists	NA	NA	NA	34,180	35,430	NA	NA	NA	74.22	75.81
Nurse midwives	NA	NA	NA	5,710	5,460	NA	NA	NA	43.78	44.34
Nurse practitioners	NA	NA	NA	105,780	113,370	NA	NA	NA	43.97	45.71
Occupational therapists	77,080	87,430	97,840	105,540	108,410	25.10	28.41	33.98	36.73	37.45
Opticians, dispensing	63,120	70,090	60,840	64,930	68,390	13.49	14.80	16.73	16.83	17.17
Pharmacists	223,630	229,740	267,860	281,560	287,420	35.02	42.62	51.27	55.27	56.01
Pharmacy technicians	207,140	266,790	331,890	353,340	362,690	10.82	12.19	13.92	14.63	14.83
Physical therapists	126,450	151,280	174,490	191,460	195,670	28.43	31.42	36.64	38.99	39.51
Physician assistants	56,200	63,350	76,900	83,640	88,110	30.00	34.17	40.78	44.45	45.36
Psychiatric technicians	59,750	62,040	70,730	67,760	66,760	12.94	14.04	14.77	15.93	16.09
Radiation therapists	13,460	14,120	15,570	18,230	16,950	25.71	30.59	37.18	38.66	39.30
Radiologic technologists[3]	168,240	184,580	213,560	194,790	194,000	18.68	22.60	26.05	27.14	27.29
Recreational therapists	26,830	23,260	21,960	19,180	18,640	14.92	16.90	19.84	21.29	21.88
Registered nurses[4]	2,217,990	2,368,070	2,583,770	2,633,980	2,661,890	23.19	27.35	31.99	32.66	33.13
Respiratory therapists	82,930	95,320	107,270	116,960	118,640	19.17	22.24	26.06	27.50	27.83
Respiratory therapy technicians	28,700	22,060	15,100	13,460	12,070	16.93	18.57	21.96	22.84	23.01
Speech-language pathologists	83,110	94,660	111,640	121,690	125,050	24.20	27.89	32.86	34.97	35.56
Health Care Support Occupations										
Dental assistants	267,840	270,720	294,020	300,160	309,540	13.29	14.41	16.35	16.86	17.13
Home health aides	560,190	663,280	955,220	839,930	806,710	8.90	9.34	10.39	10.49	10.60
Massage therapists	26,440	37,670	55,920	71,040	79,040	15.93	19.33	19.13	19.40	19.42
Medical assistants	345,930	382,720	495,970	553,140	571,690	11.71	12.58	14.16	14.69	14.80
Medical equipment preparers	33,540	41,790	47,070	50,230	51,300	11.29	12.42	14.32	15.51	16.02
Medical transcriptionists	94,090	90,380	82,810	74,810	68,350	12.99	14.36	16.03	16.66	16.95
Nursing assistants[5]	1,307,600	1,391,430	1,438,010	1,420,020	1,427,830	9.54	10.67	12.01	12.32	12.51
Occupational therapy aides	7,560	6,220	8,040	7,950	8,710	11.70	13.20	13.89	14.36	13.90
Occupational therapy assistants	17,520	22,160	26,680	29,500	30,450	17.39	19.13	24.44	25.52	26.56
Pharmacy aides	58,130	46,610	52,230	42,600	42,250	9.22	9.76	10.74	11.28	11.78
Physical therapist aides	35,250	41,930	44,160	48,700	48,630	10.45	11.01	12.01	12.22	12.50
Physical therapist assistants	47,810	58,670	63,750	69,810	72,640	17.18	18.98	23.36	25.15	25.63
Psychiatric aides	59,640	56,150	62,610	77,880	75,340	11.42	11.47	13.19	12.83	12.98

NOTE: This table excludes occupations such as dentists, physicians, and chiropractors, which have a large percentage of workers who are self-employed.   1 Employment is the number of filled positions. This table includes both full-time and part-time wage and salary positions. Estimates do not include business establishments where persons are self-employed, owners and partners in unincorporated firms, household workers, or unpaid family workers and were rounded to the nearest 10.   2 The mean hourly wage rate for an occupation is the total wages that all workers in the occupation earn in an hour divided by the total employment of the occupation. More information is available from: http://www.bls.gov/oes/current/oes_tec.htm.   3 2012 and 2013 data are not comparable to earlier data. Starting with 2012 data, the radiologic technologists and technicians occupation category was split into two occupations as part of the 2010 SOC revision: Radiologic technologists (29–2034) and Magnetic resonance imaging technologists (29–2035).   4 2012 and 2013 data are not comparable to earlier data. Starting with 2012 data, the registered nurses occupation category was split into four occupations as part of the 2010 SOC revision: Registered nurses (29–1141), plus three advanced practice nursing occupations: Nurse anesthetists (29–1151), Nurse midwives (29–1161), and Nurse practitioners (29–1171).   5 2012 and 2013 data are not comparable to earlier data. Starting with 2012 data, the nursing aides, orderlies, and attendants occupation category was split into two occupations as part of the 2010 SOC revision: Nursing assistants (31–1014) and Orderlies (31–1015).

Table 3-54. Employment and Wages in the Health Care Industry, by Selected Occupation, May 2014

(Number; dollars.)

Occupation	Employment	Median hourly wage (dollars)	Mean hourly wage (dollars)	Annual mean wage (dollars)
Healthcare Practitioners and Technical Occupations	7,854,380	29.67	36.54	76,010
Chiropractors	29,830	32.08	38.35	79,760
Dentists, General	97,990	71.90	80.20	166,810
Oral and Maxillofacial Surgeons	5,120	#	105.58	219,600
Orthodontists	6,190	#	96.65	201,030
Prosthodontists	630	48.21	68.67	142,830
Dentists, All Other Specialists	5,450	81.78	81.05	168,580
Dietitians and Nutritionists	59,490	27.38	27.62	57,440
Optometrists	33,340	48.76	54.33	113,010
Pharmacists	290,780	58.15	56.96	118,470
Anesthesiologists	30,060	#	118.42	246,320
Family and General Practitioners	124,810	86.63	89.58	186,320
Internists, General	48,390	#	91.60	190,530
Obstetricians and Gynecologists	21,740	#	103.25	214,750
Pediatricians, General	31,010	78.53	84.33	175,400
Psychiatrists	25,080	87.44	87.84	182,700
Surgeons	41,070	#	115.60	240,440
Physicians and Surgeons, All Other	311,320	#	91.23	189,760
Physician Assistants	91,670	46.07	46.77	97,280
Podiatrists	8,910	58.03	66.10	137,480
Therapists	609,870	34.76	35.76	74,390
Occupational Therapists	110,520	37.89	38.46	80,000
Physical Therapists	200,670	39.61	40.35	83,940
Radiation Therapists	16,380	38.51	40.25	83,710
Recreational Therapists	17,950	21.15	22.14	46,060
Respiratory Therapists	119,410	27.27	28.12	58,490
Speech-Language Pathologists	126,500	34.40	36.01	74,900
Therapists, All Other	11,770	26.87	28.46	59,190
Veterinarians	62,470	42.11	47.23	98,230
Registered Nurses	2,687,310	32.04	33.55	69,790
Nurse Anesthetists	36,590	73.93	76.40	158,900
Nurse Midwives	5,110	46.62	46.97	97,700
Nurse Practitioners	122,050	45.84	47.11	97,990
Audiologists	12,250	35.13	36.92	76,790
Miscellaneous Health Diagnosing and Treating Practitioners	35,310	35.29	40.89	85,050
Health Technologists and Technicians	2,876,000	19.92	21.66	45,060
Clinical Laboratory Technologists and Technicians	322,170	23.71	24.37	50,690
Medical and Clinical Laboratory Technologists	161,710	28.57	29.12	60,560
Medical and Clinical Laboratory Technicians	160,460	18.45	19.59	40,750
Dental Hygienists	196,520	34.38	34.60	71,970
Diagnostic Related Technologists and Technicians	357,690	28.64	29.23	60,800
Cardiovascular Technologists and Technicians	51,080	26.12	26.54	55,210
Diagnostic Medical Sonographers	59,760	32.47	32.88	68,390
Nuclear Medicine Technologists	20,320	34.66	35.21	73,230
Radiologic Technologists	193,400	26.86	27.65	57,510
Emergency Medical Technicians and Paramedics	235,760	15.24	16.88	35,110
Health Practitioner Support Technologists and Technicians	700,820	15.41	16.36	34,040
Dietetic Technicians	28,690	12.39	13.75	28,600
Pharmacy Technicians	368,760	14.33	14.95	31,090
Psychiatric Technicians	64,540	14.97	16.91	35,160
Respiratory Therapy Technicians	10,610	22.98	23.46	48,800
Surgical Technologists	98,450	20.84	21.64	45,010
Veterinary Technologists and Technicians	93,300	14.94	15.56	32,350
Licensed Practical and Licensed Vocational Nurses	695,610	20.43	20.87	43,420
Medical Records and Health Information Technicians	184,740	17.26	18.68	38,860
Opticians, Dispensing	73,110	16.48	17.43	36,260
Orthotists and Prosthetists	7,830	30.79	33.99	70,690
Hearing Aid Specialists	5,570	20.68	22.99	47,820
Health Technologists and Technicians, All Other	96,170	19.91	21.93	45,620
Other Healthcare Practitioners and Technical Occupations	144,540	27.50	29.21	60,760
Occupational Health and Safety Specialists and Technicians	79,120	31.42	32.25	67,070
Occupational Health and Safety Specialists	65,130	33.27	33.88	70,470

Table 3-54. Employment and Wages in the Health Care Industry, by Selected Occupation, May 2014 — continued

(Number; dollars.)

Occupation	Employment	Median hourly wage (dollars)	Mean hourly wage (dollars)	Annual mean wage (dollars)
Occupational Health and Safety Technicians	13,990	23.14	24.65	51,270
Athletic Trainers	22,400	^	^	45,730
Genetic Counselors	2,180	32.45	33.43	69,540
Healthcare Practitioners and Technical Workers, All Other	40,840	23.76	27.07	56,300
Healthcare Support Occupations	3,940,500	12.71	13.86	28,820
Home Health Aides	799,080	10.28	10.77	22,400
Psychiatric Aides	72,860	12.61	13.67	28,430
Nursing assistants	1,427,740	12.07	12.62	26,250
Orderlies	52,420	11.85	12.82	26,670
Occupational Therapy Assistants	32,230	27.38	27.53	57,260
Occupational Therapy Aides	8,570	12.76	13.96	29,040
Physical Therapist Assistants	76,910	26.16	26.12	54,330
Physical Therapist Aides	48,730	11.85	12.82	26,660
Massage Therapists	87,670	17.88	20.09	41,790
Dental Assistants	314,330	17.02	17.43	36,260
Medical Assistants	584,970	14.41	15.01	31,220
Medical Equipment Preparers	50,550	15.51	16.28	33,850
Medical Transcriptionists	61,210	16.71	17.11	35,580
Pharmacy Aides	41,240	11.15	12.28	25,540
Veterinary Assistants and Laboratory Animal Caretakers	71,060	11.44	12.20	25,370
Phlebotomists	111,950	14.74	15.33	31,890
Healthcare Support Workers, All Other	98,980	16.64	17.04	35,440

= This wage is equal to or greater than $90.00 per hour or $187,199 per year.   ^ = Wages for some occupations that do not generally work year-round, full time, are reported either as hourly wages or annual salaries depending on how they are typically paid.

Table 3-55. Employment and Wages for the Highest- and Lowest-Paying Detailed Health Sector Occupations, by Annual Mean Wage, May 2014

(Dollars; number.)

Occupation title	Annual mean wage (dollars)	Median hourly wage (dollars)	Employment
Highest-Paying Positions			
Anesthesiologists	246,320	118.42	30,060
Surgeons	240,440	115.60	41,070
Oral and Maxillofacial Surgeons	219,600	105.58	5,120
Obstetricians and Gynecologists	214,750	103.25	21,740
Orthodontists	201,030	96.65	6,190
Physicians and Surgeons	194,990	93.74	633,480
Internists, General	190,530	91.60	48,390
Physicians and Surgeons, All Other	189,760	91.23	311,320
Family and General Practitioners	186,320	89.58	124,810
Psychiatrists	182,700	87.84	25,080
Lowest-Paying Positions			
Home Health Aides	22,400	10.77	799,080
Veterinary Assistants and Laboratory Animal Caretakers	25,370	12.20	71,060
Pharmacy Aides	25,540	12.28	41,240
Nursing Assistants	26,250	12.62	1,427,740
Orderlies	26,670	12.82	52,420
Physical Therapist Aides	26,660	12.82	48,730
Psychiatric Aides	28,430	13.67	72,860
Dietetic Technicians	28,600	13.75	28,690
Occupational Therapy Aides	29,040	13.96	8,570
Pharmacy Technicians	31,090	14.95	368,760

Table 3-56. Industries with the Highest Levels of Employment and Highest Concentration of Employment in Health Care and Practitioner and Technical Occupations, May 2014

(Number; dollars.)

Industry	Employment[1]	Percent of industry employment	Hourly mean wage (dollars)	Annual mean wage (dollars)[2]
Industries with the Highest Levels of Employment in Health Care and Practitioner and Technical Occupations				
General Medical and Surgical Hospitals	2,892,130	55.11	34.43	71,600
Offices of Physicians	1,034,900	42.13	56.92	118,390
Nursing Care Facilities (Skilled Nursing Facilities)	428,460	25.86	25.76	53,590
Health and Personal Care Stores	358,620	35.14	30.53	63,510
Home Health Care Services	307,220	24.46	31.54	65,610
Industries with the Highest Concentration of Employment in Health Care and Practitioner and Technical Occupations				
General Medical and Surgical Hospitals	2,892,130	55.11	34.43	71,600
Other Ambulatory Health Care Services	152,210	54.78	18.42	38,310
Specialty (Except Psychiatric and Substance Abuse) Hospitals	124,650	50.55	35.80	74,470
Offices of Physicians	1,034,900	42.13	56.92	118,390
Medical and Diagnostic Laboratories	104,150	41.75	30.92	64,320

1 Estimates for detailed occupations do not sum to the totals because the totals include occupations not shown separately. Estimates do not include self-employed workers.   2 Annual wages have been calculated by multiplying the hourly mean wage by a "year-round, full-time" hours figure of 2,080 hours; for those occupations where there is not an hourly mean wage published, the annual wage has been directly calculated from the reported survey data.

Table 3-57. States with the Highest Level of Employment and Highest Concentration of Jobs in Health Care Practitioner and Technical Occupations, May 2014

(Number, dollar.)

State	Employment[1]	Employment per thousand jobs	Location quotient[2]	Hourly mean wage (dollars)	Annual mean wage (dollars)[3]
States with the Highest Employment Level in This Occupation					
California	737,820	48.80	0.84	44.56	92,690
Texas	584,740	52.07	0.90	35.34	73,510
New York	504,800	57.29	0.99	40.72	84,690
Florida	475,220	62.00	1.07	34.56	71,880
Pennsylvania	366,220	64.77	1.11	34.77	72,330
States with the Highest Concentration of Jobs and Location Quotients in This Occupation					
West Virginia	56,350	79.62	1.37	30.23	62,870
Massachusetts	235,250	70.81	1.22	41.27	85,840
Maine	40,930	69.81	1.20	37.10	77,160
South Dakota	28,470	69.56	1.20	30.78	64,030
Mississippi	75,140	68.68	1.18	29.92	62,230

1 Estimates for detailed occupations do not sum to the totals because the totals include occupations not shown separately. Estimates do not include self-employed workers.   2 The location quotient is the ratio of the area concentration of occupational employment to the national average concentration. A location quotient greater than one indicates the occupation has a higher share of employment than average, and a location quotient less than one indicates the occupation is less prevalent in the area than average.   3 Annual wages have been calculated by multiplying the hourly mean wage by a "year-round, full-time" hours figure of 2,080 hours; for those occupations where there is not an hourly mean wage published, the annual wage has been directly calculated from the reported survey data.

Table 3-58. Top Paying Metropolitan Areas for Health Care Practitioner and Technical Occupations, May 2014

(Number, dollar.)

Metropolitan area	Employment[1]	Employment per thousand jobs	Location quotient[2]	Hourly mean wage (dollars)	Annual mean wage (dollars)[3]
San Jose-Sunnyvale-Santa Clara, CA	40,260	41.35	0.71	53.01	110,260
San Francisco-San Mateo-Redwood City, CA Metropolitan Division	40,340	37.12	0.64	52.80	109,820
Santa Cruz-Watsonville, CA	4,450	50.30	0.87	51.86	107,870
Oakland-Fremont-Hayward, CA Metropolitan Division	54,990	53.59	0.92	50.92	105,920
Santa Barbara-Santa Maria-Goleta, CA	7,620	43.13	0.74	47.62	99,050
Sacramento–Arden-Arcade–Roseville, CA	43,300	50.47	0.87	47.20	98,170
Bethesda-Rockville-Frederick, MD Metropolitan Division	38,540	68.05	1.17	46.84	97,430
Corvallis, OR	2,290	68.34	1.18	46.83	97,400
Vallejo-Fairfield, CA	7,420	61.58	1.06	46.51	96,740
Danbury, CT	4,440	63.80	1.10	46.33	96,360

1 Estimates for detailed occupations do not sum to the totals because the totals include occupations not shown separately. Estimates do not include self-employed workers.   2 The location quotient is the ratio of the area concentration of occupational employment to the national average concentration. A location quotient greater than one indicates the occupation has a higher share of employment than average, and a location quotient less than one indicates the occupation is less prevalent in the area than average.   3 Annual wages have been calculated by multiplying the hourly mean wage by a "year-round, full-time" hours figure of 2,080 hours; for those occupations where there is not an hourly mean wage published, the annual wage has been directly calculated from the reported survey data.

Table 3-59. Top Paying Nonmetropolitan Areas for Health Care Practitioner and Technical Occupations, May 2014

(Number, dollar.)

Metropolitan area	Employment[1]	Employment per thousand jobs	Location quotient[2]	Hourly mean wage (dollars)	Annual mean wage (dollars)[3]
Southeast Alaska nonmetropolitan area	1,530	43.41	0.75	46.37	96,450
Los Alamos County, New Mexico nonmetropolitan area	420	28.27	0.49	44.36	92,270
Railbelt/Southwest Alaska nonmetropolitan area	2,930	38.75	0.67	43.86	91,230
Mother Lode Region of California nonmetropolitan area	2,330	59.95	1.03	43.55	90,580
Other Nevada nonmetropolitan area	1,600	28.69	0.49	42.22	87,830

1 Estimates for detailed occupations do not sum to the totals because the totals include occupations not shown separately. Estimates do not include self-employed workers.   2 The location quotient is the ratio of the area concentration of occupational employment to the national average concentration. A location quotient greater than one indicates the occupation has a higher share of employment than average, and a location quotient less than one indicates the occupation is less prevalent in the area than average.   3 Annual wages have been calculated by multiplying the hourly mean wage by a "year-round, full-time" hours figure of 2,080 hours; for those occupations where there is not an hourly mean wage published, the annual wage has been directly calculated from the reported survey data.

HEALTH EXPENDITURES

Figure 3-13. Percent Distribution of Personal Health Care Expenditures, by Type, 2013

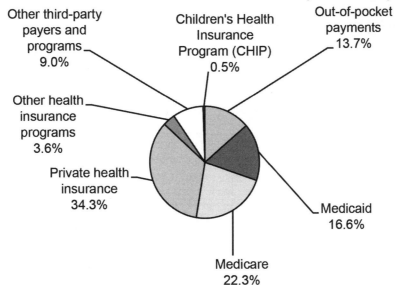

Other third-party payers and programs 9.0%

Other health insurance programs 3.6%

Private health insurance 34.3%

Children's Health Insurance Program (CHIP) 0.5%

Out-of-pocket payments 13.7%

Medicaid 16.6%

Medicare 22.3%

Table 3-60. Gross Domestic Product, National Health Expenditures, Per Capita Amounts, Percent Distribution, and Average Annual Percent Change, Selected Years, 1960–2013

(Number; dollars.)

Gross domestic product and national health expenditures	1960	1970	1980	1990	2000	2009	2010	2012	2013
Gross domestic product (GDP)	$543	$1,076	$2,863	$5,980	$10,285	$14,419	$14,964	$16,163	$16,768
Price deflator for GDP[1]	17.5	22.8	44.5	66.8	81.9	100.0	101.2	105.2	106.7
Amount (in Billions)									
National health expenditures	$27.4	$74.9	$255.8	$724.3	$1,378.0	$2,505.8	$2,604.1	$2,817.3	$2,919.1
Health consumption expenditures	24.8	67.1	235.7	675.6	1,290.0	2,359.5	2,454.5	2,653.6	2,754.5
Personal health care	23.4	63.1	217.2	616.8	1,165.7	2,117.9	2,196.2	2,379.3	2,468.6
Administration and net cost of private health insurance	1.1	2.6	12.0	38.8	81.3	167.6	182.8	199.5	210.6
Public health	0.4	1.4	6.4	20.0	43.0	74.0	75.5	74.8	75.4
Investment[2]	2.6	7.8	20.1	48.7	88.0	146.3	149.7	163.7	164.6
Chain-weighted national health expenditure deflator[1]	NA	NA	NA	NA	NA	100.0	102.7	106.9	108.3
Per Capita Amount (in Dollars)									
National health expenditures	$147	$356	$1,110	$2,855	$4,881	$8,175	$8,428	$8,996	$9,255
Health consumption expenditures	133	319	1,023	2,663	4,570	7,698	7,943	8,473	8,733
Personal health care	125	300	943	2,431	4,129	6,909	7,107	7,597	7,826
Administration and net cost of private health insurance	6	12	52	153	288	547	592	637	668
Public health	2	6	28	79	152	242	244	239	239
Investment[2]	14	37	87	192	312	477	484	523	522
Percent									
National health expenditures as percent of GDP	5.0	7.0	8.9	12.1	13.4	17.4	17.4	17.4	17.4
Percent Distribution									
National health expenditures	100.0	100.0	100.0	100.0	100.0	100.0	100.0	100.0	100.0
Health consumption expenditures	90.6	89.6	92.1	93.3	93.6	94.2	94.3	94.2	94.4
Personal health care	85.4	84.3	84.9	85.2	84.6	84.5	84.3	84.5	84.6
Administration and net cost of private health insurance	3.9	3.5	4.7	5.4	5.9	6.7	7.0	7.1	7.2
Public health	1.4	1.8	2.5	2.8	3.1	3.0	2.9	2.7	2.6
Investment[2]	9.4	10.4	7.9	6.7	6.4	5.8	5.7	5.8	5.6
Average Annual Percent Change from Previous Year Shown									
GDP	X	7.1	10.3	7.6	5.6	3.8	3.8	3.9	3.7
National health expenditures	X	10.6	13.1	11.0	6.6	6.9	3.9	4.0	3.6
Health consumption expenditures	X	10.5	13.4	11.1	6.7	6.9	4.0	4.0	3.8
Personal health care	X	10.4	13.2	11.0	6.6	6.9	3.7	4.1	3.8
Administration and net cost of private health insurance	X	9.4	16.4	12.4	7.7	8.4	9.1	4.5	5.6
Public health	X	13.8	16.9	12.0	8.0	6.2	1.9	-0.4	0.8
Investment[2]	X	11.7	10.0	9.2	6.1	5.8	2.3	4.6	0.5
National health expenditures	X	9.2	12.0	9.9	5.5	5.9	3.1	3.3	2.9
Health consumption expenditures	X	9.1	12.4	10.0	5.5	6.0	3.2	3.3	3.1
Personal health care	X	9.1	12.1	9.9	5.4	5.9	2.9	3.4	3.0
Administration and net cost of private health insurance	X	7.2	15.8	11.4	6.5	7.4	8.2	3.7	4.9
Public health	X	11.6	16.7	10.9	6.8	5.3	0.8	-1.0	0.0
Investment[2]	X	10.2	8.9	8.2	5.0	4.8	1.5	4.0	-0.2

NOTE: Dollar amounts are in current dollars. The data reflect preliminary annual estimates of the resident population for the United States, as of July 1, 2010, excluding the Armed Forces overseas.   NA = Not available.   X = Not applicable.   1 Year 2009 = 100.   2 Investment consists of research and structures and equipment.

Table 3-61. National Health Expenditures, Average Annual Percent Change and Percent Distribution, by Type of Expenditure, Selected Years, 1960–2013

(Dollars; percent.)

Type of national health expenditure	1960	1970	1980	1990	2000	2009	2012	2013
Amount (in Billions of Dollars)								
National health expenditures	$27.4	$74.9	$255.8	$724.3	$1,378.0	$2,505.8	$2,817.3	$2,919.1
Health consumption expenditures	24.8	67.1	235.7	675.6	1,290.0	2,359.5	2,653.6	2,754.5
Personal health care	23.4	63.1	217.2	616.8	1,165.7	2,117.9	2,379.3	2,468.6
Hospital care	9.0	27.2	100.5	250.4	415.5	776.8	898.5	936.9
Professional services	8.0	19.8	64.6	208.1	390.2	672.4	752.0	777.9
Physician and clinical services	5.6	14.3	47.7	158.9	290.9	503.2	565.3	586.7
Other professional services	0.4	0.7	3.5	17.4	37.0	66.8	76.8	80.2
Dental services	2.0	4.7	13.4	31.7	62.3	102.5	110.0	111.0
Other health, residential, and personal care	0.5	1.3	8.5	24.3	64.5	122.5	140.1	148.2
Home health care[1]	0.1	0.2	2.4	12.6	32.4	67.2	77.1	79.8
Nursing care facilities and continuing care retirement communities[1]	0.8	4.0	15.3	44.9	85.1	138.5	152.2	155.8
Retail outlet sales of medical products	5.0	10.6	25.9	76.5	177.9	340.3	359.4	370.0
Prescription drugs	2.7	5.5	12.0	40.3	121.2	255.0	264.4	271.1
Durable medical equipment	0.7	1.7	4.1	13.8	25.2	35.0	41.3	43.0
Other nondurable medical products	1.6	3.3	9.8	22.4	31.6	50.3	53.7	55.9
Government administration[2]	0.1	0.7	2.8	7.2	17.1	29.8	34.2	37.0
Net cost of health insurance[3]	1.0	1.9	9.3	31.6	64.2	137.8	165.3	173.6
Government public health activities[4]	0.4	1.4	6.4	20.0	43.0	74.0	74.8	75.4
Investment	2.6	7.8	20.1	48.7	88.0	146.3	163.7	164.6
Research[5]	0.7	2.0	5.4	12.7	25.5	45.2	48.0	46.7
Structures and equipment	1.9	5.8	14.7	36.0	62.5	101.1	115.7	117.9
Average Annual Percent Change from Previous Year Shown								
National health expenditures	X	10.6	13.1	11.0	6.6	6.9	4.0	3.6
Health consumption expenditures	X	10.5	13.4	11.1	6.7	6.9	4.0	3.8
Personal health care	X	10.4	13.2	11.0	6.6	6.9	4.0	3.8
Hospital care	X	11.7	14.0	9.6	5.2	7.2	5.0	4.3
Professional services	X	9.5	12.6	12.4	6.5	6.2	3.8	3.4
Physician and clinical services	X	9.8	12.8	12.8	6.2	6.3	4.0	3.8
Other professional services	X	6.4	17.0	17.5	7.8	6.8	4.7	4.5
Dental services	X	9.0	11.0	9.0	7.0	5.7	2.4	0.9
Other health, residential, and personal care	X	11.4	20.4	11.1	10.2	7.4	4.6	5.8
Home health care[1]	X	14.5	26.9	18.1	9.9	8.4	4.7	3.4
Nursing care facilities and continuing care retirement communities[1]	X	17.4	14.2	11.4	6.6	5.6	3.2	2.4
Retail outlet sales of medical products	X	7.7	9.4	11.4	8.8	7.5	1.8	2.9
Prescription drugs	X	7.5	8.2	12.8	11.6	8.6	1.2	2.5
Durable medical equipment	X	9.0	8.8	13.0	6.2	3.7	5.6	4.2
Other nondurable medical products	X	7.4	11.4	8.6	3.5	5.3	2.2	4.0
Government administration[2]	X	29.9	14.1	10.0	9.1	6.4	4.7	8.2
Net cost of health insurance[3]	X	6.4	17.3	13.1	7.3	8.9	6.3	5.0
Government public health activities[4]	X	13.8	16.9	12.0	8.0	6.2	0.3	0.8
Investment	X	11.7	10.0	9.2	6.1	5.8	3.8	0.5
Research[5]	X	10.9	10.8	8.9	7.2	6.6	2.1	-2.6
Structures and equipment	X	12.0	9.7	9.4	5.7	5.5	4.6	1.9
Percent Distribution								
National health expenditures	100.0	100.0	100.0	100.0	100.0	100.0	100.0	100.0
Health consumption expenditures	90.6	89.6	92.1	93.3	93.6	94.2	94.2	94.4
Personal health care	85.4	84.3	84.9	85.2	84.6	84.5	84.5	84.6
Hospital care	32.8	36.3	39.3	34.6	30.2	31.0	31.9	32.1
Professional services	29.3	26.4	25.3	28.7	28.3	26.8	26.7	26.6
Physician and clinical services	20.6	19.1	18.7	21.9	21.1	20.1	20.1	20.1
Other professional services	1.4	1.0	1.4	2.4	2.7	2.7	2.7	2.7
Dental services	7.3	6.3	5.2	4.4	4.5	4.1	3.9	3.8
Other health, residential, and personal care	1.6	1.8	3.3	3.4	4.7	4.9	5.0	5.1
Home health care[1]	0.2	0.3	0.9	1.7	2.4	2.7	2.7	2.7
Nursing care facilities and continuing care retirement communities[1]	3.0	5.4	6.0	6.2	6.2	5.5	5.4	5.3
Retail outlet sales of medical products	18.4	14.1	10.1	10.6	12.9	13.6	12.8	12.7
Prescription drugs	9.8	7.3	4.7	5.6	8.8	10.2	9.4	9.3
Durable medical equipment	2.7	2.3	1.6	1.9	1.8	1.4	1.5	1.5
Other nondurable medical products	5.9	4.4	3.8	3.1	2.3	2.0	1.9	1.9
Government administration[2]	0.2	1.0	1.1	1.0	1.2	1.2	1.2	1.3
Net cost of health insurance[3]	3.7	2.5	3.6	4.4	4.7	5.5	5.9	5.9
Government public health activities[4]	1.4	1.8	2.5	2.8	3.1	3.0	2.7	2.6
Investment	9.4	10.4	7.9	6.7	6.4	5.8	5.8	5.6
Research[5]	2.5	2.6	2.1	1.8	1.8	1.8	1.7	1.6
Structures and equipment	6.8	7.8	5.7	5.0	4.5	4.0	4.1	4.0
Per cent Distribution								
Personal health care	100.0	100.0	100.0	100.0	100.0	100.0	100.0	100.0
Hospital care	38.5	43.1	46.3	40.6	35.6	36.7	37.8	38.0
Professional services	34.3	31.3	29.8	33.7	33.5	31.8	31.6	31.5
Physician and clinical services	24.1	22.7	22.0	25.8	25.0	23.8	23.8	23.8
Other professional services	1.7	1.2	1.6	2.8	3.2	3.2	3.2	3.3

Table 3-61. National Health Expenditures, Average Annual Percent Change and Percent Distribution, by Type of Expenditure, Selected Years, 1960–2013— continued

(Dollars; percent.)

Type of national health expenditure	1960	1970	1980	1990	2000	2009	2012	2013
Dental services	8.5	7.5	6.2	5.1	5.3	4.8	4.6	4.5
Other health, residential, and personal care	1.9	2.1	3.9	3.9	5.5	5.8	5.9	6.0
Home health care[1]	0.2	0.3	1.1	2.0	2.8	3.2	3.2	3.2
Nursing care facilities and continuing care retirement communities[1]	3.5	6.4	7.0	7.3	7.3	6.5	6.4	6.3
Retail outlet sales of medical products	21.6	16.8	11.9	12.4	15.3	16.1	15.1	15.0
Prescription drugs	11.5	8.7	5.5	6.5	10.4	12.0	11.1	11.0
Durable medical equipment	3.2	2.8	1.9	2.2	2.2	1.7	1.7	1.7
Other nondurable medical products	7.0	5.3	4.5	3.6	2.7	2.4	2.3	2.3

X = Not applicable.   1 Includes expenditures for care in freestanding facilities only. Additional services of this type are provided in hospital-based facilities and are considered hospital care.   2 Includes all administrative costs (federal and state and local employees' salaries; contracted employees, including fiscal intermediaries; rent and building costs; computer systems and programs; other materials and supplies; and other miscellaneous expenses) associated with insuring individuals enrolled in the following health insurance programs: Medicare, Medicaid, Children's Health Insurance Program, Department of Defense, Department of Veterans Affairs, Indian Health Service, workers' compensation, maternal and child health, vocational rehabilitation, Substance Abuse and Mental Health Services Administration, and other federal programs.   3 Net cost of health insurance is calculated as the difference between calendar year incurred premiums earned and benefits incurred for private health insurance. This includes administrative costs, and in some cases additions to reserves, rate credits and dividends, premium taxes, and net underwriting gains or losses. Also included in this category is the difference between premiums earned and benefits incurred for the private health insurance companies that insure the enrollees of the following programs: Medicare, Medicaid, Children's Health Insurance Program, and workers' compensation (health portion only).   4 Includes personal care services delivered by government public health agencies.   5 Research and development expenditures of drug companies and other manufacturers and providers of medical equipment and supplies are excluded. These are included in the expenditure class in which the product falls because such expenditures are covered by the payment received for that product.

Table 3-62. Personal Health Care Expenditures, by Source of Funds and Type of Expenditure, Selected Years 1960–2013

(Number; percent.)

Type of personal health care expenditures and source of funds	1960	1970	1980	1990	2000	2005	2008	2009	2010	2011	2012	2013
Amount in Billions												
Per capita	$125	$300	$943	$2,431	$4,129	$5,757	$6,638	$6,909	$7,107	$7,337	$7,597	$7,826
Amount in Billions												
All personal health care expenditures[1]	$23.4	$63.1	$217.2	$616.8	$1,165.7	$1,700.9	$2,017.3	$2,117.9	$2,196.2	$2,281.8	$2,379.3	$2,468.6
Out-of-pocket payments	13.1	25.0	58.4	138.6	201.5	267.2	300.9	300.9	306.2	317.3	328.8	339.4
Health insurance	6.6	29.6	131.9	403.2	845.5	1,281.3	1,544.5	1,639.2	1,701.4	1,769.9	1,842.0	1,907.9
Private health insurance	4.9	14.0	61.4	205.1	407.3	606.5	706.2	736.1	755.4	788.2	822.9	846.0
Medicare	X	7.3	36.3	107.3	216.3	326.3	442.1	471.2	489.2	511.9	532.2	550.5
Medicaid	X	5.0	24.7	69.7	186.9	287.7	317.9	346.4	366.2	374.4	389.0	410.8
Federal	X	2.7	13.7	40.3	109.3	165.5	188.3	230.7	247.5	228.7	224.0	236.7
State and local	X	2.3	11.0	29.4	77.6	122.2	129.6	115.6	118.6	145.7	165.0	174.1
CHIP[2]	X	X	X	X	2.5	6.5	8.7	9.5	9.7	10.1	10.6	11.3
Federal	X	X	X	X	1.8	4.5	6.1	6.7	6.8	7.0	7.4	7.8
State and local	X	X	X	X	0.8	2.0	2.6	2.8	2.9	3.0	3.2	3.5
Other health insurance programs[3]	1.7	3.3	9.6	21.2	32.4	54.3	69.6	76.1	80.9	85.4	87.2	89.3
Other third-party payers and programs[4]	3.7	8.5	26.9	74.9	118.7	152.4	171.9	177.8	188.6	194.6	208.5	221.2
Amount in Billions												
Chain-weighted personal health care deflator (2009 = 100.0)[5]	9.3	13.5	28.5	56.4	75.7	89.1	97.3	100.0	102.7	104.8	106.8	108.4
Percent Distribution												
All sources of funds	100.0	100.0	100.0	100.0	100.0	100.0	100.0	100.0	100.0	100.0	100.0	100.0
Out-of-pocket payments	55.9	39.6	26.9	22.5	17.3	15.7	14.9	14.2	13.9	13.9	13.8	13.7
Health insurance	28.3	46.9	60.7	65.4	72.5	75.3	76.6	77.4	77.5	77.6	77.4	77.3
Private health insurance	21.1	22.2	28.3	33.2	34.9	35.7	35.0	34.8	34.4	34.5	34.6	34.3
Medicare	X	11.5	16.7	17.4	18.6	19.2	21.9	22.2	22.3	22.4	22.4	22.3
Medicaid	X	8.0	11.4	11.3	16.0	16.9	15.8	16.4	16.7	16.4	16.3	16.6
Federal	X	4.3	6.3	6.5	9.4	9.7	9.3	10.9	11.3	10.0	9.4	9.6
State and local	X	3.7	5.1	4.8	6.7	7.2	6.4	5.5	5.4	6.4	6.9	7.1
CHIP[2]	X	X	X	X	0.2	0.4	0.4	0.5	0.4	0.4	0.4	0.5
Federal	X	X	X	X	0.2	0.3	0.3	0.3	0.3	0.3	0.3	0.3
State and local	X	X	X	X	0.1	0.1	0.1	0.1	0.1	0.1	0.1	0.1
Other health insurance programs[3]	7.2	5.2	4.4	3.4	2.8	3.2	3.5	3.6	3.7	3.7	3.7	3.6
Other third-party payers and programs[4]	15.8	13.5	12.4	12.1	10.2	9.0	8.5	8.4	8.6	8.5	8.8	9.0
Amount in Billions												
Hospital expenditures[6]	$9.0	$27.2	$100.5	$250.4	$415.5	$609.4	$728.9	$776.8	$814.9	$849.9	$898.5	$936.9
Percent Distribution												
All sources of funds	100.0	100.0	100.0	100.0	100.0	100.0	100.0	100.0	100.0	100.0	100.0	100.0
Out-of-pocket payments	20.6	9.0	5.4	4.5	3.2	3.2	3.2	3.2	3.3	3.3	3.4	3.5
Health insurance	50.7	71.4	79.6	82.6	86.2	87.4	87.8	87.6	87.2	87.2	86.8	86.3
Private health insurance	35.6	32.5	36.7	38.7	34.1	35.7	36.4	36.1	35.9	36.6	37.2	37.1
Medicare	X	19.7	26.1	26.9	29.7	29.0	28.2	27.8	27.1	26.8	26.3	25.9
Medicaid	X	9.7	9.2	10.6	17.1	17.2	17.2	17.6	18.0	17.6	17.4	17.5
Federal	X	5.2	5.0	6.3	10.3	10.0	10.2	11.7	12.2	10.8	10.1	10.1
State and local	X	4.5	4.2	4.3	6.8	7.2	7.0	6.0	5.9	6.8	7.3	7.4
CHIP[2]	X	X	X	X	0.2	0.4	0.4	0.4	0.4	0.4	0.4	0.4
Federal	X	X	X	X	0.2	0.3	0.3	0.3	0.3	0.3	0.3	0.3
State and local	X	X	X	X	0.1	0.1	0.1	0.1	0.1	0.1	0.1	0.1
Other health insurance programs[3]	15.1	9.5	7.7	6.3	5.0	5.1	5.5	5.7	5.8	5.7	5.5	5.4
Other third-party payers and programs[4]	28.7	19.5	15.0	13.0	10.6	9.4	9.0	9.2	9.5	9.5	9.7	10.2
Amount in Billions												
Physician and clinical expenditures	$5.6	$14.3	$47.7	$158.9	$290.9	$417.2	$486.5	$503.2	$519.0	$540.8	$565.3	$586.7
Percent Distribution												
All sources of funds	100.0	100.0	100.0	100.0	100.0	100.0	100.0	100.0	100.0	100.0	100.0	100.0
Out-of-pocket payments	60.1	45.1	29.8	18.9	11.2	10.2	10.0	9.5	9.8	9.9	9.6	9.4
Health insurance	32.6	48.8	59.8	67.8	76.6	79.2	80.3	81.4	81.0	81.0	80.7	80.5
Private health insurance	28.3	29.4	34.8	42.2	47.4	48.5	47.8	47.3	46.5	46.2	45.9	45.6
Medicare	X	11.5	17.4	19.2	20.2	20.5	21.3	22.2	22.2	22.4	22.5	22.2
Medicaid	X	4.5	5.1	4.4	6.6	7.1	7.3	7.9	8.2	8.2	8.1	8.5
Federal	X	2.4	2.9	2.6	3.9	4.3	4.5	5.5	5.7	5.2	4.9	5.3
State and local	X	2.1	2.2	1.8	2.7	2.9	2.8	2.5	2.5	3.0	3.1	3.2
CHIP[2]	X	X	X	X	0.3	0.4	0.6	0.6	0.6	0.6	0.6	0.6
Federal	X	X	X	X	0.2	0.3	0.4	0.4	0.4	0.4	0.4	0.4
State and local	X	X	X	X	0.1	0.1	0.2	0.2	0.2	0.2	0.2	0.2
Other health insurance programs[3]	4.3	3.4	2.4	2.1	2.1	2.6	3.2	3.5	3.5	3.6	3.6	3.5
Other third-party payers and programs[4]	7.3	6.1	10.4	13.3	12.3	10.6	9.7	9.1	9.2	9.1	9.8	10.1

Table 3-62. Personal Health Care Expenditures, by Source of Funds and Type of Expenditure, Selected Years 1960–2013— continued

(Number; percent.)

Type of personal health care expenditures and source of funds[1]	1960	1970	1980	1990	2000	2005	2008	2009	2010	2011	2012	2013
Amount in Billions												
Home health care expenditures[7]	$2.0	$4.7	$13.4	$31.7	$62.3	$87.0	$102.4	$102.5	$105.4	$107.6	$110.0	$111.0
Percent Distribution												
All sources of funds	100.0	100.0	100.0	100.0	100.0	100.0	100.0	100.0	100.0	100.0	100.0	100.0
Out-of-pocket payments	96.0	90.0	65.8	48.1	44.4	44.0	44.4	42.0	41.5	41.8	42.1	42.5
Health insurance	3.2	9.5	33.3	51.3	55.0	55.6	55.2	57.5	57.9	57.7	57.4	57.0
Private health insurance	1.9	4.5	28.4	48.1	50.2	49.3	47.9	48.7	48.5	48.4	48.1	47.4
Medicare	X	X	X	0.0	0.1	0.1	0.2	0.3	0.2	0.3	0.3	0.4
Medicaid	X	3.4	3.7	2.4	3.7	4.8	5.3	6.6	7.0	6.8	6.6	6.8
Federal	X	1.8	2.0	1.3	2.1	2.7	3.2	4.5	4.8	4.2	3.8	3.9
State and local	X	1.6	1.7	1.0	1.6	2.0	2.1	2.1	2.2	2.6	2.8	2.8
CHIP[2]	X	X	X	X	0.4	0.5	0.7	0.7	1.0	1.1	1.2	1.3
Federal	X	X	X	X	0.3	0.4	0.5	0.5	0.7	0.7	0.8	0.9
State and local	X	X	X	X	0.1	0.2	0.2	0.2	0.3	0.3	0.4	0.4
Other health insurance programs[3]	1.3	1.6	1.2	0.9	0.6	0.9	1.0	1.1	1.2	1.2	1.1	1.1
Other third-party payers and programs[4]	0.8	0.4	0.8	0.6	0.6	0.4	0.4	0.5	0.5	0.5	0.5	0.5
Amount in Billions												
Nursing care facilities and continuing care retirement communities expenditures[7]	$0.1	$0.2	$2.4	$12.6	$32.4	$48.7	$62.3	$67.2	$71.2	$73.8	$77.1	$79.8
Percent Distribution												
All sources of funds	100.0	100.0	100.0	100.0	100.0	100.0	100.0	100.0	100.0	100.0	100.0	100.0
Out-of-pocket payments	12.3	9.5	15.3	17.9	19.6	12.8	8.9	7.6	7.5	7.7	7.9	8.1
Health insurance	5.3	37.7	53.7	66.1	71.4	81.5	87.3	89.1	89.5	89.3	88.9	88.9
Private health insurance	1.8	3.2	14.7	22.9	23.8	12.6	7.9	7.0	6.8	6.8	7.4	7.9
Medicare	X	26.8	26.8	26.0	26.4	37.4	43.4	45.1	44.6	43.6	43.6	43.1
Medicaid	X	6.8	11.6	17.1	20.9	31.0	35.2	36.2	37.0	37.6	36.7	36.5
Federal	X	3.2	6.2	9.1	11.3	16.8	20.0	23.5	24.3	22.0	20.0	20.1
State and local	X	3.2	5.4	7.9	9.6	14.3	15.3	12.6	12.6	15.6	16.6	16.4
CHIP[2]	X	X	X	X	0.0	0.0	0.0	0.0	0.0	0.0	0.0	0.0
Federal	X	X	X	X	0.0	0.0	0.0	0.0	0.0	0.0	0.0	0.0
State and local	X	X	X	X	0.0	0.0	0.0	0.0	0.0	0.0	0.0	0.0
Other health insurance programs[3]	3.5	1.4	0.5	0.3	0.3	0.5	0.7	0.9	1.2	1.2	1.3	1.4
Other third-party payers and programs[4]	80.7	52.7	31.1	16.0	9.0	5.6	3.8	3.2	3.0	3.0	3.1	3.0
Amount in Billions												
Prescription drug expenditures	$0.8	$4.0	$15.3	$44.9	$85.1	$112.5	$132.6	$138.5	$143.0	$149.2	$152.2	$155.8
Percent Distribution												
All sources of funds	100.0	100.0	100.0	100.0	100.0	100.0	100.0	100.0	100.0	100.0	100.0	100.0
Out-of-pocket payments	74.7	49.5	40.7	40.3	31.9	29.7	29.6	28.9	28.1	27.5	29.1	29.4
Health insurance	X	28.5	51.9	48.8	61.1	63.8	63.8	64.5	64.7	65.5	63.5	63.2
Private health insurance	X	0.2	1.3	6.2	8.8	6.5	7.3	7.5	7.6	7.6	8.0	8.1
Medicare	X	3.5	2.0	3.8	12.7	18.3	20.8	21.7	22.5	23.9	22.2	22.2
Medicaid	X	23.3	46.2	36.6	37.4	36.6	33.0	32.4	31.8	31.1	30.4	30.1
Federal	X	12.5	26.1	20.6	21.7	20.6	19.3	21.6	21.5	18.8	17.3	17.1
State and local	X	10.8	20.1	16.0	15.7	15.9	13.6	10.9	10.3	12.2	13.1	12.9
CHIP[2]	X	X	X	X	0.0	0.0	0.0	0.0	0.0	0.0	0.0	0.0
Federal	X	X	X	X	0.0	0.0	0.0	0.0	0.0	0.0	0.0	0.0
State and local	X	X	X	X	0.0	0.0	0.0	0.0	0.0	0.0	0.0	0.0
Other health insurance programs[3]	0.0	1.5	2.4	2.2	2.2	2.5	2.7	2.8	2.8	2.9	2.9	2.9
Other third-party payers and programs[4]	25.3	21.9	7.4	10.9	6.9	6.5	6.6	6.7	7.2	7.0	7.4	7.4
Amount in Billions												
Dental services expenditures	$2.7	$5.5	$12.0	$40.3	$121.2	$205.3	$242.7	$255.0	$256.2	$263.0	$264.4	$271.1
Percent Distribution												
All sources of funds	100.0	100.0	100.0	100.0	100.0	100.0	100.0	100.0	100.0	100.0	100.0	100.0
Out-of-pocket payments	96.0	82.4	71.3	56.8	27.8	25.1	20.5	19.4	18.0	17.8	17.6	16.9
Health insurance	1.5	16.5	26.9	40.3	70.3	73.0	77.9	79.2	80.6	81.1	81.4	82.1
Private health insurance	1.3	8.8	15.0	27.0	50.5	49.8	45.7	46.4	46.4	46.0	44.8	43.5
Medicare	X	X	X	0.5	1.7	1.9	20.9	21.4	23.0	24.0	25.5	27.5
Medicaid	X	7.6	11.7	12.6	16.3	17.7	7.9	7.9	7.8	7.6	7.6	7.8
Federal	X	4.1	6.8	7.2	9.3	10.1	4.7	5.3	5.3	4.5	4.1	4.3
State and local	X	3.5	4.9	5.4	7.0	7.6	3.2	2.6	2.5	3.1	3.5	3.5
CHIP[2]	X	X	X	X	0.2	0.5	0.5	0.5	0.6	0.5	0.5	0.5
Federal	X	X	X	X	0.2	0.4	0.3	0.4	0.4	0.4	0.4	0.4
State and local	X	X	X	X	0.1	0.1	0.1	0.2	0.2	0.2	0.2	0.2
Other health insurance programs[3]	0.1	0.1	0.2	0.2	1.5	3.1	3.0	2.9	2.8	2.9	2.9	2.8
Other third-party payers and programs[4]	2.5	1.1	1.8	3.0	1.9	1.9	1.5	1.4	1.3	1.1	1.0	0.9
Amount in Billions												
All other personal health care expenditures[8]	$3.2	$7.1	$25.8	$77.9	$158.3	$220.9	$261.9	$274.6	$286.6	$297.5	$311.9	$327.4

Table 3-62. Personal Health Care Expenditures, by Source of Funds and Type of Expenditure, Selected Years 1960–2013— continued

(Number; percent.)

Type of personal health care expenditures and source of funds	1960	1970	1980	1990	2000	2005	2008	2009	2010	2011	2012	2013
Percent Distribution												
All sources of funds	100.0	100.0	100.0	100.0	100.0	100.0	100.0	100.0	100.0	100.0	100.0	100.0
Out-of-pocket payments	84.9	74.5	57.1	49.9	38.3	34.2	33.9	32.9	32.6	32.7	32.3	32.4
Health insurance	3.4	8.3	25.0	33.3	44.3	49.2	49.5	50.6	51.1	51.1	52.0	52.5
Private health insurance	2.0	3.4	6.7	12.0	12.6	12.7	12.7	12.5	12.5	12.7	12.6	12.5
Medicare	X	1.0	2.8	5.5	8.0	9.7	10.4	10.4	10.4	10.5	10.7	10.2
Medicaid	X	2.9	14.7	14.9	22.6	25.5	25.5	26.7	27.0	26.5	27.2	28.2
Federal	X	1.6	8.1	8.5	12.9	14.5	15.0	17.7	18.2	16.0	15.4	16.0
State and local	X	1.3	6.7	6.4	9.7	11.0	10.5	8.9	8.8	10.5	11.8	12.3
CHIP[2]	X	X	X	X	0.2	0.3	0.4	0.4	0.4	0.4	0.4	0.4
Federal	X	X	X	X	0.1	0.2	0.3	0.3	0.3	0.3	0.3	0.3
State and local	X	X	X	X	0.1	0.1	0.1	0.1	0.1	0.1	0.1	0.1
Other health insurance programs[3]	1.4	0.9	0.8	0.9	0.8	1.0	0.5	0.6	0.8	1.0	1.0	1.1
Other third-party payers and programs[4]	11.7	17.2	17.9	16.9	17.5	16.5	16.6	16.5	16.4	16.2	15.7	15.1

X = Not applicable.   0.0 = Quantity more than zero but less than 0.05.   1 Includes all expenditures for specified health services and supplies other than expenses for government administration, net cost of health insurance, public health activities, research, and structures and equipment.   2 Children's Health Insurance Program (CHIP). Medicaid CHIP expansions are included.   3 Includes Department of Defense and Department of Veterans Affairs.   4 Includes worksite health care, other private revenues, Indian Health Service, workers' compensation, general assistance, maternal and child health, vocational rehabilitation, other federal programs, Substance Abuse and Mental Health Services Administration, other state and local programs, and school health.   5 The personal health care deflator is calculated as a chain-weighted price index using the Producer Price Indexes for hospitals, offices of physicians, medical and diagnostic laboratories, home health care services, and nursing care facilities; and Consumer Price Indices specific to each of the remaining personal health care components.   6 Includes expenditures for hospital-based nursing home and home health agency care.   7 Includes expenditures for care in freestanding nursing homes. Expenditures for care in hospital-based nursing homes are included with hospital care.   8 Includes expenditures for other professional services, other nondurable medical products, durable medical equipment, and other health, residential, and personal care, not shown separately.

Table 3-63. Cost of Hospital Discharges with Common Hospital Operating Room Procedures in Nonfederal Community Hospitals, by Age and Selected Principal Procedure, Selected Years, 2000–2012

(Dollars.)

Age and principal operating room procedure[1]	Mean inflation-adjusted cost per hospitalization: 2012 dollars[2]			Number of discharges with operating room principal procedure			Total inflation-adjusted national costs: 2012 dollars (in millions of dollars)		
	2000	2005	2012	2000	2005	2012	2000	2005	2012
All Ages									
Hospital discharges with an operating room principal procedure[3]	$13,317	$15,980	$18,521	8,743,631	9,964,151	8,870,290	$115,725	$159,370	$164,141
Laminectomy (back surgery)	8,207	9,293	13,384	285,636	248,800	184,060	2,354	2,313	2,478
Heart valve procedures	43,107	52,827	52,625	79,719	93,802	104,200	3,430	4,975	5,481
Coronary artery bypass graft (CABG)	31,425	38,266	40,142	337,972	221,325	153,635	10,657	8,483	6,170
Percutaneous coronary angioplasty (PTCA) (balloon angioplasty of heart)	15,063	18,559	19,225	581,183	727,912	455,635	8,753	13,516	8,767
Insertion, revision, replacement, removal of cardiac pacemaker or cardioverter/defibrillator	27,789	35,585	35,028	66,286	160,629	100,270	1,856	5,709	3,509
Colorectal resection (removal of part of the bowel)	19,560	22,789	23,204	253,780	274,599	249,415	5,067	6,266	5,783
Appendectomy	7,359	8,542	9,649	269,089	298,829	226,210	1,959	2,552	2,188
Cholecystectomy (gall bladder removal)	10,447	12,152	12,846	389,079	376,158	337,575	4,030	4,572	4,344
Hysterectomy	6,562	7,300	9,799	580,019	550,659	266,400	3,779	4,027	2,612
Cesarean section	5,456	5,487	5,892	898,859	1,258,990	1,159,970	4,789	6,913	6,839
Treatment, fracture or dislocation of hip and femur	12,633	15,353	17,309	237,615	251,071	233,705	3,052	3,852	4,045
Arthroplasty knee (knee replacement)	13,873	15,691	16,556	318,854	533,216	671,374	4,398	8,370	11,117
Hip replacement	15,045	17,171	17,486	295,940	369,634	436,815	4,507	6,340	7,637
Spinal fusion	17,509	24,954	28,190	204,320	322,610	406,995	3,492	8,060	11,484
Under 18 Years									
Hospital discharges with an operating room principal procedure[3]	13,366	19,442	25,470	382,455	535,472	343,670	4,940	10,365	8,697
Incision and excision of CNS (a type of brain surgery)	29,016	35,228	43,217	6,352	11,436	7,600	177	405	327
Tonsillectomy and/or adenoidectomy	4,443	5,748	7,041	12,045	16,288	11,145	55	95	79
Small bowel resection (removal of part of the small bowel)	36,440	50,816	46,904	1,712	2,993	2,125	62	150	99
Appendectomy	6,603	8,160	9,158	75,481	85,790	60,045	485	700	551
Cesarean section	6,058	5,756	6,118	23,690	28,609	15,945	130	165	98
Spinal fusion	29,437	46,330	56,398	7,463	12,880	10,170	217	591	571
18 to 44 Years	8,800	9,960	11,819	2,806,078	3,101,461	2,571,636	24,163	30,922	30,371
Hospital discharges with an operating room principal procedure[3]	25,586	30,692	37,981	19,510	18,229	17,890	480	563	678
Incision and excision of CNS (a type of brain surgery)	7,385	8,654	12,342	95,687	67,321	37,080	712	583	459
Laminectomy	6,779	7,773	8,721	133,662	135,504	97,850	894	1,053	855
Appendectomy	8,556	9,458	10,287	132,538	128,987	119,540	1,089	1,221	1,232
Cholecystectomy (gall bladder removal)	6,379	7,427	10,150	38,252	33,384	20,150	247	248	205
Oophorectomy (removal of one or both ovaries)	4,717	4,544	6,016	75,221	74,449	61,305	335	338	369
Ligation of fallopian tubes ("tying" of fallopian tubes)	6,084	6,628	8,856	291,704	255,025	108,685	1,749	1,692	963
Hysterectomy	5,439	5,477	5,884	873,231	1,226,170	1,140,550	4,647	6,721	6,715
Cesarean section	9,376	11,904	15,044	68,015	59,527	47,940	627	708	722
Treatment, fracture or dislocation of lower extremity (other than hip or femur)	16,460	23,113	26,096	73,228	87,276	73,515	1,165	2,018	1,919
Spinal fusion									
45 to 64 Years									
Hospital discharges with an operating room principal procedure[3]	14,568	17,528	20,776	2,435,212	2,909,930	2,806,265	35,322	51,076	58,220
Laminectomy	8,279	9,174	14,122	107,720	96,084	73,155	893	883	1,038
Heart valve procedures	40,489	48,406	50,948	22,849	26,650	28,145	920	1,298	1,434
Coronary artery bypass graft (CABG)	29,362	35,053	38,570	139,897	94,742	67,190	4,127	3,328	2,594
Percutaneous coronary angioplasty (PTCA)	14,578	17,923	18,892	252,151	318,811	202,975	3,668	5,718	3,837
Insertion, revision, replacement, removal of cardiac pacemaker or cardioverter/defibrillator	34,034	38,618	37,351	15,957	44,029	29,575	539	1,699	1,103
Colorectal resection	17,594	20,300	21,803	76,604	95,108	95,070	1,374	1,933	2,071
Cholecystectomy	9,853	11,700	12,891	117,432	117,636	108,565	1,157	1,379	1,402
Oophorectomy	7,637	8,738	12,333	21,232	22,459	22,780	162	196	280
Hysterectomy	6,693	7,443	9,941	231,498	242,030	123,495	1,546	1,805	1,228
Arthroplasty knee (knee replacement)	14,193	15,744	16,710	95,902	199,682	281,825	1,355	3,144	4,710
Hip replacement	15,635	17,416	17,364	65,118	105,138	152,480	1,026	1,828	2,647
Spinal fusion	16,805	23,196	26,806	87,388	150,313	195,235	1,431	3,490	5,237
65 to 74 Years									
Hospital discharges with an operating room principal procedure[3]	16,321	19,492	21,488	1,511,467	1,602,345	1,630,700	24,797	31,284	35,019
Laminectomy	8,673	9,264	12,894	45,976	45,731	41,735	399	424	543
Heart valve procedures	44,119	53,721	51,726	23,236	24,774	27,895	1,016	1,335	1,444
Coronary artery bypass graft (CABG)	31,979	39,029	39,725	112,652	70,404	51,505	3,600	2,750	2,047
Percutaneous coronary angioplasty (PTCA)	14,996	18,386	19,340	166,497	196,855	122,225	2,493	3,621	2,364
Insertion, revision, replacement, removal of cardiac pacemaker or cardioverter/defibrillator	30,360	36,723	36,133	19,096	44,900	27,275	583	1,646	985
Endarterectomy (plaque removal from artery lining of brain, head, neck)	8,740	9,377	10,395	51,292	40,715	31,305	460	383	326
Colorectal resection	19,670	23,087	23,429	63,693	62,337	60,115	1,291	1,442	1,407
Cholecystectomy	11,542	13,864	14,866	65,953	55,566	50,890	774	771	758
Arthroplasty knee	14,130	15,643	16,372	110,961	177,306	233,810	1,553	2,776	3,829
Hip replacement	14,986	16,885	17,322	71,986	86,918	115,385	1,094	1,467	1,998
Spinal fusion	18,507	26,788	29,263	23,419	47,031	88,200	432	1,260	2,584

Table 3-63. Cost of Hospital Discharges with Common Hospital Operating Room Procedures in Nonfederal Community Hospitals, by Age and Selected Principal Procedure, Selected Years, 2000–2012— continued

(Dollars.)

Age and principal operating room procedure[1]	Mean inflation-adjusted cost per hospitalization: 2012 dollars[2]			Number of discharges with operating room principal procedure			Total inflation-adjusted national costs: 2012 dollars (in millions of dollars)		
	2000	2005	2012	2000	2005	2012	2000	2005	2012
75 to 84 Years									
Hospital discharges with an operating room principal procedure[3]	16,567	20,146	21,475	1,224,573	1,360,428	1,094,565	20,583	27,442	23,513
Laminectomy	9,358	10,164	12,818	31,059	31,945	25,285	293	325	326
Heart valve procedures	45,508	56,607	52,882	21,004	25,070	28,010	967	1,425	1,480
Coronary artery bypass graft (CABG)	34,672	43,386	44,119	68,750	45,187	27,290	2,403	1,962	1,203
Percutaneous coronary angioplasty (PTCA)	15,877	19,647	19,715	111,169	144,906	81,495	1,776	2,847	1,609
Insertion, revision, replacement, removal of cardiac pacemaker or cardioverter/defibrillator	24,903	34,513	34,021	19,975	48,557	25,735	507	1,673	875
Endarterectomy (plaque removal from artery lining of brain, head, neck)	9,079	9,721	10,813	45,337	38,073	24,980	425	372	270
Colorectal resection	21,451	25,600	25,201	62,096	61,238	44,120	1,368	1,568	1,111
Cholecystectomy	13,229	16,353	16,298	52,448	49,823	38,025	709	814	620
Treatment, fracture or dislocation of hip and femur	11,895	14,308	15,892	73,332	72,878	61,615	898	1,044	980
Arthroplasty knee	14,124	15,743	16,370	79,138	121,865	123,025	1,119	1,919	2,015
Hip replacement	14,806	17,041	17,538	92,715	105,580	96,635	1,395	1,797	1,695
Spinal fusion	19,256	27,950	29,264	11,770	22,902	35,875	226	640	1,052
85 Years and Over									
Hospital discharges with an operating room principal procedure[3]	$15,190	$18,535	$19,622	382,341	434,936	421,815	$5,898	$8,069	8,289
Heart valve procedures	47,840	60,719	49,972	2,985	3,957	9,215	143	240	460
Coronary artery bypass graft (CABG)	39,005	49,965	49,855	5,280	4,174	2,960	204	209	147
Percutaneous coronary angioplasty (PTCA)	18,019	21,913	20,570	16,682	28,942	23,985	298	633	494
Insertion, revision, replacement, removal of cardiac pacemaker or cardioverter/defibrillator	14,779	25,124	25,449	7,071	13,675	10,355	107	343	264
Colorectal resection	23,180	27,405	25,980	20,729	20,456	16,990	491	561	441
Cholecystectomy	16,099	18,157	17,693	15,698	16,732	15,045	256	303	267
Treatment, fracture or dislocation of hip and femur	11,582	13,738	15,361	76,900	77,692	74,205	917	1,069	1,141
Arthroplasty knee	14,320	16,536	17,241	10,122	15,784	17,245	146	261	297
Hip replacement	14,397	17,111	17,843	50,005	53,975	54,755	731	923	977
Amputation of lower extremity (amputation of leg, foot or toe)	13,289	17,178	17,269	12,855	10,029	7,610	173	173	132

Note: Excludes newborn infants.   1 Data are based on valid operating room procedures. Operating room procedures were identified using the Centers for Medicare & Medicaid Services' Diagnosis Related Groups (DRGs). For DRGs, physician panels identified International Classification of Diseases (ICD-9-CM) procedure codes, which would be performed in operating rooms in most hospitals. Operating room procedures, as defined by DRGs, are classified by the Clinical Classifications Software (CCS) into 1 of 231 clinically meaningful categories. Mean costs per hospitalization are based on the principal procedure as determined by the CCS. The number of discharges is based on the first-listed (principal) major procedure.   2 Charges (the amount billed by the hospital) were converted to costs using cost-charge ratios from the Centers for Medicare & Medicaid Services. Costs are for the entire hospitalization including the principal procedure. Costs were adjusted to 2010 dollars for inflation using the gross domestic product deflator. 3 Includes discharges for operating room principal procedures not shown separately.

Table 3-64. Out-of-Pocket Health Care Expenses Among Persons with Medical Expenses, by Age, Selected Years 1987–2011

(Percent.)

| Age and year | Percent of persons with expenses | Amount paid out of pocket among persons with expenses[1] | | | | | |
		Total	$0	$1 to 99	$100 to 499	$500 to 999	$1,000 to 1,999	$2,000+
All Ages								
1987	84.5	100.0	10.4	19.9	36.6	15.3	10.0	7.7
1997	84.1	100.0	8.5	26.1	35.1	14.3	9.4	6.6
1998	83.8	100.0	7.7	26.6	35.6	14.0	9.5	6.5
1999	84.3	100.0	7.4	27.1	34.2	14.5	9.5	7.3
2000	83.5	100.0	6.9	26.6	34.4	14.4	9.8	7.8
2001	85.4	100.0	7.1	24.6	33.8	14.6	11.0	8.8
2002	85.2	100.0	7.8	23.4	32.5	15.1	11.9	9.4
2003	85.6	100.0	7.6	21.9	32.1	15.8	12.1	10.4
2004	84.7	100.0	8.8	22.1	31.2	14.9	12.0	11.1
2005	84.7	100.0	8.7	21.2	31.5	15.8	11.9	10.8
2006	84.6	100.0	8.7	21.4	31.6	15.8	12.2	10.2
2007	84.9	100.0	9.8	22.6	31.6	15.3	11.5	9.2
2008	84.4	100.0	9.9	22.9	32.1	14.8	11.2	9.1
2009	84.6	100.0	11.0	22.3	31.3	15.4	11.2	8.7
2010	84.6	100.0	12.6	22.7	31.0	14.2	10.8	8.7
2011	84.6	100.0	12.1	22.2	31.8	14.8	11.0	8.2
Under 6 Years								
1987	88.9	100.0	19.2	28.0	39.8	8.5	2.5	2.0
1997	88.0	100.0	20.0	44.5	28.7	4.0	2.2	0.7
1998	87.6	100.0	17.4	48.0	28.7	4.0	1.5	0.3
1999	87.9	100.0	17.7	50.7	26.0	4.2	0.7	0.7
2000	86.7	100.0	16.7	51.4	25.9	4.1	1.4	0.5
2001	88.8	100.0	18.5	49.0	27.9	3.0	1.3	0.3
2002	88.8	100.0	21.5	42.8	28.8	4.9	1.4	0.5
2003	91.3	100.0	20.6	42.4	29.6	5.4	1.4	0.6
2004	90.0	100.0	26.0	40.5	26.0	4.8	2.1	0.7
2005	88.9	100.0	27.2	36.6	27.5	6.1	1.9	0.7
2006	89.2	100.0	27.1	39.3	26.4	4.3	1.9	1.0
2007	88.7	100.0	30.2	36.5	24.7	5.1	2.0	1.4
2008	88.8	100.0	31.4	36.1	25.9	3.9	1.9	0.8
2009	88.7	100.0	34.2	33.7	24.1	5.3	1.9	*0.8
2010	88.9	100.0	40.0	33.8	21.1	3.2	1.5	*0.5
2011	89.6	100.0	40.1	31.5	22.5	3.9	1.4	*0.7
6 to 17 Years								
1987	80.2	100.0	15.5	27.4	37.4	9.0	5.7	5.0
1997	81.7	100.0	16.5	36.2	32.1	7.5	3.6	4.1
1998	80.6	100.0	16.3	36.3	32.7	7.9	3.9	3.0
1999	81.5	100.0	15.0	38.0	31.6	7.9	3.8	3.8
2000	80.0	100.0	14.7	37.2	33.0	6.5	4.1	4.5
2001	83.2	100.0	15.0	36.5	32.3	7.3	3.8	5.2
2002	83.6	100.0	16.6	35.8	31.8	7.9	3.7	4.3
2003	84.1	100.0	16.1	32.8	33.1	8.9	5.4	3.8
2004	83.9	100.0	18.7	33.8	30.2	8.3	4.7	4.4
2005	83.0	100.0	18.6	32.4	31.1	9.2	4.6	4.0
2006	83.6	100.0	19.2	32.8	29.9	8.7	4.1	5.3
2007	84.0	100.0	21.6	33.0	29.4	7.6	4.2	4.1
2008	82.5	100.0	22.4	33.0	28.3	7.4	4.0	4.9
2009	85.3	100.0	24.5	30.4	28.5	7.6	4.9	4.1
2010	84.4	100.0	28.4	29.8	26.7	7.3	3.3	4.4
2011	84.9	100.0	28.5	30.2	26.1	7.1	3.7	4.4

18 to 44 Years

Table 3-64. Out-of-Pocket Health Care Expenses Among Persons with Medical Expenses, by Age, Selected Years 1987–2011—continued

(Percent.)

Age and year	Percent of persons with expenses	Amount paid out of pocket among persons with expenses[1]					
		Total	$0	$1 to 99	$100 to 499	$500 to 999	$1,000 to 1,999	$2,000+
1987	81.5	100.0	10.1	22.0	39.4	14.9	8.3	5.4
1997	78.3	100.0	7.3	28.4	39.4	14.0	6.9	3.9
1998	78.0	100.0	6.4	29.1	40.3	13.1	7.0	4.1
1999	78.9	100.0	6.4	29.6	39.2	13.3	7.1	4.4
2000	77.7	100.0	5.8	29.4	39.8	13.8	6.9	4.4
2001	79.3	100.0	6.0	26.4	39.7	15.1	8.4	4.5
2002	78.5	100.0	6.7	26.3	38.3	14.6	8.8	5.3
2003	79.0	100.0	6.4	24.5	38.8	15.4	9.2	5.7
2004	77.0	100.0	7.2	24.8	37.6	14.8	9.4	6.2
2005	77.1	100.0	7.0	24.8	37.9	15.0	9.0	6.2
2006	76.9	100.0	6.8	24.2	38.3	15.2	8.9	6.5
2007	77.3	100.0	7.7	26.7	37.1	14.2	8.8	5.5
2008	76.5	100.0	7.9	27.1	36.6	14.0	8.3	6.1
2009	76.2	100.0	8.5	25.8	35.9	15.1	8.8	5.9
2010	76.0	100.0	9.5	28.0	36.2	13.1	7.9	5.4
2011	75.6	100.0	8.7	26.7	37.6	13.2	8.1	5.6
45 to 64 Years								
1987	87.0	100.0	5.7	12.5	35.7	20.9	14.7	10.5
1997	89.2	100.0	3.4	16.8	36.3	19.6	14.8	9.2
1998	89.2	100.0	2.9	17.2	36.3	19.7	14.5	9.5
1999	88.9	100.0	2.7	16.6	35.9	20.2	14.7	9.9
2000	88.5	100.0	2.6	15.7	35.2	20.4	15.1	11.0
2001	89.9	100.0	2.4	14.3	33.8	19.9	17.2	12.4
2002	90.0	100.0	2.3	14.0	31.2	21.1	18.3	13.1
2003	89.6	100.0	2.4	12.9	29.9	21.2	18.1	15.6
2004	88.9	100.0	2.7	13.1	30.8	20.8	17.3	15.2
2005	89.7	100.0	2.4	12.9	29.5	21.7	18.6	14.8
2006	89.2	100.0	2.7	12.9	30.4	21.1	17.9	15.0
2007	89.2	100.0	2.9	14.3	30.6	21.2	17.0	14.1
2008	89.1	100.0	2.8	15.2	33.2	20.0	16.4	12.3
2009	88.4	100.0	3.4	15.9	32.5	19.0	16.6	12.6
2010	89.2	100.0	4.0	16.3	32.1	18.9	15.6	13.1
2011	88.8	100.0	3.7	16.6	32.2	19.4	16.2	11.9
65 to 74 Years								
1987	92.8	100.0	5.3	10.0	27.3	21.8	19.4	16.2
1997	94.6	100.0	3.2	10.7	31.6	23.6	17.0	14.0
1998	94.3	100.0	2.0	9.8	33.6	21.6	19.5	13.6
1999	95.3	100.0	1.4	10.0	27.4	23.8	19.4	17.9
2000	94.7	100.0	1.5	10.0	27.2	22.1	21.0	18.3
2001	95.6	100.0	1.5	9.9	27.0	21.5	20.6	19.5
2002	96.1	100.0	1.8	6.3	25.4	21.4	24.1	21.1
2003	95.3	100.0	1.7	6.5	21.0	23.8	23.3	23.8
2004	96.6	100.0	1.5	8.0	23.2	19.3	20.6	27.3
2005	95.9	100.0	1.7	6.5	24.8	20.8	21.5	24.6
2006	95.7	100.0	1.7	7.3	23.7	22.0	25.6	19.7
2007	95.8	100.0	2.7	8.8	28.9	23.0	20.8	15.9
2008	95.8	100.0	1.5	9.6	28.8	22.0	20.4	17.7
2009	95.7	100.0	2.0	11.6	28.3	24.2	18.7	15.2
2010	95.8	100.0	2.4	9.1	28.8	22.5	21.3	15.8
2011	96.2	100.0	2.6	9.8	30.1	23.9	20.0	13.6
75 Years and Over								
1987	95.1	100.0	5.6	7.6	24.7	20.0	19.7	22.4
1997	95.8	100.0	2.4	9.8	27.5	19.5	21.2	19.7
1998	96.3	100.0	3.0	9.6	26.6	20.3	21.0	19.4
1999	95.3	100.0	2.7	8.9	26.3	22.4	19.7	20.0
2000	96.5	100.0	2.6	10.0	25.2	21.5	19.8	20.9
2001	97.0	100.0	1.7	7.0	22.1	19.5	23.0	26.7
2002	96.5	100.0	2.2	6.2	20.1	18.5	24.9	28.2
2003	97.5	100.0	1.9	6.2	19.0	19.5	23.5	29.9
2004	97.7	100.0	1.8	6.1	19.2	16.9	24.8	31.1

Table 3-64. Out-of-Pocket Health Care Expenses Among Persons with Medical Expenses, by Age, Selected Years 1987–2011—continued

(Percent.)

Age and year	Percent of persons with expenses	Amount paid out of pocket among persons with expenses[1]						
		Total	$0	$1 to 99	$100 to 499	$500 to 999	$1,000 to 1,999	$2,000+
2005	97.4	100.0	1.6	6.3	21.2	19.7	19.7	31.4
2006	97.6	100.0	1.7	6.8	22.1	22.8	24.0	22.6
2007	97.3	100.0	1.9	8.7	25.9	19.8	21.8	21.9
2008	97.6	100.0	1.9	10.0	25.9	20.5	22.0	19.7
2009	97.5	100.0	2.7	10.1	24.3	23.4	19.7	19.9
2010	97.0	100.0	3.0	9.7	27.6	19.9	22.1	17.7
2011	96.7	100.0	2.4	11.1	29.7	22.1	19.3	15.5

*Estimates are considered unreliable. Data preceded by an asterisk have a relative standard error equal to or greater than 30 percent.   1 Estimates of expenses were converted to 2011 dollars using the Consumer Price Index (all items).

Table 3-65. Expenditures for Health Services and Supplies and Percent Distribution, by Sponsor, Selected Years, 1987–2013

(Dollars in billions, percent.)

Type of sponsor	1987	1990	1995	2000	2010	2013
NATIONAL HEALTH EXPENDITURES	$519.1	$724.3	$1,027.4	$1,378.0	$2,604.1	$2,919.1
Business, Households, and Other Private Revenues	354.0	488.2	642.3	888.4		
Private business	122.3	178.3	243.7	346.5	533.7	610.9
Employer contribution to private health insurance premiums[1]	84.3	129.5	176.3	255.1	413.5	471.1
Employer contribution to Medicare hospital insurance trust fund[2]	24.6	29.4	43.1	62.3	79.7	91.7
Workers compensation and temporary disability insurance and worksite health care	13.4	19.3	24.3	29.1	40.5	48.2
Household	189.9	253.0	318.9	434.0	738.3	823.8
Employee contribution to private health insurance premiums and individual policy premiums[3]	44.0	68.5	100.3	133.6	270.8	300.2
Employee and self-employment contributions and voluntary premiums paid to Medicare hospital insurance trust fund[4]	29.5	35.7	56.0	82.6	112.1	124.8
Premiums paid by individuals to Medicare supplementary medical insurance trust fund[5]	6.2	10.2	16.4	16.3	49.2	59.4
Out-of-pocket health spending	110.2	138.6	146.2	201.5	306.2	339.4
Other private revenues	41.9	56.9	79.7	107.9	174.6	218.1
Governments	165.1	236.1	385.2	489.6	1,157.5	1,266.3
Federal government	86.2	125.3	217.3	261.9	733.1	757.5
Employer contributions to private health insurance premiums	4.9	9.9	11.4	14.3	28.5	32.4
Employer contributions to Medicare hospital insurance trust fund	1.7	2.0	2.3	2.7	4.1	4.0
Adjusted Medicare[6]	17.4	27.7	57.6	49.2	250.2	274.0
Health program expenditures (excluding Medicare)	62.2	85.8	146.0	195.8	450.3	447.1
Medicaid[7]	28.2	43.3	87.9	119.4	275.9	267.1
Other programs[8]	34.0	42.5	58.1	76.4	174.5	180.0
State and local government	78.9	110.8	167.9	227.7	424.5	508.8
Employer contributions to private health insurance premiums[9]	16.0	26.4	38.9	56.9	142.9	156.0
Employer contributions to Medicare hospital insurance trust fund	3.1	4.1	5.6	7.5	11.2	11.4
Health expenditures by program	59.8	80.3	123.3	163.4	270.4	341.5
Medicaid[7]	22.7	31.5	60.3	85.3	135.0	196.3
Other programs[10]	37.1	48.8	63.1	78.0	135.3	145.2
PERCENT DISTRIBUTION						
NATIONAL HEALTH EXPENDITURES	100.0	100.0	100.0	100.0	100.0	100.0
Business, Households, and Other Private Revenues	68.2	67.4	62.5	64.5	55.6	56.6
Private business	23.6	24.6	23.7	25.1	20.5	20.9
Employer contribution to private health insurance premiums[1]	16.2	17.9	17.2	18.5	15.9	16.1
Employer contribution to Medicare hospital insurance trust fund[2]	4.7	4.1	4.2	4.5	3.1	3.1
Workers compensation and temporary disability insurance and worksite health care	2.6	2.7	2.4	2.1	1.6	1.7
Household	36.6	34.9	31.0	31.5	28.4	28.2
Employee contribution to private health insurance premiums and individual policy premiums[3]	8.5	9.5	9.8	9.7	10.4	10.3
Employee and self-employment contributions and voluntary premiums paid to Medicare hospital insurance trust fund[4]	5.7	4.9	5.5	6.0	4.3	4.3
Premiums paid by individuals to Medicare supplementary medical insurance trust fund[5]	1.2	1.4	1.6	1.2	1.9	2.0
Out-of-pocket health spending	21.2	19.1	14.2	14.6	11.8	11.6
Other private revenues	8.1	7.9	7.8	7.8	6.7	7.5
Governments	31.8	32.6	37.5	35.5	44.4	43.4
Federal government	16.6	17.3	21.2	19.0	28.2	25.9
Employer contributions to private health insurance premiums	0.9	1.4	1.1	1.0	1.1	1.1
Employer contributions to Medicare hospital insurance trust fund	0.3	0.3	0.2	0.2	0.2	0.1
Adjusted Medicare[6]	3.4	3.8	5.6	3.6	9.6	9.4
Health program expenditures (excluding Medicare)	12.0	11.8	14.2	14.2	17.3	15.3
Medicaid[7]	5.4	6.0	8.6	8.7	10.6	9.2
Other programs[8]	6.5	5.9	5.7	5.5	6.7	6.2
State and local government	15.2	15.3	16.3	16.5	16.3	17.4
Employer contributions to private health insurance premiums[9]	3.1	3.6	3.8	4.1	5.5	5.3
Employer contributions to Medicare hospital insurance trust fund	0.6	0.6	0.5	0.5	0.4	0.4
Health expenditures by program						
Medicaid[7]	4.4	4.3	5.9	6.2	5.2	6.7
Other programs[10]	7.1	6.7	6.1	5.7	5.2	5.0

1 Excludes Medicare Retiree Drug Subsidy (RDS) payments to private plans beginning in 2006, small-business tax credits beginning in 2010 and Early Retirement Reinsurance Program (ERRP) payments for 2010–2011.   2 Includes one-half of self-employment contribution to the Medicare Hospital Insurance (HI) Trust Fund.   3 Excludes government-subsidized Consolidated Omnibus Budget Reconciliation Act (COBRA) payments in 2009–2011.   4 Includes one-half of self-employment contribution to Medicare HI Trust Fund and trust fund revenues from the income taxation of Social Security benefits.   5 Includes premiums paid for the Pre-Existing Condition Insurance Plan (PCIP) beginning in 2010.   6 Federal government Medicare expenditures equal Trust Fund interest income and Federal general revenue contributions to Medicare less the net change in Trust Fund balances. Includes Medicare RDS paid to private and state and local government employer plans beginning in 2006. Excludes Part D state phase-down payments to Medicare beginning in 2006 and Medicare premium buy-in programs by Medicaid for people eligible for both Medicaid and Medicare (dual eligibles).   7 Includes Medicare Premium buy-in programs by Medicaid for people eligible for both Medicaid and Medicare (dual eligibles).   8 Includes maternal and child health, vocational rehabilitation, Substance Abuse and Mental Health Services Administration, Indian Health Service, federal workers' compensation, and other federal programs, public health activities, Department of Defense, Department of Veterans Affairs, Children's Health Insurance Program (CHIP), and investment (research, structures and equipment). Also includes government-subsidized COBRA payments in 2009–2011, small business tax credits beginning in 2006, and ERRP payments in 2010–2011. Excludes premiums paid for the Pre-Existing Condition Insurance Plan (PCIP) premiums beginning in 2010.   9 Excludes Medicare RDS payments to state and local government employer plans beginning in 2006 and ERRP payments in 2010–2011.   10 Includes maternal and child health, vocational rehabilitation, general assistance, school health, CHIP, public health activities, other state and local programs, investment (research, structures and equipment). Also includes Part D state phase-down payments to Medicare beginning in 2006.

Table 3-66. Department of Veterans Affairs Health Care Expenditures and Use, and Persons Treated, by Selected Characteristics, Selected Fiscal Years, 2000–2013

(Dollars; numbers in thousands; percent.)

Type of expenditure and use	2000	2005[1]	2006[1]	2007[1]	2008[1]	2009[1]	2010[1]	2011[1]	2012[1]	2013[1]
All Expenditures (Amount in Millions) [2]	$19,327	$30,291	$31,909	$34,025	$38,282	$42,955	$47,280	$50,575	$51,880	$54,738
Percent Distribution										
All services	100.0	100.0	100.0	100.0	100.0	100.0	100.0	100.0	100.0	100.0
Inpatient hospital	37.3	24.3	24.0	24.0	23.5	22.7	21.4	20.6	20.1	19.8
Outpatient care	45.7	53.4	55.2	53.5	53.2	53.5	52.5	52.6	53.8	53.2
Nursing home care	8.2	8.4	8.2	8.3	8.1	7.8	7.4	7.2	7.3	7.0
All other[3]	8.8	13.9	12.6	14.2	15.2	16.0	18.8	19.6	18.8	20.0
Health Care Use										
Inpatient hospital discharges[4,5]	579	614	601	607	622	640	656	653	646	632
Outpatient visits[6]	38,370	57,169	59,132	62,234	66,484	73,969	79,457	83,146	87,370	90,226
Nursing home discharges[5,7]	91	61	59	63	64	65	67	63	67	69
Inpatients [8]	417	488	467	477	492	512	532	540	546	545
Percent Distribution										
Total	100.0	100.0	100.0	100.0	100.0	100.0	100.0	100.0	100.0	100.0
Veterans with service-connected disability	34.4	37.6	38.8	39.9	41.1	42.6	43.5	44.9	46.5	48.3
Veterans without service-connected disability	64.7	61.5	60.2	59.1	58.0	56.4	55.6	54.3	52.6	50.8
Low income	41.7	39.9	37.9	36.9	35.4	34.8	34.6	33.4	32.1	30.4
Veterans receiving aid and attendance or housebound benefits or who are catastrophically disabled[9]	16.0	12.1	11.6	11.3	11.1	10.5	10.1	9.8	9.6	9.4
Veterans receiving medical care subject to copayments[10]	5.2	8.6	9.7	9.8	10.0	9.5	9.3	9.3	9.2	9.3
Other and unknown[11]	1.8	1.0	1.0	1.0	1.6	1.6	1.6	1.7	1.7	1.7
Nonveterans	0.9	0.9	0.9	0.9	0.9	1.0	0.9	0.9	0.9	0.9
Outpatients [8]	3,657	5,077	5,180	5,221	5,291	5,439	5,631	5,789	5,903	6,009
Percent Distribution										
Total	100.0	100.0	100.0	100.0	100.0	100.0	100.0	100.0	100.0	100.0
Veterans with service-connected disability	30.7	31.6	32.4	33.8	34.7	37.1	38.6	39.8	41.7	44.0
Veterans without service-connected disability	60.8	62.7	62.0	60.8	59.7	57.2	56.4	55.1	53.3	51.1
Low income	37.6	31.8	30.3	28.9	27.2	25.9	25.7	24.9	24.0	22.6
Veterans receiving aid and attendance or housebound benefits or who are catastrophically disabled[9]	3.8	3.5	3.4	3.5	3.5	3.4	3.4	3.3	3.2	3.2
Veterans receiving medical care subject to copayments[10]	15.4	25.4	25.7	25.5	25.2	23.8	23.0	22.3	21.4	20.7
Other and unknown[11]	4.0	2.0	2.6	3.0	3.8	4.0	4.3	4.6	4.6	4.6
Nonveterans	8.5	5.7	5.6	5.4	5.7	5.7	5.1	5.1	5.1	4.9

1 Starting with FY2005, the cost report data are taken from a different report than earlier years. The major impact of this change was to assign more cost to outpatient care than inpatient hospital. Also in FY2005, the responsibility for residential rehabilitation programs including domiciliary care was reassigned from extended care to mental health care.   2 Health care expenditures exclude construction, medical administration, and miscellaneous operating expenses at Department of Veterans Affairs headquarters.   3 Includes miscellaneous benefits and services, contract hospitals, education and training, subsidies to state veterans hospitals, nursing homes and residential rehabilitation treatment programs (formerly domiciliaries), and the Civilian Health and Medical Program of the Department of Veterans Affairs.   4 Discharges from medicine, surgery, psychiatry, rehabilitation medicine, spinal cord, and neurology units. Starting with FY2005 data, includes domiciliary care. Does not include long-term stays.   5 Until FY2004, includes Department of Veterans Affairs nursing home and residential rehabilitation treatment programs (formerly domiciliary) stays, and community nursing home care stays.   6 Hospital outpatient care. Includes the following services: physicians, laboratory tests, home-based primary care, or outpatient fee-basis care. 7 Includes state nursing home veteran patients.   8 Individuals receiving services. Individuals with multiple discharges or visits are only counted once in the inpatient or outpatient category. The inpatient and outpatient totals are not additive because most inpatients are also treated as outpatients.   9 Includes veterans who are receiving aid and attendance or housebound benefit and veterans who have been determined by the Department of Veterans Affairs to be catastrophically disabled.   10 Includes veterans who receive medical care subject to copayments according to income level, based on financial means testing.   11 Includes expenditures for services for veterans who were prisoners of war, exposed to Agent Orange, and other. Veterans reporting Agent Orange exposure but not treated for it were means tested and placed in the low income or other group depending on income.

HEALTH INSURANCE

Figure 3-14. Number in Millions of Persons with NO Health Insurance, Selected Years, 1984–2013

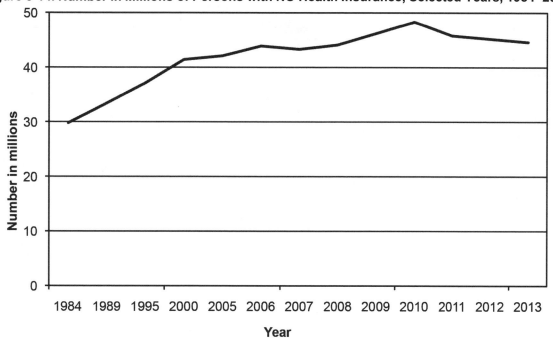

Figure 3-15. Medicaid Coverages Among Persons Under 65 Years of Age, Selected Years, 1984–2013

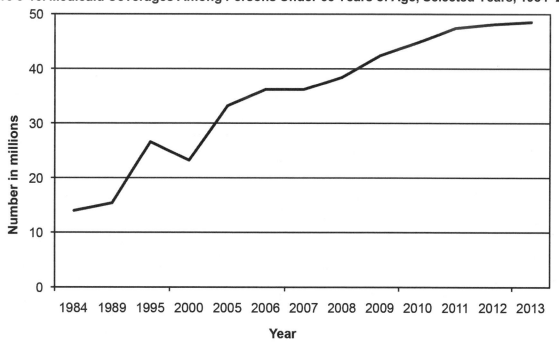

Table 3-67. Private Health Insurance[1] Coverage Among Persons Under 65 Years of Age, by Selected Characteristics, Selected Years, 1984–2011

(Numbers in millions; percent.)

Characteristic	1984[2]	1989[2]	1995[2]	2000[3]	2005	2010	2011	2012	2013
Total (number in millions)[4]	157.5	162.7	164.2	174.0	174.7	163.9	164.5	164.9	165.3
Total (percent of population)[4]	76.8	75.9	71.3	71.5	68.2	61.7	61.8	61.8	61.8
Age									
Under 19 years	72.6	71.9	65.4	66.7	62.3	54.3	53.9	53.6	53.5
Under 6 years	68.1	67.9	59.5	62.7	56.6	48.3	47.8	48.4	47.3
6 to 18 years	74.8	73.9	68.3	68.5	64.9	57.2	56.9	56.0	56.3
Under 18 years	72.6	71.8	65.2	66.6	62.1	54.1	53.7	53.4	53.2
6 to 17 years	74.9	74.0	68.3	68.5	64.7	57.2	56.7	55.8	56.0
18 to 64 years	78.6	77.6	73.9	73.5	70.7	64.7	65.0	65.1	65.1
18 to 44 years	76.5	75.5	70.9	70.5	66.6	60.0	60.9	61.4	61.8
18 to 24 years	67.4	64.5	60.8	60.3	58.0	52.3	57.2	58.1	59.0
19 to 25 years	67.4	63.8	60.1	59.1	56.3	51.8	56.9	58.1	58.9
25 to 34 years	77.4	75.9	70.1	70.1	65.1	58.7	58.6	58.7	59.0
35 to 44 years	83.9	82.7	77.7	77.0	73.7	66.9	66.0	66.7	67.0
45 to 64 years	83.3	82.5	80.1	78.7	76.9	71.3	70.6	70.0	69.5
45 to 54 years	83.3	83.4	80.9	80.0	77.4	70.9	70.1	69.6	69.8
55 to 64 years	83.3	81.6	79.0	76.7	76.2	71.8	71.2	70.4	69.1
Sex									
Male	77.3	76.1	71.6	71.6	68.0	61.1	61.4	61.8	61.9
Female	76.2	75.7	70.9	71.3	68.4	62.4	62.2	61.9	61.7
Sex and Marital Status [5]									
Male									
Married	85.0	84.2	80.2	81.5	79.6	75.1	74.5	74.9	74.8
Divorced, separated, widowed	65.5	64.6	62.4	62.2	56.7	50.6	50.5	51.0	50.9
Never married	71.3	68.3	65.4	63.8	60.2	52.5	55.1	54.7	55.8
Female									
Married	83.8	83.5	79.3	81.0	79.3	75.6	75.1	75.0	74.3
Divorced, separated, widowed	63.1	63.6	61.7	63.2	59.9	53.9	52.6	51.8	52.1
Never married	72.2	70.0	66.2	64.2	61.5	54.1	55.9	56.2	56.2
Race [6]									
White only	79.9	79.1	74.5	75.7	70.9	64.9	64.9	64.8	64.7
Black or African American only	58.1	57.7	53.0	55.9	52.9	44.8	45.9	45.8	45.4
American Indian or Alaska Native only	49.1	45.5	45.3	43.7	43.0	31.7	33.7	34.9	36.0
Asian only	69.9	71.9	68.4	72.1	72.2	68.1	65.9	67.6	69.4
Native Hawaiian or Other Pacific Islander only	---	---	---	*	*	*	*	*	*
Two or more races	---	---	---	61.4	57.6	52.4	52.3	52.9	50.0
Hispanic Origin and Race [6]									
Hispanic or Latino	55.7	51.5	46.4	47.8	42.4	36.8	36.4	36.7	37.3
Mexican	53.3	46.8	42.6	45.4	39.7	33.4	33.9	34.1	34.9
Puerto Rican	48.4	45.6	47.6	51.1	48.5	46.0	45.5	43.7	42.1
Cuban	72.5	70.3	63.6	63.9	58.1	53.8	51.1	49.1	45.3
Other Hispanic or Latino	61.6	61.0	51.4	50.7	45.6	40.9	38.1	39.5	41.2
Not Hispanic or Latino	78.7	78.5	74.4	75.2	73.0	67.0	67.3	67.5	67.4
White only	82.4	82.5	78.6	79.5	77.3	72.0	72.2	72.6	72.4
Black or African American only	58.2	57.7	53.4	56.0	53.1	45.1	46.5	46.4	45.7
Age and Percent of Poverty Level [7]									
Under 65 years									
Below 100 percent	32.2	27.0	22.6	25.2	21.4	16.0	17.2	16.5	15.5
100 percent to 199 percent	70.3	64.3	55.3	50.1	44.7	34.8	35.1	36.7	35.1
100 percent to 133 percent	59.4	52.8	41.7	39.3	36.0	24.4	24.1	26.9	25.3
134 percent to 199 percent	75.2	69.5	62.7	55.3	49.4	40.3	41.1	42.4	40.8
200 percent to 399 percent	89.3	89.2	86.4	78.1	74.8	70.7	71.1	71.3	71.3
400 percent or more	95.4	94.6	93.2	91.9	90.6	89.9	90.7	90.6	90.4
Under 19 years									
Below 100 percent	29.6	24.1	19.0	20.3	15.0	9.8	10.6	10.0	9.3
100 percent to 199 percent	73.6	68.5	55.8	49.5	41.6	31.5	31.2	32.4	29.2
100 percent to 133 percent	63.8	56.9	42.5	37.1	32.6	20.1	19.1	22.3	18.3
134 percent to 199 percent	78.4	74.0	64.4	56.1	47.0	38.1	38.0	38.4	36.2
200 percent to 399 percent	91.1	92.1	89.1	80.8	76.6	72.6	72.4	72.5	71.8
400 percent or more	96.2	96.2	93.3	93.0	92.5	91.2	92.7	91.2	92.3
Under 18 years									
Below 100 percent	28.5	22.3	16.9	19.5	14.2	9.2	9.7	9.1	8.4
100 percent to 199 percent	73.9	68.9	56.1	49.4	41.4	31.5	31.0	32.1	28.5
100 percent to 133 percent	63.9	57.3	42.3	36.8	32.0	19.9	19.0	21.6	17.8
134 percent to 199 percent	78.6	74.5	64.9	56.2	47.0	38.3	37.7	38.4	35.3
200 percent to 399 percent	91.3	92.3	89.2	81.1	76.6	72.6	72.5	72.5	71.9
400 percent or more	96.1	96.5	93.1	93.1	92.5	91.4	92.8	91.4	92.2
18 to 64 years									
Below 100 percent	35.0	30.8	27.0	29.1	25.9	20.4	21.8	20.9	19.9
100 percent to 199 percent	68.3	61.5	54.8	50.5	46.5	36.4	37.2	38.9	38.2
100 percent to 133 percent	56.6	50.0	41.4	40.9	38.3	26.9	26.7	29.6	29.2

Table 3-67. Private Health Insurance[1] Coverage Among Persons Under 65 Years of Age, by Selected Characteristics, Selected Years, 1984–2011— continued

(Numbers in millions; percent.)

Characteristic	1984[2]	1989[2]	1995[2]	2000[3]	2005	2010	2011	2012	2013
134 percent to 199 percent	73.3	66.6	61.5	54.9	50.7	41.3	42.8	44.2	43.2
200 percent to 399 percent	88.3	87.6	85.0	76.7	74.0	70.0	70.5	70.8	71.1
400 percent or more	95.2	94.4	93.2	91.6	90.1	89.5	90.2	90.4	89.9
Disability Measure among Adults 18 to 64 Years [8]									
Any basic actions difficulty or complex activity limitation	---	---	---	63.1	58.1	53.0	49.3	50.8	48.6
Any basic actions difficulty	---	---	---	63.9	58.8	53.8	49.6	51.7	49.2
Any complex activity limitation	---	---	---	48.4	44.0	38.6	35.7	36.0	34.8
No disability	---	---	---	77.2	73.7	69.3	70.5	70.2	70.7
Geographic Region									
Northeast	80.5	82.0	75.4	76.3	74.0	68.2	66.8	67.2	66.1
Midwest	80.6	81.5	77.3	78.8	74.6	66.7	67.9	68.4	68.0
South	74.3	71.4	66.9	66.8	62.5	57.5	57.8	57.3	57.4
West	71.9	71.2	67.5	66.5	65.6	58.9	58.4	58.5	59.6
Location of Residence									
Within MSA[9]	77.5	76.5	72.1	72.3	69.0	62.9	63.2	63.0	63.0
Outside MSA[9]	75.2	73.8	67.9	67.8	64.6	55.1	54.1	55.3	54.7

NA = Not available.   * = Figure does not meet standards of reliability or precision. Data not shown have a relative standard error of greater than 30 percent.   1 Any private insurance at the time of interview that was originally obtained through a present or former employer or union, or, starting with 1997 data, through the workplace, self-employment, or a professional association; includes those who also had another type of coverage.   2 Data prior to 1997 are not strictly comparable with data for later years due to the 1997 questionnaire redesign.   3 Estimates for 2000–2002 were calculated using 2000-based sample weights and may differ from estimates in other reports that used 1990-based sample weights for 2000-2002 estimates.   4 Includes all other races not shown separately, those with unknown marital status, unknown disability status, and, in 1984 and 1989, persons with unknown poverty level.   5 Includes persons 14 to 64 years of age.   6 The race groups White, Black, American Indian or Alaska Native, Asian, Native Hawaiian or Other Pacific Islander, and two or more races include persons of Hispanic and non-Hispanic origin. Persons of Hispanic origin may be of any race.   7 Percent of poverty level is based on family income and family size and composition using U.S. Census Bureau poverty thresholds. Poverty level was unknown for 10 to 11 percent of persons under 65 years of age in 1984 and 1989. Missing family income data were imputed for 1995 and beyond.   8 Any basic actions difficulty or complex activity limitation is defined as having one or more of the following limitations or difficulties: movement difficulty, emotional difficulty, sensory (seeing or hearing) difficulty, cognitive difficulty, self-care (activities of daily living or instrumental activities of daily living) limitation, social limitation, or work limitation.   9 MSA = metropolitan statistical area.

Table 3-68. Private Health Insurance[1] Coverage Obtained Through the Workplace Among Persons Under 65 Years of Age, by Selected Characteristics, Selected Years, 1984–2011

(Numbers in millions; percent.)

Characteristic	1984[2]	1995[2]	2000[3]	2005	2010	2011	2012	2013
Total Population (in Millions) [4]	141.8	150.7	160.8	160.1	147.6	146.4	148.6	148.3
Percent of Population, Total [4]	69.1	65.4	67.1	63.6	56.6	56.4	56.9	56.6
Age								
Under 19 years	66.4	60.5	63.1	58.7	50.9	49.9	50.1	49.6
Under 6 years	62.1	55.1	58.9	53.4	44.9	44.3	45.0	44.2
6 to 18 years	68.4	63.1	64.9	61.1	53.8	52.5	52.4	52.0
Under 18 years	66.5	60.4	63.0	58.6	50.7	49.7	49.9	49.3
6 to 17 years	68.7	63.3	65.0	61.1	53.8	52.4	52.3	51.8
18 to 64 years	70.3	67.6	68.8	65.7	58.9	59.1	59.6	59.5
18 to 44 years	69.6	65.3	66.5	62.2	54.6	55.6	56.7	56.9
18 to 24 years	58.7	53.5	55.5	52.1	45.3	51.0	52.7	53.1
19 to 25 years	59.0	53.0	54.2	50.6	44.1	50.5	52.7	53.0
25 to 34 years	71.2	65.0	66.4	61.1	53.3	53.0	53.8	53.8
35 to 44 years	77.4	72.7	73.2	69.9	62.8	61.6	62.7	63.1
45 to 64 years	71.8	72.2	72.9	70.9	64.8	63.9	63.6	62.9
45 to 54 years	74.6	74.7	75.6	72.6	65.9	64.7	64.4	64.3
55 to 64 years	69.0	68.4	68.6	68.6	63.4	63.0	62.6	61.3
Sex								
Male	69.8	65.9	67.3	63.6	56.1	56.1	57.1	56.9
Female	68.4	64.9	66.9	63.6	57.1	56.7	56.8	56.4
Sex and Marital Status [5]								
Male								
Married	77.9	74.9	77.5	75.3	70.1	69.3	69.9	69.8
Divorced, separated, widowed	58.0	56.4	57.4	51.9	45.3	45.0	46.2	45.3
Never married	61.5	58.2	58.8	54.9	46.2	48.4	49.6	50.0
Female								
Married	76.1	73.2	76.3	74.2	69.8	69.2	69.3	68.5
Divorced, separated, widowed	51.9	54.6	57.8	54.3	48.1	46.5	46.3	46.3
Never married	63.5	59.2	60.1	56.3	48.2	50.0	50.9	50.6
Race [6]								
White only	72.0	68.4	71.0	66.1	59.3	59.0	59.6	59.2
Black or African American only	52.4	49.3	53.4	50.6	42.3	43.5	43.2	42.9
American Indian or Alaska Native only	45.8	40.2	41.7	39.9	*29.4	32.4	34.0	34.2
Asian only	59.0	59.6	65.8	64.4	60.6	58.7	60.1	61.4
Native Hawaiian or Other Pacific Islander only	NA	NA	*	*	*	*	*	*
Two or more races	NA	NA	59.8	54.8	49.5	48.3	48.8	46.9
Hispanic Origin and Race [6]								
Hispanic or Latino	52.0	43.4	45.3	40.0	34.6	34.1	34.6	34.9
Mexican	50.5	40.9	43.6	37.6	31.6	32.0	32.5	32.5
Puerto Rican	45.9	44.5	49.4	46.2	43.6	42.8	41.6	40.8
Cuban	57.4	54.0	53.6	53.5	47.4	45.0	42.8	41.2
Other Hispanic or Latino	57.4	46.7	47.3	42.6	37.8	35.1	36.7	38.6
Not Hispanic or Latino	70.7	68.2	70.6	68.0	61.3	61.3	62.0	61.7
White only	74.0	72.1	74.5	71.9	65.7	65.5	66.6	66.1
Black or African American only	52.5	49.8	53.6	50.9	42.6	44.1	43.6	43.2
Age and Percent of Poverty Level [7]								
Under 65 years								
Below 100 percent	24.1	17.5	21.0	17.8	12.4	13.6	13.6	12.2
100 percent to 199 percent	61.7	49.3	45.4	40.1	30.2	30.4	32.2	31.0
100 percent to 133 percent	50.0	36.0	35.0	31.3	20.6	19.7	23.0	21.7
134 percent to 199 percent	66.9	56.6	50.5	44.8	35.3	36.2	37.5	36.3
200 percent to 399 percent	82.8	80.5	73.4	69.8	65.3	65.0	65.9	65.6
400 percent or more	88.8	86.7	87.9	86.1	84.2	85.0	85.1	84.6
Under 19 years								
Below 100 percent	23.6	15.1	17.1	13.3	8.2	9.1	8.7	7.8
100 percent to 199 percent	67.0	50.5	45.8	38.3	28.8	27.9	29.7	26.6
100 percent to 133 percent	56.1	37.4	33.6	29.1	17.9	16.3	20.5	16.4
134 percent to 199 percent	72.3	58.8	52.2	43.7	35.1	34.4	35.2	33.1
200 percent to 399 percent	85.7	83.9	76.9	72.4	68.7	67.0	68.0	66.7
400 percent or more	90.8	87.5	89.5	88.3	86.5	87.5	86.3	86.9
Under 18 years								
Below 100 percent	23.0	13.6	16.6	12.5	7.8	8.4	8.1	7.2
100 percent to 199 percent	67.5	50.9	45.8	38.2	28.8	27.7	29.4	26.0
100 percent to 133 percent	56.3	37.2	33.5	28.6	17.8	16.1	19.8	16.0
134 percent to 199 percent	72.8	59.6	52.4	43.9	35.2	34.1	35.2	32.4
200 percent to 399 percent	85.9	84.1	77.1	72.4	68.7	67.0	68.1	66.8
400 percent or more	90.7	87.1	89.7	88.5	86.6	87.7	86.4	86.8
18 to 64 years								
Below 100 percent	24.8	20.5	24.0	21.2	15.4	16.8	16.9	15.2
100 percent to 199 percent	58.3	48.4	45.2	41.1	30.9	31.8	33.6	33.3
100 percent to 133 percent	46.0	35.3	35.9	32.9	22.1	21.5	24.6	24.7

Table 3-68. Private Health Insurance[1] Coverage Obtained Through the Workplace Among Persons Under 65 Years of Age, by Selected Characteristics, Selected Years, 1984–2011 — continued

(Numbers in millions; percent.)

Characteristic	1984[2]	1995[2]	2000[3]	2005	2010	2011	2012	2013
134 percent to 199 percent	63.6	55.0	49.5	45.3	35.3	37.2	38.7	38.0
200 percent to 399 percent	81.4	78.8	71.7	68.7	63.9	64.3	65.0	65.2
400 percent or more	88.5	86.7	87.5	85.4	83.6	84.2	84.7	84.0
Disability Measure among Adults 18 to 64 Years[8]								
Any basic actions difficulty or complex activity limitation	NA	NA	58.5	53.3	48.0	44.4	45.8	44.0
Any basic actions difficulty	NA	NA	59.1	54.0	48.9	44.9	46.7	44.6
Any complex activity limitation	NA	NA	43.5	38.9	32.8	30.3	30.5	29.6
No disability	NA	NA	72.5	68.5	63.5	64.6	64.7	64.7
Geographic Region								
Northeast	74.0	69.8	72.5	70.6	64.4	63.0	63.4	62.3
Midwest	72.0	71.2	74.9	70.1	61.8	62.2	63.8	62.6
South	66.2	61.8	62.5	58.0	52.2	52.3	52.2	52.4
West	64.7	60.4	61.1	59.7	52.7	52.2	52.8	53.6
Location of Residence								
Within MSA[9]	70.9	66.6	68.2	64.5	57.9	57.8	58.1	57.8
Outside MSA[9]	65.3	60.7	62.6	59.6	49.4	48.7	50.3	49.4

NA = Not available.   * = Figure does not meet standards of reliability or precision. Data not shown have a relative standard error of greater than 30 percent.   1 Any private insurance at the time of interview that was originally obtained through a present or former employer or union, or, starting with 1997 data, through the workplace, self-employment, or a professional association; includes those who also had another type of coverage.   2 Data prior to 1997 are not strictly comparable with data for later years due to the 1997 questionnaire redesign.   3 Estimates for 2000–2002 were calculated using 2000-based sample weights and may differ from estimates in other reports that used 1990-based sample weights for 2000-2002 estimates.   4 Includes all other races not shown separately, those with unknown marital status, unknown disability status, and, in 1984 and 1989, persons with unknown poverty level.   5 Includes persons 14 to 64 years of age.   6 The race groups White, Black, American Indian or Alaska Native, Asian, Native Hawaiian or Other Pacific Islander, and two or more races include persons of Hispanic and non-Hispanic origin. Persons of Hispanic origin may be of any race.   7 Percent of poverty level is based on family income and family size and composition using U.S. Census Bureau poverty thresholds. Poverty level was unknown for 10 to 11 percent of persons under 65 years of age in 1984 and 1989. Missing family income data were imputed for 1995 and beyond.   8 Any basic actions difficulty or complex activity limitation is defined as having one or more of the following limitations or difficulties: movement difficulty, emotional difficulty, sensory (seeing or hearing) difficulty, cognitive difficulty, self-care (activities of daily living or instrumental activities of daily living) limitation, social limitation, or work limitation.   9 MSA = metropolitan statistical area.

Table 3-69. No Health Insurance Coverage Among Persons Under 65 Years of Age, by Selected Characteristics, Selected Years, 1984–2013

(Numbers in millions; percent.)

Characteristic	1984[1]	1995[1]	2000[2]	2005[3]	2010[3]	2011[3]	2012[3]	2013[3]
Total (number in millions)[4]	29.8	37.1	41.4	42.1	48.3	45.8	45.2	44.6
Total (percent of population)[4]	14.5	16.1	17.0	16.4	18.2	17.2	16.9	16.7
Age								
Under 19 years	14.1	13.7	12.9	9.7	8.3	7.4	7.0	7.1
Under 6 years	14.9	11.8	11.8	7.7	6.3	5.0	4.6	5.0
6 to 18 years	13.8	14.6	13.4	10.6	9.2	8.5	8.1	8.0
Under 18 years	13.9	13.4	12.6	9.3	7.8	7.0	6.6	6.6
6 to 17 years	13.4	14.3	13.0	10.1	8.6	8.0	7.6	7.4
18 to 64 years	14.8	17.3	18.9	19.3	22.3	21.2	20.9	20.5
18 to 44 years	17.1	20.4	22.4	23.5	27.1	25.4	24.8	24.2
18 to 24 years	25.0	28.0	30.4	29.1	31.4	25.9	24.5	24.6
19 to 25 years	25.1	28.8	32.3	31.7	33.8	27.9	26.3	26.7
25 to 34 years	16.2	21.1	23.3	25.6	28.3	28.1	28.1	27.1
35 to 44 years	11.2	15.1	16.9	17.9	22.6	22.2	21.7	21.0
45 to 64 years	9.6	10.9	12.6	12.9	15.7	15.4	15.6	15.4
45 to 54 years	10.5	11.6	12.8	14.2	17.9	17.4	17.7	17.1
55 to 64 years	8.7	9.9	12.4	11.1	12.8	13.0	13.2	13.5
Sex								
Male	15.3	17.4	18.1	17.9	20.3	18.8	18.5	18.1
Female	13.8	14.8	15.9	15.0	16.1	15.6	15.4	15.2
Sex and Marital Status [5]								
Male								
Married	11.1	15.0	14.1	14.4	17.2	16.5	16.2	15.9
Divorced, separated, widowed	24.9	24.0	25.8	28.6	31.4	30.0	29.3	28.1
Never married	22.4	25.6	27.2	27.6	31.1	28.0	27.5	26.9
Female								
Married	11.2	13.6	13.3	13.0	14.7	14.4	14.6	14.6
Divorced, separated, widowed	19.2	18.1	21.3	22.1	23.6	24.0	24.2	22.8
Never married	16.3	17.5	21.1	20.0	21.9	20.5	19.6	19.6
Race [6]								
White only	13.6	15.5	15.4	15.9	17.6	16.7	16.7	16.3
Black or African American only	19.9	18.0	19.5	18.4	20.6	19.0	18.0	18.9
American Indian or Alaska Native only	22.5	34.3	38.4	32.2	44.0	34.2	27.0	29.4
Asian only	18.5	18.6	17.6	17.1	17.1	16.5	16.8	14.2
Native Hawaiian or Other Pacific Islander only	NA	NA	*	*	*	*	*	*
Two or more races	NA	NA	16.8	16.5	15.8	16.0	14.5	15.3
Hispanic Origin and Race [6]								
Hispanic or Latino	29.5	31.4	35.6	33.0	32.0	31.1	30.4	30.7
Mexican	33.8	35.6	39.9	36.0	34.8	33.0	33.2	33.4
Puerto Rican	18.3	17.6	16.4	16.3	13.7	15.8	14.4	15.6
Cuban	21.6	22.3	25.4	23.2	26.5	28.1	24.3	26.6
Other Hispanic or Latino	27.4	30.2	33.4	32.6	32.4	31.8	30.1	28.8
Not Hispanic or Latino	13.2	14.2	14.0	13.4	15.2	14.2	13.9	13.4
White only	11.9	13.0	12.5	12.0	13.7	12.9	12.7	12.2
Black or African American only	19.7	17.9	19.5	18.3	20.7	18.8	17.8	18.8
Age and Percent of Poverty Level [7]								
Under 65 years								
Below 100 percent	33.9	29.6	34.2	30.6	30.3	28.4	28.2	28.0
100 percent to 199 percent	21.8	28.3	31.0	28.6	32.4	30.0	29.3	29.3
100 percent to 133 percent	28.8	34.1	35.7	30.1	34.9	32.0	31.1	30.4
134 percent to 199 percent	18.7	25.1	28.7	27.8	31.0	28.9	28.4	28.6
200 percent to 399 percent	7.6	10.0	15.4	15.7	17.4	16.5	16.2	16.1
400 percent or more	3.2	5.4	5.9	6.3	5.6	5.2	4.9	4.8
Under 19 years								
Below 100 percent	29.0	20.4	22.6	15.2	11.3	9.4	8.3	8.9
100 percent to 199 percent	18.0	22.6	22.1	15.6	13.5	12.1	11.1	11.7
100 percent to 133 percent	24.4	26.4	26.5	15.6	15.9	12.5	9.6	11.6
134 percent to 199 percent	14.9	20.1	19.7	15.6	12.0	11.9	12.0	11.7
200 percent to 399 percent	5.1	6.7	9.6	8.2	7.4	6.8	6.8	6.7
400 percent or more	1.8	4.4	3.5	3.3	2.3	2.1	2.2	1.9
Under 18 years								
Below 100 percent	28.9	20.0	22.0	14.3	10.6	8.8	7.6	8.2
100 percent to 199 percent	17.5	22.0	21.7	15.0	12.7	11.4	10.4	11.1
100 percent to 133 percent	24.0	26.1	26.4	15.1	15.1	11.5	9.0	11.2
134 percent to 199 percent	14.4	19.5	19.1	15.0	11.3	11.3	11.3	11.1
200 percent to 399 percent	4.9	6.6	9.3	7.8	7.0	6.4	6.7	6.3
400 percent or more	1.8	4.6	3.3	3.2	2.1	2.0	2.1	1.8
18 to 64 years								
Below 100 percent	37.6	37.0	42.4	40.9	42.7	40.4	40.5	40.0
100 percent to 199 percent	24.4	32.0	36.4	35.9	42.1	39.3	38.6	37.8
100 percent to 133 percent	31.9	39.7	41.7	38.9	45.7	42.5	42.2	40.4
134 percent to 199 percent	21.1	28.2	34.0	34.4	40.3	37.6	36.5	36.4

Table 3-69. No Health Insurance Coverage Among Persons Under 65 Years of Age, by Selected Characteristics, Selected Years, 1984–2013— continued

(Numbers in millions; percent.)

Characteristic	1984[1]	1995[1]	2000[2]	2005[3]	2010[3]	2011[3]	2012[3]	2013[3]
200 percent to 399 percent	8.9	11.7	18.2	19.0	21.3	20.4	19.8	19.7
400 percent or more	3.4	5.5	6.6	7.1	6.5	6.1	5.6	5.6
Disability Measure among Adults 18 to 64 Years[6]								
Any basic actions difficulty or complex activity limitation	NA	NA	17.6	19.6	20.8	22.0	20.4	20.4
Any basic actions difficulty	NA	NA	17.6	19.8	20.9	22.3	20.3	20.4
Any complex activity limitation	NA	NA	16.1	16.9	17.2	18.2	18.3	17.1
No disability	NA	NA	18.5	19.5	21.6	20.2	20.4	19.9
Geographic Region								
Northeast	10.2	13.3	12.2	11.3	12.4	11.8	11.5	11.2
Midwest	11.3	12.2	12.3	11.9	14.1	13.4	13.6	13.1
South	17.7	19.4	20.5	21.0	21.9	20.4	20.3	19.9
West	18.2	17.9	20.7	18.4	20.6	20.0	19.0	18.9
Location of Residence								
Within MSA[9]	13.6	15.5	16.6	16.1	17.8	16.7	16.4	16.2
Outside MSA[9]	16.6	18.6	18.6	17.8	20.4	19.8	19.9	19.3

NA = Not available.   * = Figure does not meet standards of reliability or precision. Data not shown have a relative standard error of greater than 30 percent.   1 Data prior to 1997 are not strictly comparable with data for later years due to the 1997 questionnaire redesign.   2 Estimates for 2000-2002 were calculated using 2000-based sample weights and may differ from estimates in other reports that used 1990-based sample weights for 2000-2002 estimates.   3 Beginning in quarter 3 of the 2004 NHIS, persons under 65 years of age with no reported coverage were asked explicitly about Medicaid coverage. Estimates were calculated without and with the additional information from this question in the columns labeled 2004(1) and 2004(2), respectively, and estimates were calculated with the additional information starting with 2005 data.   4 Includes all other races not shown separately, those with unknown marital status, unknown disability status, and, in 1984 and 1989, persons with unknown poverty level.   5 Includes persons 14 to 64 years of age.   6 The race groups White, Black, American Indian or Alaska Native, Asian, Native Hawaiian or Other Pacific Islander, and two or more races include persons of Hispanic and non-Hispanic origin. Persons of Hispanic origin may be of any race.   7 Percent of poverty level is based on family income and family size and composition using U.S. Census Bureau poverty thresholds. Poverty level was unknown for 10 to 11 percent of persons under 65 years of age in 1984 and 1989. Missing family income data were imputed for 1995 and beyond.   8 Any basic actions difficulty or complex activity limitation is defined as having one or more of the following limitations or difficulties: movement difficulty, emotional difficulty, sensory (seeing or hearing) difficulty, cognitive difficulty, self-care (activities of daily living or instrumental activities of daily living) limitation, social limitation, or work limitation.   9 MSA = metropolitan statistical area.

Table 3-70A. Health Insurance Coverage of Noninstitutionalized Medicare Beneficiaries 65 Years of Age and Over, by Type of Coverage and Selected Characteristics, Selected Years, 1992–2012

(Numbers in millions; percent.)

Characteristic	Medicare Risk Health Maintenance Organization[1]					Medicaid[2]				
	1992	1995	2000	2005	2012	1992	1995	2000	2005	2012
Age										
65 years and over (number in millions)	1.1	2.6	5.9	4.6	12.4	2.7	2.8	2.7	3.2	3.6
65 years and over (percent of population)	3.9	8.9	19.3	14.5	21.9	9.4	9.6	9.0	10.1	8.5
65 to 74 years	4.2	9.5	20.6	13.9	29.1	7.9	8.8	8.5	9.9	7.6
75 to 84 years	3.7	8.3	18.5	15.3	30.1	10.6	9.6	8.9	9.9	9.2
85 years and over	*	7.3	16.3	13.9	26.3	16.6	13.6	11.2	11.9	10.3
Sex										
Male	4.6	9.2	19.3	13.5	28.9	6.3	6.2	6.3	7.2	5.6
Female	3.4	8.6	19.3	15.2	29.2	11.6	12.0	10.9	12.3	10.7
Race and Hispanic Origin										
White, not Hispanic or Latino	3.6	8.4	18.4	13.2	26.9	5.6	5.4	5.1	6.1	5.1
Black, not Hispanic or Latino	*	7.9	20.7	17.1	30.3	28.5	30.3	23.6	23.6	19.0
Hispanic	*	15.5	27.5	27.2	45.5	39.0	40.5	28.7	29.2	20.2
Percent of Poverty Level [3]										
Below 100 percent	3.6	7.7	18.4	NA	NA	22.3	17.2	15.9	NA	NA
100 percent to less than 200 percent	3.7	9.5	23.4	NA	NA	6.7	6.3	8.4	NA	NA
200 percent or more	4.2	10.1	18.0	NA	NA	*	*	*	NA	NA
Marital Status										
Married	4.6	9.5	18.7	13.8	28.6	4.0	4.3	4.3	5.4	3.9
Widowed	2.3	7.7	19.4	15.0	28.6	14.9	15.0	13.6	14.9	13.8
Divorced	*	9.7	24.4	17.1	32.4	23.4	24.5	20.2	20.0	15.7
Never married	*	*	15.8	13.9	27,4	19.2	19.0	17.0	21.3	14.5

Table 3-70B. Health Insurance Coverage of Noninstitutionalized Medicare Beneficiaries 65 Years of Age and Over, by Type of Coverage and Selected Characteristics, Selected Years, 1992–2012

(Numbers in millions; percent.)

Characteristic	Employer-sponsored plan[4]					Medigap[5]				
	1992	1995	2000	2005	2012	1992	1995	2000	2005	2012
Age										
65 years and over (number in millions)	12.5	11.3	10.7	11.6	12.0	9.9	9.5	7.6	8.2	8.0
65 years and over (percent of population)	42.8	38.6	35.2	36.4	28.1	33.9	32.5	25.0	25.7	18.9
65 to 74 years	46.9	41.1	36.6	38.1	29.8	31.4	29.9	21.7	23.2	17.5
75 to 84 years	38.2	37.1	35.0	35.5	25.9	37.5	35.2	27.8	27.3	20.2
85 years and over	31.6	30.2	29.4	31.8	26.1	38.3	37.6	31.1	30.8	22.1
Sex										
Male	46.3	42.1	37.7	39.4	30.2	30.6	30.0	23.4	23.8	17.2
Female	40.4	36.0	33.4	34.2	26.4	36.2	34.4	26.2	27.1	20.3
Race and Hispanic Origin										
White, not Hispanic or Latino	45.9	41.3	38.6	39.5	30.6	37.2	36.2	28.3	29.1	22.4
Black, not Hispanic or Latino	25.9	26.7	22.0	27.9	27.4	13.6	10.2	7.5	9.5	5.7
Hispanic	20.7	16.9	15.8	18.6	13.1	15.8	10.1	11.3	11.1	6.3
Percent of Poverty Level [3]										
Below 100 percent	29.0	32.1	28.1	NA	NA	30.8	29.8	22.6	NA	NA
100 percent to less than 200 percent	37.5	32.0	27.0	NA	NA	39.3	39.1	28.4	NA	NA
200 percent or more	58.4	52.8	49.0	NA	NA	32.8	32.2	26.2	NA	NA
Marital Status										
Married	49.9	44.6	41.0	41.7	32.9	33.0	32.6	25.6	27.0	20.1
Widowed	34.1	30.3	28.7	30.4	22.6	37.5	35.2	26.7	26.2	19.9
Divorced	27.3	26.6	22.4	25.1	19.7	27.9	24.1	16.9	19.8	13.0
Never married	38.0	35.1	28.5	29.1	29.1	29.1	26.2	21.9	15.4	16.7

Table 3-70C. Health Insurance Coverage of Noninstitutionalized Medicare Beneficiaries 65 Years of Age and Over, by Type of Coverage and Selected Characteristics, Selected Years, 1992–2012

(Numbers in millions; percent.)

Characteristic	Medicare fee-for-service only or other[6]				
	1992	1995	2000	2005	2012
Age					
65 years and over (number in millions)	2.9	3.1	3.5	4.3	6.6
65 years and over (percent of population)	9.9	10.5	11.5	13.3	15.5
65 to 74 years	9.7	10.7	12.6	14.9	16.0
75 to 84 years	10.1	9.9	9.9	11.9	14.6
85 years and over	10.8	11.3	12.1	11.6	15.1
Sex					
Male	12.2	12.6	13.3	16.2	18.0
Female	8.3	8.9	10.2	11.2	13.4
Race and Hispanic Origin					
White, not Hispanic or Latino	7.7	8.7	9.6	12.2	15.1
Black, not Hispanic or Latino	26.7	25.0	26.1	21.9	17.6
Hispanic	18.3	17.1	16.7	13.9	14.9
Percent of Poverty Level[3]					
Below 100 percent	14.3	13.3	15.1	NA	NA
100 percent to less than 200 percent	12.9	13.1	12.7	NA	NA
200 percent or more	4.0	4.5	6.3	NA	NA
Marital Status					
Married	8.5	9.0	10.5	12.1	14.6
Widowed	11.2	11.9	11.6	13.5	15.1
Divorced	15.7	15.1	16.1	17.9	19.3
Never married	*	13.1	16.8	20.4	17.2

NA = Not available.   * = Figure does not meet standards of reliability or precision. Estimates are considered unreliable if the sample cell size is 50 or fewer.   --- = Data not available.   1 Enrollee has Medicare risk Health Maintenance Organization (HMO) regardless of other insurance.   2 Enrolled in Medicaid and not enrolled in a Medicare risk HMO.   3 Percent of poverty level is based on family income and family size and composition using U.S. Census Bureau poverty thresholds.   4 Private insurance plans purchased through employers (own, current, or former employer, family business, union, or former employer or union of spouse) and not enrolled in a Medicare risk HMO or Medicaid.   5 Supplemental insurance purchased privately or through organizations such as American Association of Retired Persons or professional organizations, and not enrolled in a Medicare risk HMO, Medicaid, or employer-sponsored plan.   6 Medicare fee-for-service only or other public plans (except Medicaid).

Table 3-71. Persons Under 65 Years of Age Without Health Insurance Coverage, by State, Territory, and Age, 2009–2013

(Percent.)

Characteristic	2009	2010	2011	2012	2013
Under 65 Years					
United States[1]	17.2	17.6	17.2	16.9	16.7
Alabama	16.0	16.9	16.3	15.4	15.9
Alaska	22.0	19.4	21.7	22.0	20.3
Arizona	19.8	19.5	19.9	20.3	20.3
Arkansas	19.3	20.2	19.7	19.0	18.8
California	20.1	20.7	20.3	20.0	19.3
Colorado	17.4	17.6	17.0	16.3	15.7
Connecticut	10.1	10.3	9.8	10.6	10.8
Delaware	11.9	11.5	10.2	9.9	11.7
District of Columbia	7.8	8.4	8.3	6.1	7.1
Florida	24.8	25.4	25.0	24.0	24.2
Georgia	21.0	21.9	21.8	20.8	21.1
Hawaii	7.9	8.7	8.4	7.7	8.3
Idaho	19.1	20.3	17.8	18.3	18.5
Illinois	14.9	15.7	14.5	14.6	14.4
Indiana	15.8	17.0	16.6	16.6	16.2
Iowa	10.1	10.8	10.4	9.7	10.2
Kansas	14.5	15.6	14.4	14.6	14.3
Kentucky	16.5	17.5	16.6	15.8	16.8
Louisiana	19.5	20.1	19.9	19.0	19.2
Maine	11.9	12.5	13.1	12.4	13.3
Maryland	12.5	12.7	11.5	11.5	11.4
Massachusetts	4.9	4.9	4.8	4.5	4.4
Michigan	14.1	14.3	13.6	13.4	12.8
Minnesota	10.2	10.1	9.9	9.4	9.5
Mississippi	20.0	20.7	20.2	19.7	19.6
Missouri	15.3	15.2	15.7	16.1	15.2
Montana	21.9	19.6	21.8	21.4	19.7
Nebraska	13.1	13.4	13.6	12.7	12.2
Nevada	24.6	25.4	24.7	25.0	23.4
New Hampshire	12.0	12.7	11.4	12.8	12.6
New Jersey	14.2	15.0	14.7	14.5	15.3
New Mexico	23.1	22.8	22.8	21.6	22.2
New York	13.0	13.5	13.0	12.5	12.4
North Carolina	18.2	19.2	18.7	18.9	18.0
North Dakota	11.4	11.5	11.5	12.4	11.9
Ohio	14.0	14.1	13.9	13.4	12.8
Oklahoma	21.3	22.0	21.3	21.1	20.4
Oregon	19.8	19.7	18.0	16.9	17.4
Pennsylvania	11.3	11.9	11.8	11.3	11.3
Rhode Island	12.8	13.7	12.6	13.3	13.9
South Carolina	19.2	20.2	19.4	19.3	18.4
South Dakota	15.6	13.6	13.4	12.3	14.3
Tennessee	16.3	16.4	17.0	16.1	16.2
Texas	26.3	26.3	25.5	24.8	24.5
Utah	15.7	17.0	16.5	15.3	14.7
Vermont	9.9	9.0	8.3	7.7	8.1
Virginia	13.3	14.5	14.1	14.2	14.1
Washington	15.3	16.1	16.0	15.7	16.1
West Virginia	16.7	17.2	18.2	16.9	16.1
Wisconsin	10.4	10.9	10.6	10.6	10.4
Wyoming	17.5	16.6	17.5	18.3	14.6
Puerto Rico[2]	9.4	9.4	8.9	8.5	7.7

Table 3-71. Persons Under 65 Years of Age Without Health Insurance Coverage, by State, Territory, and Age, 2009–2013— continued

(Percent.)

Characteristic	2009	2010	2011	2012	2013
Under 18 Years					
United States[1]	8.5	8.0	7.5	7.1	7.1
Alabama	6.1	5.9	5.2	4.0	4.5
Alaska	12.8	9.3	13.9	13.3	11.7
Arizona	12.1	13.0	12.8	12.8	12.1
Arkansas	6.2	6.3	5.5	5.4	5.7
California	9.4	9.0	8.0	8.0	7.3
Colorado	9.8	9.8	9.3	8.1	8.4
Connecticut	3.9	2.9	2.5	3.7	4.1
Delaware	5.7	5.6	3.5	3.6	5.1
District of Columbia	*	*2.0	*4.1	*	*2.2
Florida	14.7	12.7	11.9	10.8	11.0
Georgia	10.7	9.8	9.5	8.9	9.5
Hawaii	2.4	3.7	3.9	2.9	3.2
Idaho	10.7	10.6	8.5	7.6	8.3
Illinois	4.4	4.8	3.4	3.2	4.3
Indiana	8.5	8.9	8.4	8.0	8.4
Iowa	4.4	4.3	4.6	4.3	4.8
Kansas	8.1	7.7	6.1	6.9	6.6
Kentucky	5.8	5.8	5.9	5.9	5.9
Louisiana	6.4	5.6	5.7	5.3	5.6
Maine	5.7	3.8	5.5	4.2	5.1
Maryland	4.7	4.9	4.5	3.8	4.3
Massachusetts	1.7	1.4	1.6	1.3	1.5
Michigan	4.3	4.2	3.9	4.2	4.2
Minnesota	7.0	6.3	6.1	5.7	6.1
Mississippi	10.1	8.2	7.4	7.2	7.3
Missouri	7.2	6.3	6.7	7.2	7.3
Montana	13.4	12.7	12.8	10.9	10.4
Nebraska	6.3	5.2	7.3	5.4	5.9
Nevada	18.0	17.9	16.1	16.5	13.9
New Hampshire	4.6	4.9	3.2	4.2	3.5
New Jersey	6.2	6.0	5.2	5.1	5.7
New Mexico	12.0	9.9	9.1	8.1	9.0
New York	4.8	4.8	4.4	4.0	4.1
North Carolina	7.9	8.1	7.8	7.3	5.9
North Dakota	6.3	6.6	7.6	7.4	7.7
Ohio	6.4	5.9	6.1	5.4	5.1
Oklahoma	11.1	10.4	10.9	9.9	10.5
Oregon	10.8	8.8	7.0	5.6	6.3
Pennsylvania	5.0	5.2	5.4	5.1	5.0
Rhode Island	4.9	4.8	3.9	5.1	6.0
South Carolina	9.5	9.8	8.7	7.8	7.0
South Dakota	6.8	7.2	5.6	3.9	7.2
Tennessee	5.7	5.3	5.8	5.6	5.7
Texas	16.3	14.7	13.3	12.3	12.5
Utah	10.2	11.1	11.1	9.3	9.0
Vermont	*3.3	*2.7	*	*3.0	*
Virginia	6.7	6.4	5.8	5.6	5.7
Washington	7.0	6.4	6.1	5.5	6.3
West Virginia	5.4	4.7	5.0	3.9	4.0
Wisconsin	4.6	5.2	4.6	4.7	4.4
Wyoming	9.0	7.4	8.7	9.9	6.3
Puerto Rico[2]	4.2	4.5	4.0	4.3	3.5
18 to 64 Years					
United States[1]	20.6	21.4	21.0	20.6	20.3

Table 3-71. Persons Under 65 Years of Age Without Health Insurance Coverage, by State, Territory, and Age, 2009–2013— continued

(Percent.)

Characteristic	2009	2010	2011	2012	2013
Alabama	19.8	21.2	20.5	19.7	20.2
Alaska	25.8	23.6	24.8	25.5	23.9
Arizona	23.3	22.3	22.8	23.4	23.7
Arkansas	24.6	25.8	25.4	24.5	24.0
California	24.5	25.3	25.1	24.7	23.8
Colorado	20.3	20.5	19.9	19.4	18.5
Connecticut	12.4	13.0	12.4	13.1	13.1
Delaware	14.3	13.7	12.7	12.2	14.1
District of Columbia	9.2	9.9	9.3	7.1	8.3
Florida	28.6	29.9	29.5	28.6	28.8
Georgia	25.4	26.9	26.8	25.6	25.8
Hawaii	9.9	10.5	10.1	9.4	10.1
Idaho	22.8	24.7	22.0	23.1	23.1
Illinois	19.0	20.0	18.8	19.0	18.1
Indiana	18.8	20.3	19.8	20.0	19.2
Iowa	12.2	13.3	12.6	11.8	12.3
Kansas	17.1	18.9	17.9	17.8	17.4
Kentucky	20.6	22.0	20.7	19.5	20.8
Louisiana	24.8	25.8	25.6	24.4	24.5
Maine	14.0	15.4	15.5	15.1	15.8
Maryland	15.4	15.5	14.0	14.3	14.0
Massachusetts	5.9	6.1	5.8	5.5	5.3
Michigan	17.8	18.1	17.3	16.8	16.0
Minnesota	11.4	11.6	11.3	10.9	10.8
Mississippi	24.3	26.0	25.6	25.0	24.6
Missouri	18.4	18.7	19.2	19.5	18.2
Montana	25.0	22.1	25.0	25.1	23.0
Nebraska	15.9	16.8	16.2	15.7	14.8
Nevada	27.3	28.4	28.1	28.4	27.1
New Hampshire	14.4	15.3	14.1	15.6	15.6
New Jersey	17.2	18.3	18.2	17.9	18.7
New Mexico	27.8	28.2	28.5	27.2	27.6
New York	16.0	16.6	16.0	15.4	15.2
North Carolina	22.2	23.5	22.9	23.3	22.6
North Dakota	13.2	13.3	12.9	14.1	13.4
Ohio	16.9	17.2	16.8	16.4	15.6
Oklahoma	25.6	26.8	25.6	25.6	24.5
Oregon	23.1	23.6	21.9	20.9	21.2
Pennsylvania	13.6	14.2	14.0	13.4	13.5
Rhode Island	15.5	16.7	15.5	16.0	16.4
South Carolina	23.0	24.2	23.5	23.6	22.5
South Dakota	19.1	16.3	16.6	15.7	17.2
Tennessee	20.4	20.7	21.2	20.0	20.1
Texas	30.9	31.5	30.9	30.4	29.7
Utah	18.6	20.1	19.3	18.4	17.7
Vermont	12.0	11.1	10.3	9.2	9.6
Virginia	15.8	17.4	17.1	17.3	17.1
Washington	18.4	19.7	19.6	19.4	19.8
West Virginia	20.5	21.5	22.7	21.2	20.2
Wisconsin	12.5	13.1	12.8	12.8	12.7
Wyoming	20.7	20.2	20.7	21.5	17.8
Puerto Rico[2]	11.5	11.3	10.9	10.0	9.2

*Estimates are considered unreliable. Data preceded by an asterisk have a relative standard error of 20 percent to 30 percent. Data not shown have an RSE greater than 30 percent.   1 Excludes data for Puerto Rico.   2 Data for Puerto Rico are collected in the Puerto Rico Community Survey. Data are not collected for the other territories.

Table 3-72. Medicaid Coverage Among Persons Under 65 Years of Age, by Selected Characteristics, Selected Years, 1984–2013

(Percent.)

Characteristic	1984[1]	1989[1]	1995[1]	2000[2]	2005[3]	2006[3]	2007[3]	2008[3]	2009[3]	2010[3]	2011[3]	2012[3]	2013[3]
Total (number in millions)[4]	14.0	15.4	26.6	23.2	33.2	36.2	36.2	38.4	42.4	44.8	47.4	48.1	48.5
Total (percent of population)[4]	6.8	7.2	11.5	9.5	12.9	14.0	13.9	14.7	16.1	16.9	17.8	18.0	18.1
Age													
Under 19 years	11.7	12.2	21.1	19.2	26.6	29.4	29.3	30.6	33.9	35.7	37.5	38.1	38.1
Under 6 years	15.5	15.7	29.3	24.7	34.0	36.6	36.6	38.1	41.4	43.7	46.1	45.7	45.9
6 to 18 years	9.8	10.5	17.0	16.8	23.3	26.1	25.9	27.1	30.3	31.8	33.4	34.7	34.6
Under 18 years	11.9	12.6	21.5	19.6	27.2	29.9	29.8	31.3	34.5	36.4	38.2	38.9	38.9
6 to 17 years	10.1	10.9	17.4	17.2	23.9	26.7	26.4	27.9	30.9	32.5	34.1	35.5	35.5
18 to 64 years	4.5	4.9	7.1	5.2	7.2	7.7	7.5	8.1	8.9	9.2	9.9	10.0	10.2
18 to 44 years	5.1	5.2	7.8	5.6	8.3	8.6	8.7	9.2	10.3	10.9	11.6	11.6	11.6
18 to 24 years	6.4	6.8	10.4	8.1	11.3	11.4	11.4	12.2	14.0	14.5	15.2	15.4	14.2
19 to 25 years	6.3	6.6	10.2	7.3	10.3	9.7	9.9	10.6	12.2	12.6	13.4	13.4	12.1
25 to 34 years	5.3	5.2	8.2	5.5	8.0	8.3	8.5	9.3	10.1	11.1	11.5	11.4	11.7
35 to 44 years	3.5	4.0	5.9	4.3	6.6	7.1	7.0	7.1	7.7	8.1	9.0	8.8	9.6
45 to 64 years	3.4	4.3	5.6	4.5	5.5	6.3	5.9	6.4	6.9	6.8	7.5	8.0	8.4
45 to 54 years	3.2	3.8	5.1	4.2	5.2	6.4	6.0	6.2	7.0	7.0	8.0	8.2	8.6
55 to 64 years	3.6	4.9	6.4	4.9	5.8	6.1	5.7	6.8	6.8	6.6	6.9	7.7	8.2
Sex													
Male	5.4	5.7	9.6	8.2	11.6	12.6	12.5	13.4	14.4	15.2	16.3	16.3	16.5
Female	8.1	8.6	13.4	10.8	14.3	15.5	15.2	15.9	17.8	18.5	19.3	19.7	19.8
Sex and Marital Status [5]													
Male													
Married	1.9	1.8	2.9	2.2	3.5	3.7	3.5	3.6	4.1	4.0	4.9	4.8	5.3
Divorced, separated, widowed	4.9	5.4	7.7	6.1	7.0	7.9	7.8	8.1	8.3	9.3	9.8	9.7	10.3
Never married	4.8	5.6	8.1	7.2	10.4	11.6	11.3	12.1	13.1	13.5	14.5	15.1	14.8
Female													
Married	2.6	3.0	5.2	3.1	4.7	4.6	4.7	5.2	5.3	5.7	6.4	6.2	6.9
Divorced, separated, widowed	16.0	16.1	19.0	12.7	14.6	16.2	16.3	17.2	18.7	17.6	18.0	18.8	18.8
Never married	10.7	11.9	16.5	13.2	17.3	19.0	18.1	18.7	20.9	22.2	21.9	22.6	22.2
Race [6]													
White only	4.6	5.1	8.9	7.1	11.0	11.8	11.4	12.1	13.7	14.5	15.4	15.5	15.6
Black or African American only	20.5	19.0	28.5	21.2	24.9	26.6	27.7	28.3	29.5	30.4	30.9	31.6	31.6
American Indian or Alaska Native only	*28.2	29.7	19.0	15.1	24.2	24.3	21.2	37.0	29.7	21.6	29.0	36.5	32.0
Asian only	*8.7	*8.8	10.5	7.5	8.2	9.7	8.7	9.2	9.9	12.0	14.7	13.0	13.2
Native Hawaiian or Other Pacific Islander only	NA	NA	NA	*	*	*	*	*	*	*	*	*	*
Two or more races	NA	NA	NA	19.1	22.0	24.0	27.9	24.7	30.1	27.4	27.2	29.1	30.4
Hispanic Origin and Race [6]													
Hispanic or Latino	13.3	13.5	21.9	15.5	22.9	23.1	24.7	24.9	27.6	28.6	30.1	30.5	29.5
Mexican	12.2	12.4	21.6	14.0	23.0	23.0	25.9	25.4	28.4	29.5	31.0	31.0	29.8
Puerto Rican	31.5	27.3	33.4	29.4	31.9	35.7	28.0	31.0	32.1	35.7	33.0	35.3	36.9
Cuban	*4.8	*7.7	13.4	9.2	17.7	*11.3	13.3	13.0	16.7	17.3	20.0	22.9	23.3
Other Hispanic or Latino	7.9	11.1	18.2	14.5	19.7	20.2	21.4	22.3	24.6	24.5	27.7	28.3	27.0
Not Hispanic or Latino	6.2	6.5	10.2	8.5	11.1	12.3	11.7	12.6	13.7	14.4	15.2	15.2	15.5
White only	3.7	4.1	7.1	6.1	8.5	9.5	8.5	9.2	10.4	11.0	11.8	11.5	11.9
Black or African American only	20.7	19.0	28.1	21.0	24.8	26.2	27.3	27.9	29.1	30.0	30.5	31.3	31.3
Age and Percent of Poverty Level [7]													
Under 65 years													
Below 100 percent	33.0	37.6	48.4	38.4	45.7	45.8	47.6	49.1	51.2	50.8	51.4	52.5	53.7
100 percent to 199 percent	5.3	7.5	14.4	16.2	23.4	23.8	26.1	27.4	29.0	28.5	30.6	30.1	30.8
100 percent to 133 percent	8.7	11.9	23.1	22.4	30.6	30.8	34.8	36.1	39.3	36.3	38.8	38.0	38.8
134 percent to 199 percent	3.7	5.6	9.7	13.1	19.5	20.0	21.7	22.9	23.6	24.4	26.1	25.5	26.2
200 percent to 399 percent	0.8	1.3	2.3	4.0	6.6	7.0	6.8	7.8	8.0	8.4	8.9	9.0	9.0
400 percent or more	0.2	0.5	0.4	0.9	1.5	1.7	1.5	1.6	1.7	2.0	1.7	1.7	1.9
Under 19 years													
Below 100 percent	42.0	45.8	63.5	56.9	69.4	70.4	72.7	73.4	77.5	78.4	79.9	82.1	82.1
100 percent to 199 percent	6.5	8.6	21.3	27.8	41.7	44.1	47.2	48.5	52.7	53.5	56.7	56.3	58.9
100 percent to 133 percent	10.3	13.4	32.4	36.4	51.0	51.3	57.5	60.0	65.6	63.5	69.1	68.8	70.3
134 percent to 199 percent	4.7	6.3	14.3	23.3	36.2	39.4	41.3	42.3	45.3	47.7	49.9	48.8	51.6
200 percent to 399 percent	1.0	1.7	3.5	7.6	13.0	13.5	13.3	16.4	16.4	17.7	18.3	18.8	19.1
400 percent or more	*	*1.2	*	2.1	2.9	3.5	3.0	3.5	3.6	4.3	3.5	3.6	3.2
Under 18 years													
Below 100 percent	43.3	47.8	66.0	58.5	71.2	72.0	75.0	75.3	78.3	79.8	81.4	83.7	83.9
100 percent to 199 percent	6.6	8.7	21.6	28.4	42.5	44.7	48.1	49.5	53.5	54.3	57.6	57.3	60.1
100 percent to 133 percent	10.4	13.5	32.9	36.9	52.0	51.7	58.4	61.1	66.9	64.6	70.1	70.1	71.2
134 percent to 199 percent	4.8	6.4	14.4	23.8	36.9	40.1	42.2	43.2	45.9	48.2	50.6	49.6	52.9
200 percent to 399 percent	1.0	1.7	3.5	7.6	13.3	13.8	13.3	16.8	16.8	18.0	18.6	19.1	19.5
400 percent or more	*	*1.1	*	2.2	2.9	3.4	3.0	3.6	3.7	4.3	3.6	3.6	3.3
18 to 64 years													
Below 100 percent	25.3	29.1	34.8	24.9	29.6	28.9	30.6	33.0	33.6	32.4	33.0	34.0	35.4
100 percent to 199 percent	4.5	6.8	10.2	9.1	13.1	13.0	14.0	15.3	16.2	15.7	17.1	16.8	17.1
100 percent to 133 percent	7.6	10.8	16.3	13.2	17.9	17.8	20.2	21.9	23.7	21.0	22.7	21.8	22.0
134 percent to 199 percent	3.1	5.1	7.2	7.2	10.7	10.5	11.0	11.8	12.4	13.0	14.1	13.9	14.4
200 percent to 399 percent	0.7	1.1	1.7	2.4	3.8	4.2	4.0	4.1	4.6	4.8	5.2	5.1	5.1
400 percent or more	0.2	0.4	0.4	0.6	1.1	1.2	1.1	1.1	1.2	1.3	1.2	1.2	1.6

Table 3-72. Medicaid Coverage Among Persons Under 65 Years of Age, by Selected Characteristics, Selected Years, 1984–2013—continued

(Percent.)

Characteristic	1984[1]	1989[1]	1995[1]	2000[2]	2005[3]	2006[3]	2007[3]	2008[3]	2009[3]	2010[3]	2011[3]	2012[3]	2013[3]
Disability Measure among Adults 18 to 64 Years [8]													
Any basic actions difficulty or complex activity limitation	NA	NA	NA	12.8	16.4	16.2	16.5	18.6	18.2	17.8	19.6	19.3	21.1
Any basic actions difficulty	NA	NA	NA	12.2	15.5	15.3	15.9	17.7	17.8	16.7	19.1	18.4	20.6
Any complex activity limitation	NA	NA	NA	23.2	28.5	28.7	28.7	31.0	30.2	30.0	30.8	30.8	32.3
No disability	NA	NA	NA	3.0	4.9	5.1	5.2	4.9	6.4	6.8	6.9	7.0	6.8
Geographic Region													
Northeast	8.6	6.6	11.7	10.6	13.3	16.8	15.4	16.1	17.3	17.9	19.6	19.3	20.8
Midwest	7.4	7.6	10.5	8.0	12.3	13.9	13.7	14.5	16.4	17.3	16.7	16.3	16.9
South	5.1	6.5	11.3	9.4	12.7	12.9	12.9	13.5	14.8	16.0	17.3	17.8	17.8
West	7.0	8.5	12.9	10.4	13.8	13.8	14.5	15.7	16.8	17.1	18.4	19.1	18.0
Location of Residence													
Within MSA[9]	7.1	7.0	11.3	8.9	12.4	13.3	13.3	14.2	15.2	16.1	17.0	17.4	17.4
Outside MSA[9]	6.1	7.9	12.3	11.9	15.5	17.7	17.1	17.2	20.8	21.4	22.1	21.4	22.5

NA = Not available.   * = Figure does not meet standards of reliability or precision. Data not shown have a relative standard error of greater than 30 percent.   1 Data prior to 1997 are not strictly comparable with data for later years due to the 1997 questionnaire redesign.   2 Estimates for 2000-2002 were calculated using 2000-based sample weights and may differ from estimates in other reports that used 1990-based sample weights for 2000-2002 estimates.   3 Beginning in quarter 3 of the 2004 NHIS, persons under 65 years of age with no reported coverage were asked explicitly about Medicaid coverage. Estimates were calculated with the additional information starting with 2005 data.   4 Includes all other races not shown separately, those with unknown marital status, unknown disability status, and, in 1984 and 1989, persons with unknown poverty level.   5 Includes persons 14 to 64 years of age.   6 The race groups White, Black, American Indian or Alaska Native, Asian, Native Hawaiian or Other Pacific Islander, and two or more races include persons of Hispanic and non-Hispanic origin. Persons of Hispanic origin may be of any race.   7 Percent of poverty level is based on family income and family size and composition using U.S. Census Bureau poverty thresholds. Poverty level was unknown for 10 to 11 percent of persons under 65 years of age in 1984 and 1989. Missing family income data were imputed for 1995 and beyond.   8 Any basic actions difficulty or complex activity limitation is defined as having one or more of the following limitations or difficulties: movement difficulty, emotional difficulty, sensory (seeing or hearing) difficulty, cognitive difficulty, self-care (activities of daily living or instrumental activities of daily living) limitation, social limitation, or work limitation.   9 MSA = metropolitan statistical area.

Table 3-73. Medicaid Beneficiaries and Payments, by Basis of Eligibility, and Race and Hispanic Origin, Selected Fiscal Years, 1999–2011

(Number, percent, dollar.)

Characteristic	1999	2000	2004	2005	2007	2008	2009	2010	2011
Beneficiaries (Number in Millions) [1]									
All beneficiaries	40.1	42.8	55.6	57.7	56.8	58.8	56.0	65.7	68.8
Percent of Beneficiaries									
Basis of eligibility									
Aged (65 years and over)	9.4	8.7	7.8	7.6	7.1	7.1	6.5	6.5	6.2
Blind and disabled	16.7	16.1	14.6	14.2	14.8	14.8	14.0	14.3	14.1
Adults in families with dependent children[2]	18.7	20.5	22.5	21.5	21.8	21.8	22.6	23.7	23.7
Children under age 21[3]	46.9	46.1	47.8	47.5	48.4	48.0	48.4	48.3	47.2
Other Title XIX[4]	8.4	8.6	7.3	9.1	7.8	8.4	8.5	7.2	8.8
Race and Hispanic Origin [5]									
White	NA	NA	41.1	39.3	38.6	38.1	36.5	38.9	38.3
Black or African American	NA	NA	22.1	21.5	21.6	21.1	21.1	20.6	20.5
American Indian or Alaska Native	NA	NA	1.3	1.2	1.2	1.3	1.3	1.2	1.1
Asian or Pacific Islander	NA	NA	3.3	3.5	3.5	3.5	3.5	3.6	3.7
Asian	NA	NA	2.4	2.5	2.6	2.6	2.6	2.7	2.9
Pacific Islander	NA	NA	0.9	0.9	0.9	0.9	0.8	0.9	0.9
Hispanic or Latino	NA	NA	19.4	20.6	21.6	21.7	23.6	22.3	22.3
Multiple race or unknown	NA	NA	12.7	13.9	13.5	14.3	14.1	13.3	14.0
Payments (Billions of Dollars) [6]									
All payments	154	168	258	275	276	294	287	339	365
Percent Distribution	100.0	100.0	100.0	100.0	100.0	100.0	100.0	100.0	100.0
Basis of eligibility									
Age (65 years and over)	27.7	26.4	23.1	23.1	20.7	20.6	19.2	19.4	18.2
Blind and disabled	42.9	43.2	43.3	43.4	43.3	43.5	43.5	43.4	42.4
Adults in families with dependent children[2]	10.3	10.6	12.0	11.7	12.4	12.6	13.9	14.2	14.8
Children under age 21[3]	15.7	15.9	17.2	17.3	19.4	19.4	19.9	19.8	19.6
Other Title XIX[4]	3.4	3.9	4.5	4.6	4.2	4.0	3.5	3.1	5.0
Race and Hispanic Origin [5]									
White	NA	NA	53.4	53.0	50.7	50.2	48.6	50.2	48.7
Black or African American	NA	NA	19.8	19.8	20.8	20.6	21.3	20.5	20.6
American Indian or Alaska Native	NA	NA	1.2	1.2	1.2	1.3	1.3	1.3	1.2
Asian or Pacific Islander	NA	NA	2.5	2.7	2.8	2.9	3.0	3.0	3.2
Asian	NA	NA	1.7	1.9	2.0	2.1	2.2	2.3	2.4
Pacific Islander	NA	NA	0.8	0.8	0.8	0.8	0.8	0.7	0.8
Hispanic or Latino	NA	NA	10.7	12.2	13.1	13.7	15.2	14.2	14.2
Multiple race or unknown	NA	NA	12.3	11.1	11.4	11.4	10.5	10.8	12.1
Payments per Beneficiary (Dollars) [6]									
All beneficiaries	3,819	3,936	4,639	4,768	4,862	5,051	5,122	5,160	5,304
Basis of eligibility									
Age (65 years and over)	11,268	11,929	13,687	14,427	14,141	14,742	15,141	15,286	15,489
Blind and disabled	9,832	10,559	13,714	14,531	14,194	14,843	15,921	15,695	15,982
Adults in families with dependent children[2]	2,104	2,030	2,471	2,587	2,753	2,917	3,156	3,095	3,306
Children under age 21[3]	1,282	1,358	1,664	1,735	1,951	2,038	2,107	2,122	2,198
Other Title XIX[4]	1,532	1,778	2,896	2,380	2,622	2,407	2,087	2,219	3,020
Race and Hispanic Origin [5]									
White	NA	NA	6,026	6,422	6,390	6,657	6,832	6,663	6,741
Black or African American	NA	NA	4,158	4,397	4,669	4,928	5,184	5,142	5,333
American Indian or Alaska Native	NA	NA	4,320	4,626	4,826	5,218	5,439	5,421	5,544
Asian or Pacific Islander	NA	NA	3,513	3,710	3,863	4,133	4,445	4,300	4,531
Asian	NA	NA	3,198	3,624	3,847	4,123	4,389	4,307	4,528
Pacific Islander	NA	NA	4,366	3,947	3,907	4,161	4,619	4,275	4,540
Hispanic or Latino	NA	NA	2,563	2,822	2,960	3,175	3,298	3,276	3,381
Multiple race or unknown	NA	NA	4,493	3,816	4,106	4,014	3,804	4,173	4,575

NOTE: Data are for fiscal years ending September 30.   NA = Not available.   1 Beneficiaries include those who received services through Medicaid.   2 Includes adults who meet the requirements for the Aid to Families with Dependent Children (AFDC) program that were in effect in their state on July 16, 1996, or, at state option, more liberal criteria (with some exceptions). Includes adults in the Temporary Assistance for Needy Families (TANF) program. Starting with 2001 data, includes women in the Breast and Cervical Cancer Prevention and Treatment Program and unemployed adults.   3 Includes children (including those in the foster care system) in the TANF program.   4 Includes some participants in the Supplemental Security Income program and other people deemed medically needy in participating states. Prior to 2001, includes unemployed adults. Excludes foster care children and includes unknown eligibility.   5 Race and Hispanic origin are as determined on initial Medicaid application. Categories are mutually exclusive. Starting with 2001 data, the Hispanic category included Hispanic persons, regardless of race. Persons indicating more than one race were included in the multiple race category.   6 Medicaid payments exclude disproportionate share hospital (DSH) payments ($14.7 billion in FY2009) and DSH mental health facility payments ($3.1 billion in FY2009).

Table 3-74. Medicaid Beneficiaries and Payments, by Type of Service, Selected Fiscal Years, 1999–2011

(Number; percent.)

Type of service	1999	2000	2004	2005	2007	2008	2009	2010	2011
Beneficiaries (Number in Millions) [1]									
All beneficiaries	40.2	42.8	55.6	57.7	56.8	58.8	62.6	65.7	68.8
Percent									
Inpatient hospital	11.2	11.5	9.8	9.5	9.0	8.9	8.7	6.9	7.5
Mental health facility	0.2	0.2	0.2	0.2	0.2	0.2	0.2	0.2	0.2
Intermediate care facility for the mentally retarded	0.3	0.3	0.2	0.2	0.2	0.2	0.2	0.2	0.1
Nursing facility	4.0	4.0	3.1	3.0	2.9	2.7	2.6	2.4	2.3
Physician	45.7	44.7	43.1	42.0	38.8	36.9	36.9	36.9	34.9
Dental	14.0	13.8	16.2	16.2	16.8	16.7	17.8	19.1	19.5
Other practitioner	9.9	11.1	10.7	10.2	9.5	8.8	8.8	9.2	8.3
Outpatient hospital	30.9	30.9	28.7	28.2	26.2	25.2	26.4	24.2	23.7
Clinic	16.8	17.9	20.0	20.7	20.6	20.2	20.6	20.7	20.9
Laboratory and radiological	25.4	26.6	28.9	27.7	27.8	26.6	26.2	25.8	24.5
Home health	2.0	2.3	2.1	2.1	2.1	1.9	1.7	1.7	1.6
Prescribed drugs	49.4	48.0	50.3	49.2	42.1	41.8	42.6	44.7	44.0
Capitated care	51.5	49.7	54.2	58.1	64.5	64.9	66.6	70.8	71.2
Primary care case management	9.7	13.0	15.4	15.1	12.5	14.9	13.1	13.3	13.7
Personal support	10.1	10.6	11.3	11.8	11.6	10.8	10.7	11.0	10.3
Other care [2]	21.6	21.4	22.9	21.9	21.5	21.3	20.6	19.9	19.8
Payments (Billions of Dollars) [3]									
All payments	$153.5	$168.3	$257.7	$274.9	$276.2	$296.8	$326.0	$339.0	$365.2
Percent Distribution	100.0	100.0	100.0	100.0	100.0	100.0	100.0	100.0	100.0
Inpatient hospital	14.5	14.4	13.5	12.8	13.4	12.5	11.8	9.9	10.1
Mental health facility	1.1	1.1	0.9	0.8	0.9	0.8	0.8	0.7	0.7
Intermediate care facility for the mentally retarded	6.1	5.6	4.3	4.3	4.3	4.2	3.9	3.7	3.6
Nursing facility	21.7	20.5	16.3	16.3	16.8	16.1	14.9	14.4	13.2
Physician	4.3	4.0	4.0	4.1	3.6	3.5	3.5	3.5	3.3
Dental	0.8	0.8	1.1	1.1	1.2	1.3	1.4	1.6	1.6
Other practitioner	0.3	0.4	0.4	0.4	0.3	0.3	0.3	0.3	0.5
Outpatient hospital	4.0	4.2	4.0	3.6	3.7	3.7	3.7	3.8	3.6
Clinic	3.8	3.7	3.2	3.2	3.1	3.1	3.1	3.2	3.4
Laboratory and radiological	0.8	0.8	1.0	1.1	1.1	1.0	1.0	1.0	1.0
Home health	1.9	1.9	1.8	2.0	2.3	2.2	2.2	2.1	2.0
Prescribed drugs	10.8	11.9	15.3	15.6	8.0	7.9	7.8	8.0	8.1
Capitated care	14.0	14.5	16.5	16.9	21.2	23.0	25.5	27.2	29.8
Primary care case management	0.3	0.1	0.2	0.1	0.1	0.1	0.1	0.1	0.1
Personal support	6.9	6.9	7.2	7.5	8.4	8.3	8.0	7.7	6.9
Other care [2]	8.6	8.8	10.3	10.2	11.6	12.0	11.9	12.7	12.3
Payments per Beneficiary (Dollars) [3]									
All beneficiaries	$3,819	$3,936	$4,639	$4,768	$4,862	$5,051	$5,209	$5,160	$5,304
Inpatient hospital	4,943	4,919	6,424	6,411	7,191	7,083	7,070	7,347	7,186
Mental health facility	18,094	17,800	19,928	19,252	21,407	21,975	21,404	20,782	20,074
Intermediate care facility for the mentally retarded	76,443	79,330	97,497	107,028	113,735	123,053	127,837	125,851	139,149
Nursing facility	20,568	20,220	24,475	26,185	28,282	29,533	29,551	31,617	29,843
Physician	357	356	426	465	457	485	496	492	502
Dental	214	238	318	326	340	389	423	432	424
Other practitioner	118	139	160	200	170	171	171	190	291
Outpatient hospital	491	533	639	617	695	736	735	803	804
Clinic	860	805	750	749	741	772	792	791	857
Laboratory and radiological	114	113	168	183	185	188	198	205	208
Home health	3,571	3,135	3,978	4,487	5,334	5,789	6,628	6,375	6,568
Prescribed drugs	837	975	1,411	1,509	926	957	951	926	974
Capitated care	1,040	1,148	1,415	1,386	1,598	1,786	1,991	1,983	2,220
Primary care case management	119	30	58	27	33	32	41	49	45
Personal support	2,583	2,543	2,946	3,035	3,534	3,852	3,903	3,593	3,553
Other care [2]	1,508	1,600	2,086	2,228	2,611	2,856	3,015	3,289	3,287

1 Beneficiaries include those who received services through Medicaid.   2 Unknown services (0.2 percent of beneficiaries and 0.9 percent of payments in 2011) are included with Other Care.   3 Medicaid payments exclude disproportionate share hospital (DSH) payments ($14.3 billion in FY2011) and DSH mental health facility payments ($2.9 billion in FY2011).

Table 3-75. Medicare Enrollees and Expenditures and Percent Distribution, by Medicare Program and Type of Service, Selected Years, 1970–2013

(Number; dollars; percent.)

Medicare program and type of service	1970	1980	1990	1995	2000	2005	2009	2010	2011	2012	2013[1]
Enrollees (Numbers in Millions)											
Total Medicare[2]	20.4	28.4	34.3	37.6	39.7	42.6	46.6	47.7	48.9	50.9	52.3
Hospital insurance	20.1	28.0	33.7	37.2	39.3	42.2	46.3	47.4	48.5	50.5	51.9
Supplementary medical insurance (SMI)[3]	19.5	27.3	32.6	35.6	37.3	NA	NA	NA	NA	NA	NA
Part B	19.5	27.3	32.6	35.6	37.3	39.8	42.9	43.9	44.9	46.5	47.9
Part D[4]	NA	NA	NA	NA	NA	1.8	33.6	34.8	35.7	37.4	39.1
Expenditures (Dollars in Billions)											
Total Medicare	$7.5	$36.8	$111.0	$184.2	$221.8	$336.4	$509.0	$522.9	$549.1	$574.2	$582.9
Total hospital insurance (HI)	5.3	25.6	67.0	117.6	131.1	182.9	242.5	247.9	256.7	266.8	266.2
HI payments to managed care organizations[5]	NA	0.0	2.7	6.7	21.4	24.9	59.4	60.7	64.6	70.2	74.2
HI payments for fee-for-service utilization	5.1	25.0	63.4	109.5	105.1	156.6	179.5	183.3	187.0	189.2	187.0
Inpatient hospital	4.8	24.1	56.9	82.3	87.1	123.3	133.8	135.9	133.7	138.4	135.2
Skilled nursing facility	0.2	0.4	2.5	9.1	11.1	19.3	26.3	27.1	32.1	28.7	28.8
Home health agency	0.1	0.5	3.7	16.2	4.0	6.0	7.1	7.2	7.1	6.9	6.9
Hospice	NA	NA	0.3	1.9	2.9	8.0	12.3	13.1	14.0	15.2	16.1
Other programs and sequestration[6]	NA	NA	NA	NA	NA	NA	NA	NA	0.9	2.8	0.0
Home health agency transfer[7]	NA	NA	NA	NA	1.7	NA	NA	NA	NA	NA	NA
Medicare Advantage premiums[8]	NA	NA	NA	NA	NA	NA	0.1	0.2	0.2	0.2	0.3
Accounting error (CY 2005-2008)[9]	NA	NA	NA	NA	NA	-1.9	NA	NA	NA	NA	NA
Administrative expenses[10]	0.2	0.5	0.9	1.4	2.9	3.3	3.5	3.8	4.0	4.3	4.7
Total supplementary medical insurance (SMI)[3]	2.2	11.2	44.0	66.6	90.7	153.5	266.5	274.9	292.5	307.4	316.7
Total Part B	2.2	11.2	44.0	66.6	90.7	152.4	205.7	212.9	225.3	240.5	247.1
Part B payments to managed care organizations[5]	0.0	0.2	2.8	6.6	18.4	22.0	53.4	55.2	59.1	66.0	72.7
Part B payments for fee-for-service utilization[11]	1.9	10.4	39.6	58.4	72.2	125.0	149.0	154.3	162.3	170.3	170.8
Physician/supplies[12]	1.8	8.2	29.6	NA	NA	NA	NA	NA	NA	NA	NA
Outpatient hospital[13]	0.1	1.9	8.5	NA	NA	NA	NA	NA	NA	NA	NA
Independent laboratory[14]	0.0	0.1	1.5	NA	NA	NA	NA	NA	NA	NA	NA
Physician fee schedule	NA	NA	NA	31.7	37.0	57.7	61.8	63.9	67.5	69.5	68.6
Durable medical equipment	NA	NA	NA	3.7	4.7	8.0	8.2	8.3	8.2	8.2	7.1
Laboratory[15]	NA	NA	NA	4.3	4.4	6.9	8.7	8.9	9.0	9.8	9.7
Other[16]	NA	NA	NA	9.9	13.6	26.7	32.4	33.2	34.2	36.6	36.6
Hospital[17]	NA	NA	NA	8.7	8.1	18.7	26.2	28.0	31.4	34.7	37.2
Home health agency	0.0	0.2	0.1	0.2	4.5	7.1	11.7	12.0	12.1	11.5	11.5
Home health agency transfer[7]	NA	NA	NA	NA	-1.7	NA	NA	NA	NA	NA	NA
Medicare Advantage premiums[8]	NA	NA	NA	NA	NA	NA	0.1	0.2	0.2	0.2	0.3
Accounting error (CY 2005-2008)[9]	NA	NA	NA	NA	NA	1.9	NA	NA	NA	NA	NA
Administrative expenses[10]	0.2	0.6	1.5	1.6	1.8	2.8	3.2	3.2	3.7	4.0	3.4
Part D start-up costs[18]	NA	NA	NA	NA	NA	0.7	NA	NA	NA	NA	NA
Total Part D[4]	NA	NA	NA	NA	NA	1.1	60.8	62.1	67.1	66.9	69.7
Percent Distribution of Expenditures											
Total hospital insurance (HI)	100.0	100.0	100.0	100.0	100.0	100.0	100.0	100.0	100.0	100.0	100.0
HI payments to managed care organizations[5]	NA	0.0	4.0	5.7	16.3	13.6	24.5	24.5	25.2	26.3	27.9
HI payments for fee-for-service utilization	97.0	97.9	94.6	93.1	80.2	85.6	74.0	73.9	72.8	70.9	70.3
Inpatient hospital	91.4	94.3	85.0	70.0	66.4	67.4	55.2	54.8	52.1	51.9	50.8
Skilled nursing facility	4.7	1.5	3.7	7.8	8.5	10.6	10.9	10.9	12.5	10.8	10.8
Home health agency	1.0	2.1	5.5	13.8	3.1	3.3	2.9	2.9	2.8	2.6	2.6
Hospice	NA	NA	0.5	1.6	2.2	4.4	5.1	5.3	5.5	5.7	6.1
Other[6]	NA	NA	NA	NA	NA	NA	NA	NA	0.3	1.1	0.0
Home health agency transfer[7]	NA	NA	NA	NA	1.3	NA	NA	NA	NA	NA	NA
Medicare Advantage premiums[8]	NA	NA	NA	NA	NA	NA	0.1	0.1	0.1	0.1	0.1
Accounting error (CY 2005-2008)[9]	NA	NA	NA	NA	NA	-1.0	NA	NA	NA	NA	NA
Administrative expenses[10]	3.0	2.1	1.4	1.2	2.2	1.8	1.4	1.5	1.6	1.6	1.8
Total supplementary medical insurance (SMI)[3]	100.0	100.0	100.0	100.0	100.0	100.0	100.0	100.0	100.0	100.0	100.0
Total Part B	100.0	100.0	100.0	100.0	100.0	99.3	77.2	77.4	77.1	78.2	78.0
Part B payments to managed care organizations[5]	1.2	1.8	6.4	9.9	20.2	14.3	20.0	20.1	20.2	21.5	22.9
Part B payments for fee-for-service utilization[11]	88.1	92.8	90.1	87.6	79.6	81.5	55.9	56.1	55.5	55.4	53.9
Physician/supplies[12]	80.9	72.8	67.3	NA	NA	NA	NA	NA	NA	NA	NA
Outpatient hospital[13]	5.2	16.9	19.3	NA	NA	NA	NA	NA	NA	NA	NA
Independent laboratory[14]	0.5	1.0	3.4	NA	NA	NA	NA	NA	NA	NA	NA
Physician fee schedule	NA	NA	NA	47.5	40.8	37.6	23.2	23.2	23.1	22.6	21.6
Durable medical equipment	NA	NA	NA	5.5	5.2	5.2	3.1	3.0	2.8	2.7	2.3
Laboratory[15]	NA	NA	NA	6.4	4.8	4.5	3.2	3.2	3.1	3.2	3.1
Other[16]	NA	NA	NA	14.8	15.0	17.4	12.1	12.1	11.7	11.9	11.5
Hospital[17]	NA	NA	NA	13.0	8.9	12.2	9.8	10.2	10.7	11.3	11.7
Home health agency	1.5	2.1	0.2	0.3	4.9	4.6	4.4	4.4	4.1	3.7	3.6

Table 3-75. Medicare Enrollees and Expenditures and Percent Distribution, by Medicare Program and Type of Service, Selected Years, 1970–2013— continued

(Number; dollars; percent.)

Medicare program and type of service	1970	1980	1990	1995	2000	2005	2009	2010	2011	2012	2013[1]
Home health agency transfer[7]	NA	NA	NA	NA	-1.9	NA	NA	NA	NA	NA	NA
Medicare Advantage premiums[8]	NA	NA	NA	NA	NA	NA	0.0	0.1	0.1	0.1	0.1
Accounting error (CY 2005-2008)[9]	NA	NA	NA	NA	NA	1.2	NA	NA	NA	NA	NA
Administrative expenses[10]	10.7	5.4	3.5	2.4	2.0	1.8	1.2	1.2	1.3	1.3	1.1
Part D start-up costs[18]	NA	NA	NA	NA	NA	0.4	NA	NA	NA	NA	NA
Total Part D[4]	NA	NA	NA	NA	NA	0.7	22.8	22.6	22.9	21.8	22.0

NA = Not available.   0.0 = Quantity more than zero but less than 0.05.   1 Preliminary estimates.   2 Average number enrolled in the hospital insurance (HI) and/or supplementary medical insurance (SMI) programs for the period.   3 Starting with 2004 data, the SMI trust fund consists of two separate accounts: Part B (which pays for a portion of the costs of physicians' services, outpatient hospital services, and other related medical and health services for voluntarily enrolled individuals) and Part D (Medicare Prescription Drug Account, which pays private plans to provide prescription drug coverage).   4 The Medicare Modernization Act, enacted on December 8, 2003, established within SMI two Part D accounts related to prescription drug benefits: the Medicare Prescription Drug Account and the Transitional Assistance Account.   5 Medicare-approved managed care organizations.   6 Includes Community-Based Care Transitions Program ($0.1 billion in each of 2011, 2012, and 2013), Electronic Health Records Incentive Program ($0.7 billion in 2011, $2.7 billion in 2012, and $3.4 billion in 2013), and Sequestration per the Budget Control Act of 2011 (-$3.5 billion in 2013).   7 For 1998 to 2003 data, reflects annual home health HI to SMI transfer amounts.   8 When a beneficiary chooses a Medicare Advantage plan whose monthly premium exceeds the benchmark amount, the additional premiums (that is, amounts beyond those paid by Medicare to the plan) are the responsibility of the beneficiary.   9 Represents misallocation of benefit payments between the HI trust fund and the Part B account of the SMI trust fund from May 2005 to September 2007, and the transfer made in June 2008 to correct the misallocation.   10 Includes expenditures for research, experiments and demonstration projects, peer review activity (performed by Peer Review Organizations from 1983 to 2001 and by Quality Review Organizations from 2002 to present), and to combat and prevent fraud and abuse.   11 Type-of-service reporting categories for fee-for-service reimbursement differ before and after 1991.   12 Includes payment for physicians, practitioners, durable medical equipment, and all suppliers other than independent laboratory through 1990. Starting with 1991 data, physician services subject to the physician fee schedule are shown. Payments for laboratory services paid under the laboratory fee schedule and performed in a physician office are included under Laboratory beginning in 1991.   13 Includes payments for hospital outpatient department services, skilled nursing facility outpatient services, Part B services received as an inpatient in a hospital or skilled nursing facility setting, and other types of outpatient facilities.   14 Starting with 1991 data, those independent laboratory services that were paid under the laboratory fee schedule (most of the independent laboratory category) are included in the Laboratory line; the remaining services are included in the Physician fee schedule and Other lines.   15 Payments for laboratory services paid under the laboratory fee schedule performed in a physician office, independent laboratory, or in a hospital outpatient department.   16 Includes payments for physician-administered drugs; freestanding ambulatory surgical center facility services; ambulance services; supplies; freestanding end-stage renal disease (ESRD) dialysis facility services; rural health clinics; outpatient rehabilitation facilities; psychiatric hospitals; and federally qualified health centers.   17 Includes the hospital facility costs for Medicare Part B services that are predominantly in the outpatient department, with the exception of hospital outpatient laboratory services, which are included on the Laboratory line. Physician reimbursement is included on the Physician fee schedule line.   18 Part D start-up costs were funded through the SMI Part B account in 2004-2008.

Table 3-76. Medicare Enrollees and Program Payments Among Fee-for-Service Medicare Beneficiaries, by Sex and Age, Selected Years, 1994–2010

(Number; percent; dollars.)

Characteristic	1994	1995	2000	2005	2006	2007	2008	2009	2010
Fee-for-Service Enrollees (Numbers in Thousands)									
Total	34,076	34,062	32,740	36,685	35,847	35,490	35,320	35,360	35,910
Sex									
Male	14,533	14,563	14,195	16,251	15,958	15,879	15,890	15,968	16,281
Female	19,543	19,499	18,545	20,433	19,890	19,611	19,430	19,392	19,629
Age									
Under 65 years	4,031	4,239	4,907	6,286	6,225	6,318	6,359	6,435	6,619
65 to 74 years	16,713	16,373	14,230	15,587	15,179	15,041	15,182	15,336	15,648
75 to 84 years	9,845	9,911	9,919	10,689	10,298	9,947	9,592	9,335	9,291
85 years and over	3,486	3,540	3,684	4,123	4,146	4,184	4,187	4,254	4,352
Fee-for-Service Program Payments (Billions of Dollars)									
Total	147	159	174	274	281	289	301	318	331
Sex									
Male	63.9	68.8	76.2	121.0	123.6	126.5	131.5	139.1	145.4
Female	82.6	90.2	98.0	153.2	157.0	162.1	169.7	178.9	185.7
Age									
Under 65 years	18.8	21.0	25.8	46.7	48.4	50.9	54.2	59.7	63.7
65 to 74 years	55.1	58.1	57.5	86.6	87.4	89.1	92.9	98.1	102.5
75 to 84 years	50.7	55.3	62.7	95.2	96.2	96.4	97.9	100.2	101.8
85 years and over	21.8	24.6	28.3	45.6	48.7	52.1	56.1	60.0	63.2
Percent Distribution of Fee-for-Service Program Payments									
Total	100.0	100.0	100.0	100.0	100.0	100.0	100.0	100.0	100.0
Sex									
Male	43.6	43.2	43.7	44.1	44.0	43.8	43.7	43.7	43.9
Female	56.4	56.8	56.3	55.9	56.0	56.2	56.3	56.3	56.1
Age									
Under 65 years	12.9	13.2	14.8	17.0	17.2	17.6	18.0	18.8	19.2
65 to 74 years	37.6	36.5	33.0	31.6	31.1	30.9	30.9	30.9	31.0
75 to 84 years	34.6	34.8	36.0	34.7	34.3	33.4	32.5	31.5	30.7
85 years and over	14.9	15.5	16.2	16.6	17.3	18.0	18.6	18.9	19.1
Average Fee-for-Service Payment Per Enrollee (Dollars)									
Total	4,301	4,667	5,323	7,473	7,830	8,129	8,526	8,993	9,221
Sex									
Male	4,397	4,721	5,370	7,443	7,747	7,964	8,274	8,711	8,931
Female	4,229	4,627	5,286	7,497	7,896	8,263	8,732	9,226	9,461
Age									
Under 65 years	4,673	4,960	5,252	7,435	7,774	8,058	8,530	9,280	9,616
65 to 74 years	3,300	3,548	4,040	5,558	5,756	5,924	6,119	6,398	6,550
75 to 84 years	5,152	5,576	6,320	8,904	9,345	9,696	10,206	10,731	10,953
85 years and over	6,267	6,950	7,684	11,061	11,742	12,440	13,396	14,103	14,527

NOTE: Table includes data for Medicare enrollees residing in Puerto Rico, U.S. Virgin Islands, Guam, other outlying areas, foreign countries, and unknown residence.   1 Medicare enrollees in managed care plans are not included in the denominator used to calculate average payments.

Table 3-77. Medicare Beneficiaries, by Race, Hispanic Origin, and Selected Characteristics, Selected Years, 1992–2009

(Number; percent; dollars.)

Characteristic	All			White			African American			Hispanic or Latino (of any race)		
	1992	2000	2009	1992	2000	2009	1992	2000	2009	1992	2000	2009
All Medicare beneficiaries (number in millions)	36.8	40.6	47.2	30.9	32.4	36.5	3.3	3.7	4.6	1.9	2.8	3.9
All Medicare beneficiaries (percent distribution)	100.0	100.0	100.0	84.2	80.1	77.3	8.9	9.1	9.8	5.2	7.0	8.2
Medical Care Use												
All Medicare beneficiaries												
Long–term care facility stay	7.7	9.3	8.1	8.0	9.7	8.7	6.2	8.8	8.6	4.2	6.0	4.4
Community-only residents												
Inpatient hospital	17.9	19.2	17.6	18.1	19.2	17.8	18.4	22.8	18.4	16.6	16.2	16.9
Outpatient hospital	57.9	69.8	72.7	57.8	70.7	73.2	61.1	69.0	72.2	53.1	63.7	70.0
Physician/supplier[1]	92.4	94.9	95.9	93.0	95.4	96.3	89.1	92.8	93.4	87.9	92.9	93.3
Dental	40.4	43.5	44.6	43.1	46.9	49.0	23.5	24.1	23.9	29.1	33.9	33.5
Prescription medicine	85.2	91.1	94.3	85.5	91.5	94.4	83.1	89.5	93.0	84.6	90.1	94.6
Expenditures												
All Medicare beneficiaries												
Total health care[2]	6,716	10,490	16,068	6,816	10,475	15,938	7,043	12,328	19,211	5,784	9,089	14,860
Long–term care facility[3]	1,581	2,310	2,438	1,674	2,406	2,533	1,255	2,438	2,598	*758	1,799	1,758
Community-only residents												
Total personal health care	5,054	7,911	12,295	4,988	7,814	12,031	5,530	9,419	14,210	4,938	6,934	12,754
Inpatient hospital	2,098	2,664	2,363	2,058	2,605	2,222	2,493	3,465	3,454	1,999	2,133	2,496
Outpatient hospital	504	875	1,385	478	796	1,312	668	1,523	1,873	511	915	1,414
Physician/supplier[1]	1,524	2,491	3,336	1,525	2,503	3,476	1,398	2,621	2,763	1,587	2,234	2,836
Dental	142	258	408	153	278	460	70	101	204	97	193	220
Prescription medicine	468	1,163	3,013	481	1,182	2,891	417	1,135	3,565	389	1,014	3,316
Long-term care facility residents only												
Long–term care facility[4]	23,054	32,442	42,103	23,177	31,795	41,174	21,272	36,132	44,326	*25,026	*39,057	*50,851
Sex												
Both sexes	100.0	100.0	100.0	100.0	100.0	100.0	100.0	100.0	100.0	100.0	100.0	100.0
Male	42.9	43.4	45.1	42.7	43.3	45.2	42.0	40.0	45.1	46.7	46.9	44.8
Female	57.1	56.6	54.9	57.3	56.7	54.8	58.0	60.0	54.9	53.3	53.1	55.2
Eligibility Criteria and Age												
All Medicare beneficiaries[5]	100.0	100.0	100.0	100.0	100.0	100.0	100.0	100.0	100.0	100.0	100.0	100.0
Disabled	10.2	13.6	16.0	8.6	11.5	13.2	19.1	23.3	31.4	16.5	21.7	23.6
Under 45 years	3.5	3.9	3.7	2.9	3.2	3.0	7.6	7.5	8.0	6.9	5.5	5.6
45 to 64 years	6.5	9.8	12.3	5.8	8.3	10.2	11.5	15.8	23.4	9.6	16.3	18.0
Aged	89.8	86.4	84.0	91.4	88.5	86.9	81.0	76.7	68.5	83.5	78.3	76.4
65 to 74 years	51.5	45.4	45.1	52.0	46.7	45.5	48.0	41.7	39.3	49.4	45.5	47.2
75 to 84 years	28.8	30.0	26.8	29.5	31.4	28.3	24.0	25.9	20.8	27.1	22.9	21.6
85 years and over	9.7	10.9	12.1	9.9	11.5	13.2	9.0	9.0	8.4	6.9	9.9	7.6
Living Arrangement												
All living arrangements	100.0	100.0	100.0	100.0	100.0	100.0	100.0	100.0	100.0	100.0	100.0	100.0
Alone	27.0	29.3	29.1	27.5	29.8	30.1	27.7	32.5	31.1	20.2	22.9	21.7
With spouse	51.2	49.0	48.7	53.3	51.0	51.0	33.3	30.0	30.8	50.4	49.2	48.6
With children	9.1	9.5	10.2	7.7	7.6	8.2	16.8	18.6	17.9	16.6	14.8	15.4
With others	7.6	7.1	7.9	6.2	6.2	6.5	18.1	13.7	16.4	10.8	9.9	11.7
Long-term care facility	5.1	5.1	4.1	5.3	5.4	4.3	4.0	5.2	3.8	*2.0	*3.3	*2.7
Age and Limitation of Activity[6]												
Disabled, under age 65 years	100.0	100.0	100.0	100.0	100.0	100.0	100.0	100.0	100.0	100.0	100.0	100.0
None	22.7	27.3	40.9	21.8	25.2	42.8	26.2	35.7	37.5	21.2	30.1	38.3
IADL only	39.0	35.1	32.1	38.9	35.5	31.5	35.8	33.2	36.8	46.1	37.3	28.5
1 or 2 IADL	21.2	21.8	16.8	21.5	23.2	16.6	21.2	17.7	15.0	*20.9	*16.8	*17.9
3 to 5 IADL	17.2	15.9	10.3	17.9	16.1	9.1	*16.8	*13.5	*10.8	*11.9	*15.8	*15.4
65 to 74 years	100.0	100.0	100.0	100.0	100.0	100.0	100.0	100.0	100.0	100.0	100.0	100.0
None	67.0	71.5	72.5	68.7	72.6	74.5	55.1	64.8	68.9	59.2	69.4	61.1
IADL only	17.8	15.4	15.3	17.0	15.1	14.3	22.9	18.0	14.1	*20.9	*13.6	23.0
1 or 2 IADL	10.4	8.6	7.7	9.6	8.2	7.3	14.4	10.8	*9.5	*15.7	*13.2	*10.1
3 to 5 IADL	4.8	4.5	4.5	4.6	4.2	3.9	*7.6	*6.3	*7.5	*4.2	*4.0	*5.8
75 to 84 years	100.0	100.0	100.0	100.0	100.0	100.0	100.0	100.0	100.0	100.0	100.0	100.0
None	46.6	52.2	52.8	47.5	53.1	54.2	42.0	46.2	44.9	44.3	48.3	51.9
IADL only	23.9	23.0	23.1	23.6	22.7	22.9	26.7	20.9	25.7	*27.8	24.9	*20.3

Table 3-77. Medicare Beneficiaries, by Race, Hispanic Origin, and Selected Characteristics, Selected Years, 1992–2009— continued

(Number; percent; dollars.)

Characteristic	All			White			African American			Hispanic or Latino (of any race)		
	1992	2000	2009	1992	2000	2009	1992	2000	2009	1992	2000	2009
1 or 2 IADL	16.5	14.3	13.6	16.8	13.8	13.5	15.3	17.7	*13.3	*14.9	*18.6	*13.8
3 to 5 IADL	13.0	10.6	10.5	12.2	10.4	9.4	*15.9	15.2	*16.2	*13.0	*8.2	*14.1
85 years and over	100.0	100.0	100.0	100.0	100.0	100.0	100.0	100.0	100.0	100.0	100.0	100.0
None	19.9	24.9	27.0	20.2	25.1	27.7	*19.6	*25.9	*18.0	*19.7	*23.4	*24.7
IADL only	20.9	22.6	26.6	20.2	22.4	26.3	*22.1	*19.7	*33.6	*24.7	*24.7	*21.7
1 or 2 IADL	23.5	22.2	19.7	23.5	22.3	20.4	*24.3	*19.3	*12.5	*23.7	*28.1	*16.7
3 to 5 IADL	35.8	30.4	26.8	36.1	30.2	25.6	*34.0	35.1	*35.9	*31.8	*23.8	*37.0

* = Figure does not meet standards of reliability or precision. Estimates are based on 50 persons or fewer or with a relative standard error of 30 percent or higher and are considered unreliable.   1 Physician/supplier services include medical and osteopathic doctor and health practitioner visits, diagnostic laboratory and radiology services, medical and surgical services, and durable medical equipment and nondurable medical supplies.   2 Total health care expenditures by Medicare beneficiaries, including expenses paid by Medicare and all other sources of payment for the following services: inpatient hospital, outpatient hospital, physician/supplier, dental, prescription medicine, home health, and hospice and long-term care facility care. Does not include health insurance premiums.   3 Expenditures for long-term care in facilities for all beneficiaries include facility room and board expenses for beneficiaries who resided in a facility for the full year, for beneficiaries who resided in a facility for part of the year and in the community for part of the year, and expenditures for short-term facility stays for full-year or part-year community residents.   4 Expenditures for facility-based long-term care for facility-based beneficiaries include facility room and board expenses for beneficiaries who resided in a facility for the full year and for beneficiaries who resided in a facility for part of the year and in the community for part of the year. They do not include expenditures for short-term facility stays for full-year community residents.   5 Medicare beneficiaries with end-stage renal disease (ESRD) are included within the subgroups Aged and Disabled. In 2007, less than 1 percent of Medicare beneficiaries qualified because of ESRD.   6 IADL is instrumental activities of daily living; ADL is activities of daily living. Includes data for both community and long-term care facility residents.

Table 3-78. Medicare-Certified Providers and Suppliers, Selected Years, 1975–2010

(Number of providers or suppliers.)

Providers or suppliers	1975	1980	1985	1990	2000	2005	2010
Skilled nursing facilities	NA	5,052	6,451	8,937	14,841	15,006	15,084
Home health agencies	2,242	2,924	5,679	5,730	7,857	8,090	10,914
Clinical Laboratory Improvement Amendments facilities	NA	NA	NA	NA	171,018	196,296	224,679
End-stage renal disease facilities	NA	999	1,393	1,937	3,787	4,755	5,631
Outpatient physical therapy	117	419	854	1,195	2,867	2,962	2,536
Portable X-ray	132	216	308	443	666	553	561
Rural health clinics	NA	391	428	551	3,453	3,661	3,845
Comprehensive outpatient rehabilitation facilities	NA	NA	72	186	522	634	354
Ambulatory surgical centers	NA	NA	336	1,197	2,894	4,445	5,316
Hospices	NA	NA	164	825	2,326	2,872	3,509
Critical access hospitals	NA	NA	NA	NA	NA	NA	1,325

NA = Not available.

NOTES AND DEFINITIONS

SOURCES OF DATA

The principal source for data presented in this part is from National Center for Health Statistics. *Health, United States, 2013: With Special Feature on Prescription Drugs.* Hyattsville, MD, 2014, an annual report on trends in health statistics compiled by the National Center of Health Statistics (NCHS), a component of the Centers for Disease Control and Prevention (CDC). Updated tables for this publication can be found at http://www.cdc.gov/nchs/hus/contents2014.htm.

The data for Tables 3-54 through 3-59 are from the Bureau of Labor Statistics (BLS), Occupational Employment Statistics. For more detailed information, see Occupational Employment and Wages news release. OES can be accessed at http://www.bls.gov/oes/.

CONCEPTS AND DEFINITIONS

Age-adjustment —used to compare risks of two or more populations at one point in time or one population at two or more points in time. Age-adjusted rates are computed by the direct method by applying age-specific rates in a population of interest to a standardized age distribution, to eliminate differences in observed rates that result from age differences in population composition. Age-adjusted rates should be viewed as relative indexes rather than actual measures of risk. Age-adjusted estimates from other age-adjusted estimates based on the same data and presented elsewhere if different age groups are used in the adjustment procedure.

Body mass index (BMI) —a measure that adjusts bodyweight for height. It is calculated as weight in kilograms divided by height in meters squared. Overweight for children and adolescents is defined as BMI at or above the sex- and age-specific 95th percentile BMI cut points from the 2000 CDC Growth Charts. Healthy weight for adults is defined as a BMI of 18.5 to less than 25; overweight, as greater than or equal to a BMI of 25; and obesity, as greater than or equal to a BMI of 30.

Cholesterol, serum—a measure of the total blood cholesterol. Elevated total blood cholesterol—a combination of high-density lipoproteins (HDL), low-density lipoproteins (LDL), and very-low density lipoproteins (VLDL)—is a risk factor for cardiovascular disease. According to the National Cholesterol Education Program, high serum cholesterol is defined as greater than or equal to 240 mg/dL (6.20 mmol/L). Borderline high serum cholesterol is defined as greater than or equal to 200 mg/dL and less than 240 mg/dL. Assessments of the components of total cholesterol or lower thresholds for high total cholesterol may be used for individuals with other risk factors for cardiovascular disease.

Condition—A health condition is a departure from a state of physical or mental well being. In the National Health Interview Survey, each condition reported as a cause of an individual's activity limitation has been classified as chronic, not chronic, or unknown if chronic, based on the nature and duration of the condition.

Dental caries—evidence of tooth decay on any surface of the tooth. Untreated dental caries are determined by an oral examination conducted by a trained dentist.

Diagnosis—the act or process of identifying or determining the nature and cause of a disease or injury through evaluation of patient history, examination, and review of laboratory data.

Gross domestic product (GDP) —the market value of the goods and services produced by labor and property located in the United States. As long as the labor and property are located in the United States, the suppliers (i.e., the workers and, for property, the owners) may be U.S. residents or residents of other countries.

Health expenditures, national—estimated by the Centers for Medicare & Medicaid Services (CMS) it measures spending for health care in the United States by type of service delivered (e.g., hospital care, physician services, nursing home care) and source of funding for those services (e.g., private health insurance, Medicare, Medicaid, out-of-pocket spending). CMS produces both historical and projected estimates of health expenditures by category.

Health insurance coverage—broadly defined to include both public and private payers who cover medical expenditures incurred by a defined population in a variety of settings.

Health maintenance organization (HMO)—a health care system that assumes or shares both the financial risks and the delivery risks associated with providing comprehensive medical services to a voluntarily enrolled population in a particular geographic area, usually in return for a fixed, prepaid fee. Pure HMO enrollees use only the prepaid capitated health services of the HMO panel of medical care providers. Open-ended HMO enrollees use the prepaid HMO health services but, in addition, may receive medical care from providers who are not part of the HMO panel. There is usually a substantial deductible, co-payment, or co-insurance associated with use of non-panel providers.

Hispanic origin—includes persons of Mexican, Puerto Rican, Cuban, Central and South American, and other or unknown Latin American or Spanish origins. Persons of Hispanic origin may be of any race.

Hypertension—elevated blood pressure or hypertension is defined as having an average systolic blood pressure reading of at least 140mmHg or diastolic pressure of at least 90 mmHg, which is consistent with the Seventh Report of the

Joint National Committee on Prevention, Detection, Evaluation, and Treatment of High Blood Pressure. People are also considered to have hypertension if they report that they are taking a prescription medicine for high blood pressure, even if their blood pressure readings are within normal range.

Incidence—the number of cases of disease having their onset during a prescribed period of time. It is often expressed as a rate (e.g., the incidence of measles per 1,000 children 5–15 years of age during a specified year). Incidence is a measure of morbidity or other events that occur within a specified period of time. Measuring incidence may be complicated because the population at risk for the disease may change during the period of interest, for example, due to births, deaths, or migration. In addition, determining that a case is new—that is, that its onset occurred during the prescribed period of time—may be difficult. Because of these difficulties in measuring incidence, many health statistics are measured using prevalence.

Instrumental activities of daily living (IADL) —activities related to independent living and include preparing meals, managing money, shopping for groceries or personal items, performing light or heavy housework, and using a telephone. In the National Health Interview Survey (NHIS) respondents are asked whether they or family members 18 years of age and over need the help of another person for handling routine IADL needs because of a physical, mental, or emotional problem. Persons are considered to have an IADL limitation in the NHIS if any causal condition is chronic.

Limitation of activity—may be defined different ways, depending on the conceptual framework. In the National Health Interview Survey, limitation of activity refers to a long-term reduction in a person's capacity to perform the usual kind or amount of activities associated with his or her age group as a result of a chronic condition. Limitation of activity is assessed by asking persons a series of questions about limitations in their or household members' ability to perform activities usual for their age group because of a physical, mental, or emotional problem. Persons are asked about limitations in activities of daily living, instrumental activities of daily living, play, school, work, difficulty walking or remembering, and any other activity limitations. For reported limitations, the causal health conditions are determined, and persons are considered limited if one or more of these conditions is chronic. Children under 18 years of age who receive special education or early intervention services are considered to have a limitation of activity.

Mammography—an x-ray image of the breast used to detect irregularities of the breast tissue.

Managed care—a term originally used to refer to the prepaid health care sector (health maintenance organizations or HMOs) where care is provided under a fixed budget and costs are therein capable of being managed. Increasingly, the term is being used to include preferred provider organizations (PPOs) and even forms of indemnity.

Medicare —the federal program which helps pay health care costs for people 65 and older and for certain people under 65 with long-term disabilities.

Medicaid —a program authorized by the Social Security Act in 1965 as a jointly funded cooperative venture between the federal and state governments to assist states in the provision of adequate medical care to eligible needy persons. Families with dependent children, the aged, blind, and disabled who are in financial need are eligible for Medicaid.

Notifiable disease—a disease, that when diagnosed, health providers are required, usually by law, to report to state or local public health officials. Notifiable diseases are those of public interest by reason of their contagiousness, severity, or frequency.

Pap smear—a microscopic examination of cells scraped from the cervix that is used to detect cancerous or precancerous conditions of the cervix or other medical conditions.

Physical activity, leisure-time—starting with 1998 data, leisure-time physical activity is assessed in the National Health Interview Survey by asking adults a series of questions about how often they do vigorous or light/moderate physical activity of at least 10 minutes duration and for about how long these sessions generally last. Vigorous physical activity is described as causing heavy sweating or a large increase in breathing or heart rate and light/moderate as causing light sweating or a slight to moderate increase in breathing or heart rate. Adults classified as inactive did not report any sessions of light/moderate or vigorous leisure-time physical activity of at least 10 minutes duration or reported they were unable to perform leisure-time physical activity. Adults classified with some leisure-time activity reported at least one session of light/moderate or vigorous activity of at least 10 minutes duration but did not meet the requirement for regular leisure-time activity. Adults classified with regular leisure-time activity reported at least three sessions per week of vigorous leisure-time physical activity lasting at least 20 minutes in duration or at least five sessions per week of light/moderate physical activity lasting at least 30 minutes in duration.

Poverty—based on definitions originally developed by the Social Security Administration. These include a set of money income thresholds that vary by family size and composition. Families or individuals with income below their appropriate thresholds are classified as below poverty. These thresholds are updated annually by the U.S. Census Bureau to reflect changes in the Consumer Price Index for all urban consumers (CPI-U). For example, the average poverty threshold for a family of four was $24,230 in 2014, $22,314 in 2010, $17,603 in 2000, and $13,359 in 1990.

Preferred provider organization (PPO) —a type of medical plan where coverage is provided to participants through a network of selected health care providers (such as hospitals and physicians). The enrollees may go outside the network, but they would pay a greater percentage of the cost of coverage than within the network.

Prevalence—the number of cases of a disease, infected persons, or persons with some other attribute present during a particular interval of time. It is often expressed as a rate (e.g., the prevalence of diabetes per 1,000 persons during a year).

Short-stay hospital—hospitals that provide general (rather than specialized) care and have an average length of stay of less than 30 days.

Specialty hospital—hospitals that provide a particular type of service to the majority of their patients such as psychiatric, tuberculosis, chronic disease, rehabilitation, maternity, and alcoholic or narcotic.

State Children's Health Insurance Program (SCHIP) —Title XXI of the Social Security Act, known as the State Children's Health Insurance Program (SCHIP), is a program initiated by the Balanced Budget Act of 1997 (BBA). SCHIP provides more federal funds for states to provide health care coverage to low-income, uninsured children. SCHIP gives states broad flexibility in program design while protecting beneficiaries through federal standards. Funds from SCHIP may be used to expand Medicaid or to provide medical assistance to children during a presumptive eligibility period for Medicaid. This is one of several options from which states may select to provide health care coverage for more children, as prescribed within the BBA's Title XXI program.

Substance use—the use of selected substances including alcohol, tobacco products, drugs, inhalants, and other substances that can be consumed, inhaled, injected, or otherwise absorbed into the body with possible detrimental effects.

Suicidal ideation—having thoughts of suicide or of taking action to end one's own life. Suicidal ideation includes all thoughts of suicide, both when the thoughts include a plan to commit suicide and when they do not include a plan. Suicidal ideation is measured in the Youth Risk Behavior Survey by the question ''During the past 12 months, did you ever seriously consider attempting suicide?''

Uninsured—in the Current Population Survey (CPS) persons are considered uninsured if they do not have coverage through private health insurance, Medicare, Medicaid, State Children's Health Insurance Program, military or Veterans coverage, another government program, a plan of someone outside the household, or other insurance. Persons with only Indian Health Service coverage are considered uninsured. In addition, if the respondent has missing Medicaid information but has income from certain low-income public programs, then Medicaid coverage is imputed. The questions on health insurance are administered in March and refer to the previous calendar year.

PART 4

MARRIAGE

Figure 4-1. Marriage and Divorce Rates, United States, Selected States, 2000–2014

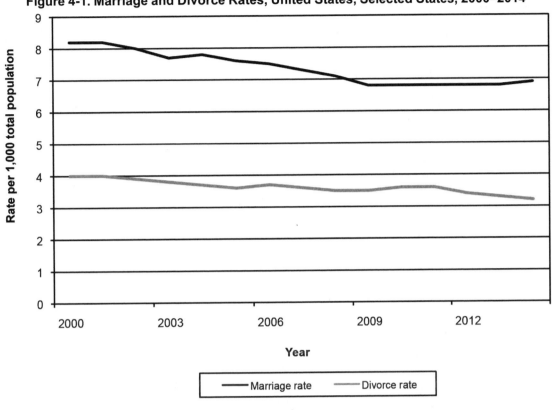

HIGHLIGHTS

- In 2014, Nevada had the highest rate of marriage per 1,000 resident population at 31.9, significantly greater than the next-highest states (Hawaii, 17.7; the District of Columbia, 11.8; and Arkansas, 10.1). New Jersey and Connecticut had the lowest marriage rates, at 5.4 each, followed by Massachusetts at 5.6, Wisconsin at 5.7, and Pennsylvania, Ohio, Michigan, and Arizona, at 5.8 each.

- Among reporting states (California, Georgia, Hawaii, Indiana, and Minnesota did not have available information) in 2014, Iowa had the lowest divorce rate, at 1.5 per 1,000 resident population, followed by Illinois (2.2), Louisiana (2.3), Maryland (2.5), and Connecticut and the District of Columbia (2.6 each). Nevada, which had the highest marriage rate, also had the highest divorce rate at 5.3, followed by Arkansas (4.8), Wyoming (4.6), Oklahoma (4.2), and Idaho and West Virginia (4.2 each).

- The median age at first marriage for all races and origins in the United States was 29.5 years for males and 27.6 years for females in 2014. Male median ages ranged from 28.6 for Native Hawaiian and Other Pacific Islanders to 31.6 for Black or African American alone males. Ages for females ranged from 27.0 for Some Other Race alone to 30.8 for Black or African American alone.

- In the United States, the median duration of current marriages was 19.5 years in 2014. The District of Columbia had the shortest median duration, at 11.0 years, while Maine had the longest median duration, at 23.2 years.

Table 4-1. Marriages in the Last Year for the Population Age 15 Years and Over, American Community Survey 1-Year Estimates, by Sex and State, 2014

(Number.)

State	Total, age 15 years and over	Male					Female				
		Total	Never married	Ever married			Total	Never married	Ever married		
				Total, ever married	Married last year	Not married last year			Total, ever married	Married last year	Not married last year
United States	257,770,670	125,664,923	45,864,923	79,800,000	2,280,174	77,519,826	132,105,747	39,943,973	92,161,774	2,241,036	89,920,738
Alabama	3,931,966	1,878,536	621,776	1,256,760	36,382	1,220,378	2,053,430	566,426	1,487,004	35,000	1,452,004
Alaska	579,778	305,440	117,205	188,235	8,966	179,269	274,338	83,733	190,605	7,860	182,745
Arizona	5,381,925	2,655,529	986,840	1,668,689	47,133	1,621,556	2,726,396	810,874	1,915,522	47,087	1,868,435
Arkansas	2,381,476	1,157,713	367,542	790,171	22,806	767,365	1,223,763	305,010	918,753	25,070	893,683
California	31,206,124	15,387,827	6,217,072	9,170,755	281,222	8,889,533	15,818,297	5,280,301	10,537,996	270,045	10,267,951
Colorado	4,309,301	2,153,568	760,603	1,392,965	47,678	1,345,287	2,155,733	601,891	1,553,842	45,169	1,508,673
Connecticut	2,967,896	1,433,554	539,976	893,578	20,254	873,324	1,534,342	485,371	1,048,971	20,639	1,028,332
Delaware	765,491	366,631	132,545	234,086	6,481	227,605	398,860	123,172	275,688	7,733	267,955
District of Columbia	559,363	262,074	150,865	111,209	7,958	103,251	297,289	165,425	131,864	7,013	124,851
Florida	16,544,829	8,013,533	2,819,903	5,193,630	123,325	5,070,305	8,531,296	2,409,539	6,121,757	116,815	6,004,942
Georgia	8,019,982	3,862,111	1,444,653	2,417,458	75,491	2,341,967	4,157,871	1,315,258	2,842,613	76,995	2,765,618
Hawaii	1,158,752	583,110	220,895	362,215	12,179	350,036	575,642	166,862	408,780	10,580	398,200
Idaho	1,274,423	632,611	194,809	437,802	14,337	423,465	641,812	148,957	492,855	14,310	478,545
Illinois	10,412,161	5,061,711	1,930,523	3,131,188	83,564	3,047,624	5,350,450	1,730,603	3,619,847	80,913	3,538,934
Indiana	5,284,811	2,572,431	865,086	1,707,345	51,224	1,656,121	2,712,380	751,182	1,961,198	52,230	1,908,968
Iowa	2,503,309	1,232,864	394,855	838,009	23,271	814,738	1,270,445	330,276	940,169	22,335	917,834
Kansas	2,299,146	1,136,728	370,573	766,155	23,581	742,574	1,162,418	299,323	863,095	22,583	840,512
Kentucky	3,569,190	1,740,854	555,037	1,185,817	31,707	1,154,110	1,828,336	457,294	1,371,042	31,624	1,339,418
Louisiana	3,716,740	1,797,076	694,903	1,102,173	33,118	1,069,055	1,919,664	625,735	1,293,929	34,601	1,259,328
Maine	1,119,690	541,803	170,892	370,911	8,119	362,792	577,887	150,136	427,751	9,452	418,299
Maryland	4,854,750	2,322,878	884,012	1,438,866	37,268	1,401,598	2,531,872	834,587	1,697,285	37,313	1,659,972
Massachusetts	5,604,860	2,687,387	1,074,332	1,613,055	39,328	1,573,727	2,917,473	1,004,940	1,912,533	41,865	1,870,668
Michigan	8,089,154	3,933,762	1,424,877	2,508,885	58,783	2,450,102	4,155,392	1,258,179	2,897,213	58,777	2,838,436
Minnesota	4,386,934	2,166,462	766,344	1,400,118	38,760	1,361,358	2,220,472	636,833	1,583,639	37,565	1,546,074
Mississippi	2,383,607	1,141,338	415,131	726,207	23,634	702,573	1,242,269	385,898	856,371	23,904	832,467
Missouri	4,909,194	2,378,868	794,587	1,584,281	40,879	1,543,402	2,530,326	703,820	1,826,506	42,345	1,784,161
Montana	835,422	417,444	131,905	285,539	6,874	278,665	417,978	107,164	310,814	6,920	303,894
Nebraska	1,488,730	733,769	242,745	491,024	13,186	477,838	754,961	200,086	554,875	12,600	542,275
Nevada	2,287,984	1,144,209	429,417	714,792	24,387	690,405	1,143,775	342,521	801,254	24,277	776,977
New Hampshire	1,111,188	545,435	177,905	367,530	10,085	357,445	565,753	151,360	414,393	10,549	403,844
New Jersey	7,282,046	3,518,889	1,328,240	2,190,649	56,111	2,134,538	3,763,157	1,196,420	2,566,737	51,523	2,515,214
New Mexico	1,667,854	820,542	308,918	511,624	14,629	496,995	847,312	265,986	581,326	14,310	567,016
New York	16,248,072	7,787,815	3,207,375	4,580,440	130,009	4,450,431	8,460,257	3,045,518	5,414,739	122,086	5,292,653
North Carolina	8,029,973	3,863,351	1,332,169	2,531,182	72,682	2,458,500	4,166,622	1,188,823	2,977,799	71,350	2,906,449
North Dakota	598,037	305,227	112,831	192,396	5,724	186,672	292,810	78,241	214,569	5,406	209,163
Ohio	9,422,595	4,562,386	1,610,302	2,952,084	73,606	2,878,478	4,860,209	1,417,330	3,442,879	73,853	3,369,026
Oklahoma	3,080,740	1,510,864	480,122	1,030,742	35,447	995,295	1,569,876	389,663	1,180,213	35,415	1,144,798
Oregon	3,258,094	1,601,320	547,721	1,053,599	29,489	1,024,110	1,656,774	452,271	1,204,503	30,256	1,174,247
Pennsylvania	10,562,571	5,117,508	1,878,338	3,239,170	82,673	3,156,497	5,445,063	1,675,810	3,769,253	81,673	3,687,580
Rhode Island	882,072	422,664	165,692	256,972	7,021	249,951	459,408	152,890	306,518	6,394	300,124
South Carolina	3,929,135	1,889,452	667,180	1,222,272	36,933	1,185,339	2,039,683	605,264	1,434,419	34,266	1,400,153
South Dakota	675,764	337,200	115,307	221,893	7,666	214,227	338,564	91,746	246,818	7,159	239,659
Tennessee	5,309,334	2,556,919	832,587	1,724,332	50,754	1,673,578	2,752,415	751,194	2,001,221	51,188	1,950,033
Texas	21,001,527	10,339,954	3,693,020	6,646,934	218,175	6,428,759	10,661,573	3,117,291	7,544,282	207,999	7,336,283
Utah	2,178,253	1,085,912	356,153	729,759	26,403	703,356	1,092,341	284,780	807,561	28,787	778,774
Vermont	528,064	256,941	86,611	170,330	3,914	166,416	271,123	75,506	195,617	4,045	191,572
Virginia	6,772,134	3,297,416	1,144,868	2,152,548	64,669	2,087,879	3,474,718	1,019,938	2,454,780	65,654	2,389,126
Washington	5,722,255	2,845,066	982,876	1,862,190	55,652	1,806,538	2,877,189	784,563	2,092,626	57,086	2,035,540
West Virginia	1,532,355	751,800	240,214	511,586	13,599	497,987	780,555	184,876	595,679	13,274	582,405
Wisconsin	4,682,400	2,307,821	804,084	1,503,737	37,178	1,466,559	2,374,579	678,969	1,695,610	39,045	1,656,565
Wyoming	469,219	238,620	72,507	166,113	5,860	160,253	230,599	54,138	176,461	6,098	170,363

Table 4-2. Marriages Ending in Widowhood for the Population Age 15 Years and Over, American Community Survey 1-Year Estimates, by Sex and State, 2014

(Number.)

State	Total, age 15 years and over	Male					Female				
		Total	Never married	Ever married			Total	Never married	Ever married		
				Total, ever married	Widowed last year	Not widowed last year			Total, ever married	Widowed last year	Not widowed last year
United States	257,770,670	125,664,923	45,864,923	79,800,000	438,484	79,361,516	132,105,747	39,943,973	92,161,774	1,003,598	91,158,176
Alabama	3,931,966	1,878,536	621,776	1,256,760	8,146	1,248,614	2,053,430	566,426	1,487,004	19,316	1,467,688
Alaska	579,778	305,440	117,205	188,235	763	187,472	274,338	83,733	190,605	1,281	189,324
Arizona	5,381,925	2,655,529	986,840	1,668,689	7,354	1,661,335	2,726,396	810,874	1,915,522	20,564	1,894,958
Arkansas	2,381,476	1,157,713	367,542	790,171	4,508	785,663	1,223,763	305,010	918,753	13,306	905,447
California	31,206,124	15,387,827	6,217,072	9,170,755	41,585	9,129,170	15,818,297	5,280,301	10,537,996	101,868	10,436,128
Colorado	4,309,301	2,153,568	760,603	1,392,965	5,910	1,387,055	2,155,733	601,891	1,553,842	9,160	1,544,682
Connecticut	2,967,896	1,433,554	539,976	893,578	5,669	887,909	1,534,342	485,371	1,048,971	10,524	1,038,447
Delaware	765,491	366,631	132,545	234,086	1,505	232,581	398,860	123,172	275,688	2,538	273,150
District of Columbia	559,363	262,074	150,865	111,209	347	110,862	297,289	165,425	131,864	1,067	130,797
Florida	16,544,829	8,013,533	2,819,903	5,193,630	30,528	5,163,102	8,531,296	2,409,539	6,121,757	76,601	6,045,156
Georgia	8,019,982	3,862,111	1,444,653	2,417,458	12,095	2,405,363	4,157,871	1,315,258	2,842,613	33,864	2,808,749
Hawaii	1,158,752	583,110	220,895	362,215	1,653	360,562	575,642	166,862	408,780	5,562	403,218
Idaho	1,274,423	632,611	194,809	437,802	2,493	435,309	641,812	148,957	492,855	3,277	489,578
Illinois	10,412,161	5,061,711	1,930,523	3,131,188	16,051	3,115,137	5,350,450	1,730,603	3,619,847	39,991	3,579,856
Indiana	5,284,811	2,572,431	865,086	1,707,345	9,230	1,698,115	2,712,380	751,182	1,961,198	21,159	1,940,039
Iowa	2,503,309	1,232,864	394,855	838,009	4,833	833,176	1,270,445	330,276	940,169	10,909	929,260
Kansas	2,299,146	1,136,728	370,573	766,155	4,094	762,061	1,162,418	299,323	863,095	7,965	855,130
Kentucky	3,569,190	1,740,854	555,037	1,185,817	9,557	1,176,260	1,828,336	457,294	1,371,042	14,851	1,356,191
Louisiana	3,716,740	1,797,076	694,903	1,102,173	7,317	1,094,856	1,919,664	625,735	1,293,929	19,490	1,274,439
Maine	1,119,690	541,803	170,892	370,911	2,043	368,868	577,887	150,136	427,751	5,079	422,672
Maryland	4,854,750	2,322,878	884,012	1,438,866	6,684	1,432,182	2,531,872	834,587	1,697,285	17,418	1,679,867
Massachusetts	5,604,860	2,687,387	1,074,332	1,613,055	8,664	1,604,391	2,917,473	1,004,940	1,912,533	22,744	1,889,789
Michigan	8,089,154	3,933,762	1,424,877	2,508,885	16,100	2,492,785	4,155,392	1,258,179	2,897,213	34,607	2,862,606
Minnesota	4,386,934	2,166,462	766,344	1,400,118	6,923	1,393,195	2,220,472	636,833	1,583,639	14,650	1,568,989
Mississippi	2,383,607	1,141,338	415,131	726,207	5,040	721,167	1,242,269	385,898	856,371	11,461	844,910
Missouri	4,909,194	2,378,868	794,587	1,584,281	10,034	1,574,247	2,530,326	703,820	1,826,506	20,431	1,806,075
Montana	835,422	417,444	131,905	285,539	1,525	284,014	417,978	107,164	310,814	2,427	308,387
Nebraska	1,488,730	733,769	242,745	491,024	2,646	488,378	754,961	200,086	554,875	4,689	550,186
Nevada	2,287,984	1,144,209	429,417	714,792	3,278	711,514	1,143,775	342,521	801,254	9,083	792,171
New Hampshire	1,111,188	545,435	177,905	367,530	2,022	365,508	565,753	151,360	414,393	3,707	410,686
New Jersey	7,282,046	3,518,889	1,328,240	2,190,649	10,404	2,180,245	3,763,157	1,196,420	2,566,737	25,251	2,541,486
New Mexico	1,667,854	820,542	308,918	511,624	2,490	509,134	847,312	265,986	581,326	7,275	574,051
New York	16,248,072	7,787,815	3,207,375	4,580,440	25,028	4,555,412	8,460,257	3,045,518	5,414,739	56,105	5,358,634
North Carolina	8,029,973	3,863,351	1,332,169	2,531,182	16,142	2,515,040	4,166,622	1,188,823	2,977,799	32,391	2,945,408
North Dakota	598,037	305,227	112,831	192,396	1,201	191,195	292,810	78,241	214,569	2,267	212,302
Ohio	9,422,595	4,562,386	1,610,302	2,952,084	18,967	2,933,117	4,860,209	1,417,330	3,442,879	39,277	3,403,602
Oklahoma	3,080,740	1,510,864	480,122	1,030,742	6,401	1,024,341	1,569,876	389,663	1,180,213	13,951	1,166,262
Oregon	3,258,094	1,601,320	547,721	1,053,599	5,554	1,048,045	1,656,774	452,271	1,204,503	12,361	1,192,142
Pennsylvania	10,562,571	5,117,508	1,878,338	3,239,170	21,124	3,218,046	5,445,063	1,675,810	3,769,253	46,690	3,722,563
Rhode Island	882,072	422,664	165,692	256,972	899	256,073	459,408	152,890	306,518	2,877	303,641
South Carolina	3,929,135	1,889,452	667,180	1,222,272	8,439	1,213,833	2,039,683	605,264	1,434,419	16,999	1,417,420
South Dakota	675,764	337,200	115,307	221,893	1,133	220,760	338,564	91,746	246,818	2,429	244,389
Tennessee	5,309,334	2,556,919	832,587	1,724,332	10,957	1,713,375	2,752,415	751,194	2,001,221	23,171	1,978,050
Texas	21,001,527	10,339,954	3,693,020	6,646,934	32,194	6,614,740	10,661,573	3,117,291	7,544,282	79,250	7,465,032
Utah	2,178,253	1,085,912	356,153	729,759	3,740	726,019	1,092,341	284,780	807,561	6,968	800,593
Vermont	528,064	256,941	86,611	170,330	899	169,431	271,123	75,506	195,617	1,742	193,875
Virginia	6,772,134	3,297,416	1,144,868	2,152,548	12,849	2,139,699	3,474,718	1,019,938	2,454,780	28,292	2,426,488
Washington	5,722,255	2,845,066	982,876	1,862,190	8,515	1,853,675	2,877,189	784,563	2,092,626	19,389	2,073,237
West Virginia	1,532,355	751,800	240,214	511,586	3,074	508,512	780,555	184,876	595,679	9,395	586,284
Wisconsin	4,682,400	2,307,821	804,084	1,503,737	8,992	1,494,745	2,374,579	678,969	1,695,610	16,311	1,679,299
Wyoming	469,219	238,620	72,507	166,113	885	165,228	230,599	54,138	176,461	1,618	174,843

Table 4-3. Divorces in the Last Year for the Population Age 15 Years and Over, American Community Survey 1-Year Estimates, by Sex and State, 2014

(Number.)

State	Total, age 15 years and over	Male					Female				
		Total	Never married	Ever married			Total	Never married	Ever married		
				Total, ever married	Divorced last year	Not divorced last year			Total, ever married	Divorced last year	Not divorced last year
United States	257,770,670	125,664,923	45,864,923	79,800,000	1,017,815	78,782,185	132,105,747	39,943,973	92,161,774	1,145,110	91,016,664
Alabama	3,931,966	1,878,536	621,776	1,256,760	17,639	1,239,121	2,053,430	566,426	1,487,004	21,358	1,465,646
Alaska	579,778	305,440	117,205	188,235	2,775	185,460	274,338	83,733	190,605	2,823	187,782
Arizona	5,381,925	2,655,529	986,840	1,668,689	19,883	1,648,806	2,726,396	810,874	1,915,522	24,070	1,891,452
Arkansas	2,381,476	1,157,713	367,542	790,171	13,902	776,269	1,223,763	305,010	918,753	14,187	904,566
California	31,206,124	15,387,827	6,217,072	9,170,755	102,669	9,068,086	15,818,297	5,280,301	10,537,996	113,803	10,424,193
Colorado	4,309,301	2,153,568	760,603	1,392,965	21,128	1,371,837	2,155,733	601,891	1,553,842	22,569	1,531,273
Connecticut	2,967,896	1,433,554	539,976	893,578	10,490	883,088	1,534,342	485,371	1,048,971	12,320	1,036,651
Delaware	765,491	366,631	132,545	234,086	3,779	230,307	398,860	123,172	275,688	3,518	272,170
District of Columbia	559,363	262,074	150,865	111,209	1,520	109,689	297,289	165,425	131,864	2,547	129,317
Florida	16,544,829	8,013,533	2,819,903	5,193,630	61,235	5,132,395	8,531,296	2,409,539	6,121,757	81,300	6,040,457
Georgia	8,019,982	3,862,111	1,444,653	2,417,458	33,632	2,383,826	4,157,871	1,315,258	2,842,613	46,661	2,795,952
Hawaii	1,158,752	583,110	220,895	362,215	4,041	358,174	575,642	166,862	408,780	3,421	405,359
Idaho	1,274,423	632,611	194,809	437,802	4,710	433,092	641,812	148,957	492,855	9,235	483,620
Illinois	10,412,161	5,061,711	1,930,523	3,131,188	35,117	3,096,071	5,350,450	1,730,603	3,619,847	38,953	3,580,894
Indiana	5,284,811	2,572,431	865,086	1,707,345	25,944	1,681,401	2,712,380	751,182	1,961,198	30,688	1,930,510
Iowa	2,503,309	1,232,864	394,855	838,009	9,307	828,702	1,270,445	330,276	940,169	8,442	931,727
Kansas	2,299,146	1,136,728	370,573	766,155	11,298	754,857	1,162,418	299,323	863,095	12,551	850,544
Kentucky	3,569,190	1,740,854	555,037	1,185,817	18,443	1,167,374	1,828,336	457,294	1,371,042	20,024	1,351,018
Louisiana	3,716,740	1,797,076	694,903	1,102,173	14,921	1,087,252	1,919,664	625,735	1,293,929	13,115	1,280,814
Maine	1,119,690	541,803	170,892	370,911	5,794	365,117	577,887	150,136	427,751	6,351	421,400
Maryland	4,854,750	2,322,878	884,012	1,438,866	15,866	1,423,000	2,531,872	834,587	1,697,285	20,692	1,676,593
Massachusetts	5,604,860	2,687,387	1,074,332	1,613,055	17,492	1,595,563	2,917,473	1,004,940	1,912,533	20,553	1,891,980
Michigan	8,089,154	3,933,762	1,424,877	2,508,885	33,626	2,475,259	4,155,392	1,258,179	2,897,213	38,065	2,859,148
Minnesota	4,386,934	2,166,462	766,344	1,400,118	16,395	1,383,723	2,220,472	636,833	1,583,639	17,268	1,566,371
Mississippi	2,383,607	1,141,338	415,131	726,207	12,898	713,309	1,242,269	385,898	856,371	12,439	843,932
Missouri	4,909,194	2,378,868	794,587	1,584,281	23,188	1,561,093	2,530,326	703,820	1,826,506	21,249	1,805,257
Montana	835,422	417,444	131,905	285,539	5,098	280,441	417,978	107,164	310,814	2,883	307,931
Nebraska	1,488,730	733,769	242,745	491,024	6,276	484,748	754,961	200,086	554,875	6,745	548,130
Nevada	2,287,984	1,144,209	429,417	714,792	11,263	703,529	1,143,775	342,521	801,254	11,885	789,369
New Hampshire	1,111,188	545,435	177,905	367,530	4,953	362,577	565,753	151,360	414,393	4,999	409,394
New Jersey	7,282,046	3,518,889	1,328,240	2,190,649	23,170	2,167,479	3,763,157	1,196,420	2,566,737	20,600	2,546,137
New Mexico	1,667,854	820,542	308,918	511,624	6,939	504,685	847,312	265,986	581,326	8,202	573,124
New York	16,248,072	7,787,815	3,207,375	4,580,440	46,042	4,534,398	8,460,257	3,045,518	5,414,739	53,686	5,361,053
North Carolina	8,029,973	3,863,351	1,332,169	2,531,182	30,164	2,501,018	4,166,622	1,188,823	2,977,799	37,370	2,940,429
North Dakota	598,037	305,227	112,831	192,396	1,532	190,864	292,810	78,241	214,569	2,237	212,332
Ohio	9,422,595	4,562,386	1,610,302	2,952,084	35,740	2,916,344	4,860,209	1,417,330	3,442,879	42,121	3,400,758
Oklahoma	3,080,740	1,510,864	480,122	1,030,742	17,458	1,013,284	1,569,876	389,663	1,180,213	19,562	1,160,651
Oregon	3,258,094	1,601,320	547,721	1,053,599	13,920	1,039,679	1,656,774	452,271	1,204,503	17,270	1,187,233
Pennsylvania	10,562,571	5,117,508	1,878,338	3,239,170	36,609	3,202,561	5,445,063	1,675,810	3,769,253	39,266	3,729,987
Rhode Island	882,072	422,664	165,692	256,972	2,763	254,209	459,408	152,890	306,518	3,930	302,588
South Carolina	3,929,135	1,889,452	667,180	1,222,272	16,757	1,205,515	2,039,683	605,264	1,434,419	18,236	1,416,183
South Dakota	675,764	337,200	115,307	221,893	2,388	219,505	338,564	91,746	246,818	2,590	244,228
Tennessee	5,309,334	2,556,919	832,587	1,724,332	28,092	1,696,240	2,752,415	751,194	2,001,221	26,212	1,975,009
Texas	21,001,527	10,339,954	3,693,020	6,646,934	101,128	6,545,806	10,661,573	3,117,291	7,544,282	108,770	7,435,512
Utah	2,178,253	1,085,912	356,153	729,759	10,331	719,428	1,092,341	284,780	807,561	13,021	794,540
Vermont	528,064	256,941	86,611	170,330	1,716	168,614	271,123	75,506	195,617	1,813	193,804
Virginia	6,772,134	3,297,416	1,144,868	2,152,548	26,776	2,125,772	3,474,718	1,019,938	2,454,780	30,206	2,424,574
Washington	5,722,255	2,845,066	982,876	1,862,190	24,995	1,837,195	2,877,189	784,563	2,092,626	25,068	2,067,558
West Virginia	1,532,355	751,800	240,214	511,586	7,126	504,460	780,555	184,876	595,679	9,702	585,977
Wisconsin	4,682,400	2,307,821	804,084	1,503,737	17,262	1,486,475	2,374,579	678,969	1,695,610	18,660	1,676,950
Wyoming	469,219	238,620	72,507	166,113	1,625	164,488	230,599	54,138	176,461	1,874	174,587

SOURCES OF DATA

Tables 4-1 through 4-3 are from the 1-year estimates from the 2014 American Community Survey, which is conducted by the U.S. Census Bureau. Additional information and reports can be found at http://www.census.gov/hhes/socdemo/marriage/data/acs/index.html.

NOTES AND DEFINITIONS

Accuracy of the data—Data are based on a sample and are subject to sampling variability. The degree of uncertainty for an estimate arising from sampling variability is represented through the use of a margin of error. The margin of error can be interpreted roughly as providing a 90 percent probability that the interval defined by the estimate minus the margin of error and the estimate plus the margin of error (the lower and upper confidence bounds) contains the true value. In addition to sampling variability, the ACS estimates are subject to nonsampling error. The effect of nonsampling error is not represented in these tables.

Foreign born—Foreign born excludes people born outside the United States to a parent who is a U.S. citizen.

Population—ACS population comprises individuals age 15 to 54 years.

Widowhood—Widowhood estimates may vary from the mortality data released by the National Center for Health Statistics (NCHS) because of differences in methodology and data collection. NCHS uses information collected on death certificates from each state that record the current marital status of the decedent at the time of death. From these administrative records, NCHS then publishes information about men and women who died in that calendar year by their marital status. By inference, people who were married at their time of death were survived by a widowed spouse. In contrast, the ACS collects survey-based reports from individuals as to whether or not they were widowed in the last 12 months. We recommend using caution when comparing the NCHS estimates to the ACS estimates of widowhood.

INDEX

BOCA RATON PUBLIC LIBRARY, FLORIDA

3 3656 0643781 2